L. Kanerva · P. Elsner · J. E. Wahlberg · H. I. Maibach (Eds.)

Condensed Handbook of Occupational Dermatology

Springer-Verlag Berlin Heidelberg GmbH

Lasse Kanerva
Peter Elsner
Jan E. Wahlberg
Howard I. Maibach (Eds.)

Condensed Handbook
of Occupational Dermatology

With 40 Figures and 107 Tables

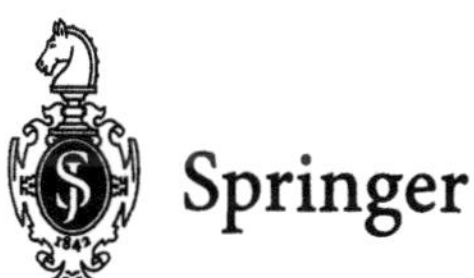 Springer

Prof. Lasse Kanerva, M.D., Ph.D.
Section of Dermatology
Finnish Institute of Occupational Health
Topeliuksenkatu 41 aA
00250 Helsinki, Finland

Prof. Dr. med. Peter Elsner
Department of Dermatology
and Allergology
Friedrich-Schiller University
Erfurter Str. 35, 07743 Jena, Germany

Prof. Jan E. Wahlberg, M.D., Ph.D.
Karolinska Hospital
Department of Occupational Dermatology
and the National Institute for Working Life
11776 Stockholm, Sweden

Prof. Howard I. Maibach, M.D.
University of California
School of Medicine
Box 0989, Surge 100
San Francisco, CA 94143-0989, USA

ISBN 978-3-540-44348-3

Library on Congress Cataloging-in-Publication Data
Condensed handbook of occupational dermatology / L. Kanerva ... [et al.].
    p.; cm.
    Includes bibliographical references and index.
    ISBN 978-3-540-44348-3   ISBN 978-3-642-18556-4 (eBook)
    DOI 10.1007/978-3-642-18556-4
    1. Occupational dermatitis–Handbooks, manuals, etc. 2. Skin–Diseases–Handbooks,
    manuals, etc. I. Kanerva, L. (Lasse), 1943–
    [DNLM: 1. Dermatitis, Occupational–etiology–Handbooks. 2. Skin
    Diseases–chemically induced–Handbooks. WR 39 C745 2004]

The use of general descriptive names, registered names, trademarks, etc. in this publication does not imply, even in the absence of a specific statement, that such names are exempt from the relevant protective laws and regulations and therefore free for general use.

Production: PRO Edit GmbH, 69126 Heidelberg, Germany
Typesetting: K+V Fotosatz GmbH, 64743 Beerfelden, Germany
Cover design: Erich Kirchner, 69121 Heidelberg, Germany
24/3150/göh – 5 4 3 2 1 0 – Printed on acid-free paper

Preface

The *Handbook of Occupational Dermatology*, published in 2000, attracted widespread interest and acceptance by general and occupational dermatologists and occupational physicians. At 1300 pages, it remains the most extensive and up-to-date textbook in the field. However, for the benefit of a wide audience of physicians and safety engineers who cannot go into the detail provided by the *Handbook*, it was decided to produce a compact version. We the editors are now pleased to present the *Condensed Handbook of Occupational Dermatology*. In this new volume, the central chapters have been revised and abridged by the authors. Some background information has been omitted, but all of the most important messages have been retained. New information has been added as deemed necessary. We hope that the *Condensed Handbook* will be useful in the care of patients with occupational skin problems in daily life, while at the same time providing information to help prevent these problems in the workplace.

We would like to thank the authors for their additional work and support and the staff of Springer-Verlag for their help.

Autumn 2003   The Editors

Contents

Part 2
Substances, Products, Occupations, Concentrations

List of Contributors

ALANKO, KRISTIINA
Section of Dermatology
Finnish Institute of Occupational Health
Topeliuksenkatu 41 aA
00250 Helsinki, Finland

ALE, IRIS
University of Uruguay
Department of Dermatology
Arazati 1194, 11300 Montevideo
Uruguay

ANGELINI, GIOVANNI
University of Bari
Section of Dermatology
Dept. of Internal Medicine,
Immunology and Infectious Diseases
Piazza Guilio Cesare 11, 70124 Bari, Italy

ANIGBOGU, A.
University of California
Dept. of Dermatology
School of Medicine
San Fransisco, CA 94143-0989, USA

AVNSTORP, CHRISTIAN
Dermatologic Clinic
Roskildevej 264
2610 Roedovre, Denmark

BARAN, ROBERT
Nail Disease Center
"Le Grand Palais"
42, Rue des Serbes
06400 Cannes, France

BASKETTER, DAVID A.
Unilever Environment Safety Laboratory
Colworth House, Sharnbrook
Bedford MK44 1LW, UK

BELSITO, DONALD V.
University of Kansas Medical Center
Division of Dermatology
3901 Rainbow Boulevard
Kansas City, KS 66160-7319, USA

BIGARDI, ANDREA STEFANO
Department of Dermatology
University of Milan
IRCCS Ospedale Maggiore of Milan
Milan, Italy

BOMAN, ANDERS
Department of Occupational
and Environmental Dermatology
Stockholm Country Council, Norrbacka
17176 Stockholm, Sweden

BRUZE, MAGNUS
Department of Occupational
and Environmental Dermatology
University Hospital
20502 Malmö, Sweden

BURROWS, DESMOND
11 Broomhill Park
Belfast BT9 5JB, Ireland

COENRAADS, PIETER JAN
Ziekenhuis Groningen
9713 GZ Groningen, The Netherlands

DE GROOT, ANTON C.
Spurkstraat 45
5275 JB Den Dungen
The Netherlands

Diepgen, Thomas L.
Universitätsklinikum Heidelberg
Institut und Poliklinik
für Arbeits- und Sozialmedizin
Abt. Klinische Sozialmedizin
Bergheimerstr. 58
69115 Heidelberg, Germany

Elsner, Peter
Department of Dermatology
and Allergology
Friedrich-Schiller University
Erfurter Str. 35
07743 Jena, Germany

Engasser, Patricia G.
34 Ashfield Road
Atherton, CA 94027, USA

Estlander, Tuula
Mäntypaadentie 13 as 5
00830 Helsinki, Finland

Flyvholm, Mari-Ann
National Institute of Occupational Health
Lersø Parkallé 105
2100 Copenhagen, Denmark

Francalanci, Stefano
Department of Dermatology
Unit of Allergological, Occupational,
and Environmental Dermatologies
University of Florence
Via Alfani, 37
50121 Florence, Italy

Frank, Udine
Department of Dermatology
Friedrich Schiller University
Erfurter Str. 35
07740 Jena, Germany

Gebhardt, M.
Leipziger Str. 90
08058 Zwickau, Germany

Goh, Chee Leok
National University of Singapore
Institute of Dermatology
National Skin Centre
1 Mandalay Road
Singapore 308205, Singapore

Guin, Jere D.
18 Corporate Hill, Suite 100
Little Rock, AR 72205, USA

Haustein, Uwe-Frithjof
Universitätsklinikum Leipzig AöR
Klinik und Poliklinik für Hautkrankheiten
Stephanstr. 11
04103 Leipzig, Germany

Hewitt, Philip
Merck KGaA
Frankfurter Str. 250
64293 Darmstadt, Germany

Jolanki, Riitta
Finnish Institute of Occupational Health
Section of Dermatology
Department of Occupational Medicine
Topeliuksenkatu 41 aA
00250 Helsinki, Finland

Kalimo, Kirsti
University of Turku
Department of Dermatology
20520 Turku, Finland

Kanerva, Lasse
Chief, Section of Dermatology
Finnish Institute of Occupational Health
Topeliuksenkatu 41 aA
00250 Helsinki, Finland

Karlberg, Ann-Therese
Göteborg University
Dermatochemistry and Skin Allergy
Department of Chemistry
41296 Göteborg, Sweden

Lammintausta, Kaija
University of Turku
Department of Dermatology
Kiinamyllynkatu 8
20520 Turku

Lidén, Caroline
Dept. of Occupational
and Environmental Dermatology
Stockholm Country Council
Norrbacka, 17176 Stockholm, Sweden

MAIBACH, HOWARD J.
University of California, San Francisco
School of Medicine
Department of Dermatology
Box 0989, Surge 100
San Francisco, CA 04143-0989, USA

MELLSTRÖM, GUNH A.
Medical Products Agency
P.O. Box 26, 751 03 Uppsala, Sweden

PIGATTO, PAOLO DANIELE
Department of Dermatology
University of Milan
IRCCS Ospedale Maggiore
of Milan, Via Pace 9
20122 Milan, Italy

SEIDENARI, STEFANIA
Universita Degli Studi di Modena
e Reggio Emilia
Clinica Dermatologica
Largo del Pozzo 71
41100 Modena, Italy

SERTOLI, ACHILLE
Department of Dermatology
Unit of Allergological, Occupational,
and Environmental Dermatologies
University of Florence
Via Alfani, 37
50121 Florence, Italy

SPOO, JULIA
Universitätsklinikum Jena
Klinik für Dermatologie
und dermatologische Allergie
Erfurter Str. 35
07743 Jena, Germany

TAYLOR, JAMES S.
Department of Dermatology
The Cleveland Clinic Foundation
9500 Euclid Avenue
Cleveland, OH 44195-5032, USA

UTER, WOLFGANG
Institut für Medizininformatik,
Biometrie und Epidemiologie
der Universität Erlangen-Nürnberg
Waldstr. 6
91054 Erlangen, Germany

VAN DER WALLE, HENK
Centrum voor Huid en Arbeid
Wagnerlaan 55
6815 AD Arnhem, The Netherlands

WAHLBERG, JAN E.
National Institute for Working life
Vanadisvigen 9
11391 Stockholm, Sweden

WIGGER-ALBERTI, W.
ProDERM
Institut für Angewandte Dermatologische
Forschung GmbH
Industriestr. 1
22869 Schenefeld, Germany

ZHAI, H.
University of California,
Department of Dermatology
School of Medicine
Box 0989, Surge 110
San Francisco, CA 94143-0989, USA

ZIMERSON, ERIK
Department of Occupational
and Environmental Dermatology
University Hospital
20502 Malmö, Sweden

Part 1
Epidemiology, Treatment, and Prognosis

CHAPTER 1

The Epidemiology of Occupational Contact Dermatitis

T. L. DIEPGEN, P. J. COENRAADS

Introduction

Work-related dermatoses, in particular hand dermatitis, are still among the most prevalent occupational diseases. There is a vast literature on work-related dermatoses, particularly case reports and investigative clinical studies; their epidemiology, however, has received little attention. Understanding the epidemiology of occupational contact dermatitis (OCD) is essential to determine the etiologic and contributing factors of the disease and to make recommendations for its prevention. Only a few truly epidemiological studies of OCD have been published, and most of our knowledge about OCD is derived from clinical case reports, clinical studies of groups consisting of in- and out-patients, statistical compilations of patch test reports, official occupational disease reports based on workers' compensation agencies and state labor and health departments, or from studies of small outbreaks of skin diseases at the work place. All these data sources have their limitations and must be interpreted carefully. In this chapter the methodological aspects of the available data on the distribution and determinants of OCD will be discussed.

The majority of work-related dermatoses (more than 95%) are subtypes of contact dermatitis; the rest are other dermatoses such as skin cancer, contact urticaria, oil acne, chloracne, chemically-induced leucoderma, and infections. Contact dermatitis is a pattern of inflammatory response of the skin that may occur as a result of contact with external factors (allergens, irritants). The clinical picture is a polymorphic pattern of inflammation of the skin characterized by a wide range of clinical features like itching, redness, scaling, erythema, vesiculation, and clustered papulovesicles. In chronic cases, fissuring, hyperkeratosis, and lichenification occur. On etiological grounds the two most important types of OCD are irritant contact dermatitis (ICD) and allergic contact dermatitis (ACD). ICD results from contact with irritant substances, while ACD is a delayed-type immunological reaction in response to contact with an allergen in sensitized individuals. In the pathogenesis of contact dermatitis, irritants and allergens are simultaneously interwoven and endogenous and environmental factors are often additionally involved. In many instances of allergic contact dermatitis, simultaneous exposure to different irritant factors plays an essential part in its development. The distinction from other types of eczematous disorders may sometimes be difficult because the classifications are based upon a combination of morphological, etiological, constitutional and other factors. The variety of morphology and natural history of contact dermatitis makes it difficult to define a widely accepted, standardized definition which is needed to compare epidemiological studies.

A special subtype of contact allergy is mediated by IgE, resulting in an immediate-type contact reaction presenting itself as contact urticaria. The clinical picture of urticaria is different from eczema/dermatitis, but after repeated episodes on the hands this contact urticaria can eczematize, i.e. gradually progress to hand eczema. In the past decade, this disease has gained increasing attention because of the rising prevalence of contact urticaria due to latex proteins among health care workers (Turjanmaa et al. 1996).

Case Ascertainment, Misclassification, and Bias

The accuracy of the diagnosis depends on the experience, knowledge and skill level of the physician who makes the diagnosis, and on the difficulties in confirming the relationship with an exposure. Detailed patch testing or provocation tests are necessary to determine whether sensitization to certain agents has occurred, but even then it is sometimes not certain whether the contact dermatitis is of allergic origin. Therefore, these patch tests or provocation tests are helpful in diagnosing ACD, but they carry the risk of high false positive rates, irritant reactions or difficulties in interpretation. It is often a matter of subjectivity to establish a positive patch test result as a clinically or occupationally relevant reaction, in addition to deciding whether the test result is false-positive or not.

False positive reactions are common. It was reported by Nethercott (Nethercott 1990) that the sensitivity and specificity of patch testing are approximately 70% with a 50% relevance for positive tests (i.e., in only half the cases can the substance inducing a patch test response be established as the cause of the patient's skin disease). In order to ascertain the validity of a used instrument like patch testing, the terms "sensitivity," "specificity" and "predictive value" are used. The sensitivity stands for the chance that cases with ACD are correctly diagnosed, the specificity that the non-ACD cases are correctly stated. From a statistical point of view, however, it is more essential to calculate the positive predictive value (PPV), which is the proportion of those individuals diagnosed by the instrument used, who actually have ACD. The PPV is a function of the true prevalence of ACD in the population, the sensitivity and the specificity (Diepgen and Coenraads 2000). If, for example, the prevalence of ACD to nickel were 10% and the specificity and sensitivity of patch testing 90%, then a positive reaction would diagnose only 50% of the cases correctly. Therefore, nearly always, individuals are missed who do carry an ACD, while others are wrongly designated as cases of ACD. In summary, patch testing is less than the ideal gold standard, while in ICD there are no additional confirmatory tests.

There are other sources of systematic errors in samples of patients with OCD (Table 1). The lack of a standard case definition of OCD leads to difficulties in obtaining accurate epidemiological data; case definition can vary from one data source to another.

Table 1. Reasons for systematic errors in samples of patients with occupational contact dermatitis (OCD)

Type of errors	Reasons
Misclassification	Overlap between allergic and irritant contact dermatitis
	Sensitivity and specificity of patch testing is approximately 70%
	Lack of standard case definition
Information bias	Ascertainment of cases varied from dermatological examination to self-administered questionnaires
	Instruments are not standardized or evaluated ($\rightarrow$ over- or underestimation)
Selection bias	Samples of OCD are not selected at random
	Samples are not population based
	Less than one third of cases with work-related skin complains result in medical attention

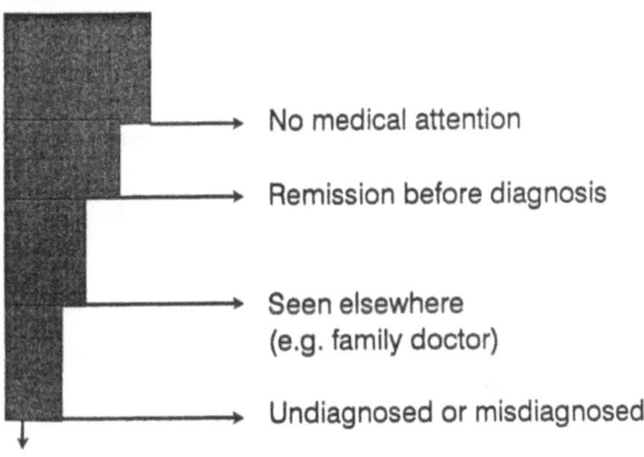

Fig. 1. Selection bias in epidemiological studies of contact dermatitis

Classical epidemiological sources of data are morbidity statistics or observational studies. Mortality statistics are unhelpful because contact dermatitis is never fatal. In morbidity statistics, case ascertainment usually involves registration of persons with dermatitis who fulfill additional criteria for registration, such as hospital admission, sickness leave or referral to a specialist. This restriction in the definition of a case will probably result in selective inclusion of the more severe cases, since a large proportion of individuals suffering from contact dermatitis do not come to medical attention or are seen elsewhere (Fig. 1).

In an epidemiological study on the prevalence of hand eczema (HE) in different occupational groups it was noted that in population-based studies the symptoms of contact dermatitis are relatively mild in the majority of cases, judged from the proportion of cases that resulted in sick leave or medical attention (Smit et al. 1993). Out of all persons with work-related hand dermatitis only between

15% and 36% had consulted a physician for treatment, and sick leave due to their symptoms occurred in only 4% to 9%.

In observational studies on contact dermatitis the ascertainment of cases varies from intensive efforts by medical examination of the complete study population to the relatively easy-to-apply method of self-administered questionnaires or by a combination of both. The advantage of observational studies is that case ascertainment can be performed using uniform criteria for the definition of cases. However, the frequency of cases obtained by questionnaire may be quite different from those ascertained by clinical examination. The size of the differences in prevalence estimates that may arise as a result of differences in the definition and method of diagnosing hand eczema (information bias) has been investigated by Smit et al. (1992). Two types of questionnaire diagnoses, a "symptom-based" and a "self-reported" diagnosis were compared with the medical diagnosis of hand eczema. The prevalence of HE according to the medical diagnosis was 18%, but according to the symptom-based diagnosis 48%, and to the self-reported diagnosis 17%. The sensitivity and specificity of the symptom-based diagnosis were 100% and 64%, and of the self-reported 65% and 93%. That means that the symptom-based diagnosis of HE overestimated, and the self-reported diagnosis underestimated the prevalence of HE according to the medical diagnosis.

An adaptation of the same questionnaire to a study among workers in the rubber industry showed different findings: sensitivity was moderate (71%), with a low positive predictive value of 18% (Vermeulen 2000). A Swedish study indicates that questionnaires based on self reports of clinical symptoms are not necessarily better (Svensson 2002). A recently developed extensive questionnaire, also available in English, is currently being evaluated in Scandinavian countries (Tuohilampi questionnaire, no date).

Incidence and Prevalence

Data on the incidence and prevalence of occupational dermatoses are scarce. The most important sources of data are occupational disease registries, case series of patients visiting dermatology clinics, and a limited number of cross-sectional studies in one or more occupational groups. There is a huge amount of data on patch-tested patients in different countries (Storrs et al. 1989; Frosch et al. 1993; Schnuch et al 1998) (Table 2).

Nevertheless, all measures of disease frequency need, in addition to the number of cases in the numerator, an estimate of the size of the population under study in the denominator. As mentioned above, in case series the numerator is often biased. And with few exceptions the size of the denominator is unknown in many publications presenting the frequency of occupational contact dermatitis. This is the reason why studies among patient populations from dermatology clinics are not adequate for estimating prevalence or incidence rates.

The point prevalence includes only subjects with actual OCD. Since OCD is often a chronically relapsing disease, the point prevalence is therefore less informative than the period prevalence. On the other hand, the accuracy of recall will decrease with time, because persons who have not had recent complaints are more

Table 2. Incidence of notified occupational skin diseases per 1000 per year

Occupation or occupational sector	Geographical entity		
	United States	Bavaria, Germany	Denmark
Cooks, bakers		6	10
Hairdressers		24	11
Services	0.6		
Cleaners, household			13.2
Hospitals	3.1		
Nurses		1.5	1.5
Machinery	2.3		
Mechanics		3.4	6.6
Meat products	5.7		
Meat/fish industry			10.1
Grand average of total workforce	0.8	0.8	0.8

likely to forget to report their earlier contact dermatitis. The period prevalence includes subjects with long-lasting contact dermatitis as well as relatively recent cases and thus poses analytical difficulties. No association can be made between exposure and contact dermatitis because the exposure may have changed over time, past exposure may be over- or underestimated, and preventive measures may have been taken after symptoms occurred. Given these considerations, incidence figures are preferred for analyzing risk factors for OCD.

A large-scale survey on hand eczema in an industrial city was repeated a decade later (Meding 1987; Meding 2002). Although it was not strictly a cohort-study, the data gave some indication of secular changes and of a decrease in occupationally related hand eczema.

In many countries occupational contact dermatitis ranks first among all notified occupational diseases and constitutes up to 30% of all occupational diseases for which compensation is payable.

Occupational disease registries provide national data based on the notification of occupational skin diseases and are available in many countries. Although the comparison of national data is hampered by differences across countries in reporting occupational diseases, the average incidence rate of registered occupational contact dermatitis in some countries lies roughly between 0.5 and 1.9 cases per 1000 full-time workers per year (Mathias et al. 1990; Roche 1993; Halkier-Sorensen 1996; Dickel et al. 2002). For a summary of some of these incidence rates, see Fig. 2.

National registries are usually incomplete as a result of underdiagnosis and underreporting of the disease (Taylor 1988). It has been estimated that the incidence of occupational skin diseases in the United States is underestimated by a factor of 10 to 50 (Mathias et al. 1988; BLS 1993), with the milder cases of skin disease not being registered at all. The extent of underreporting is likely to differ between countries, because each country has its own system of notification. The registration of occupational diseases in several countries is based on the notification of occupational diseases for which compensation is payable.

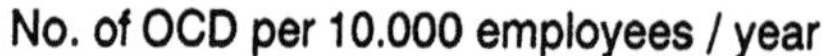

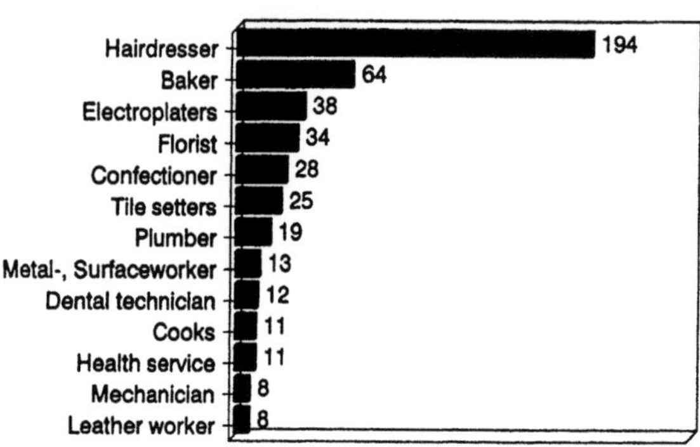

Fig. 2. Incidence rates (per 10,000 employees/3 years) of occupational contact dermatitis (OCD) in North Bavaria (according to Dickel et al. 2001)

In the United States, the occupational disease statistics originate from an annual survey by the Bureau of Labor Statistics among a representative random sample of employees in private industry (Mathias et al. 1988; BLS 1993; Tuohilampi questionnaire, no date).

In the United Kingdom the EPIDERM project for recording occupational dermatoses requires dermatologists in a number of centers to report confirmed or suspected cases of occupational skin disease, including the occupation of the patient concerned (Cherry et al 1994). It is a voluntary system, and operates on the principle of simplicity (ensuring compliance). The system can detect previously unreported hazards. The epidemiological limitations are well recognized, but the system corrects the virtual absence of meaningful official statistics in the UK since 1983.

A fairly active nationwide notification program operates in Denmark: the incidence is 17,700 cases in a workforce of about 2.6 million, i.e., about 0.8 per 1000 per year (Halkier-Sorensen 1996).

In Germany, occupational skin diseases without skin cancer mostly fall under "BK 5101," which is the German code number for those occupational diseases defined as "severe or recurrent skin diseases that force the discontinuation of any activity that causes or that could be causing the development, the worsening, or the recurrence of the skin disease." In the year 2000, out of 81,542 notified occupational diseases, 20,931 were skin disease according to BK 5101 (Diepgen 2002). In Northern Bavaria (Germany), a detailed population-based prospective study was performed to classify all cases of occupational skin diseases without skin cancer (BK 5101) (Diepgen et al. 1994; Tacke et al. 1995; Dickel et al. 2001, 2002). From 1990 to 1999, a total 5,285 cases were closed and recorded. In cooperation with the State Institute of Labor and Occupation (Bundesanstalt für Arbeit) the numbers of all persons employed in different occupations during the same time period were collected. Since the number of employees in the different occupations was known, a population-based study was performed to investigate incidences and demographic characteristics in occupations classified into 24 groups. In the occupational groups, a work-related skin disease was found in 3,097 cases. In Fig. 2 the annual incidence rates are given for different professions. The estimated overall incidence was 6.7 cases per 10,000 workers per year. The highest incidence was in hairdressers (97.4), bakers (33.2), and florists (23.9), while the largest number of cases was in hairdressers (856), health services (481), and metal-surface workers (260). The median age of all cases was 25 years. The induction period was very short: about 2 years in hairdressers, 3 years in the food industry, and about 4 years in health services and in metalworkers. Females had a considerably higher risk of developing OCD than men. The IR of contact dermatitis was highest between the ages of 15 and 24 years. In 1,611 cases (52%) a delayed-type sensitization with occupational relevance was perceived. The results demonstrate the rank of occupations hazardous for the skin and are helpful for defining target groups for prevention.

Social and Economic Impact of OCD

Although contact dermatitis does not commonly lead to hospitalization, and minor degrees of contact dermatitis are often accepted as a normal hazard of life, the occupational, domestic, social and psychological implications of OCD may be considerable. It must be assumed that the total economic impact of OCD is very high (Table 3). OCD interacts with numerous allergens and irritants that are present in daily household activities, in many hobbies and sports. Additionally, contact dermatitis is often localized on the hands, a highly visible area of the body, thus drawing attention and causing difficulties in social interaction. Jowett and Ryan (1985) found that, in general, 38% of patients with eczema noticed interference with their social life.

There are only a few studies about the costs of OCD. About 20 years ago, the total annual costs of OCD may have ranged from $222 million to $1 billion in the US (Mathias 1985). These estimates do not include costs of occupational retraining. In Germany, retraining costs about 100,000 to 200,000 DM per case; in the year 1993, 3,150 individuals attended such a retraining program (Diepgen et al. 1995).

The Netherlands government (Ministry of Social Affairs and Employment) published a report about the cost of work-related diseases and injuries (Ministry 1997). The direct medical costs, i.e. not the costs in terms of loss of income, loss of productivity etc., due to work-related skin diseases was estimated to be 92 million guilders for the year 1995. This is about 42 million Euro for a Netherlands population of about 15 million inhabitants.

Table 3. The total economic impact of occupational contact dermatitis is very high according to the following costs

- Direct cost of medical care, workers' compensation or disability payments
- Indirect costs associated with lost workdays and loss of productivity
- Costs of occupational retraining
- Costs attributable to the effects on the quality of life

In spite of the poor clinical prognosis of OCD, there are no recent studies on the costs attributable to the effects on the quality of life or activities of daily living.

Determinants of OCD

The development of OCD is determined by a combination of individual susceptibility (endogenous factors) and exposure characteristics (exogenous factors). Skin contact with irritants and/or allergens is a necessary condition of contact dermatitis and the probability and severity of a reaction depend on the type and intensity of exposure. Additionally, apart from exposure to hazardous substances there are many endogenous factors that may influence the development of contact dermatitis, such as atopic constitution, the condition of the epidermal barrier, sensitization, psychological factors, age, and gender. Environmental factors may play a role in this process by influencing the individual susceptibility and the characteristics of exposure. If these factors are not properly controlled for, either in the design or in the analysis, they may act as confounders in the study.

Exposure to Irritants and Allergens

The most important risk factor for OCD is the exposure to irritants. Well known irritants are water (wet work), detergents and cleansing agents, hand cleaners, chemicals, cutting fluids, and abrasives. In a study on hand eczema (HE) (Diepgen and Fartasch 1993) at least one of those irritants were always involved in ICD but also in 84% of ACD, and in 60% of atopic HE. Out of 145 grouped exposure sources, the 5 most frequently stated substances were detergents, water, metals, foodstuff and rubber in notified occupational skin diseases in Denmark (Halkier-Sorensen 1996). These substances caused approximately half of the eczema cases. The most important irritant seems to be wet work. According to the German regulation of hazardous substances at the work place, "wet work" is defined if individuals have their skin exposed to liquids longer than 2 h per day, or use occlusive gloves longer than 2 h per day, or clean their hands very often (e.g. 20 times per day or less if the cleaning procedure is more aggressive).

The highest priority in the cascade of prevention measures has the elimination or replacement of harmful exposures. Therefore it is important to know the prevalence and distribution of sensitizations in different profession.

In hairdressing there is detailed knowledge about work related allergens. A study in North Bavaria (Diepgen et al. 1994) showed that glycerylmonothioglycolate (GMTG), p-phenylendiamin, ammonium persulphate and toluylendiaminsulphate are the most frequent sensitizers and the most frequent occupationally relevant allergens in hairdressers with OCD. Sensitization to nickel is frequent, but nickel very rarely plays an occupationally relevant role in hairdressers, and is usually not occupationally related to the contact dermatitis in many other professions (Diepgen and Drexler 2000). In metalworkers on the contrary, occupational contact dermatitis is mostly caused by irritants, and in metalworkers with OCD, occupationally important allergens as contributing factor are rarely detected. In the North Bavarian study, the sensitizations diagnosed in this group were mostly caused by substances that are included in the "European standard series" (a standard panel of patch tests) but only a few of these sensitizers were occupationally relevant.

Nickel is a commonly used industrial product (Kanerva et al. 2000), which can be found as an alloy component in most metals as well as precious metals, including stainless steel, silver, and 14 karat gold (Liden 1994). A nickel layer is even found underneath chromium plated metal. Sweating dissolves more nickel out of the metal and will do so even through a layer of cloth, paint, nail polish, or other barriers. McDonagh et al. (1992) confirmed that ear piercing is likely to induce nickel sensitivity in women, whereas men are more likely to be sensitized by occupational exposure. The first report on a contact dermatitis caused by nickel ions was published in 1889 by Blaschko (1889) as "galvanizer eczema." Workers at risk of acquiring a nickel sensitization are platers, due to direct nickel exposure; electronic workers, due to nickel-plated earthing straps and tools; metalworkers, due to cutting fluids with dissolved nickel; hairdressers, due to nickel-containing tools and equipment; car mechanics, due to nickel-plated tools; and cleaners, due to nickel-plated handles, tools, and other equipment. The role of nickel-releasing metal tools and equipment can be easily checked by the dimethylglyoxime test (Liden et al. 1998; Liden and Johnsson 2001). Notwithstanding the occurrence of nickel in numerous work environments, it should be emphasized that a nickel allergy is predominantly non-occupationally related, normally induced by personal nickel-plated objects, such as costume jewelry, eyeglass frames, buttons, and catches (Diepgen and Drexler 2000). In 2001, the EU Nickel Directive passed in 1994, which aimed to lower nickel sensitization rates in Europe, became fully operative.

Chromium sensitization is still a problem in occupational and non-occupational contact dermatitis. Irvine et al. 1994 have described OCD among 1138 construction workers employed in the Channel Tunnel project. Out of 180 patch tested workers with OCD, 53% had a positive reaction to chromate. We have analyzed the distribution of sensitizations against chromium and the percentage of occupationally relevant sensitizations in different groups of patients with notified occupational contact dermatitis (Fig. 3). The highest percentages were found in tile setters, bricklayers, electroplaters, and the leather industry. Only through such a population-based investigation can it be clearly demonstrated which occupational groups are running a mild, moderate or high risk of ACD due to specific allergens.

There are, however, limitations and problems in epidemiological studies examining the risk of sensitizing or irritant agents. A high ranking agent in a case series is not automatically a strong sensitizer or irritant. A wide application of a weak allergen or irritant is more likely to result in a high proportion of cases than the use of a particular strong but rare agent. It should be noted that exposure is characterized by concentration and duration. Without doubt, exposure is the most important determinant of risk, but exposure quantification techniques are underdeveloped in occupational dermatology. Exposure changes with time, and the affected worker may continue to have eczema yet no longer be exposed

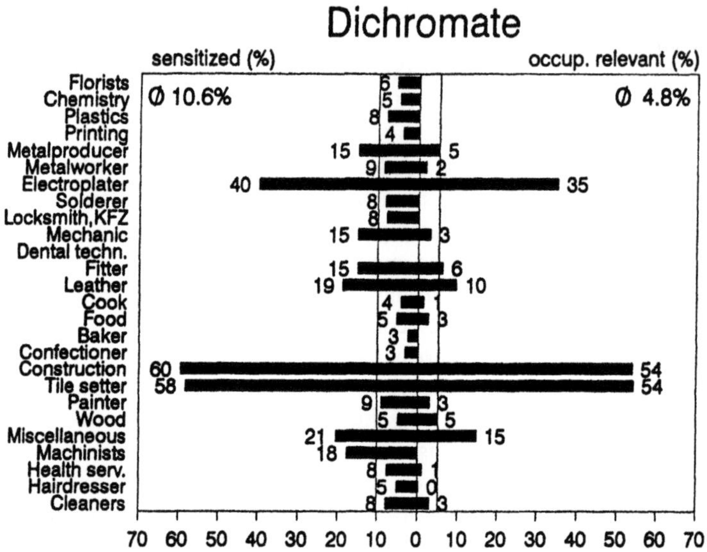

Fig. 3. Distribution of delayed-type sensitization and occupationally relevant allergy against chromium in different occupational groups of individuals with notified occupational contact dermatitis in North Bavaria

to the causative agent. The evaluation of past exposure may be exceedingly difficult which leads to recall and information bias. Because of unique exposures, the results of a study may not be generalizable. Cross-sectional studies are subject to survivor bias because subjects with severe skin diseases and/or contact allergy may leave the work force (healthy worker effect). The reverse has also been observed: in a study of hand eczema among office workers there were a number of subjects with hand eczema who had chosen this occupation because of their handicap (Uter 1998).

Atopy and Atopic Skin Diathesis

Individuals with a personal history of atopy seems to run a considerable risk of developing hand eczema when exposed to occupational agents that are a burden to the skin. (Coenraads and Diepgen 1998). In comparing the figures quoted in the literature one is faced with the same difficulties of selection and interpretation that have been mentioned before. Additionally, the definition of atopy itself differs considerably. Some authors include a family history as well as a personal history of atopy, others divide their subjects into those with atopic eczema and those with respiratory allergy; some would only accept positive prick-tests as evidence for the atopic diathesis.

Individuals with an atopic disposition can develop atopic eczema, allergic rhinitis or allergic asthma. Presently there is sufficient evidence that these different atopic manifestations, especially respiratory atopy, are not always associated with an increased risk for occupational contact dermatitis. Two important issues have to be distinguished:

1. A personal history of atopy is a well known factor influencing irritant but not allergic contact dermatitis. An allergic contact dermatitis based on a type IV contact allergy to occupational sensitizers does not seem to be more prevalent among atopics (Rystedt 1985; Klas et al. 1996). With respect to type I (IgE-mediated) contact urticarial reactions, which can proceed to hand eczema, the situation is different. Immediate-type contact reactions to latex (gloves used by health-care personnel) or alpha-amylase (in yeast used by bakers) or food proteins (in caterers) are more common among atopics (Rycroft 1995; Lahti 1995).
2. Mucosal atopy (asthma, hay fever) must be distinguished from atopic skin diathesis with regard to the risk of developing occupational contact dermatitis. Nowadays there is sufficient evidence that mucosal atopy, without skin manifestations, is not associated with increased risk of irritant contact dermatitis (Rystedt 1985; Diepgen and Fartasch 1993; Diepgen et al. 1993; Majoie et al. 1996).

In bakers, we can demonstrate that atopic skin diathesis is the most important endogenous risk factor (Tacke et al. 1995). Assuming different frequency figures of atopic skin diathesis in the general population the relative risk for atopic subjects of developing occupational contact dermatitis differs between 4.6 and 18.8%. The attributable risk or etiologic fraction, representing the proportion of OSD that can be explained by this risk factor, was between 42% and 51% in this population.

Atopic eczema (AE) in childhood seems to be a risk factor for hand eczema in adults (Lammintausta and Kalimo 1981; Rystedt 1985). However, theses studies also found that a considerable number of subjects with a personal history of AE managed to work in risk occupations without developing HE. Therefore a reduced resistance to irritants does not occur in all subjects with AE and may occur in subjects with respiratory atopy and in non-atopics.

In a prospective study among 1,564 new employees of an automobile manufacturing industry, on average 4.4% acquired hand eczema during the first year of employment (Kristensen et al. 1992). The risk was significantly higher in individuals with previous hand eczema (21%), atopic dermatitis (14%), wool intolerance (11%), and hay fever (9%).

Smit et al. (1994) followed 74 apprentice hairdressers and 111 apprentice nurses from the start of first occupational exposure until the end of their apprenticeship. The average incidence rate of hand dermatitis was 32.8 cases/100 person-years in hairdressers and 14.5 cases/100 person-years in nurses. The relative risk on hand eczema of having a dry versus normal skin type was 7.3 in hairdressers and 1.7 in nurses. Apprentice nurses with a history of (atopic) mucosal symptoms had a 3.4-fold increased risk of hand dermatitis, in apprentice hairdressers this was 2.2.

Prognosis of OCD

The prognosis of OCD is notoriously poor (Rycroft 1995). A review of the studies about the prognosis of contact dermatitis showed that only half or less than half of the patients had healed after several years of follow-up (Hogan et al. 1990). Depending on the severity of the symptoms, the period of follow-up, and the intensity of exposure, recurring symptoms of contact dermatitis in working-populations varied widely in eczema patients (35–80%).

The prognosis for allergic contact dermatitis is thought to be worse than for irritant contact dermatitis (Fregert 1975; Meding and Swanbeck 1990). Not all studies show this effect, but the greater tendency for medical consultation, sick leave, and permanent disability in persons with allergic contact dermatitis is consistent with the observation that symptoms in these patients are generally more persistent than in patients with irritant dermatitis (Fregert 1975; Meding and Swanbeck 1990). It should be kept in mind, however, that information bias and selection bias may have caused the discrepancies; contact allergy to chromate in men, and to nickel in women have probably "contaminated" the statistics. A persistent and troublesome type of dermatitis is more likely to be subject to additional skin testing, creating a greater chance of a positive test result. The relevance of these common allergies with respect to persistence is uncertain; it can be questioned whether people with such an allergy have allergic contact dermatitis, or rather a subtype of dermatitis that is complicated by allergy to the metals, chromate and nickel. Moreover, for specific contact allergies, it may be relatively easy to avoid the causative agent.

Some recent retrospective studies found a better prognosis: In a questionnaire study with a response rate of 68%, out of 201 workers with OCD, 76% noted improvement and 40% reported that they were currently free of any eruption (Nethercott and Holness 1994). Approximately one third noted that their skin disease interfered with household, work, or recreational activities. It is notable that 37% of this group still had ongoing problems with their skin at the time of follow-up. In a Swiss study, out of 88 construction workers with occupational dichromate contact dermatitis 72% healed in the first few years after being recognized as medically unfit to continue their job (Lips et al. 1996). These workers mostly changed industry and strictly avoided all contact with cement or chromium salts. The authors conclude that strict allergen avoidance and financial support in the case of job change are important factors in improving the prognosis of OCD. In contrast to these findings, Shah et al. (1996) reported that hand eczema in metal-workers carries a poor prognosis, with most workers remaining symptomatic even if they no longer had occupational exposure to metals or oils. Out of a former 51 patients, 82% still had HE.

A follow-up among a sample of the cases notified in the EPIDERM project in the UK indicated that 16% still had persistent dermatitis (Adisesh 2002).

Prevention Studies in OCD

Approaches to the prevention of work-related dermatoses are analogous to the prevention of other work-related diseases. In Table 4 the principles and range of prevention measures for OCD are presented. The highest priority should be given to measures "at the source," such as elimination or replacement of harmful expo-

Table 4. Principles and range of prevention measures for occupational contact dermatitis

1. Elimination or replacement of harmful substances (irritants, allergens)
2. Technical measures (e.g. encapsulation of the process, automation)
3. Organization (e.g. wet work distributed to all employees)
4. Personal protection (e.g. gloves, barrier creams, after-work creams, soaps)
5. Pre-employment screening

sures to irritants and allergens. Strategies in the prevention of occupational contact dermatitis include identifying allergens and irritants, substituting chemicals that are less irritating or allergenic, establishing engineering controls to reduce exposure, and organizing the work in a way that all employees are exposed at the same degree. Personal protection, such as gloves or barrier cream, has to be the last choice, but is often resorted to in the first place. Selection of less susceptible individuals is an undesirable option.

Presently, epidemiological intervention studies that evaluate the relative impact of various measures to prevent contact dermatitis, have rarely been published. Clinical observations indicate that many personal protective measures do not have the desired effect, but epidemiological evidence for or against is lacking. Protective gloves, for example, are widely recommended, but may well contribute to increased risk of contact dermatitis: inside gloves the micro-environment is drastically changed and faulty gloves are worse than no gloves at all. In some working processes (machine operating) the use of gloves can cause accidents. Barrier creams are also widely prescribed, although the effect in terms of reduction of incidence or prevalence of dermatitis has not yet been documented. Emollient creams and ointments used during and after work are also supposed to be effective in preventing contact dermatitis of the irritant type, but the epidemiological evidence is scant (Berndt 2000; Goh and Gan 1994; Halkier-Sorensen and Thestrup-Pedersen 1993; McCormick et al. 2001; Perrenoud et al. 2000). The misuse of soaps and detergents can directly provoke irritant contact dermatitis of the hands. Therefore, additional interventions are needed, which include providing advice on the proper use of gloves and barrier creams, and educating the workforce about exposure and skin care (Uter 1999).

Scandinavian countries introduced the addition of ferrous sulfate to cement as mandatory to reduce the prevalence of chromate allergy in bricklayers (Fregert et al. 1979). However, chromate allergy seems to have decreased in countries that did not introduce this measure (Burrows and Corbett 1977) and in Sweden before the change (Färm 1986). A historical cohort, studied during the transition to chromate-free cement in Denmark, was reconstructed by Avnstorp (1989) from two cross-sectional studies in the same cement factory. As the data were derived mostly from two different populations and did not give incidence-based relative risks, the evidence was indirect, but pointed towards a beneficial effect. Zachariae et al. (1996) confirm that chromium eczema due to occupational cement contact is now a rare disease in a Danish region where the chromate content in wet cement has been reduced below a level of 2 ppm, but chromium eczema from other causes, particularly from leather, is still a problem in the same area.

Recently an impressive downward trend of stated cases of occupational skin diseases in hairdressers in Northern Bavaria over the last decade was demonstrated (Dickel et al. 2002). This appears to reflect primarily improvements in working conditions due to legislation and intensified preventive measures rather than a change in the natural history of occupational skin disease. While the prognosis for recovery from occupational skin disease has not changed significantly over the past five decades, the co-operation of dermatologists, governmental physicians, employers, employees, competent workers' compensation board, hairdressers' guild, hair cosmetics manufacturers, and legislative authorities has led to a reduction of occupational skin diseases in hairdressing. However, to achieve a long-lasting reduction, interdisciplinary co-operation needs to be continued and primary prevention should start as early as possible, preferably by supplementary medical pre-employment examinations of a legally binding character.

References

Adishesh A, Meyer JD, Cherry NM (2002) Prognosis and work absence due to occupational contact dermatitis. Contact Dermatitis 46:273–279

Avnstorp C (1989) Prevalence of cement eczema in Denmark before and since addition of ferrous sulfate to Danish cement. Acta Derm Venereol (Stockh) 69:151–155

Berndt U, Wigger-Alberti W, Gabard B, Elsner P (2000) Efficacy of a barrier cream and its vehicle as protective measures against occupational irritant contact dermatitis. Contact Dermatitis 42:77–80

Blaschko A (1889) Die Berufsdermatosen der Arbeiter. Ein Beitrag zur Gewerbehygiene. I. Das Galvaniseur-Ekzem. Dtsch Med Wochenschr 15:925–927

BLS: Bureau of Labor Statistics (1993) Occupational injuries and illnesses in the United States. US Dept of Labor, Bull 2424

Burrows D, Corbett JR (1977) Industrial dermatitis in Northern Ireland. Contact Dermatitis 3:145–150

Coenraads PJ, Diepgen TL (1998) Risk of hand eczema in employees with past or present atopic dermatitis. Int Arch Occup Environ Health 71:7–13

Coenraads PJ, Diepgen TL, Smit J (2001) Epidemiology. In: Rycroft RJG, Menné T, Frosch PJ, Lepoittevin JP (eds) Textbook of contact dermatitis. 3rd edn, Springer, Berlin Heidelberg New York, pp 187–206

Cherry NM, Beck MH, Owen-Smith V (1994) Surveillance of occupational skin disease in the United Kingdom: the OCC-DERM project. In: Proceedings of the Ninth International Symposium on Epidemiology in Occupational Health. DHHS (NIOSH) Publication no 94–112, Cincinnati, 608–10

Dickel H, Kuss O, Blesius CR, Schmidt A, Diepgen TL (2001) Occupational skin diseases in Northern Bavaria between 1990 and 1999: a population based study. Br J Dermatol 145:453–462

Dickel H, Kuss O, Schmidt A, Diepgen TL (2002) Impact of preventive strategies on trend of occupational skin disease in hairdressers: population-based register study. Br Med J 324:1422–1423

Dickel H, Kuss O, Schmidt A, Diepgen TL (2002) Occupational relevance of positive standard patch test results in employed persons with an initial report of an occupational skin disease. Int Arch Occup Environ Health 75:423–434

Dickel H, Bruckner T, Berhard-Klimt C, Koch T, Scheidt R, Diepgen TL (2002) Surveillance scheme for occupational skin disease in the Saarland, FRG: first report from BKH-S. Contact Dermatitis 46:197–206

Dickel H, Kuss O, Schmidt A, Diepgen TL (2002) Impact of preventive strategies on trend of occupational skin disease in hairdressers: population-based register study. Br Med J 324:1422–1423

Diepgen TL, Fartasch M (1992) Recent epidemiological and genetic studies in atopic dermatitis. Acta Derm Venereol (Stockh) 176:13–18

Diepgen TL, Fartasch M (1993) General aspects of risk factors in hand eczema. In: Menné T, Maibach HI (eds) Hand eczema. CRC Press, Boca Raton, pp 141–156

Diepgen TL, Tepe A, Pilz B, Schmidt A, Hüner A, Huber A, Hornstein OP, Frosch PJ, Fartasch M (1993) Occupational skin diseases in hairdressers and nurses during apprenticeship: design of a prospective epidemiological study. Allergologie 10:396–403

Diepgen TL, Schmidt A, Schmidt M, Fartasch M (1994) Demographic and legal characteristics of occupational skin diseases. Allergologie 17:84–89

Diepgen TL, Schmidt A, Berg A, Plinske W (1995) Medizinische Hinweise für die berufliche Rehabilitation von hautkranken Beschäftigten. Dt Ärztebl 92:A31–A40

Diepgen TL, Coenraads PJ (1995) What can we learn from epidemiological studies on irritant contact dermatitis. In: Elsner P, Maibach HI (eds) Irritant dermatitis: new clinical and experimental aspects. Karger, Basel, pp 18–23

Diepgen TL, Sauerbrei W, Fartasch M (1996) Development and validation of diagnostic scores for atopic dermatitis incorporating criteria of data quality and practical usefulness. J Clin Epidemiology 49:1031–1038

Diepgen TL, Coenraads PJ (1999) The epidemiology of occupational contact dermatitis. Int Arch Occup Environ Health 72:496–506

Diepgen TL, Coenraads PJ (2000) The impact of sensitivity, specificity and positive predictive value of patch testing: The more you test, the more you get? Contact Dermatitis 42:315–317

Diepgen TL, Drexler H (2000) Nickel und seine arbeitsmedizinische Bedeutung als Allergen. Arbeitsmed Sozialmed Umweltmed 35:136–145

Diepgen TL (2002) Editorial. Arbeitsmed Sozialmed Umweltmed

Färm A (1986) Changing patterns in chromate allergy. Contact Dermatitis 15:298–310

Fregert S (1975) Occupational dermatitis in a 10-year material. Contact Dermatitis 1:96–107

Fregert S, Gruvberger G, Sandahl E (1979) Reduction of chromate in cement by iron sulfate. Contact Dermatitis 5:39–42

Frosch PJ, Burrows D, Camarasa JG, Dooms-Goossens A, Ducombs G, Lathi A, Menné T, Rycroft RJG, Shaw S, White IR, Wilkinson JD (1993) Allergic reactions to a hairdressers' series: results from 9 European centres. Contact Dermatitis 28:180–183

Funke U, Fartasch M, Diepgen TL (2001) Incidence of work related hand eczema in apprenticeship – first results of a prospective cohort study in the car industry. Contact Dermatitis 44:166–172

Goh CL, Gan SL (1994) Efficacies of a barrier cream and an afterwork emollient cream against fluid dermatitis in metalworkers: a prospective study. Contact Dermatitis 31:176–180

Halkier-Sorensen L (1996) Occupational skin diseases. Contact Dermatitis 35 [Suppl] 1:1–120

Halkier-Sorensen L, Thestrup-Pedersen K (1993) The efficacy of a moisturizer (Locobase) among cleaners and kitchen assistants during everyday exposure to water and detergents. Contact Dermatitis 29:1–6

Hogan DJ, Dannaker CJ, Maibach HI (1990) The prognosis of contact dermatitis. J Am Acad Dermatol 23:300–307

Irvine C, Pugh CE, Hansen EJ, Rycroft RJG (1994) Cement dermatitis in underground workers during construction of the Channel Tunnel. Occup Med 44:17–23

Johnson MLT, Roberts J (1978) Skin conditions and related need for medical care among persons 1–74 years. United States, 1971–1974. Vital Health Stat 11:i–v, 1–72

Jowett S, Ryan T (1985) Skin disease and handicap: an analysis of the impact of skin conditions. Soc Sci Med 20:425–429

Kanerva L, Toikkanen J, Jolanki R, Estlander T (1996) Statistical data on occupational contact urticaria. Contact Dermatitis 35:229–233

Kanerva L, Jolanki R, Estlander T, Alanko K, Savela A (2000) Incidence rates of occupational allergic contact dermatitis caused by metals. Am J Contact Dermatitis 11:155–160

Klas PA, Corey G, Storrs FJ, Chan SC, Hanifin JM (1996) Allergic and irritant patch test reactions and atopic disease. Contact Dermatitis 34:121–124

Kristensen O (1992) A prospective study of the development of hand eczema in an automobile manufacturing industry. Contact Dermatitis 26:341–345

Lahti A (1995) Immediate contact reactions. In: Rycroft RJG, Menné T, Frosch PJ, Benezra C (eds) Textbook of contact dermatitis. Springer, Berlin Heidelberg New York, pp 62–74

Lammintausta K, Kalimo K (1981) Atopy and hand dermatitis in hospital wet work. Contact Dermatitis 7:301–308

Lidén C (1994) Occupational contact dermatitis due to nickel allergy. Sci Total Environ 148:283–285

Lidén C, Röndell E, Skare L, Nalbanti A (1998) Nickel release from tools on the Swedish market. Contact Dermatitis 39:127–131

Lidén C, Johnsson S (2001) Nickel on the Swedish market before the Nickel Directive. Contact Dermatitis 44:7–12

Lips R, Rast H, Elsner P (1996) Outcome of job change in patients with occupational chromate dermatitis. Contact Dermatitis 34:268–271

Majoie IML, von Blomberg BME, Bruynzeel DP (1996) Development of hand eczema in junior hairdressers: an 8-year follow-up study. Contact Dermatitis 34:243–247

Mathias CGT (1985) The cost of occupational skin disease. Arch Dermatol 121:332–334

Mathias CGT, Morrison JH (1988) Occupational skin disease, United States. Results from the Bureau of Labor Statistics Annual Survey of Occupational Injuries and Illnesses, 1973 through 1984. Arch Dermatol 124:1519–1524

Mathias CGT, Sinks TH, Seligman PJ, Halperin WE (1990) Surveillance of occupational skin disease: a method utilizing worker's compensation claims. Am J Ind Med 17:363–370

McCormick R, Buchman TL, Maki DG (2000) Double-blind, randomized trial of scheduled use of a novel barrier cream and an oil-containing lotion for protecting the hands of health care workers. Am J Infect Control 28:302–310

McDonagh AJG, Wright AL, Cork MJ, Gawkrodger DJ (1992) Nickel sensitivity: the influence of ear piercing and atopy. Br J Dermatol 126:16–18

Meding B, Swanbeck G (1987) Prevalence of hand eczema in an industrial city. Br J Dermatol 116:627-634

Meding B, Swanbeck G (1990) Consequences of having hand eczema. Contact Dermatitis 23:6–14

Meding B, Jarvholm B (2002) Hand eczema in Swedish adults – changes in prevalence between 1983 and 1996. J Invest Dermatol 118:719–723

Ministry of Social Affairs and Employment, The Netherlands (1997) The cost of workplace circumstances in The Netherlands (in Dutch: Kerncijfers maatschappelijke kosten arbeidsomstandigheden). Vuga Uitgeverij, The Hague, NL. ISBN 90.5250.683.3

Nethercott JR (1990) Practical problems in the use of patch testing in the evaluation of patients with contact dermatitis. Curr Probl Dermatol 2:95–123

Nethercott JR, Holness DL (1994) Disease outcome in workers with occupational skin disease. J Am Acad Dermatol 30:569–574

Perrenoud D, Gallerot D, van Melle G (2001) The efficacy of a protective cream in a real world apprentice hairdressers environment. Contact Dermatitis 45:134–138

Roche LM (1993) Use of employer illness reports for occupational disease surveillance among public employees in New Jersey. J Occup Med 35(6):581–586

Rycroft RJG. (1995) Occupational contact dermatitis. In: Rycroft RJG, Menné T, Frosch PJ, Benezra C (eds) Textbook of contact dermatitis. Springer, Berlin Heidelberg New York, pp 343–400

Rystedt I (1985) Work-related hand eczema in atopics. Contact Dermatitis 12:167–171

Schnuch A, Uter W, Geier J, Frosch PJ, Rustemeyer T (1998) Contact allergies in healthcare workers. Results from the IVDK. Acta Derm Venereol 78:358–363

Shah M, Lewis FM, Gawkrodger DJ (1996) Prognosis of occupational hand dermatitis in metalworkers. Contact Dermatitis 34:27–30

Smit HA, Coenraads PJ, Lavrijsen APM, Nater JP (1992) Evaluation of a self-administered questionnaire on hand dermatitis. Contact Dermatitis 26:11–16

Smit HA, Burdorf A, Coenraads PJ (1993) The prevalence of hand dermatitis in different occupations. Int J Epidemiol 22:288–293

Smit HA, van Rijssen A, Vandenbroucke J, Coenraads PJ (1994) Individual susceptibility and the incidence of hand dermatitis in a cohort of apprentice hairdressers and nurses. Scand J Work Environ Health 20:113–121

Storrs FJ, Rosenthal LE, Adams RM, Clendenning W, Emmet EA, Fisher AA, Larsen WG, Maibach HI, Rietschel RL, Schorr WF, Taylor JS (1989) Prevalence and relevance of allergic reactions in patients patch tested in North America -1984 to 1985. J Am Acad Dermatol 20:1038–1045

Svensson A, Meding B, Sundberg K, Stenberg B (2002) Self reported hand eczema: symptom based reports do not increase the validity of diagnosis. Br J Dermatol 147:281–284

Tacke J, Schmidt A, Fartasch M, Diepgen TL (1995) Occupational contact dermatitis in bakers, confectioners and cooks - a population-based study. Contact Dermatitis 33:112–117

Taylor JS. (1988) Occupational disease statistics in perspective (editorial). Arch Dermatol 124:1557–1558

Tuohilampi questionnaire (no date) www.occuphealth.fi

Turjanmaa K, Alenius H, Makinen-Kiljunen S, Reunala T, Palosuo T (1996) Natural rubber latex allergy. Allergy 51:593–602

Uter W, Pfahlberg A, Gefeller O, Schwanitz HJ (1998) Hand eczema in a prospectively followed cohort of office workers. Contact Dermatitis 38:83–89

Uter W, Pfahlberg A, Gefeller O, Schwanitz HJ (1999) Hand dermatitis in a prospectively followed cohort of hairdressing apprentices: final results of the POSH study. Contact Dermatitis 41:280–286

Vermeulen R, Kromhout H, Bruynzeel DP, de Boer EM (2000) Ascertainment of hand dermatitis using a symptom-based questionnaire; applicability in an industrial population. Contact Dermatitis 42:202–206

Zachariae COC, Agner T, Menné T (1996) Chromium allergy in consecutive patients in a country where ferrous sulfate has been added to cement since 1981. Contact Dermatitis 35:83–85

CHAPTER 2

Systemic Toxicity

2

P. Hewitt, H. I. Maibach

Introduction

Human skin is exposed to a plethora of chemicals from birth to death. Following percutaneous absorption, a chemical and/or its metabolites may cause toxicity in another organ distant from the point of entry. Although not generally appreciated, some chemicals are more toxic, at least in animals, when applied topically rather than orally. Further, many compounds are absorbed to a greater degree from the skin than the gastrointestinal (GI) tract, and whole-body exposure can produce systemic absorption of grams of material. This chapter focuses on the limited epidemiologic material available, depending largely on case reports. Many drugs for topical use are capable of producing systemic side effects whose occurrence and severity depends largely on factors that affect the absorption of topically applied drugs.

Factors Affecting Percutaneous Absorption

Integrity of the Barrier

The stratum corneum layer of the epidermis is a major barrier to percutaneous absorption. Anything that alters the structure or function of the stratum corneum will affect epidermal absorption, such as inflammatory processes (dermatitis or psoriasis) or removal of the stratum corneum by stripping or damage by alkalis, acids, etc.

The Physicochemical Properties of the Substance

Absorption is affected by the relative water/lipid solubility of the drug, as well as other factors, such as molecular weight, molecular volume and melting point.

Occlusion

The penetration of some topicals may be increased by up to a factor of ten or more by the use of an occlusive covering. This can be due to increased water retention in the stratum corneum, increased blood flow, increased temperature, and increased surface area after prolonged occlusion (skin wrinkling). Occlusion also prevents accidental wiping off or evaporation (for volatile compounds), hence maintaining a higher dose on the skin surface.

Vehicle Containing the Drug

The greater the affinity of a vehicle for the drug it contains, the less the percutaneous absorption of the drug. The vehicle can also cause chemical damage to the barrier layer. Enhanced solubility produces greater thermodynamic activity, yielding greater flux. Extensive documentation on factors affecting penetration is found in Bronaugh and Maibach (1990; 1991) and Smith and Maibach (1995).

Site of Application

Regional differences in permeability of skin largely depend on the thickness of the intact stratum corneum (Wester and Maibach 1989).

Age

The greatest toxicological response to topical administration has been seen in the infant. The preterm infant does not have intact barrier function and hence is more susceptible to systemic toxicity from topically applied drugs (Greaves et al. 1975). A normal full-term infant probably has a fully developed stratum corneum with complete barrier function (Rasmussen 1979). However, the ratio of surface area to body weight in the newborn is three times that in the adult, resulting in a higher absorption per kilogram of body weight (Wester et al. 1977). Barrett and Rutter (1994) and Maibach and Boisits (1982) provide extensive documentation on this issue. Absorption of some compounds decreases in the aged. Roskos and Maibach (1992) reported that, in older subjects, absorption was decreased for steroids but unchanged for other, more hydrophilic compounds.

Temperature

Generally, increased skin temperature enhances penetration rate, due to the increased blood flow or an increase in skin hydration (Siddiqui 1989; Danon et al. 1986).

Metabolism

It has been well documented that the skin is capable of metabolizing a wide range of xenobiotics and has a full complement of phase-I and phase-II enzymes. When the total volume of the skin is taken into account, it is apparent that the skin is an efficient drug-metabolizing organ. Recent information on skin metabolism is found in Hotchkiss (1995).

Systemic Side-Effects Caused by Topically Applied Drugs and Cosmetics

Topically applied drugs and cosmetics can cause allergic or irritant contact dermatitis. However, this type of side effect, usually limited to the skin, is outside the scope of this chapter. The reader is referred to the textbooks of Fisher (1986) and Rycroft (1995) for references to contact dermatitis. Systemic side effects from topically applied chemicals can sometimes result from either a toxic (irritant) reaction or a hypersensitivity reaction. The latter can be an anaphylactic type of reaction, which is the extreme manifestation of contact urticaria syndrome (Amin et al. 1996). While anaphylactic reactions to topical medicaments are uncommon, their potentially serious nature warrants attention. However, reports of toxic (as distinct from allergic) reactions to applied drugs and cosmetics are more numerous and include many medicaments that have been safely used for many years but which can be toxic under special circumstances.

In the following, chemicals are reviewed in alphabetical order.

Agrochemicals

It has been proposed that the most serious occupational skin-exposure hazard is in agricultural workers, involved in pesticide application. Contaminated clothing, lack of adequate protection and unsafe spraying procedures have caused numerous toxic responses, mainly due to skin absorption (Hotchkiss 1995). A prime example is the insecticide Lindane, which when absorbed into the body, accumulates in the central nervous system and the brain and has been linked with cancer (Murphy 1986). Other pesticides have been found to be genotoxic after topical exposure, including aminocarb, chlordane, dichloro-diphenyl-trichloroethane (DDT) and dichlorvos (Schop et al. 1990).

Anti-acne Creams

Anti-acne creams have been shown to cause systemic toxic effects. For example, retinoic acid is a known teratogen (Steele et al. 1983) and is found in certain formulations. Other formulations contain clindamycin, which is reviewed below.

Antibiotics

Chloramphenicol

Marrow aplasia with a fatal outcome after topical application of chloramphenicol in eye ointment was described by Abrams et al. (1982).

Clindamycin

Topical clindamycin is widely used in the treatment of acne vulgaris. Several cases of topical-clindamycin-associated diarrhea have been reported (Becker et al. 1981; Milstone et al. 1981).

Gentamycin

Topical application to large thermal injuries of the skin has caused ototoxic effects, ranging from mild to severe hearing loss (Dayal et al. 1974). Use of gentamycin ear drops may also be associated with ototoxic reactions (Mittelman 1972).

Neomycin

Just as ototoxicity is a well-known hazard of parenteral neomycin administration, so has deafness been reported after local treatment, including skin infections and burns (Bamford and Jones 1978), application as an aerosol for inhalation, instillation into cavities (Masur et al. 1976), irrigation of large wounds (Kelly et al. 1969) and use of neomycin-containing eardrops (Goffinet 1977; Kellerhals 1978).

Antihistamines

Diphenylpyraline Hydrochloride

Diphenylpyraline hydrochloride has been used topically in Germany for the treatment of eczematous and other itching dermatoses. Psychomotor restlessness, followed by symptomatic psychosis has been observed in 12 patients, nine of whom were children. Other symptoms included disorientation, and optic and acoustic hallucinations. All symptoms disappeared 4 days after discontinuation of the topical medication (Cammann et al. 1971).

Promethazine

Block and Beysovec (1982) reported a 16-month-old male who, after application of 15–20 g of the cream, showed abnormal behavior, loss of balance, inability to focus, irritability, drowsiness and failure to recognize his mother. One day later, all symptoms had spontaneously disappeared.

Doxepin

Percutaneous absorption frequently leads to clinical sedation (package insert, Zonulong, Genderm, Lincolnville, Ill.).

Antimicrobials

Castellani's Solution

Castellani's solution (or paint) is an old medicament mainly used for the local treatment of fungal skin infections. It contains boric acid, fuchsin, resorcinol, water, phenol (90%), acetone, and spirit. Several cases of mild toxicity have been reported after exposure (Lundell and Nordman 1973; Rogers et al. 1978).

Hexachloraphene

Hexachlorophene has been extensively used for reducing the incidence of staphylococcal infections among the newborn (Haddad 1990b). In addition, it has been an ingredient of many medical preparations, cosmetics and other consumer goods. In 1972, as a result of the accidental addition of 6.3% hexachlorophene to baby talcum powder, 204 babies fell ill (convulsions, behavioral changes and CNS depression), and 36 died from respiratory arrest (Pines 1973). The drug was later found to be neurotoxic. Consequently, in 1972, the U.S. Food and Drug Administration (FDA) restricted use of hexachlorophene to prescription use only, or as a surgical scrub and hand wash for health-care personnel. Marzulli and Maibach (1975) have placed in perspective lessons to be learned from its toxicity.

4-Homosulfanilamide

4-Homosulfanilamide (sulfamylon) is a topical sulfonamide used for the treatment of large burns. Sulfamylon is a carbonic anhydrase inhibitor and caused hyperchloremic metabolic acidosis in patients with extensive burns (Liebman et al. 1982). Reversible pulmonary complications (Albert et al. 1982) and methemoglobinuria (Ohlgisser et al. 1978) have also been reported.

Povidone-Iodine

Povidone-iodine (Betadine) is a water-soluble iodine complex which retains the broad-range microbiocidal activity of iodine without its undesirable effects. However, toxicity still occurs from povidone-iodine, mainly when it is used on large areas of burnt skin or on neonates. This is comprehensively dealt with by Postellon and Aronow (1990).

Phenol (Carbolic Acid)

In dilutions of 0.5–2.0%, phenol is sometimes prescribed as an antipruritic in topical medicaments and is used for phenol face peels. It is readily absorbed through the skin and has been shown to have a prolonged elimination due to extensive tissue distribution (Bentur 1998; Baranowski-Dutkiewicz 1981). Phenol-induced ochronosis has been reported in patients who, for many years, treated leg ulcers with wet dressings containing phenol (Cullison 1983). Several case reports document fatal reactions to percutaneously absorbed phenol: by accidental spillage of phenol (Johnstone 1948), due to treatment of burns with a phenol-containing preparation (Cronin and Brauer1949) and due to the application of phenol to wounds (Deichmann 1949). Several cases of sudden death and intra- or post-operative complications have been reported after phenol face peels (Del and Tanski 1980; Truppman and Ellenby 1979). However, this is rather controversial, and some authors feel that, when the procedure is done over a period of more than 1 h and when the dose applied is carefully monitored, phenol face peels are not risky (Baker 1979).

Resorcinol

Resorcinol is used for its keratolytic properties in the treatment of acne vulgaris. It is also a constituent of the antifungal Castellani's solution. It has an anti-thyroid activity; consequently, several cases of myxedema caused by percutaneous absorption of resorcinol, especially from ulcerated surfaces, have been described (Thomas and Gisburn 1961). Methemoglobinemia in children, caused by absorption of resorcinol applied to wounds, has also been reported (Murray 1926). Cunningham (1956) reported many cases of infant toxicity, including cyanosis, hemolytic anemia and hemoglobinemia, and in some cases fatalities were recorded. Although the use of resorcinol in young children and for leg ulcers should be avoided, topical resorcinol, when used for acne vulgaris, has been reported to be safe (Yeung et al. 1983).

Silver Sulfadiazine

Silver sulfadiazine cream is widely used for the topical treatment of burns. Intended primarily for the control of *Pseudomonas* infections, this bactericidal agent acts on a variety of gram-positive and gram-negative bacteria, as well as on yeasts. Its relative freedom from side effects has contributed to its popularity, although there have been reports of nephrotic syndrome (Owens et al. 1974) and leukopenia (Fraser and Beaulieu 1979) following topical therapy.

Aromatic Amines

4,4'-Methylenedianiline and 4,4'-methylene-bis-chloroaniline are two widely used aromatic amines employed in the manufacture of polyurethane foams, epoxy resins and as a curing agent in rubber manufacture. These two chemicals have been shown to be carcinogenic and mutagenic in a number of animal species, and they are structurally similar to the known human bladder carcinogen benzidine (McQueen et al. 1981; Lamb et al. 1986). Both chemicals have been detected in the urine of factory workers (Cocker et al. 1988), and Hotchkiss et al. (1993) reported substantial absorption through human skin in vitro.

Carmustine

Topical carmustine has been used for the treatment of mycosis fungoides, lymphomatoid papulosis and parapsoriasis en plaques. Zackheim (1994) reported their experience of 172 patients with patch-plaque-stage mycosis fungoides treated with topical 1,3-bis(2-chloroethyl)-1-nitrosourea (BCNU) solution. Mild, reversible myelosuppression occurred in less than 10% of patients using 20 mg/day total-body application and was rare in those using 10 mg/day.

Camphor

Camphor is an ingredient of a large number of over-the-counter topical remedies (with a camphor content of 1–20%). It is readily absorbed from all sites of administration, including topical application to the skin. The compound is classified as a class-IV chemical, i.e., a very toxic substance. Many cases of intoxication have been reported, usually after accidental ingestion by children (Skoglund et al. 1977; Kopelman 1990).

Cosmetic Agents

Henna dye is used on nails, skin and hair by married women in the Islamic community and consists of the dried leaves of *Lawsonia alba* (coloring matter is lawsone, a hydroxynaphthoquinone). Sudanese women mix a "black powder" (*p*-phenylenediamine) with henna to accelerate the fixing; however, this combination is particularly toxic, and over 20 cases of such toxicity, some fatal, have been reported. Initial symptoms are those of angioneurotic edema with massive edema of the face, lips, glottis, pharynx, neck and bronchi. The symptoms may then progress on the second day to anuria and acute renal failure (renal tubular necrosis), with death occurring on the third day (D'Arcy 1982). Systemic administration of the *p*-phenylenediamine leads to similar symptoms, and several deaths due to ingestion with suicidal intent have been reported (El et al. 1983).

Spencer and Bischoff (1987) reported that after skin penetration musk ambrette (mainly used as a fragrance) causes the breakdown of cellular elements within the brain, spinal cord and peripheral nerves. These types of effects were also reported for the fragrance acetyl ethyl tetramethyl tetralin.

Crude Oil

Feuston et al. (1997) have reported systemic toxic effects after the dermal application of crude oils to rats. The major effects included reduction in body weight gain, increases in absolute and relative liver and thymus weight, and alteration in red blood cell count, hemoglobin, hematocrit and platelet count. These effects were related to concentrations of polycyclic aromatic compounds found in the crude oil.

Diethyltoluamide

N,N-Diethyl-*m*-toluamide (DEET) has been used as an effective insect repellent since 1957. Although DEET has an overall low incidence of toxicity, prolonged use in children has been discouraged because of reports of toxic encephalopathy (Edwards and Johnson 1987). Although most reports of CNS toxicity have been in children, adults and fetuses may also be at risk. Long-term occupational exposure has led to episodes of confusion, depression, insomnia and muscle cramps (Robbins and Cherniack 1986).

Dimethyl Sulfoxide

The toxicology of in vivo topical dimethyl sulfoxide (DMSO) has been investigated by Kligman (1965). Except for the appearance of cutaneous signs, such as erythema, scaling, contact urticaria, stinging and burning sensations, the drug was tolerated well by all but two individuals. These two individuals developed systemic symptoms, including diffuse erythematous and scaling rash accompanied by severe abdominal cramps, nausea, chills and chest pains. These signs, however, abated in spite of continued administration of the drug.

Dinitrochlorobenzene

Dinitrochlorobenzene (DNCB), a potent contact allergen, has been used for the treatment of recalcitrant alopecia areata. Today, however, its use has been discouraged because of suspicion that DNCB may be mutagenic. DNCB is absorbed in substantial amounts through the skin (Feldmann and Maibach 1970), and possible systemic reactions to DNCB have been reported (McDaniel et al. 1982). A 25-year-old man treated with 0.1% DNCB (daily for 2 months) after prior sensitization experienced generalized urticaria, pruritus and dyspepsia.

Ethanol

Gimenez et al. (1968) described 28 children (3–12 months old) with ethanol toxicity from percutaneous absorption. Ethanol-soaked cloths had been applied under rubber panties, and the number of applications varied from one to three (40 ml/application). All 28 children showed some degree of CNS depression, 24 showed miosis, 15 hypoglycemia, 5 convulsions and 5 respiratory depression; 2 died. Of the two who died, one was autopsied, and the findings were consistent with ethanol toxicity. Topically applied ethanol in tar gel (Ellis et al. 1979) and beer containing shampoo (Stoll and King 1980) has caused Antabuse effects (through percutaneous absorption) in patients on disulfiram for alcoholism.

Fumaric Acid Monoethyl Ester

Two psoriasis patients treated with locally applied fumaric acid ointments consisting of 3% or 5% ethyl fumarate in petrolatum developed symptoms of renal toxicity (Dubiuel and Happle 1972).

Insecticides

Lindane

Lindane is widely used in the treatment of scabies and pediculosis, usually in a 1% lotion which is applied to the entire body. The percutaneous absorption of the drug has been widely documented (Ginsburg et al. 1977; Hosler et al. 1980), as has toxicity (notably CNS) from excessive topical therapeutic application of lindane (Davies et al. 1983; Pramanik and Hansen 1979). Most authors agree that the benefits to be derived from the use of lindane as a scabicide and pediculicide outweigh the risks involved (Solomom et al. 1977).

Malathion

The detailed toxicology of malathion is dealt with by Haddad (1990 a). Malathion is used in the treatment of lice and is generally safe when applied as a 0.5% cream. Ramu et al. (1973) reported four children with toxicity following hair washing with 50% malathion in xylene for the purpose of louse control.

Local Anaesthetics

Benzocaine

Methemoglobinemia has been reported following the topical application of benzocaine (ethyl aminobenzoate) to both skin and mucous membranes, with most cases occurring in infants (Haggerty 1962; Olson and McEvoy 1981). However, toxicity is uncommon (American Medical Association 1977).

Lidocaine

Lidocaine hydrochloride is widely used for topical and local injection anesthesia. Serum lidocaine concentrations higher than 6 µg/ml are associated with toxicity (Selden and Sasahara 1967), whose signs are CNS stimulation followed by depression and later inhibition of cardiovascular function. Systemic toxicity (generalized seizures) from lidocaine applied to the oral cavity in two children has been described (Giard et al. 1983; Mofenson et al. 1983).

Mercurials

The toxicology of mercury is comprehensively dealt with by Aronow (1990). With few exceptions, the use of mercury in medicine is considered to be outdated. However, mercury may still be present in many drugs, even in over-the-counter formulations. All mercurial preparations are a potential hazard and may cause toxicity. Young (1960) examined 70 psoriatic patients treated with an ointment containing ammoniated mercury. Symptoms and signs of mercurial poisoning could be detected in 33 patients. Nephrotic syndrome has been reported after ammoniated mercury-containing ointment application (Lyons et al. 1975). There have been two case reports (Stanley and Frank 1971; Clark et al. 1982) of children who died following the treatment of an omphalocele with merbromin (an organic mercurial antiseptic).

Monobenzone

Monobenzone (monobenzyl ether of hydroquinone) is used topically by patients with extensive vitiligo to depigment their remaining normally pigmented skin. A patient who had been applying the drug for 1 year had an anterior linear deposition of pigment on both corneas. Eleven additional patients with vitiligo acquired conjunctival melanosis and pingueculae (Hedges et al. 1983).

2-Naphthol

2-Naphthol (β-naphthol) is used for the treatment of acne, and between 5% and 10% of a cutaneous dose has been recovered from the urine of subjects (Hemels 1972). Extensive application of 2-naphthol ointments has been responsible for systemic side effects, including vomiting and death (Osol and Farrar 1947).

Podophyllum

The toxicity of podophyllum was reviewed by Cassidy et al. (1982). Although there have been a significant number of case reports describing serious neurologic illness or death following the application of podophyllum, these are generally related to its use in widespread lesions. Podophyllum (20%) in tincture of benzoin is still indicated for isolated venereal warts (Chamberlain et al. 1972).

Salicylic Acid

The general toxicology and percutaneous absorption of salicylates is reviewed by Proudfoot (1990). Salicylic acid (SA) is widely used in dermatology as a topical application for its keratolytic properties. An unpublished review by the U.S. Department of Health, Education and Welfare, quoted by Rasmussen (1979), revealed 13 deaths associated with the widespread use of SA preparations, and all but three occurred in children. Von Weiss and Lever (1964) reported 13 deaths resulting from intoxication with SA following application to the skin and several nonfatal cases of intoxication. The most dramatic account is that of two plantation workers in the Solomon Islands who were painted twice daily with an alcoholic solution of 20% SA and who contracted tinea imbricata involving about 50% of the body. The victims were comatose after 6 h and dead within 28 h (Lindsey 1968).

Silver Nitrate

Ternberg and Luce (1968) observed fatal methemoglobinemia in a 3-year-old girl suffering from extensive burns who was treated with silver nitrate solution. Due to the hypotonicity of the silver nitrate dressings, hyponatremia, hypokalemia and hyperchloremia may develop, especially in children (Connelly 1970). Excessive use of silver-containing drugs has led to local and systemic argyria (Marshall and Schneider 1977) and to renal damage involving the glomeruli with proteinuria (Zech et al. 1973).

Steroids

Corticosteroids

Topically applied glucocorticosteroids are absorbed through the skin (Feldmann and Maibach 1965), resulting in sufficient quantities in the systemic circulation to replace endogenous production. Systemic side effects of topical corticosteroids occur more frequently in children (Feiwel et al. 1969) and in patients with liver disease, due to reduced metabolism of the drug (Burton et al. 1974). The two main causes of systemic side effects are hypercorticism, leading to an iatrogenic Cushing's syndrome, and suppression of the hypothalamic-pituitary-adrenal axis (May et al. 1976).

Sex Hormones

Topical application of estrogen-containing preparations leads to resorption of these hormones and, therefore, to systemic estrogenic effects. Beas et al. (1969) reported on seven children with pseudoprecocious puberty due to an ointment containing estrogens. The most important clinical signs were: intense pigmentation of mammillary areola, linea alba of the abdomen and the genitals, mammary enlargement and the presence of pubic hair. Three female patients also had vaginal discharge and bleeding. After discontinuation of the drug, all symptoms progressively disappeared in every patient. Gynecomastia has also been reported in young boys and men (Edidin and Levitsky 1982; DiRaimondo et al. 1980; Gabrilove and Luria 1978).

Transdermal Drug-Delivery Systems

Reed and Hamburg (1986) reported a case of clonidine-patch toxicity in a 9-month-old infant when a Catapres transdermal therapeutic system 1 (TTS-1) was inadvertently transferred to him from his father. When the clonidine patch was discovered, less than one-tenth of the patch's surface area was adherent to the skin. However, transdermal systems contain an excess amount of drug to maintain the needed concentration gradient for drug delivery. Upon removal, patches still retain a substantial amount of active drug (McEvoy 1989), increasing the risk of toxicity if applied to the skin of an infant or young child.

Miscellaneous

There are many other examples of systemic toxicity caused by absorption through the skin. For example, exposure to acrylamide dust in polymer factories, causing a chronic disease of the nervous system (Garland and Patterson 1967). Skin exposure to ethylene glycol dinitrate during dynamite production results in toxic effects after only a few minutes (Hogstedt and Stahl 1980). Carbon tetrachloride and 2-chloroethanol cause hepatotoxicity and hepatocarcinogenicity (Kronevi et al. 1979). Glycol ethers, in particular ethylene glycol monoethylene ether, are teratogenic and cause menstrual disorders in women (Barlow 1987). Mint (1995) showed that repeated dermal exposure of rats in vivo to dibutyl phthalate caused significant hepatic peroxisome proliferation within 14 days. Crude coal tar has been reported to cause methemogloinemia in infants (Goluboff and MacFadyen 1955). 2,4-Pentanedione, an industrial chemical with a high potential for skin contact, has been shown to cause central neurotoxicity, as well as possible immune system effects (Ballantyne 2001).

Comment

This chapter summarizes literature citations and the basic aspects of percutaneous penetration to alert the reader to the potential for systemic toxicity from topical exposure. Demonstrating causality (rather than association) requires careful documentation. Combining knowledge of the inherent molecular and animal toxicology, cutaneous penetration and metabolism with the adverse-human-reaction literature permits a more precise determination of causality. With each example presented here, the original citations combined with the further documentation noted here should permit more discriminate causality judgments. The above data focuses the need for controlled studies on the toxicity of chemicals that come into contact with the skin, either accidentally or deliberately. Recent texts emphasizing current approaches and technology are Bronaugh and Maibach (1990, 1991), Smith and Maibach (1995) and Marzulli and Maibach (1996).

References

Abrams SM, Degnan TJ, Vinciguerra V (1980) Marrow aplasia following topical application of chloramphenicol eye ointment. Arch Intern Med 140:576–577

Albert T, Lewis N, Warpeha R (1982) Late pulmonary complications with use of mafenide acetate. J Burn Care Rehabil 3

American Medical Association (1977) AMA drug evaluations. Publishing Sciences Group, Littleton

Amin S, Lahti A, Maibach H (1996) Contact urticaria and the contact urticaria syndrome (immediate contact reactions). In: Marzulli F, Maibach H (eds) Dermatoxicology, 5th edn. Hemisphere, Washington, pp 485–504

Aronow R (1990) Mercury. In: Haddad L, Winchester J (eds) Clinical management of poisoning and drug overdose. Saunders, Philadelphia, pp 1002–1009

Baker T (1979) The voice of polite dissent. Plast Reconstr Surg 63:262

Bamford MF, Jones LF (1978) Deafness and biochemical imbalance after burns treatment with topical antibiotics in young children. Report of 6 cases. Arch Dis Child 53:326–329

Baranowski-Dutkiewicz B (1981) Skin absorption of phenol from aqueous solutions in men. Int Arch Occup Environ Health 49:99

Barlow SM (1987) Reproductive hazards from chemicals absorbed through the skin. In: Marzulli FN, Maibach HI (eds) Dermatotoxicology. Hemisphere, New York, pp 597–605

Barrett DA, Rutter N (1994) Transdermal delivery and the premature neonate. Crit Rev Ther Drug Carrier Syst 11:1–30

Beas F, Vargas L, Spada RP, Merchak N (1969) Pseudoprecocious puberty in infants caused by a dermal ointment containing estrogens. J Pediatr 75:127–130

Becker LE, Bergstresser PR, Whiting DA, et al. (1981) Topical clindamycin therapy for acne vulgaris. A cooperative clinical study. Arch Dermatol 117:482–485

Block R, Beysovec L (1982) Promethazine toxicity through percutaneous absorption. Contin Pract 9:28

Bronaugh R, Maibach H (eds) (1990) Percutaneous absorption. Marcel Dekker, New York

Bronaugh R, Maibach H (eds) (1991) Percutaneous penetration in vitro. Marcel Dekker, New York

Burton T, Cunliffe W, Holti G, Wright W (1974) Complications of topical corticosteroid therapy in patients with liver disease. Br J Dermatol 9:22

Cammann R, Hennecke H, Beier R (1971) Symptomatic psychoses after application of "Kolton-Gelee". Psychiatr Neurol Med Psychol (Leipz) 23:426–431

Cassidy DE, Drewry J, Fanning JP (1982) Podophyllum toxicity: a report of a fatal case and a review of the literature. J Toxicol Clin Toxicol 19:35–44

Chamberlain MJ, Reynolds AL, Yeoman WB (1972) Medical memoranda. Toxic effect of podophyllum application in pregnancy. BMJ 3:391–392

Clark JA, Kasselberg AG, Glick AD, O'Neill JJ (1982) Mercury poisoning from merbromin (Mercurochrome) therapy of omphalocele: correlation of toxicologic, histologic, and electron microscopic findings. Clin Pediatr (Phila) 21:445–447

Cocker J, Boobis AR, Davies DS (1988) Determination of the N-acetyl metabolites of 4,4'-methylenedianiline and 4,4'-methylene-bis(2-chloroaniline) in urine. Biomed Environ Mass Spectrom 17:161–167

Connelly DM (1970) Silver nitrate. Ideal burn wound therapy? NY State J Med 70:1642–1644

Cronin T, Brauer R (1949) Death due to phenol contained in FoilleR. JAMA 139:777

Cullison D, Abele DC, O'Quinn JL (1983) Localized exogenous ochronosis. J Am Acad Dermatol 8:882–889

Cunningham A (1956) Resorcine poisoning. Arch Dis Child 31:173

Danon A, Ben-Shimon S, Ben-Zui Z (1986) Effect of exercise and heat exposure on percutaneous absorption of methyl salicylate. Eur J Clin Pharmacol 3:49–52

D'Arcy P (1982) Fatalities with the use of a henna dye. Pharm Int 3:217

Davies JE, Dedhia HV, Morgade C, Barquet A, Maibach HI (1983) Lindane poisonings. Arch Dermatol 119:142–144

Dayal VS, Smith EL, McCain WG (1974) Cochlear and vestibular gentamicin toxicity. A clinical study of systemic and topical usage. Arch Otolaryngol 100:338–340

Deichmann W (1949) Local and systemic effects following skin contact with phenol – a review of the literature. J Ind Hyg 31:146

Del PA, Tanski A (1980) Chemical face peeling-malignant therapy for benign disease? Plast Reconstr Surg 66:121–123

DiRaimondo CV, Roach AC, Meador CK (1980) Gynecomastia from exposure to vaginal estrogen cream. N Engl J Med 302:1089–1090

Drake TE (1974) Reaction to gentamicin sulfate cream. Arch Dermatol 110:638

Dubiel W, Happle R (1972) Experimental treatment with fumaric acid monoethylester in psoriasis vulgaris. Z Haut Geschlechtskr 47:545–550

Edidin DV, Levitsky LL (1982) Prepubertal gynecomastia associated with estrogen-containing hair cream. Am J Dis Child 136:587–588

Edwards DL, Johnson CE (1987) Insect-repellent-induced toxic encephalopathy in a child. Clin Pharm 6:496–498

El AE, Ahmed ME, Clague HW (1983) Systemic toxicity of p-phenylenediamine. Lancet 1:1341

Ellis CN, Mitchell AJ, Beardsley GJ (1979) Tar gel interaction with disulfiram. Arch Dermatol 115:1367–1368

Feiwel M, James VH, Barnett ES (1969) Effect of potent topical steroids on plasma cortisol levels of infants and children with eczema. Lancet 1:485–487

Feldmann RJ, Maibach HI (1965) Penetration of 14C hydrocortisone through normal skin. Arch Dermatol 91:661

Feldmann RJ, Maibach HI (1970) Absorption of some organic compounds through the skin in man. J Invest Dermatol 54:399–404

Feuston MH, Mackerer CR, Schreiner CA, Hamilton CE (1997) Systemic toxicity of dermally applied crude oils in rats. J Toxicol Environ Health 51:387–399

Fisher A (ed) (1986) Contact dermatitis. Lea and Febiger, Philadelphia

Food and Drug Administration (1976) Gamma benzene hexachloride (Kwell) and other products alert. FDA Drug Bull 6:28

Fraser GL, Beaulieu JT (1979) Leukopenia secondary to sulfadiazine silver. JAMA 241:1928–1929

Gabrilove JL, Luria M (1978) Persistent gynecomastia resulting from scalp inunction of estradiol: a model for persistent gynecomastia. Arch Dermatol 114:1672–1673

Garland TO, Patterson MW (1967) Six cases of acrylamide poisoning. BMJ 4:134–138

Giard MJ, Uden DL, Whitlock DJ, Watson DM (1983) Seizures induced by oral viscous lidocaine (letter). Clin Pharm 2:110

Gimenez ER, Vallejo NE, Izurieta EM, et al (1968) Acute alcoholic intoxication by the percutaneous route. Clinical and experimental study (in Spanish). Arch Argent Pediatr 66:121–135

Ginsburg CM, Lowry W, Reisch JS (1977) Absorption of lindane (gamma benzene hexachloride) in infants and children. J Pediatr 91:998–1000

Goffinet M (1977) Clinically presumptive toxicity of various ear-drops (in French). Acta Otorhinolaryngol Belg 31:585–590

Goluboff N, MacFadyen D (1955) Methemoglobinemia in an infant. J Pediatr 47:222

Greaves SJ, Ferry DG, McQueen EG, et al (1975) Serial hexachlorophene blood levels in the premature infant: clinical pharmacology of hexachlorophene in newborn infants. NZ Med J 81:334–336

Haddad L (1990a) Miscellany. In: Haddad L, Winchester J (eds) Clinical management of poisoning and drug overdose. Saunders, Philadelphia, pp 1474–1478

Haddad L (1990b) Organophosphates and other insecticides In: Haddad L, Winchester J (eds) Clinical management of poisoning and drug overdose. Saunders, Philadelphia, pp 1076–1087

Haggerty R (1962) Blue baby due to methemoglobinemia. N Engl J Med 267:1303

Hedges TD, Kenyon KR, Hanninen LA, Mosher DB (1983) Corneal and conjunctival effects of monobenzone in patients with vitiligo. Arch Ophthalmol 101:64–68

Hemels HG (1972) Percutaneous absorption and distribution of 2-naphthol in man. Br J Dermatol 87:614–622

Hogstedt C, Stahl R (1980) Skin absorption and protective gloves in dynamite work. Am Ind Hyg Assoc J 41:367–372

Hosler J, Tschanz C, Hignite CE, Azarnoff DL (1980) Topical application of lindane cream (Kwell) and antipyrine metabolism. J Invest Dermatol 74:51–53

Hotchkiss SAM, Hewitt PG, Caldwell J (1993) Percutaneous absorption of 4,4'-methylene-bis-2-chloroaniline and 4,4'-methylenedianiline through rat and human skin in vitro. In Vitro Toxicol 7:141–148

Hotchkiss SAM (1995) Skin absorption of occupational chemicals. In: Handbook of occupational hygiene (installment 46). Croner, Surrey, pp 1–38

Johnstone R (1948) Occupational medicine and industrial hygiene. Mosby, St. Louis

Kellerhals B (1978) Risk of inner ear damage from ototoxic eardrops (in German). HNO 26:46–52

Kelly DR, Nilo ER, Berggren RB (1969) Brief recording: deafness after topical neomycin wound irrigation. N Engl J Med 280:1338–1339

Kligman A (1965) Dimethyl sulfoxide – part 2. JAMA 193:151

Kopelman R (1990) Camphor. In: Haddad L, Winchester J (eds) Clinical management of poisoning and drug overdose. Saunders, Philadelphia, pp 1451–1455

Kronevi T, Wahlberg JE, Holmberg B (1979) Histopathology of skin, liver and kidney after epicutaneous administration of five industrial solvents to guinea pigs. Environ Res 19:56–69

Lamb JC, Huff JE, Haseman JK, Murphy ASK, Lilja H (1986) Carcinogenesis studies of 4,4'-methylene-dianiline dihydrochloride given in drinking water to F344/N rats and B6C3F1 mice. J Toxicol Environ Health 18:325–337

Liebman PR, Kennelly MM, Hirsch EF (1982) Hypercarbia and acidosis associated with carbonic anhydrase inhibition: a hazard of topical mafenide acetate use in renal failure. Burns Incl Therm Inj 8:395–398

Lindsey CP (1968) Two cases of fatal salicylate poisoning after topical application of an antifungal solution. Med J Aust 1:353–354

Lundell E, Nordman R (1973) A case of infantile poisoning by topical application of Castellani's solution. Ann Clin Res 5:404–406

Lyons TJ, Christu CN, Larsen FS (1975) Ammoniated mercury ointment and the nephrotic syndrome. Minn Med 58:383–384

Maibach H, Boisits E (eds) (1982) Neonatal skin: structure and function. Marcel Dekker, New York

Marshall JD, Schneider RP (1977) Systemic argyria secondary to topical silver nitrate. Arch Dermatol 113:1077–1079

Marzulli F, Maibach H (1975) Relevance of animal models: the hexachlorophene story. In: Maibach H (ed) Animal models in dermatology. Churchill Livingstone, Edinburgh, pp 156–167

Marzulli F, Maibach H (eds) (1996). Dermatoxicology, 5th edn. Hemisphere, Washington

Masur H, Whelton PK, Whelton A (1976) Neomycin toxicity revisited. Arch Surg 111:822–825

May P, Stein EJ, Ryter RJ, Hirsh FS, Michel B, Levy RP (1976) Cushing syndrome from percutaneous absorption of triamcinolone cream. Arch Intern Med 136:612–613

McDaniel DH, Blatchley DM, Welton WA (1982) Adverse systemic reaction to dinitrochlorobenzene. Arch Dermatol 118:371

McEvoy G (1989) American hospital formulary service drug information 89. American Society of Hospital Pharmacists, Bethesda

McQueen CAB, Maskinsky CJ, Crescenzi SB, Williams GM (1981) The genotoxicity of 4,4′-methylenebis (2-chloroaniline) in rat, mouse and hamster hepatocytes. Toxicol Appl Pharmacol 58:231–235

Milstone EB, McDonald AJ, Scholhamer CJ (1981) Pseudomembranous colitis after topical application of clindamycin. Arch Dermatol 117:154–155

Mint A (1995) Investigation into the topical disposition of the phthalic acid esters, dimethyl phthalate, diethyl phthalate and dibutyl phthalate in rat and human skin (Ph.D. thesis). Imperial College, London

Mittelman H (1972) Ototoxicity of "ototopical" antibiotics: past, present, and future. Trans Am Acad Ophthalmol Otolaryngol 76:1432–1443

Mofenson HC, Caraccio TR, Miller H, Greensher J (1983) Lidocaine toxicity from topical mucosal application. With a review of the clinical pharmacology of lidocaine. Clin Pediatr (Phila) 22:190–192

Murphy SD (1986) Toxic effects of pesticides. In: Klaasen CD, Amdur MO, Doull J (eds) The basic science of poisons, 3rd edn. Macmillan, New York, pp 519–582

Murray M (1926) An analysis of sixty cases of drug poisoning. Arch Pediatr 43:193

Ohlgisser M, Adler M, Ben-Dov D, Taitelman U, Birkhan HJ, Bursztein S (1978) Methemoglobinaemia induced by mafenide acetate in children. A report of two cases. Br J Anaesth 50:299–301

Olson ML, McEvoy GK (1981) Methemoglobinemia induced by local anesthetics. Am J Hosp Pharm 38:89–93

Osol A, Farrar GJ (1947) The dispensatory of the United States of America. Lippincott, Philadelphia

Owens CJ, Yarbrough Dd, Brackett NJ (1974) Nephrotic syndrome following topically applied sulfadiazine silver therapy. Arch Intern Med 134:332–335

Pines WL (1973) Hexachlorophene: why FDA concluded that hexachlorophene was too potent and too dangerous to be used as it once was. CAL 36:4–6

Postellon D, Aronow R (1990) Iodine. In: Haddad L, Winchester J (eds) Clinical management of poisoning and drug overdose. Saunders, Philadelphia, pp 1049–1053

Pramanik AK, Hansen RC (1979) Transcutaneous gamma benzene hexachloride absorption and toxicity in infants and children. Arch Dermatol 115:1224–1225

Proudfoot A (1990) Salicylates and salicylamide. In: Haddad L, Winchester J (eds) Clinical management of poisoning and drug overdose. Saunders, Philadelphia, pp 909–920

Ramu A, Slonim AE, London M, Eyal F (1973) Hyperglycemia in acute malathion poisoning. Isr J Med Sci 9:631–634

Rasmussen JE (1979) Percutaneous absorption in children. In: Dobson R (ed) Year book of dermatology. Year Book Medical, Chicago, pp 15–38

Reed MT, Hamburg EL (1986) Person-to-person transfer of transdermal drug-delivery systems: a case report. N Engl J Med 314:1120–1121

Robbins PJ, Cherniack MG (1986) Review of the biodistribution and toxicity of the insect repellent N,N-diethyl-m-toluamide (DEET). J Toxicol Environ Health 18:503–525

Rogers SC, Burrows D, Neill D (1978) Percutaneous absorption of phenol and methyl alcohol in Magenta Paint BPC. Br J Dermatol 98:559–560

Roskos KV, Maibach HI (1992) Percutaneous absorption and age: Implications for therapy. Drugs Aging 2:432–449

Rycroft R (ed) (1995) Textbook of dermatitis. Springer, Berlin Heidelberg New York

Schop RN, Hardy MH, Goldberg MT (1990) Comparison of the activity of topically applied pesticides and the herbicide 2,4-D in short term in vivo assays of the genotoxicity in the mouse. Fundam Appl Toxicol 15:666–675

Selden R, Sasahara AA (1967) Central nervous system toxicity induced by lidocaine. Report of a case in a patient with liver disease. JAMA 202:908–909

Siddiqui O (1989) Physicochemical, physiological and mathematical considerations in optimizing percutaneous absorption of drugs. Crit Rev Ther Drug Carrier Syst 6:1–39

Skoglund RR, Ware LL Jr, Schanberger JE (1977) Prolonged seizures due to contact and inhalation exposure to camphor. A case report. Clin Pediatr (Phila) 16:901

Smith E, Maibach HI (eds) (1995) Percutaneous penetration enhancers. CRC, Boca Raton

Solomon LM, Fahrner L, West DP (1977) Gamma benzene hexachloride toxicity: a review. Arch Dermatol 113:353–357

Spencer PS, Bischoff MC (1987) Skin as an entry for neurotoxic substances. In: Marzulli FN, Maibach HI (eds) Dermatotoxicology. Hemisphere, New York, pp 625–640

Stanley BE, Frank JE (1971) Mercury poisoning from application to omphalocele. JAMA 216:2144–2145

Steele CE, Trasler DG, New DA (1983) An in vivo/in vitro evaluation of the teratogenic action of excess vitamin A. Teratology 28:209–214

Stewart N, McHugh T (1990) Borates. In: Haddad L, Winchester J (eds) Clinical management of poisoning and drug overdose. Saunders, Philadelphia, pp 1447–1451

Stoll D, King LJ (1980) Disulfiram-alcohol skin reaction to beer-containing shampoo. JAMA 244:2045

Ternberg J, Luce E (1968) Methemoglobinemia: a complication of the silver nitrate treatment of burns. Surgery 63:328

Thomas A, Gisburn M (1961) Exogenous ochronosis and myxoedema from resorcinol. Br J Dermatol 73:378

Truppman ES, Ellenby JD (1979) Major electrocardiographic changes during chemical face peeling. Plast Reconstr Surg 63:44–48

Von Weiss J, Lever W (1964) Percutaneous salicylic acid intoxication in psoriasis. Arch Dermatl 90:614

Wester RC, Maibach HI (1989) Regional variation in percutaneous absorption. In: Bronaugh R, Maibach HI (eds) Percutaneous absorption: mechanisms – methodology – drug delivery. Marcel Dekker, New York, pp 111–120

Wester RC, Noonan PK, Cole MP, Maibach HI (1977) Percutaneous absorption of testosterone in the newborn rhesus monkey: comparison to the adult. Pediatr Res 11:737–739

Yeung D, Kantor S, Nacht S, Gans EH (1983) Percutaneous absorption, blood levels, and urinary excretion of resorcinol applied topically in humans. Int J Dermatol 22:321–324

Young E (1960) Ammoniated mercury poisoning. Br J Dermatol 72:449

Zackheim H (1994) Topical carmustine (BCNU) for patch/plaque mycosis fungoides. Semin Dermatol 13:202–206

Zech P, Colon S, Labeeuw R, Blanc BN, Richard P, Perol M (1973) Nephrotic syndrome with silver deposits in the glomerular basement membranes during argyria. Nouv Presse Med 2:161–164

CHAPTER 3

Evaluation of Barrier Function and Skin Reactivity in Occupational Dermatoses

3

S. Seidenari, F. Giusti, A. Martella

Introduction

A complex interplay of exogenous and endogenous factors is believed to be responsible for the occurrence and course of irritant contact dermatitis (ICD).

Besides identification of job-related aspects like frequent exposure to irritants, knowledge of the host-related predisposing components in risk groups represents an important tool for prevention. This can be achieved both by epidemiological observations and by employing experimental conditions reproducing environmental exposure to skin-damaging substances.

The major endogenous predisposing factor is atopic dermatitis (AD). However, a reduced resistance to irritants does not occur in all patients with atopic eczema and may also occur in non-atopics. Moreover other constitutional factors not fully identified so far may play a more important role than the atopic condition. However, skin defense mechanisms against toxic substances are not only based on personal characteristics but are also mediated by the environment, since the skin responds to environmental aggression with modifications of its barrier properties, thus modulating the response to further stimuli. Therefore, a periodical medical examination including evaluation of skin barrier conditions may represent a method suitable to identify and follow-up subjects at risk because of their intrinsic attributes, but also to evaluate the impact of environmental threats on the skin.

The induction of experimental dermatitis by means of model irritants represents a method for reproducing ICD in a standardized way and can be employed both for evaluating skin reactivity in high-risk subjects and for monitoring the response and adaptation to the occupational milieu. Transepidermal water loss (TEWL) and capacitance measurements and instrumental evaluation of skin blood flow, erythema and edema represent the methods for the quantification of different aspects of experimentally induced irritation.

Skin Lipids and the Barrier

Recently, the essential role of lipids in the regulation of stratum corneum (SC) barrier function and in the water-holding properties of the SC has been thoroughly investigated (Imokawa et al. 1989; Elias and Menon 1991). Removal of lipids from the SC by solvent extraction leads to a pronounced increase in TEWL, expressing a defect in the integrity of skin function and also representing a stimulus to barrier repair and increased synthesis of lipids by keratinocytes (Grubauer et al. 1989). The sequence of metabolic and subcellular events leading to recovery after acute barrier perturbation consists in a rapid secretion of preformed lamellar bodies by stratum granulosum, and an increase in lipid synthesis leading to further secretion of new lamellar bodies with reconstitution of SC intercellular lamellar bilayers (Elias and Feingold 1992).

The levels of SC ceramides vary according to age, sex, race and environmental factors (Rogers et al. 1996; Denda et al. 1993; Sugino et al. 1993; Halkier-Sørensen et al. 1995). In patients with AD, decreased levels of ceramides in SC and abnormalities in epidermal lipid metabolism may be responsible for the changes in the physiological parameters of the skin and barrier-function impairment (Schäfer and Kragballe 1991; Murata et al. 1996). On examining the skin of 47 patients with AD, we found an inverse correlation between ceramide-3 levels and barrier impairment, as measured by TEWL (Di Nardo et al. 1998) (Fig. 1). Patients with no active signs of eczema had a normal barrier function and intermediate values of ceramides and cholesterol when compared with normal subjects and AD patients with active lesions.

Depletion of lipids is considered a fundamental mechanism in barrier damage. Investigating the ultrastructural changes of epidermal lipids resulting from the topical application of sodium lauryl sulfate (SLS), absolute acetone, and glycolic acid, Fartasch demonstrated that different irritants induce distinct and characteristic alterations in skin lipids, reflecting the specific interaction with the epidermal permeability barrier (Fartasch 1997; Fartasch et al. 1997).

The amount of skin lipids represents an important factor in susceptibility to irritation. Di Nardo et al. studied the relationship between baseline ceramide composition and the intensity of SLS-induced ICD, and observed a correlation between colorimetric a* values and ceramide-6I and between TEWL and ceramide-

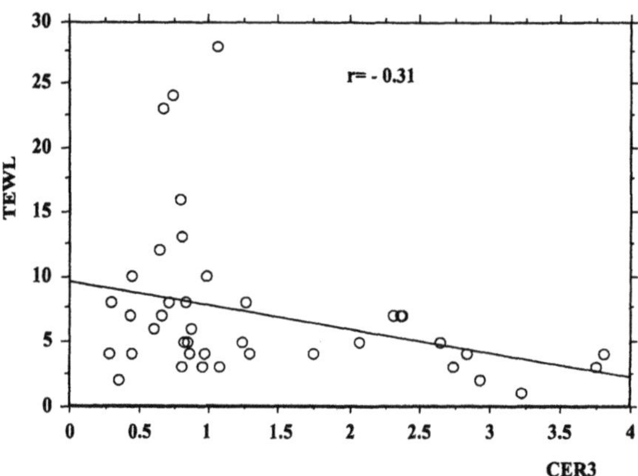

Fig. 1. Correlation between ceramide 3 (*CER3*) levels and transepidermal water loss (*TEWL*) values in 47 subjects with atopic dermatitis. Correlation coefficient $r = -0.31$

1 levels (Di Nardo et al. 1996a). The same authors employed a 24-h application of xylene and toluene to induce acute irritation (Di Nardo et al. 1996b). On comparing values of the different classes of lipids with clinical irritation parameters, a negative correlation was obtained. Based on clinical observations, two populations were selected: less reactive and hyper-reactive, which also differed in the total weight of lipids, ceramides and triglycerides. The authors concluded that skin lipids, and especially ceramide levels, may play a protective role with respect to irritant substances. Also 24h patch testing with 4% NaOH allowed a subdivision of subjects into normal and hyper-reactors (Seidenari et al. 1995). The latter showed an enhanced inflammatory response and more pronounced barrier-function damage, as assessed clinically and instrumentally. In this case, too, ceramide levels differed significantly between these two groups (A. Di Nardo et al., unpublished data). Based on the results of these studies, we can deduce that the analysis of baseline skin lipid composition may serve for the identification of subjects with a proclivity to ICD, with practical implications for workers engaged in at-risk occupations.

Time Course of Barrier Impairment in Acute and Cumulative ICD

The major factor in skin diseases caused by exogenous substances is the repeated and cumulative action on the skin of agents in weak irritant solutions. During the course of repeated exposure to surfactants, a progressively damaging clinical effect accompanied by an increase in TEWL (due to a cumulative action of these agents on the skin) is observable (Tupker et al. 1989a). After a single application of SLS simulating acute irritation, a concentration-, application-time- and skin-site-dependent impairment of the barrier is observed. If patches are re-applied on the same site, skin reactivity may vary owing to previous exposure influencing the skin. Thus, under experimental conditions, different phases follow one another, i.e. a first phase where the damage is induced, a second phase with clinical symptoms and ongoing repair, a third subclinical phase with further repair, and a final phase with barrier restitution, where the memory of the preceding aggression is preserved for a certain period.

Post-Irritation Irritant Reactivity

After irritation, time-dependent modifications in skin reactivity take place varying according to the type of irritant insult (if acute or chronic). Freeman and Maibach experimentally demonstrated that, following acute ICD, the skin is still hyper-reactive after 1 week of irritant avoidance, in spite of its clinically normal aspect and the normalization of water loss (Freeman and Maibach 1988). The repetition of the same stimulus or a combination of several different stimuli may surpass a critical level and cause a clinically detectable ICD. Tur et al. demonstrated instrumentally that very low concentrations of irritants alter the skin barrier, making the skin susceptible to a further insult with even lower concentrations (Tur et al. 1995). Persistent alterations of epidermal barrier function after cumulative irritation may be caused by changes in the composition of SC lipids (Proksch 1990). On the other hand, Widmer et al. studied post-irritation reactivity to SLS on previously irritated sites and observed a significant hypo-reactivity after a re-challenge at 6 weeks and 9 weeks (Widmer et al. 1994). The phenomenon of adaptation to environmental influences and possible recovery in spite of continuous exposure to irritant substances is called hardening and may be ascribed both to epidermal phenomena, such as a hyperkeratosis (Widmer et al. 1994) and to down-regulation of inflammation (Rietschel 1995).

Dermatitis and Skin Hyper-Irritability

Barrier Function and Skin Reactivity in Non-atopic Eczema

In non-atopic eczematous patients, basal barrier function and skin reactivity at healthy skin sites vary according to the activity of the eczema. When skin lesions are present, barrier impairment is also evident at healthy skin sites (Pasche-Koo and Hauser 1992; Seidenari 1996). Baseline barrier function and reactivity to irritants revert to normal when the dermatitis has healed: no difference in TEWL after exposure to SLS was found in patients with chronic or healed eczema as compared to controls, while patients with acute eczema showed an increased skin reactivity (Agner 1991 a).

Skin Reactivity in Eczematous Patients and Patch-Test Responses

Dermatitis localized to one skin site can have an enhancing effect on epicutaneous test reactions elsewhere and a pre-existing eczema can represent an explanation for the findings of false positive patch test reactions (Kligman and Gollhausen 1986). Moreover, a strong positive patch test reaction may induce skin hyper-reactivity and other false positive reactions during the same test session ("angry back") (Memon and Friedman 1996). The enhancement of a skin-test reaction by an adjacent strong reaction is known as spillover (Mitchell 1977). Soluble inflammatory factors that diffuse from the strong patch-test reaction into the surrounding skin are supposed to be involved. The term "excited skin syndrome" indicates that the whole skin may be involved (Maibach 1981).

Barrier Function and Skin Hyper-Reactivity in Atopic Dermatitis (AD)

Eczematous skin in atopic dermatitis patients differs from uninvolved skin, as it features higher TEWL and pH values and lower hydration values (Seidenari and Giusti 1995). Ultrasound reveals an increase in skin thickness and a decrease in skin echogenicity at affected skin areas (Seidenari 1998). At healthy skin sites, an increased TEWL, associated with decreased hydration values and impaired water-retention capacity, is observable (Berardesca et al. 1990; Conti et al. 1996). When

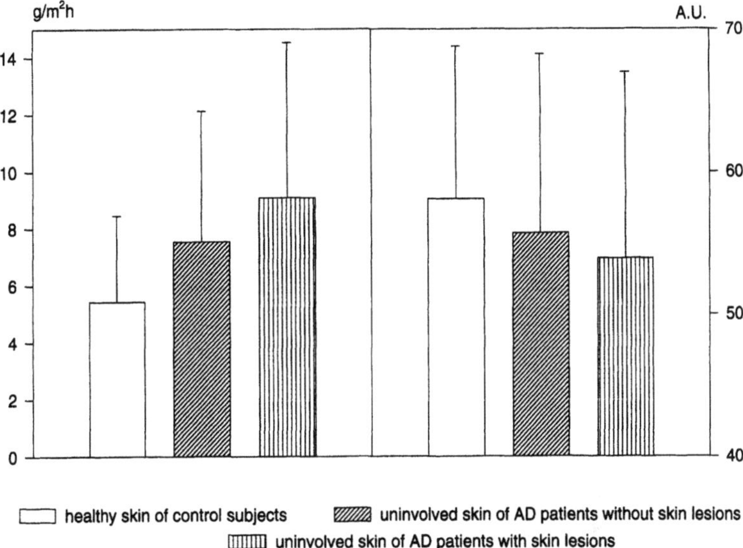

Fig. 2. Transepidermal water loss (g/m²h) and capacitance (*A.U.*, arbitrary units) mean (±SD) values in 186 children with atopic dermatitis (AD) and in 38 healthy age- and sex-matched control subjects. Values referring to uninvolved skin sites in children without skin lesions at the moment of the investigation differ from those of AD children with active dermatitis

biophysical data referring to the clinically uninvolved skin of children with AD were divided into two groups according to the presence of active dermatitis at the moment of the investigation, significant differences were observed between patients with and without skin lesions; in the former group, TEWL and pH values were higher and capacitance values lower with respect to values in the latter group (Seidenari and Giusti 1995) (Fig. 2).

Increased susceptibility to irritant stimuli has been described in AD, owing to impairment of barrier function and possibly to immune disregulation. Skin hyper-reactivity is proportional to the degree and extent of the dermatitis (Tupker et al. 1995). When we measured TEWL and capacitance values at eight different skin sites in 48 children with AD and compared these data with the SCORAD scores (for the evaluation of the extent of the dermatitis, the severity and the intensity of subjective symptoms), a fair correlation was observable between TEWL and capacitance values on one side and extension of the dermatitis and SCORAD values on the other side (Table 1) (Seidenari 2000).

Lower responses to intracutaneous bioactive agents in more severe forms of AD have been described (Giannetti and Girolomoni 1989). A negative correlation between dermatitis severity score and reactivity to intradermal injections of codeine, histamine, methacoline, and substance P was demonstrated, suggesting that down-regulation of target structures due to higher skin concentrations of inflammatory mediators may lead to increased resistance to stimuli (Tupker et al. 1995). A few studies compare skin reactivity of atopics with that of eczematous

Table 1. Correlation coefficients (r) between clinical and instrumental data

	SCORAD	% Extension
Mean capacitance (8 skin sites)	−0.392	−0.302
Capacitance on forearm skin	−0.303	−0.15
Lowest capacitance value	−0.372	−0.311
Mean TEWL (8 skin sites)	0.364	0.325
TEWL on forearm skin	0.225	0.057
Highest TEWL value	0.287	0.185

SCORAD, scoring index for atopic dermatitis; *TEWL*, transepidermal water loss.

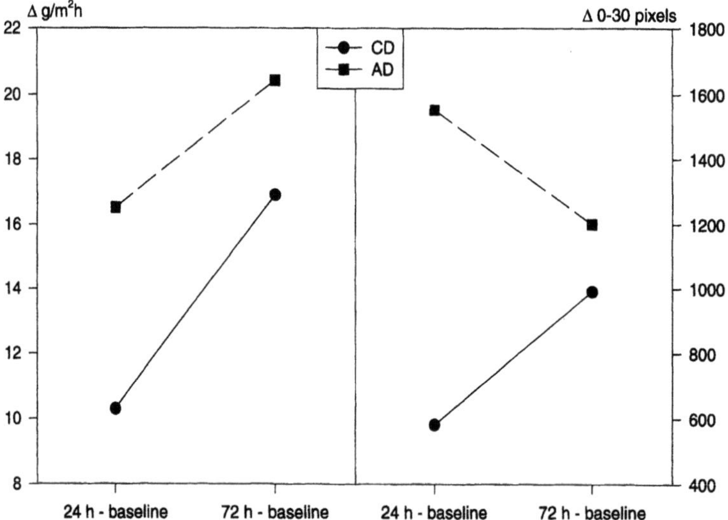

Fig. 3. Transepidermal water loss (g/m^{2}h) and echogenicity (0–30 pixels) values expressing the intensity of skin-barrier damage and inflammation on forearm skin after a 30-min 5% sodium lauryl sulfate challenge in subjects with contact dermatitis (*CD*) and with atopic dermatitis (*AD*)

non-atopics, and report a greater skin vulnerability in the former group of patients (Van der Valk et al. 1985). Comparing subjects with AD and contact eczema, capacitance values at healthy skin sites were much lower in AD patients with respect to eczematous non-atopics (CD) (Seidenari 1996). After exposure to 5% SLS, skin barrier damage, as assessed by TEWL, was greater in AD with respect to CD patients (Fig. 3). Echographic evaluation of SLS-exposed skin sites, showed that a significant hypo-reflectivity of the epidermis, expressing barrier-function damage, was present at 24 h only in atopic subjects (Seidenari 1994). Moreover, the intensity of the inflammatory response, as evaluated by dermal echogenicity variations, was greater in AD patients. These data indicate an increased reactivity to SLS in the AD group with respect to the CD group, and a specific susceptibility of atopic skin to surfactants.

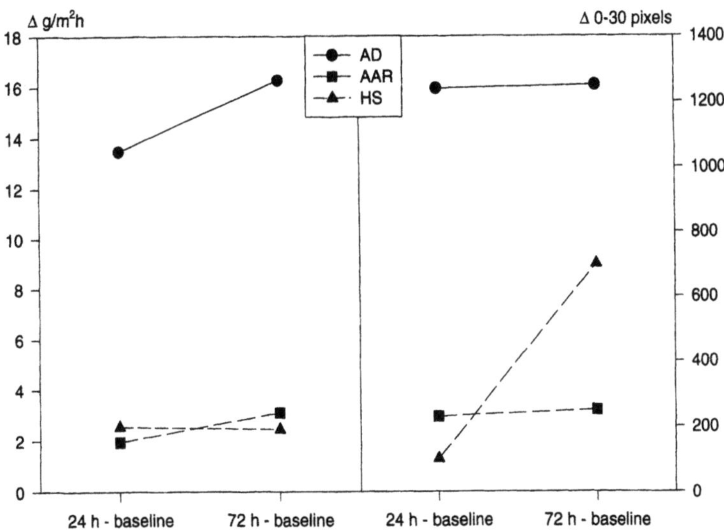

Fig. 4. Transepidermal water loss (g/m^{2}h) and echogenicity (0–30 pixels) values, expressing the intensity of skin-barrier damage and inflammation on forearm skin, after a 30-min 0.5% sodium lauryl sulfate challenge in subjects with atopic dermatitis (*AD*), allergic asthma/ rhinitis (*AAR*) and in healthy controls (*HS*)

Barrier Function and Skin Hyper-Reactivity in Atopics Without Dermatitis

Barrier-function abnormalities are characteristic of AD. Compared to that of healthy subjects (HS), the skin of patients with allergic asthma/rhinitis (AAR) does not show alterations of biophysical parameters, as in AD (Conti et al. 1996; Löffler et al. 1999). Investigating skin reactivity to detergents in AAR, AD, and HS, by means of instrumental methods, we observed an increased inflammatory response and barrier damage in AD patients, but not in AAR ones (Seidenari et al. 1996) (Fig. 4). Moreover, no difference in skin responses to SLS was found in the same subjects with AAR tested during the active phase of the disease and in winter, when no symptoms were present (Conti et al. 2000). During wintertime, post-exposure TEWL was even higher due to environmental influences on the barrier (Fig. 5), indicating that atopic skin hyper-reactivity is organ specific and is not influenced by cytokines and other mediators released by mucosal tissues during allergic inflammation. We agree with Funke et al, assuming that respiratory atopics with no signs of cutaneous atopy will behave in an occupational environment as non-atopics (Funke et al. 1996).

Barrier Impairment and Contact Sensitization

The relationship between constitutional or irritant-mediated barrier impairment and contact sensitization is complex and reciprocal. Contact-sensitive subjects, especially nickel-sensitive ones, are reported to have an increased susceptibility

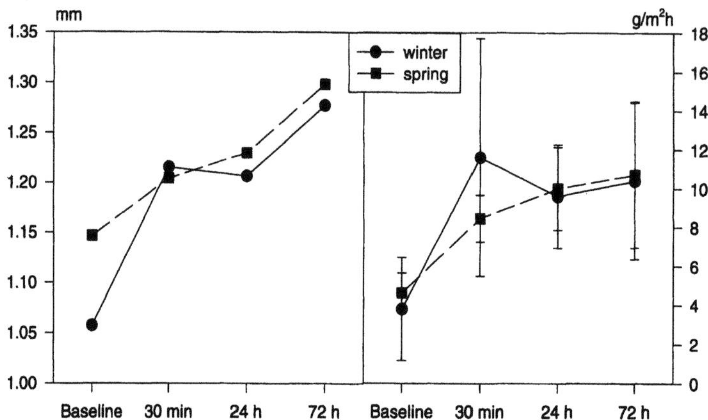

Fig. 5. Skin thickness (mm) and transepidermal water loss (g/m²h) mean (± standard deviation) values expressing the intensity of inflammation and skin-barrier damage on forearm skin after a 30-min 0.5% sodium lauryl sulfate challenge in subjects with allergic asthma/rhinitis during winter and spring

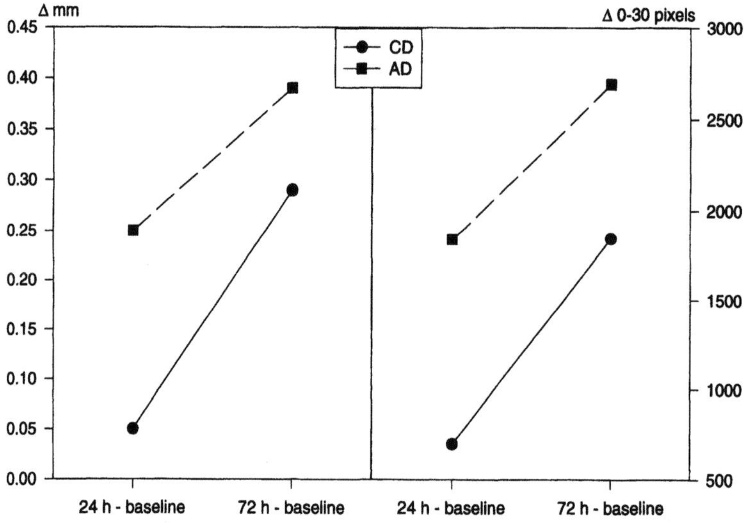

Fig. 6. Skin thickness (mm) and echogenicity (0–30 pixels) values expressing the intensity of the inflammatory response on forearm skin at nickel patch-test sites after pre-treatment with 5% sodium lauryl sulfate for 30 min in nickel-sensitive subjects with contact dermatitis (*CD*) and with atopic dermatitis (*AD*)

to irritants, suggesting that the irritancy threshold might be reduced in nickel-sensitive subjects (Van der Valk et al. 1985; Elsner and Burg 1993).

In the development of contact sensitization, irritant reactivity may well play a role, resulting in a higher frequency of ICD, with more frequent barrier perturbation and enhanced penetration of allergens. The combination of irritants and sub-eliciting doses of allergens can induce a dermatitis in sensitive patients. In order to simulate simultaneous exposure to irritants and allergens in domestic and occupational environments, pre-treatment of nickel patch-test sites was performed employing SLS in nickel-sensitive atopics and non-atopics (Seidenari 1994). With respect to non-pre-treated sites, consecutive applications of SLS and nickel sulphate induced a higher number of skin responses and more marked allergic reactions, probably depending on enhanced nickel penetration and/or summation of immune and non-immune mechanisms. In nickel-sensitive subjects with AD, an earlier inflammatory response and a more pronounced skin damage following challenge with SLS was observed, whereby the allergic response was further enhanced (Fig. 6). Thus, increased susceptibility to irritants might be responsible for augmented allergic responses in sensitized patients, especially in subjects with AD.

Monitoring of Barrier Function in Workers Exposed to Irritants

The baseline TEWL level is considered a reliable indicator of susceptibility to weak irritants (Tupker et al. 1989b; Pinnagoda et al. 1989). In fact, a high pre-exposure baseline TEWL allows SLS to penetrate and damage the skin more easily, resulting in higher TEWL values after repeated low-dose irritation. A correlation between baseline TEWL and susceptibility to SLS was confirmed by Agner (Agner 1991b), whereas it was questioned by other groups (Berardesca and Maibach 1988; Reed et al. 1995).

Only a few studies employ the assessment of skin functions to monitor the state of the barrier during occupational exposure, in order to identify at-risk subjects (Bauer et al. 1998; John SM et al. 2000). Metal workers have a high incidence of occupational skin diseases, and the risk of hand dermatitis is closely linked to metalworking-fluid exposure, especially to water-based fluids. Coenraads and Pinnagoda demonstrated that a close relationship exists between skin conditions and barrier function during follow-up of metal workers (Coenraads and Pinnagoda 1985). They undertook a 12-week study in newly recruited employees. TEWL measurements were taken from the back of the right hand and the extensor and flexor surfaces of the right forearm. The workers were subdivided into three groups according to different degrees of exposure to metalworking fluids. At the end of the study, TEWL values had increased in subjects who had developed hand dermatitis. Moreover, average TEWL values were higher for workers belonging to the workstation where continuous exposure was unavoidable. A Swiss study showed that 10% of metalworker trainees experienced minor signs of irritation 8–10 months after the beginning of their apprenticeship (Wigger-Alberti et al. 1997), whereas TEWL increased continuously during the first 3 months after the first examination, and the observed increase was significantly influenced by exposure to water-soluble metalworking fluids alone.

Occupational dermatitis is a major clinical problem and a significant cause of social disability. Many cases of contact dermatitis are multifactorial in origin, which gives rise to difficulties in both diagnosis and management. Exogenous factors frequently interact with endogenous influences. For subjects with a constitutional barrier impairment, such as patients with AD, the first work experience may be responsible for aggravation or activation of the disease. Hand eczema triggered by the occupational exposure may also represent the first manifestation of an intrinsic barrier deficiency, often appearing after the subject has undergone many months of training. If the condition is bad enough to require a job change, this represents great economic and personal loss. Therefore, recording at-risk subjects at the beginning of job training and following up their skin condition during the training may lead to the diagnosis of occupational skin disorders at an earlier stage and may enable the occupational physician to give suitable instructions on preventive measures, such as use of appropriate barrier creams, mild cleansing agents and protective gloves. Besides clinical examination, pre- and periodical post-employment instrumental evaluation of skin barrier and skin reactivity to irritants could lead to a further breakthrough for suggesting individual preventive strategies.

References

Agner T (1991a) Skin susceptibility in uninvolved skin of hand eczema patients and healthy controls. Br J Dermatol 125:140–144

Agner T (1991b) Susceptibility of atopic dermatitis patients to irritant dermatitis caused by sodium lauryl sulphate. Acta Derm Venereol 71:296–300

Bauer A, Bartsch R, Stadeler M, Schneider W, Grieshaber R, Wollina U, Gebhardt M (1998) Development of occupational skin disease during vocational training in baker and confectioner apprentices: a follow-up study. Contact Dermatitis 39:307–311

Berardesca E, Maibach HI (1988) Racial differences in sodium lauryl sulphate induced cutaneous irritation: black and white. Contact Dermatitis 18:65–70

Berardesca E, Fideli D, Borroni G, Rabbiosi G, Maibach HI (1990) In vivo hydration and water-retention capacity of stratum corneum in clinically uninvolved skin in atopic and psoriatic patients. Acta Derm Venereol 70:400–404

Coenraads PJ, Pinnagoda J (1985) Dermatitis and vapour loss in metal workers. Contact Dermatitis 13:347–348

Conti A, Di Nardo A, Seidenari S (1996) No alteration of biophysical parameters in the skin of subjects with respiratory atopy. Dermatology 192:317–320

Conti A, Seidenari S (2000) No increased skin reactivity in subjects with allergic rhinitis during the active phase of the disease. Acta Derm Venereol 80:192–195

Denda M, Koyema J, Hori J, Horii I, Takahashi M, Hara M, Tagami H (1993) Age- and sex-dependent change in stratum corneum sphyngolipids. Arch Dermatol Res 285:415–417

Di Nardo A, Sugino K, Ademola J, Wertz PW, Maibach HI (1996a) Sodium lauryl sulfate induced irritant contact dermatitis: a correlation study between ceramides and in vivo parameters of irritation. Contact Dermatitis 35:86–91

Di Nardo A, Sugino K, Ademola J, Wertz PW, Maibach HI (1996b) Role of ceramides in proclivity to toluene and xylene-induced irritation in man. Derm Beruf Umwelt 44:119–125

Di Nardo A, Wertz P, Giannetti A, Seidenari S (1998) Ceramide and cholesterol composition of the skin of patients with atopic dermatitis. Acta Derm Venereol 78:27–30

Elias PM, Feingold KR (1992) Lipids and the epidermal water barrier: metabolism, regulation and pathophysiology. Semin Dermatol 11:176–182

Elias PM, Menon GK (1991) Structural and lipid biochemical correlates of the epidermal permeability barrier. Adv Lipid Res 24:1–26

Elsner P, Burg G (1993) Irritant reactivity is a better risk marker for nickel sensitization than atopy. Acta Derm Venereol (Stockh) 73:214–216

Fartasch M (1997) Ultrastructure of the epidermis barrier after irritation. Microsc Res Tech 37:193–199

Fartasch M, Teal J, Menon GK (1997) Mode of action of glycolic acid on human stratum corneum: ultrastructural and functional evaluation of the epidermal barrier. Arch Dermatol Res 289:404–409

Freeman S, Maibach HI (1988) Study of irritant contact dermatitis produced by repeat patch test with sodium lauryl sulphate and assessed by visual methods, transepidermal water loss and laser Doppler velocimetry. J Am Acad Dermatol 19:496–502

Funke U, Diepgen T, Fartasch M (1996) Risk-group-related prevention of hand eczema at the workplace. Curr Probl Dermatol 25:123–132

Giannetti A, Girolomoni G (1989) Skin reactivity to neuropeptides in atopic dermatitis. Br J Dermatol 121:681–688

Grubauer G, Elias PM, Feingold KR (1989) Transepidermal water loss: the signal for recovery of barrier structure and function. J Lipid Res 30:323–333

Halkier-Sørensen L, Menon GK, Elias PM, Thestrup-Pedersen K, Feingold KR (1995) Cutaneous barrier function after cold exposure in hairless mice: a model to demonstrate how cold interferes with barrier homeostasis among workers in the fish-processing industry. Br J Dermatol 132:391–401

Imokawa G, Akasaki S, Minematsu Y, Kawai M (1989) Importance of intercellular lipids in water-retention properties of the stratum corneum: induction and recovery study of surfactant dry skin. Arch Dermatol Res 281:45–51

John SM, Uter W, Schwanitz HJ (2000) Relevance of multiparametric skin bioengineering in a prospectively-followed cohort of junior hairdressers. Contact Dermatitis 43(3):161–168

Kligman A, Gollhausen R (1986) The "angry back": a new concept or old confusion? Br J Dermatol 115 [Suppl 31]:93–100

Löffler H, Effendy I (1999) Skin susceptibility of atopic individuals. Contact Dermatitis 40:239–242

Maibach HI (1981) The E.S.S. - excited skin syndrome (alias the "angry back"). In: Ring J, Burg G (eds) New trends in allergy. Springer, Berlin Heidelberg New York, pp 208–221

Memon AA, Friedmann PS (1996) "Angry back syndrome": a non-reproducible phenomenon. Br J Dermatol 135:924–930

Mitchell JC (1977) Multiple concomitant positive patch test reactions. Contact Dermatitis 3:315–320

Murata Y, Ogata J, Higaki Y, Kawashima M, Yada Y, Higuchi K, Tsuchiya T, Kawaminami S, Imokawa G (1996) Abnormal expression of sphyngomyelin acylase in atopic dermatitis: an etiologic factor for ceramide deficiency? J Invest Dermatol 106:1242–1249

Pasche-Koo F, Hauser C (1992) How to understand the angry back syndrome. Dermatology 184:237–240

Pinnagoda J, Tupker RA, Coenraads PJ, Nater JP (1989) Prediction of susceptibility to an irritant response by transepidermal water loss. Contact Dermatitis 20:341–346

Proksch E (1990) Die Epidermis als metabolisch aktives Gewebe: Regelung der Lipidsynthese durch die Barrierefunktion. Z Hautkr 65:296–300

Reed JT, Ghadially R, Elias PM (1995) Skin type but neither race nor gender, influence epidermal permeability barrier function. Arch Dermatol 131:1134–1138

Rietschel RL (1995) Physiologic response of chronically inflamed and accommodated human skin. Curr Probl Dermatol 23:104–107

Rogers J, Harding C, Mayo A, Banks J, Rawlings A (1996) Stratum corneum lipids: the effect of ageing and the seasons. Arch Dermatol Res 288:765–770

Schäfer L, Kragballe K (1991) Abnormalities in epidermal lipid metabolism in patients with atopic dermatitis. J Invest Dermatol 96:10–15

Seidenari S (1994) Reactivity to nickel sulfate at sodium lauryl sulfate pretreated skin sites is higher in atopics: an echographic evaluation by means of image analysis performed on 20 MHz B-scan recordings. Acta Derm Venereol (Stockh) 74:245–249

Seidenari S, Giusti G (1995) Objective assessment of the skin of children affected by atopic dermatitis: a study of pH, capacitance and TEWL in eczematous and clinically uninvolved skin. Acta Derm Venereol (Stockh) 75:429–433

Seidenari S, Pepe P, Di Nardo A (1995) Sodium hydroxide-induced irritant dermatitis as assessed by computerized elaboration of 20 MHz B-scan images and by TEWL measurement: a method for investigating skin barrier function. Acta Derm Venereol (Stockh) 75:97–101

Seidenari S, Belletti B, Schiavi ME (1996) Skin reactivity to sodium lauryl sulfate in patients with respiratory atopy. J Am Acad Dermatol 35:47–52

Seidenari S (1996) Skin sensitivity, interindividual factors: atopy. In: van der Valk PGM, Maibach HI (eds) The irritant contact dermatitis syndrome. CRC, Boca Raton, pp 267–277

Seidenari S (1998) Biophysical methods for disease monitoring in dermatology. Curr Probl Dermatol 26:108–119

Seidenari S (2000) Evaluation of barrier functions and skin reactivity in occupational dermatoses. In: Kanerva L, Elsner P, Wahlberg JE, Maibach HI (eds) Handbook of occupational dermatology. Springer, Berlin Heidelberg New York, pp 64–75

Sugino K, Imokawa G, Maibach HI (1993) Ethnic differences of skin lipids in relation to stratum corneum barrier function. J Invest Dermatol 100:587

Tupker RA, Pinnagoda J, Coenraads PJ, Nater JP (1989a) The influence of repeated exposure to surfactants on the human skin as determined by transepidermal water loss and visual scoring. Contact Dermatitis 20:108–114

Tupker RA, Coenraads PJ, Pinnagoda J, Nater JP (1989b) Baseline transepidermal water loss (TEWL) as a prediction of susceptibility to sodium lauryl sulphate. Contact Dermatitis 20:265–269

Tupker RA, Coenraads PJ, Fidler V, De Jong MCJM, Van der Meer JB, De Monchy JGR (1995) Irritant susceptibility and weal and flare reactions to bioactive agents in atopic dermatitis. I. Influence of disease severity. Br J Dermatol 133:358–364

Tur E, Eshkol Z, Brenner S, Maibach HI (1995) Cumulative effect of subthreshold concentrations of irritants in humans. Am J Contact Dermat 6:216–220

Van der Valk PGM, Nater JP, Bleumink E (1985) Vulnerability of the skin to surfactants in different groups of eczema patients and controls as measured by water vapour loss. Clin Exp Dermatol 10:98–102

Widmer J, Elsner P, Burg G (1994) Skin irritant reactivity following experimental cumulative irritant contact dermatitis. Contact Dermatitis 30:35–39

Wigger-Alberti W, Hinnen U, Elsner P (1997) Predictive testing of metalworking fluids: a comparison of 2 cumulative human irritation models and correlation with epidemiological data. Contact Dermatitis 36:14–20

CHAPTER 4

Contact Dermatitis Due to Irritation

4

W. Wigger-Alberti, U. Frank, P. Elsner

Irritant contact dermatitis (ICD), defined as "a nonimmunologic local inflammatory reaction characterized by erythema, edema, or corrosion following single or repeated application of a chemical substance to an identical cutaneous site" (Mathias and Maibach 1994), is a leading cause of occupational disease in dermatology and causes economic damage to workers, companies, and social security systems world-wide. The perception of ICD as more trivial than the more intellectually appealing problem of allergic sensitization has recently changed dramatically. In Germany, skin diseases are the second most frequent occupational disease following musculoskeletal disorders, and most occupational dermatoses are cases of contact dermatitis. Among these ICD is probably more frequent than allergic contact dermatitis (ACD), although reliable data are still very limited. In contrast to ACD, ICD is defined as being the result of a primarily unspecific damage to the skin. It is not a clinical entity, but rather a spectrum of diseases. The clinical aspect of ICD is determined by the dose-effect relationship (Patil and Maibach 1994). The morphology of acute ICD shows erythema, edema, vesicles that may coalesce, bullae, and oozing (Figs. 1, 2). Necrosis and ulceration is seen with corrosive materials (Fig. 3). The clinical features of chronic ICD include redness, lichenification, excoriations, scaling, and hyperkeratosis (Figs. 4, 5). Any skin site may be affected. However, most frequently affected by ICD are the hands, as they are the human "tools" that interact with the environment most

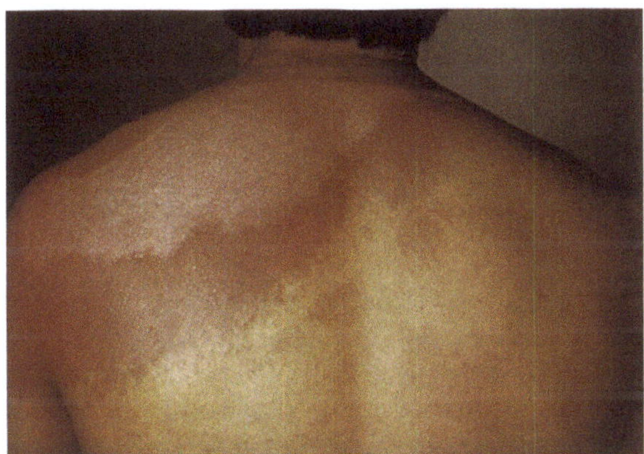

Fig. 1. Chemical burn caused by tear gas in a policeman

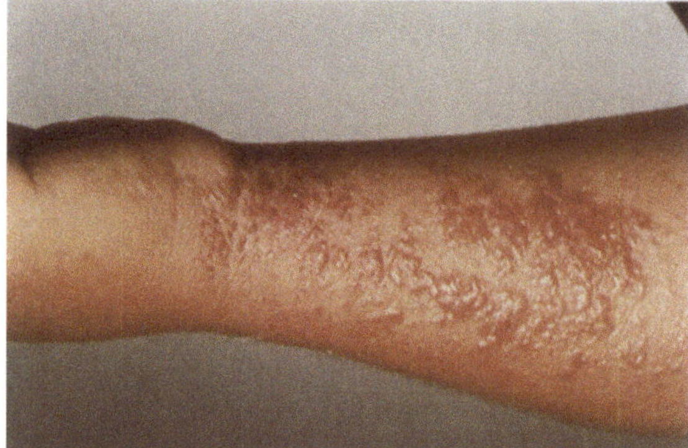

Fig. 2. Jellyfish reaction in a lifeguard

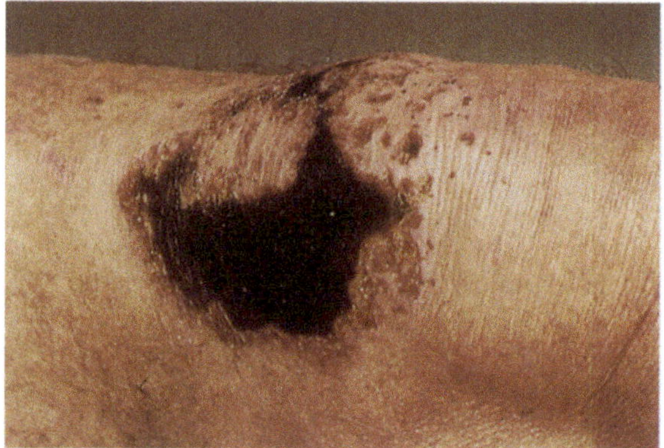

Fig. 3. Caustic reaction caused by cement

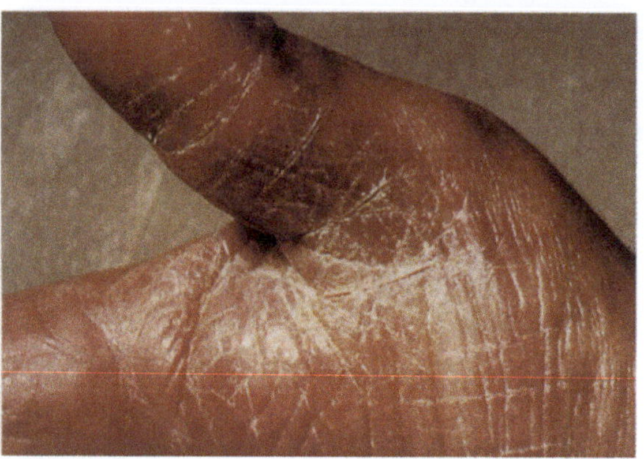

Fig. 4. Housewives' eczema due to chronic wet work

and have intensive contact with irritants. Spilling of fluids may irritate the forearms or other body sites, especially when fluids soak through work clothes. Airborne ICD develops in irritant-exposed sensitive skin, mostly the face and especially the periorbital region (Lachapelle 1986, Dooms-Goossens et al. 1986). Irritant dermatitis caused by dust may mimic textile dermatitis, with lesions most

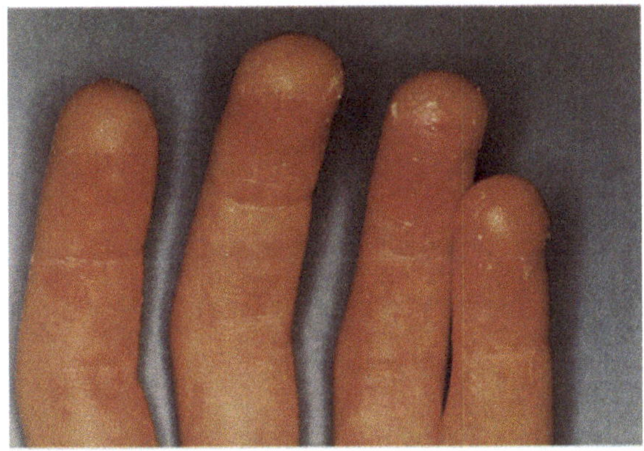

Fig. 5. Fingertip eczema due to physical trauma in a cellist

prominent in sites with close skin-garment contact, such as the axilla, the gluteal region, or the thighs (Hafner et al. 1995).

Clinical Types of Irritant Contact Dermatitis

Irritants produce a wide range of clinical features. Cutaneous responses depend on the type of irritant (detergent, acid, alkali, oil, organic solvent, oxidant, reducing agent, water), the concentration at which the irritant comes into contact with the skin, the type of exposure, and the individual response. Clinical manifestations of the ICD syndromes are also modified by external factors such as environmental factors (mechanical pressure, temperature, and humidity) and predisposing characteristics of the individual (age, sex, ethnic origin, preexisting skin disease, atopic skin diathesis, and anatomic region exposed) (Pinnagoda et al. 1989, Emtestam and Ollmar 1993, Wilkinson and Willis 1998).

Several different types of ICD have been described (based on Lammintausta and Maibach 1990, Berardesca and Distante 1995, Iliev and Elsner 1997):

Acute ICD

Acute ICD develops when the skin is exposed to a strong irritant or caustic chemical. Usually this happens as an accident at work or in special emergency situations. The irritant reaction reaches its peak quickly, and then starts to heal; this is called the decrescendo phenomenon. Because the lag-time is short (usually minutes to hours after exposure) and the association between exposure and skin symptoms is usually clear, the diagnosis is easy in most cases. It may become difficult when the patient was unaware of an exposure. Acute ACD has to be considered as a differential diagnosis, which is caused by a delayed sensitization reaction, and requires 24–48 h after allergen contact for symptoms to appear; this type of contact dermatitis is characterized by the crescendo phenomenon (i.e. a transient increase of signs and symptoms despite removal of the allergen). The clinical appearance of acute ICD is highly variable, and it may even be indistinguishable from the allergic type. There are numerous reports in the literature of even experienced dermatologists being misled into an initial assumption of ACD which later, after a careful work up, turned out to be "only irritation" (Frosch 1995). Furthermore, the combination of allergic and irritant dermatitis is frequent, e.g. "black-spot poison ivy dermatitis" (Hurwitz et al. 1984), as an acute ICD superimposed upon an ACD.

Symptoms of acute irritant dermatitis are burning, stinging, and soreness of the skin. Signs are erythema, edema, bullae, and possibly necrosis. These lesions are restricted to the area where the irritant or toxicant damaged the tissue. Borders are mostly sharply demarcated, and the asymmetrical patterns of lesions hints at an exogenous cause. The prognosis of this type is good (Elsner 1994). The most frequent potent irritants leading to acute ICD are acids and alkaline solutions (Eichmann and Amgwerd 1992). A typical accident situation is chemical burning in construction workers (Skogstad and Levy 1994) when alkaline concrete fluid soaks through garments or spills into work boots.

Chemicals burns by fluoric acid are the most dangerous of all injuries caused by acids, and need special treatment. But even substances thought to be less toxic, such as N-methyl-2-pyrrolidone, may cause acute ICD (Malten et al. 1979).

Acute Delayed ICD

Acute delayed ICD is characteristic for certain irritants, such as benzalkonium chloride, anthralin, and tretinoin that elicit a retarded inflammatory response. Clinically, acute delayed ICD resembles acute ICD. The visible inflammation is not seen until 8–24 h or more after exposure (Malten et al. 1979). Irritant patch test reactions to benzalkonium chloride may be papular and increase in intensity with time, thus imitating ACD. On the normal skin surrounding psoriatic plaques, dithranol causes redness and edema, which may become very severe on the legs because of venous stasis. Irritation due to tretinoin develops after a few days, and is characterized by mild to fiery redness followed by desquamation or large flakes of stratum corneum. The symptoms are burning rather than itching. The skin becomes sensitive to touch and to water (Frosch 1995).

Irritant Reaction ICD

Irritant reaction ICD is a type of subclinical irritant dermatitis in individuals exposed to wet work, such as hairdressers or metal workers, in their first months of training. This diagnosis is made if the clinical picture is monomorphic rather than polymorphic, and characterized by one or more of the following signs: scaling, redness, vesicles, pustules, and erosions (Frosch 1995).

On the hands it often begins under rings and then may spread over the fingers to the hands and the forearms. It usually affects the dorsum of the hands and fingers, but irritants can also cause eczema of the palmar sides of the fingers and the hands.

This distribution occurs in caterers, described as dyshidrotic eczema, and it has been reported in metal workers with an ICD from cooling lubricants (Cronin 1995). Frequently, this condition heals spontaneously, resulting in hardening of the skin; sometimes it progresses to cumulative irritant dermatitis.

Cumulative ICD

According to Malten cumulative ICD is a consequence of multiple subthreshold damage to the skin if the time between the insults is too short for complete restoration of skin barrier function (Malten 1981). It may be the result of too frequent repetition of one impairing factor, but is more commonly the result of a variety of stimuli, each beginning to be active before recovery from the foregoing stimuli has been competed. Clinical symptoms will develop only when the damage exceeds a certain "manifestation threshold", which is individually determined. Persons with sensitive skin are characterized by a decreased threshold or an increased restoration time leading to earlier development of clinical irritant dermatitis. The threshold is not a fixed value for an individual, but it may decrease with the disease. This explains why in patients with cumulative ICD even limited irritant exposure may perpetuate the condition. Cumulative ICD is not linked to exposure to a potent irritant, but to exposure to weak irritants. Very often, this exposure occurs not only at work but also in private life. Because the link between exposure and disease is often not obvious to the patient, diagnosis may be delayed considerably. This is one of the reasons for the rather doubtful prognosis of this disease (Elsner and Maibach 1993).

Symptoms of chronic irritant dermatitis are itching and pain due to cracking of hyperkeratotic skin. Signs include dryness, erythema, and vesicles, but mainly lichenification, hyperkeratosis, and chapping. In contrast to acute irritant dermatitis, the lesions are less sharply demarcated. Xerotic dermatitis is the most frequent type of cumulative toxic dermatitis (Eichmann and Amgwerd 1992).

Traumiterative ICD

In contrast to cumulative ICD resulting from a too early repetition of exposures differing in type, traumiterative ICD is a result of too early repetition of just one type of load (Malten and Arend 1985). Nevertheless, these two types are very similar clinically.

Exsiccation Eczematid

Exsiccation eczematid is a special variant of ICD that is seen mainly in elderly individuals with a history of frequent showering and bathing without remoisturizing their skin. Patients suffer from intensive itching, and their skin appears dry with ichthyosiform scaling. The condition mainly occurs during the winter months, when humidity is low.

Traumatic ICD

Traumatic ICD may develop after acute skin trauma, such as burns, lacerations and acute ICD. Patients should also be asked whether they have cleansed the skin with strong soaps or detergents. The syndrome is characterized by eczematous lesions and delayed healing. This eczematous condition persists for a considerable time period, with a minimum of 6 weeks (Frosch 1995).

The most common location is the hands. In a fully developed case, redness, infiltration, and scaling with fissuring is seen all over the affected areas.

Pustular and Acneiform ICD

Pustular and acneiform ICD is a result of exposure to certain irritants, such as croton oil, mineral oils, tars, greases, and naphthalenes. This syndrome must always be considered in conditions in which acneiform lesions develop outside the typical acne age. Those most affected are patients with seborrhoea, macroporous skin conditions, and prior acne vulgaris, as well as atopics. The pustules are sterile and transient; however, subcorneal pustular eruption may also be a manifestation of allergy to trichlorethylene, which has to be considered as a differential diagnosis in patients with appropriate history (Goh 1995).

Nonerythematous ICD

Nonerythematous ICD may be defined as a subclinical form of ICD with early stages of skin irritation characterized only by changes in the stratum corneum barrier function without a clinical correlate (van der Valk et al. 1985, Berardesca and Maibach 1988, Lammintausta et al. 1988).

Subjective ICD

Subjective or sensory ICD is characterized by the lack of clinical signs, but individuals complain of a subjective sensation of stinging, burning or smarting after contact with certain chemicals, such as lactic acid, which is also a model irritant for this type of nonvisible cutaneous irritation. This reaction may be reliably reproduced in a double-blinded exposure test. Important parameters are the quality and the concentration of the exposing agent. Also, neural pathways are considered to be responsible (Lammintausta and Maibach 1990). Immediate-type stinging caused by chemicals such as chloroform and methanol (1:1) or 95% ethanol and delayed-type stinging mostly caused by sunscreen agents, insect repellants and several dermatological therapeutic agents and vehicles that are used in cosmetics and medicaments can be differentiated (Frosch 1995, Frosch and Kligman 1977, Soschin and Kligman 1982).

Irritation or Allergy?

The distinction between irritant and allergic contact dermatitis has become increasingly blurred. Despite their different pathogenesis, ACD and ICD, especially of the chronic type, show a remarkable similarity with respect to clinical appearance, histology, and immunohistology. It is apparent that some of the same inflammatory immune mechanisms are operating both for ACD and ICD. The epidermal and dermal cell activity that produces the cascade of inflammation appears to be similar and applicable to both irritants and allergens. However, although inflammatory and immunological mediators may be activated, in contrast to ACD no memory T-cell function is involved. A review of all of the comparative studies that suggest these two entities are more alike than they are not has been presented (Gaspari 1997). Histologically, irritant contact dermatitis reactions show much greater pleomorphism than those elicited by allergens. Various alterations of epidermal cells can be observed according to the nature and concentration of the irritant applied, the type and duration of exposure and the individual reactivity of the skin. Frequently, even therapy is similar (Binnick 1981, Lauerma et al. 1994). Additionally, the concept that irritants are thought to cause symptoms and signs within minutes to hours whereas allergens take days has been disqualified for one of the most widely studied irritants. Twenty-four hours of occlusion of sodium lauryl sulfate (SLS) resulted clearly in more signs of inflammation at 48 h, a time course more characteristic of allergic reactions (Rietschel 1997).

Epidemiology

While population-based epidemiological studies on the frequency of ICD are rare, there is agreement that irritant dermatitis is more frequent than ACD, although ACD tends to have more severe consequences for the patient. Coenraads and Smit reviewed international prevalence studies for eczema due to all causes conducted with general populations in five countries (England, The Netherlands, Norway, Sweden, United States). They showed point prevalence rates of 1.7–6.3%, and 1- to 3-year-period prevalence rates of 6.2–10.6% (Coenraads and Smit 1995).

In a questionnaire study performed by Meding and Swanbeck on a random sample of 20,000 individuals from the population of the Swedish city of Gothenburg, 11.8% reported having had hand eczema within the previous 12 months (period prevalence), whereas 5.4% suffered from hand eczema at the time of investigation (point prevalence) (Meding 1990, Meding and Swanbeck 1990). The period prevalence was twice as high in women (14.6%) than in men (8.8%). The prevalence of hand eczema in the population working full-time (10.3%) was lower than in the general population. However, in the subgroup doing medical and nursing work the 1-year prevalence of hand eczema was 15.9%, and in the population doing service work it was 15.4%. The occurrence of irritant dermatitis was significantly increased in women exposed to water and detergents and in men exposed to oils and solvents, whereas the occurrence of allergic dermatitis was not significantly influenced by these exposures.

The perception that irritant dermatitis is more frequent than ACD in the occupational setting is supported by data from Singapore. Of 557 patients with occupational dermatoses, 55.7% (310) had ICD, 38.6% (215) had ACD, and 5.7% (32) had noncontact dermatitis (Goh 1987). However, the incidence rates of selected occupations according to the diagnosis of ICD and ACD in a population-based study in North Bavaria showed different preferences for ICD or ACD due to different occupational groups (Diepgen and Coenraads 1995). Since cases of irritant dermatitis tend to be less severe and chronic than those of ACD, the latter may outnumber the former in specialized occupational dermatology clinics (Kanerva et al. 1988).

Risk Factors

A number of individual factors for irritant dermatitis have been identified. Although occupational irritant hand dermatitis is more frequent in females (Meding 1990), no sex difference of irritant reactivity could be established experimentally (Hogan et al. 1990). It is suspected that increased exposure to irritants at home accounts for the higher prevalence in females. This is supported by the observation that caring for children under the age of 4 years and the lack of dishwashers significantly increased the risk of contracting hand eczema in a population of female hospital workers (Nilsson 1986). Irritant reactivity declines with increasing age. This is true not only for acute but also for cumulative irritant dermatitis (Suter-Widmer and Elsner 1994). Atopy is probably the best established risk factor for irritant hand dermatitis (Meding and Swanbeck 1990, Lammintausta et al. 1987). It has to be stressed, however, that respiratory manifestations of atopy seem to be less predictive of irritant reactivity compared with skin manifestation. On the level of the individual, there remains considerable uncertainty in the prediction of irritant reactivity. As was shown in a Swedish study, about 25% of the atopics in extreme risk occupations, such as ladies' hairdressers and nursing assistants, did not develop hand eczema (Rystedt 1985).

The incidence of ICD correlates with irritant exposure of the workers in a given profession (Goldner 1994). Some high-risk occupations are caterers (Cronin 1987, Wood and Greig 1997, Cleenewerck and Martin 1996), construction workers (Avnstorp 1996), furniture industry workers (Gan et al. 1987), hospital workers (Gawkrodger et al. 1986, Wrangsjö and Meding 1997), nurses (Kassis et al. 1984), cleaners (Singgih et al. 1986), kitchen workers, hairdressers (van der Walle and Brunsveld 1994, Uter et al. 1995), chemical industry workers (Conde Salazar et al. 1993), dry cleaners (Aoki and Kageyama 1989), warehouse workers (Ashworth et al. 1993) and metal workers (de Boer et al. 1989, Foulds and Koh 1990, Goh and Yuen 1994, Elsner et al. 1995, Rycroft 1997, Wigger-Alberti et al. 1997). Recently, apart from chemical irritants three important risk factors for the development of occupational hand dermatitis in metal worker trainees have been examined: atopic disposition, mechanical irritation, and insufficient amount of skin regeneration time (Berndt et al. 1999). Generally, occupations involving 'wet work' are especially prone to irritant dermatitis. More detailed lists of specific occupational hazards are given in the job descriptions included in Part 3 of Kanerva et al. (2000).

Diagnosis

ICD has to be diagnosed by excluding other causes for the dermatitis. Although this is more easily done on the basis of signs and symptoms for acute ICD, it is usually more difficult for cumulative irritant dermatitis. ACD, which tends to show spreading papules and vesicles, is the most important diagnosis to be excluded. It is hard to differentiate in the chronic state. Irritant dermatitis may be diagnosed if patch tests remain negative, if there is an exposure to irritants, and if the disease develops and heals, depending on the frequency and intensity of this exposure. However, many allergens are also good irritants and may confuse the interpretation of patch testing (Moshell 1997).

Since cumulative ICD may become chronic at a later stage, the relation between exposure and disease tends to weaken. Histologic examination of a biopsy cannot differentiate between chronic irritant and allergic or atopic dermatitis. However, chronic ICD differs morphologically from acute ICD (Willis 1996). Immunohistologic staining has not shown any significant differences in the inflammatory infiltrate of chronic irritant and allergic dermatitis (Brasch et al. 1992). Whereas a biopsy may be helpful to exclude palmar psoriasis, psoriasis can usually be excluded or confirmed on clinical grounds that consider sharply demarcated hyperkeratotic or pustular lesions in contrast to the fuzzy borders of eczema while searching for other features such as nail and scalp involvement.

Visual evaluation of skin erythema and surface changes is still widely used to assess irritant reactions. However, various non-invasive techniques have been developed that permit objective evaluation of skin changes compared to a visual assessment (Wilhelm et al. 1989). The new bioengineering techniques, such as measuring transepidermal water loss as an indicator of epidermal barrier function, are well suited to detect minute epidermal barrier impairment earlier than clinical examinations and to assess the grade of dermatitis quantitatively. However, they are not useful in making a safe differential diagnosis between ACD and ICD. Rather, they offer the possibility to evaluate inflammation parameters such as redness, scaling and infiltration objectively and to quantify these reactions (Iliev 1998).

Treatment and Prognosis

Avoiding the irritant(s) remains the basis of treating occupational ICD. This is achieved through technical measures (exchange of working substances, encapsulation of irritating fluids), individual skin protection (gloves, protective suits, protective creams), and, if necessary, sick leave until the epidermal barrier has completely regenerated, which may be a lengthy process, especially in cumulative irritant dermatitis.

The use of topical corticosteroids in the successful treatment of ACD has been questioned in irritant dermatitis (van der Valk and Maibach 1989). They may be effective in chronic, hyperkeratotic irritant dermatitis, but their prolonged use may lead to epidermal atrophy and consequently increased irritant sensitivity. Other therapeutic options in irritant dermatitis include topical tars and phototherapy (UVB or PUVA). In difficult cases of chronic irritant hand dermatitis, radiation may be indicated (Goldschmidt and Panizzon 1991). Bacterial superinfection may be a complication of contact dermatitis; it is treated with topical or systemic antibiotics. Potential irritants, such as irritant cleansing products, not just in the workplace but also in the home environment, must be identified and whenever possible eliminated (Frosch 1989).

Prognosis for acute ICD is good if irritant contact is avoided. Cumulative irritant dermatitis, however, has a doubtful prognosis. In a recent survey, it was stressed that the prognoses of occupational and nonoccupational contact dermatitis, ICD, and ACD are similar, and that a job change does not affect the course of the disease (Hogan et al. 1990). However, Goh summarized that most studies appear to indicate that patients with ICD have a poorer prognosis than those with ACD (Goh 1997). A reason could be that in allergic dermatitis a specific causative allergen can be identified and avoided but the cause of ICD is often unknown. Well-known factors that cause a poor prognosis for ICD are the existence of atopic dermatitis (Hogan 1996; Seidenari 1996) or what has been termed "persistant post-occupational dermatitis (PPOD)" (Wall and Gebauer 1991). In our experience, in metal workers with cutting fluid dermatitis it took up to several years despite job change and avoidance of irritants (Elsner et al. 1995). This stresses the importance of early intervention in irritant dermatitis before it reaches the chronic stage.

Prevention

Considering the high incidence of ICD at the workplace, it is clear that preventive measures play an important role. In order to increase the awareness of this health risk and to achieve optimal compliance with protective measures, employees should be adequately instructed at the start of their training. It has been shown that the risky behavior of apprentice metal workers can be linked to the fact that they are very badly informed about skin diseases, the potential risk of hand eczema at the workplace and the benefit of skin care (Itschner et al. 1996). Considering this finding, it seems a matter of urgency to intensify health and safety education.

The following types of prevention should be distinguished: Primary prevention tries to prevent the development of disease in the healthy individual; secondary prevention is targeted at the diseased individual and tries to inhibit a relapse of contact dermatitis; tertiary prevention (rehabilitation) treats a chronically diseased patient and reintegrates him into the working environment (Wigger-Alberti and Elsner 1997). Prevention of ICD requires an integrated approach that considers both the exposure and the exposed individual. The responsibility for primary prevention rests mainly with manufacturers and producers of chemicals and products, government agencies, consumer organizations, industrial physicians and nurses, and safety engineers (Wahlberg and Maibach 1994). A multidimensional approach with eight basic elements of prevention planning has been proposed by Mathias (Mathias 1990): recognition of potential cutaneous irritants and allergens, engineering controls or chemical substitution to prevent skin exposure, personal protection with appropriate clothing or protective creams, personal and environmental hygiene, regulation of potential allergens and irritants within the workplace, educational efforts to promote awareness of potential allergens and irritants, motivational techniques to promote safe work conditions and practices, and preemployment and periodic health screening.

In the prevention of exposure, the main elements are technical measures, i.e. avoidance of the irritant by its removal from the workplace or through technical shielding by the use of potent irritants in closed systems or automation, irritant replacement or removal (Lachapelle 1995), and personal protection of the workers (Wigger-Alberti and Elsner 1998). On the individual's side, screening for predisposition to irritant dermatitis and counseling of sensitive individuals may be appropriate preventive measures.

References

Aoki T, Kageyama R (1989) Three cases of dry cleaning dermatitis. Nippon Hifuka Gakkai Zasshi 9:1035–1038

Ashworth J, Rycroft RJG, Waddy RS (1993) Irritant contact dermatitis in warehouse employees. Occup Med 43:32–34

Avnstorp C (1996) Irritant cement eczema. In: van der Valk PGM, Maibach HI (eds) The irritant contact dermatitis syndrome. CRC Press, New York, pp 111–119

Berardesca E, Distante F (1995) Mechanisms of skin irritation. In: Elsner P, Maibach HI (eds) Irritant dermatitis: new clinical and experimental aspects. Karger, Basel, pp 1–8

Berardesca E, Maibach HI (1988) Racial differences in sodium lauryl sulphate induced cutaneous irritation: black and white. Contact Dermatitis 18:65–70

Berndt U, Hinnen U, Iliev D, Elsner P (1999) Role of the atopy score and of single atopic features as risk factors for the development of hand eczema in trainee metal workers. Br J Dermatol 140:922–924

Binnick AN (1981) Allergic and irritant contact dermatitis. Compr Ther 1:17–21

Brasch L, Burgard J, Sterry W (1992) Common pathogenetic pathways in allergic and irritant contact dermatitis. J Invest Dermatol 98:166–170

Bruze M, Emmett EA (1990) Occupational exposures to irritants. In: Jackson EM, Goldner P (eds) Irritant contact dermatitis. Dekker, New York, pp 81–106

Cleenewerck MB, Martin P (1996) Irritants: food. In: van der Valk PGM, Maibach HI (eds) The irritant contact dermatitis syndrome. CRC Press, New York, pp 157–184

Coenraads PJ, Smit J (1995) Epidemiology. In: Rycroft RJG, Menn T, Frosch PJ (eds) Textbook of contact dermatitis. Springer, Berlin Heidelberg New York, pp 133–150

Conde Salazar L, Gomez J, Meza B, Guimaraens D (1993) Artefactual irritant contact dermatitis. Contact Dermatitis 28:246

Cronin E (1980) Contact dermatitis. Churchill Livingston, Edinburgh

Cronin E. (1987) Dermatitis of the hands in caterers. Contact Dermatitis 17:265–269

Cronin E. (1995) Hand eczema. In: Rycroft RJG, Menn T, Frosch PJ (eds) Textbook of contact dermatitis. Springer, Berlin Heidelberg New York, pp 207–218

de Boer EM, van Ketel WG, Bruynzeel DP (1989) Dermatoses in metal workers I: Irritant contact dermatitis. Contact Dermatitis 20:212–218

Diepgen TL, Coenraads PJ (1995) What can we learn from epidemiological studies on irritant contact dermatitis? In: Elsner P, Maibach HI (eds) Irritant dermatitis: new clinical and experimental aspects. Karger, Basel, pp 18–27

Dooms-Goossens AE, Debusschere KM, Gevers DM, Dupre KM, Degreef HJ, Loncke JP, Snauwoert JE (1986) Contact dermatitis caused by airborne agent. A review and case reports. J Am Acad Dermatol 15:1–10

Eichmann A, Amgwerd D (1992) Toxische Kontaktdermatitis. Schweiz Rundsch Med Prax 19:615–617

Elsner P, Maibach HI (1993) Irritant and allergic contact dermatitis. In: Elsner P, Martius J (eds) Vulvovaginitis. Marcel Dekker, New York

Elsner P (1994) Irritant dermatitis in the workplace. Dermatol Clin 12:461–467

Elsner P, Baxmann F, Liehr HM (1995) Metal working fluid dermatitis: A comparative follow-up study in patients with irritant and non-irritant hand dermatitis. In: Elsner P, Maibach HI (eds) Irritant dermatitis: new clinical and experimental aspects. Karger, Basel, pp 77–86

Emtestam L, Ollmar S (1993) Electrical impedance index in human skin: measurements after occlusion in 5 anatomical regions and in mild irritant contact dermatitis. Contact Dermatitis 28:104–108

Foulds IS, Koh D (1990) Dermatitis from metalworking fluids. Clin Exp Dermatol 15: 157–162

Fregert S (1981) Manual of contact dermatitis, 2nd edn. Munksgaard, Copenhagen, pp 55–62

Frosch PJ (1989) Irritant contact dermatitis. In: Frosch PJ, Dooms-Goossens A, Lachapelle JM, Rycroft RJG, Scheper RJ (eds) Current topics in contact dermatitis. Springer, Berlin Heidelberg New York, pp 385–403

Frosch PJ. (1995) Cutaneous irritation. In: Rycroft RJG, Menn T, Frosch PJ (eds) Textbook of contact dermatitis. Springer, Berlin Heidelberg New York, pp 28–61

Frosch PJ, Kligman AM (1977) A method for appraising the stinging capacity of topically applied substances. Soc Cosmet Chem 28:197–209

Gan SL, Goh CL, Lee CS (1987) Occupational dermatitis among sanders in the furniture industry. Contact Dermatitis 17:237–240

Gaspari AA (1997) The role of keratinocytes in the pathophysiology of contact dermatitis. Immun Allergy Clin 17:377–405

Gawkrodger DJ, Lloyd MH, Hunter JA (1986) Occupational skin disease in hospital cleaning and kitchen workers. Contact Dermatitis 15:132–135

Goh C (1987) Occupational skin disease in Singapore: epidemiology and causative agents. Ann Acad Med Singapore 16(2):303–305

Goh CL, Yuen R (1994) A study of occupational skin disease in the metal industry (1986–1990). Ann Acad Med Singapore 23:639–644

Goh CL (1995) Noneczematous contact reactions. In: Rycroft RJG, Menn T, Frosch PJ (eds) Textbook of contact dermatitis. Springer, Berlin, Heidelberg New York, pp 221–236

Goh CL (1997) Prognosis of contact and occupational dermatitis. Clin Dermatol 15:655–659

Goldner R (1994) Work-related irritant contact dermatitis. Occup Med 9:37–44

Goldschmidt H, Panizzon RG (1991) Radiation therapy of benign tumors, hyperplasias, and dermatoses. Springer, Berlin Heidelberg New York

Hafner J, Rüegger M, Kralicek P, Elsner P (1995) Airborne irritant contact dermatitis from metal dust adhering to semisynthetic working suits. Contact Dermatitis 32:285–288

Hogan DJ, Dannaker CJ, Maibach HI (1990) The prognosis of contact dermatitis. J Am Acad Dermatol 23:300–307

Hogan DJ (1996) The prognosis of irritant contact dermatitis. In: van der Valk PGM, Maibach HI (eds) The irritant contact dermatitis syndrome. CRC Press, New York, pp 9–15

Hurwitz RM, Rivera HP, Guin JD (1984) Black-spot poison ivy dermatitis. An acute irritant contact dermatitis superimposed upon an allergic contact dermatitis. Am J Dermatopathol 6:319–322

Iliev D, Elsner P (1997) Clinical irritant contact dermatitis syndromes. Immun Allergy Clin 17:365–375

Iliev D, Hinnen U, Elsner P (1998) Skin bioengineering methods in occupational dermatology. In: Elsner P, Barel AO, Berardesca E, Gabard E, Serup J (eds) Skin bioengineering techniques and applications in dermatology and cosmetology. Karger, Basel, pp 145–150

Itschner L, Hinnen U, Elsner P (1996) Prevention of hand eczema in the metal-working industry: risk awareness and behaviour of metal worker apprentices. Dermatology 193:226–229

Kanerva L, Estlander T, Jolanki R (1988) Occupational skin disease in Finland. An analysis of 10 years of statistics from an occupational dermatology clinic. Int Arch Occup Environ Health 60:89–94

Kanerva L, Elsner P, Wahlberg JE, Maibach HI (eds) (2000) Handbook of Occupational Dermatology. Springer, Berlin Heidelberg New York

Kassis V, Vedel P, Darre E (1984) Contact dermatitis to methyl methacrylate. Contact Dermatitis 11:26–28

Lachapelle JM (1986) Industrial airborne irritant or allergic contact dermatitis. Contact Dermatitis 14:137–145

Lachapelle JM (1995) Principles of prevention and protection in contact dermatitis (with special reference to occupational dermatology). In: Rycroft RJG, Menn T, Frosch PJ (eds) Textbook of contact dermatitis. Springer, Berlin, Heidelberg New York, pp 695–702

Lammintausta K, Maibach HI (1990) Contact dermatitis due to irritation: general principles, etiology, and histology. In: Adams RM (eds) Occupational skin disease. WB Saunders, Philadelphia, pp 1–15

Lammintausta K, Maibach HI, Wilson D (1987) Irritant reactivity in males and females. Contact Dermatitis 17:276–280

Lammintausta K, Maibach HI, Wilson D (1988) Mechanisms of subjective (sensory) irritation. Propensity to non-immunologic contact urticaria and objective irritation in stingers. Derm Beruf Umwelt 36:45–49

Lauerma AI, Stein BD, Homey B, Lee CH, Bloom E, Maibach HI (1994) Topical FK506: suppression of allergic and irritant contact dermatitis in the guinea pig. Arch Dermatol Res 286:337–340

Malten KE, den Arend JA (1985) Irritant contact dermatitis: traumiterative and cumulative impairment by cosmetics, climate, and other daily loads. Derm Beruf Umwelt 33:125–132

Malten KE, den Arend JA, Wiggers RE (1979) Delayed irritation: hexanediol diacrylate and butanediol diacrylate. Contact Dermatitis 3:178–184

Malten KE (1981) Thoughts on irritant contact dermatitis. Contact Dermatitis 7:238–247

Mathias CG (1990) Prevention of occupational contact dermatitis. J Am Acad Dermatol 23:742–748

Mathias CGT, Maibach HI (1987) Dermatotoxicology monographs. 1. Cutaneous irritation: factors influencing the response to irritants. Clin Toxicol 13:333–346

Meding B, Swanbeck G (1990) Occupational hand eczema in an industrial city. Contact Dermatitis 22:13–23

Meding B (1990) Epidemiology of hand eczema in an industrial city. Acta Derm Venereol (Stockh) (Suppl) 153:1–43

Moshell AN (1997) Workshop on irritant contact dermatitis. Am J Contact Dermatitis 8:79–105

Nilsson E (1986) Individual and environmental risk factors for hand eczema in hospital workers. Acta Derm Venereol (Stockh) (Suppl) 128:1–63

Pinnagoda J, Tupker RA, Smit JA, Coenraads PJ, Nater JP (1989) The intra- and inter-individual variability and reliability of transepidermal water loss measurements. Contact Dermatitis 21:255–259

Rietschel RL (1997) Comparison of allergic and irritant dermatitis. Immun Allergy Clin 17:359–364

Rycroft RJG (1997) Metal working industry. Clin Dermatol 15:565–566

Rystedt I (1985) Work-related hand eczema in atopics. Contact dermatitis 12:164–171

Seidenari S (1996) Skin sensitivity, interindividual factors: atopy. In: van der Valk PGM, Maibach (eds) The irritant contact dermatitis syndrome. CRC Press, New York, pp 267–277

Singgih SI, Lantingha H, Nater JP, Woest TE, Kruyt-Gaspersz JA (1986) Occupational hand dermatoses in hospital cleaning personnel. Contact Dermatitis 14:14–19

Skogstad M, Levy F (1994) Occupational irritant contact dermatitis and fungal infection in construction workers. Contact dermatitis 31:28–30

Soschin D, Kligman AM (1982) Adverse subjective reactions. In: Kligman AM, Leyden JJ (eds) Safety and efficacy of topical drugs and cosmetics. Grune and Stratton, New York, pp 377–388

Suter-Widmer J, Elsner P (1994) Age and irritation. In: van der Valk PGM, Maibach HI (eds) The Irritant contact dermatitis syndrome. CRC Press, Boca Raton, pp 257–261

Uter W, Gefeller O, Schwanitz HJ (1995) Occupational dermatitis in hairdressing apprentices. In: Elsner P, Maibach HI (eds) Irritant dermatitis. New clinical and experimental aspects. Karger, Basel, pp 49–55

van der Valk PGM, Maibach HI (1989) Do topical corticosteroids modulate skin irritation in human beings? Assesment by transepidermal water loss and visual scoring. J Am Acad Dermatol 21:519–522

van der Valk PGM, Nater JP, Bleumink E (1985) Vulnerability of the skin to surfactants in different groups of eczema patients and controls as measured by water vapour loss. Clin Exp Dermatol 10:98–103

van der Walle HB, Brunsveld VM (1994) Dermatitis in hairdressers. 1. The experience of the past 4 years. Contact Dermatitis 30:217–221

Wahlberg JE, Maibach HI (1994) Prevention of contact dermatitis. In: Mellström GA, Wahlberg JE, Maibach HI (eds) Protective gloves for occupational use. CRC Press, New York, pp 7–9

Wall L, Gebauer K (1991) A follow-up study of occupational skin disease in Western Australia. Contact Dermatitis 524:241–243

Wigger-Alberti W, Elsner P (1997) Preventive measures in contact dermatitis. Clin Dermatol 15:661–665

Wigger-Alberti W, Elsner P (1998) Do barrier creams and gloves prevent or provoke contact dermatitis ? Am J Contact Dermatitis 9:100–106

Wigger-Alberti W, Hinnen U, Elsner P (1997) Predictive testing of metalworking fluids: a comparison of 2 cumulative human irritation models and correlation to epidemiological data. Contact Dermatitis 36:14–20

Wilhelm KP, Surber C, Maibach HI (1989) Quantification of sodium lauryl sulphate irritant dermatitis in man: comparison of four techniques: skin color, reflectance, transepidermal water loss, laser Doppler flow measurement and visual scores. Arch Dermatol Res 281:293–295

Wilkinson JD, Willis CM (1998) Contact dermatitis: irritant. In: Champion RH, Burton JL, Burns DA, Breathnach SM (eds) Textbook of dermatology, 6th edn. Blackwell, London, pp 709–731

Willis CM (1996) The histopathology of irritant contact dermatitis. In: van der Valk PGM, Maibach HI (eds) The irritant contact dermatitis syndrome. CRC Press, New York, pp 291–303

Wood BP, Greig DE (1997) Catering industry. Clin Dermatol 15:567–571

Wrangsjö K, Meding B (1997) Hospital workers. Clin Dermatol 15:573–578

CHAPTER 5

Fiberglass Dermatitis 5

A. Sertoli, S. Francalanci, S. Giorgini

Introduction

Glass fibers, the man-made vitreous fibers (MMVF), represent a subgroup of the so-called man-made mineral fibers (MMMF) and include glass fibers and glass wool. (TIMA 1991; Stam-Westerveld 1996). Fiberglass consists of single continuous filaments, sometimes very long, which can be processed using the techniques typical of the textile industry to produce fabrics and can be gathered together to produce felts or cut in pieces of shorter length (Björnberg 1985, Konzen 1987).

Production of Fiberglass

Glass fibers are produced exclusively from glass through fusion at temperatures ranging from 1000° to 1500°C and subsequent filtering of siliceous-based mixtures containing earthy-alkaline additives to improve their workability.

These fibers are filtered by three main methods: centrifugation, blowing with hot gasses and thinning by flame (International Labour Office 1983). Fibers are then treated with particular substances having binding, protective and lubricating effects, especially if they are to be used in the manufacture of reinforced plastic. The above-mentioned substances are: phenol-formaldehyde resins, formaldehyde-urea resins, melaminoformaldehyde resins, epoxy resins, polyester resins, polyvinylacetate, silicon, ammonium hydroxide and mineral oils (Björnberg 1985, Konzen 1987, Bruze and Almgren 1989, Jolanki et al. 1996).

Glass wool is produced from a vitreous mixture which is subsequently filtered in the shape of wool (International Labour Office 1983, Stam-Westerveld 1996).

Use of Fiberglass

Due to their ever-increasing applications, glass fibers are the most widespread artificial mineral fibers (Meneghini 1977, Lammintausta and Maibach 1990, Lachapelle et al. 1992, Sertoli et al. 1992, Rietschel and Fowler 1995, Stam-Westerveld 1996). They have become more and more important because they can replace asbestos fibers which are particularly dangerous (Ruegger 1996).

World production of glass fibers used in various kinds of insulation, assessed in 1973 at 3,600,000 tons, reached 4,800,000 tons in 1989 and represents about

80% of the whole production of MMVF (Patroni 1989). The production of glass fibers for special purposes, such as aircraft insulation and highly efficient paper filters, was estimated at 60,000 tons in 1989 and accounts for 1% of the whole production of mineral fibers.

Acoustic Insulators

Glass wool finds application in the internal setting of public buildings (offices, theatres, schools, hospitals etc.) usually in the form of panels (Verbeck at al. 1981, Wang et al. 1993).

Thermal Insulators

Glass wool in mattresses, felts and fiber glass tissues is used to insulate steam or water piping, stoves, under-roof coverings in houses with wave-form ceiling boards and in the aircraft industry. A more recent and peculiar application is in the production of printed circuit boards, (PRCB) (Koh et al. 1992, Marks and De-Leo 1992, Wang et al. 1993, Koh and Khoo 1994). They are composed of several layers, the core (fire-proof) consisting of fiberglass fabric soaked with brominated epoxy resin: the outer layers consisted of copper sheets (Bruze and Almgren 1989).

Electrical Insulators

Glass fibers are used in various forms to insulate motors, wires and electric cables (Sertoli et al. 1992).

Reinforcing Material

Tissues in glass fibers and glass wool are used with polyester, epoxy and melaminic resins to produce a large number of reinforced plastic-manufactured articles to strengthen their mechanical resistance; they are mainly used in aircraft, automotive, naval and railway industries (doors, hulls, boards etc.) and to produce sportswear and printed material in general (Sertoli et al. 1982, Carrino 1988, Sertoli et al. 1992, Tarvainen et al. 1995). In the epoxy composite materials (e.g. those used to produce skis), plastic sheets reinforced with glass fibers are laminated one by one with sheets in epoxy resins (Jolanki et al. 1996).

Filtering Material

Very thin glass fibers are mainly used in the shape of tissues for scientific purposes (chemistry laboratories, food and beverage industries) like filters for air, gases and liquid material (Sertoli and Farli 1991, Lachapelle et al. 1992).

Health Hazards

The most frequent health hazards due to glass-fiber exposure are represented by skin lesions, commonly known as fiberglass dermatitis described for the first time at the beginning of the 1940s (Sulzberger and Baer 1942). We also have to remember the potential bronchopneumopathy hazard due to glass-fiber inhalation which seems to be inversely proportional to their diameter and length: evidence exists that only fibers with length fluctuating between 80 μm and 5 μm, whose diameter is lower than 3 μm can reach peripheral areas of the lung, from which, in any case, they are expelled much more quickly than asbestos fibers.

Relative to the current levels of exposure it does not seem to be a clear-cut cancer risk for those workers handling glass fibers (Ruegger 1996).

Pathogenesis of Fiberglass Dermatitis

The basic pathogenetic mechanism of fiberglass dermatitis (Table 1) is represented by penetration (supported by pressure, rub and scraping) of fine sharp particles into the skin causing mechanical irritation (Stam-Westerveld et al. 1994, Stam-Westerveld 1996). Fibers are usually found in the horny layer but, occasionally, they can also penetrate more deeply into the skin. The pathogenic activity of fiberglass on the skin is directly proportional to its diameter and inversely proportional to its length (Konzen 1987). Only fiberglass featuring a rated diameter superior to 4.5 μm is commonly considered to be injurious. Penetration of fiberglass into derma, rather uncommon indeed, can cause the formation of foreign-body reactions (Lechner and Hartmann 1979, Lachapelle et al. 1992).

The risk of sensitization by contact is mainly due to professional exposure to the resins used for the finishing of glass fibers: allergic contact dermatitis has been reported in those workers coming into contact with resins not completely cured, in particular epoxy and formaldehyde resins (Cuypers et al. 1975b, Dahlquist et al. 1979, Kalimo et al. 1980, Conde-Salazar et al. 1985, Bruze and Almgren 1989, Holness and Nethercott 1989, Jolanki et al. 1996).

Table 1. Pathogenetic mechanism of fiberglass dermatitis

Direct, indirect (through clothing) or airborne (irritant contact dermatitis, ICD) followed by:
Simple mechanical trauma by sting
Fibers penetration and permanence into derma and subcutaneous
Sensitization (allergic contact dermatitis, ACD) by finishing resins

Fiberglass Irritant Contact Dermatitis

Fiberglass dermatitis is one of the most common professional mechanic irritant contact dermatitis (ICD) (Heisel and Mitchell 1957, Fisher and Warkentin 1969, Lachapelle 1986, Konzen 1987, Okano et al. 1987, Adams 1990, Fleming and Bergfeld 1990, Tarvainen et al. 1994, Adams 1995, Rietschel and Fowler 1995, Stam-Westerveld 1996).

Generally speaking, dermatitis arises in subjects exposed to glass fibers for a short period, while those who routinely come into contact with it seem to develop a sort of hardening and can continue working without any difficulty (Björnberg 1985).

Diagnosis is not always easy because of the different aspects conditioning the clinical picture of this kind of dermatitis:

1. *Individual characteristics.* The presence of personal and/or family atopy, and altered dermographic reactivity, which, together with clear skin, are important promoting factors (Björnberg 1985).
2. *Environmental conditions.* High temperatures and humidity characterizing the microclimate in the working environment; in the summer – but also winter time – during which the relative humidity dramatically decreases because of the heating systems,and/or inadequate ventilation; concentration of fibers also due to incorrect or inadequate cleaning (Sertoli et al. 1982, Adams 1990).
3. *Mechanisms of contact.* Direct contact of fibers with the skin or indirect contact due to accumulation on clothing, presence of fibers in the dust from the floor and/or on working surfaces; contact with airborne fibers; duration of exposure (Lachapelle 1986, Sertoli et al. 1992, Rietschel and Fowler 1995);
4. *Pathogenetic mechanisms.* Simple mechanical trauma by fibers on the skin or their permanence in derma and hypodermis after penetration; sensitization to the resins used for the finishing of fibers or the manufacture of reinforced plastics (Konzen 1987, Tarvainen et al. 1993, Stam-Westerveld 1996).

Epidemiology

Few data are available regarding the predominance of fiberglass dermatitis and they pertain solely to professional exposure. In factories where fibers and glass wool are produced, non-updated studies report on percentages ranging from 11% to 58% (Heisel and Mitchell 1957, Björnberg et al. 1979a). Within an establishment of the Ferrovie dello Stato (Italian Railways Company), Sertoli and his colleagues found percentages equal to 20.3% in personnel directly exposed to the hazard, 19.9% in those indirectly exposed, and 1.1% in other personnel apparently not directly exposed; ex-clerks who worked in areas far from the departments where glass fibers were processed (Sertoli et al. 1982). In the building industry, where the hazard appears to be high, dermatitis prevalence among the personnel has been reported as being higher than 60% (Björnberg, 1985). The PRCB industry is another field at risk in which micro-epidemics (more exactly pseudo-epidemics) have been reported; this being when the percentage of afflicted personnel is higher than 17% (Bruze and Almgren 1989, Koh et al. 1992). This percentage is much lower in industries (like that producing skis), which use laminated plastics reinforced with glass fibers (Jolanki et al. 1996). In Finland during the period 1975–1991 fiberglass dermatitis represented 1.7% of occupational dermatoses concerning 58 different activities (Tarvainen et al. 1994).

The most widespread glass-fiber field of application, insulation and ventilation used in public and private buildings, exposes an ever-growing number of people who are not professionally involved in the working activities of production and application of glass fibers (Verbeck et al. 1981, Farkas 1983).

This kind of pollution does not concern secluded areas only (offices), but also open spaces, above all those in the neighborhood of factories producing glass fibers.

Clinical Picture

Itching (of different intensity, but usually very strong) and a tingling sensation, above all at the skin fold or where clothing is in contact with the skin, usually represent the early symptoms characterizing fiberglass dermatitis. Their sudden manifestation can be the cause of serious apprehension in affected patients (Adams 1990). Afterwards, a diffused eruption of small erythematous patches together with papules of a small diameter can be observed – as in the case of papular urticaria – but not showing the typical vesicle in the center. Sometimes the patch is excoriated, with follicular localization diffused through the exposed areas where fibers come into contact with the skin via the airborne mechanism (airborne fiberglass contact dermatitis; Fig. 1) or on the portions of skin, above all the forearms, which came into contact with surfaces contaminated by glass fibers such as, in the professional environment, a work bench or, in the case of non-professional environments, clothing.

Dermatitis heals as soon as the contact stop (Erwin 1947), rarely becoming chronic with the formation of nodular elements.

This dermatitis also has the following particular characteristics: excoriated folliculitis, acute paronychia (caused by the penetration of fibers into the perionychium), nummular eczema-like lesions, eye-burning sensation and conjunctivitis, lichenification, contact urticaria, erythema multiforme-like dermatitis; granuloma anulare-like folliculitis and acneiform lesions with follicular pustules due to oils

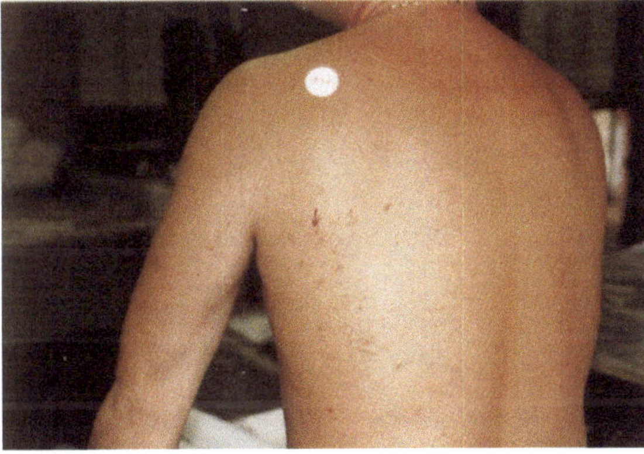

Fig. 1. Antonio T., 35 years old – airborne fiberglass dermatitis: rash in small itching papules at the trunk and upper limbs in an office worker employed in the textile industry

and emulsions used for the finishing of glass fibers can also be observed (Björnberg et al. 1979b, Lechner and Hartmann 1979, Fisher 1982, Camarasa and Moreno 1984, Fisher 1986, Konzen 1987, Sertoli et al. 1992, Beyer and Vossmann 1996).

The penetration of glass fragments into the skin of the hands of employees working in the department which produces fibers causes the so-called glass hand's syndrome described by Grzegorczyk in 1982. This syndrome is characterized by the absence of skin lesions and sometimes by the presence of a painful sensation. Later, the same author produced evidence by X-ray, and, in some cases, computed axial tomography (CAT), the penetration of glass fibers into the skin of workers in a factory producing fluorescent glass lamps (Grzegorczyk 1987).

Recently an itch with minimal redness caused by damaged plastic trays reinforced with fiberglass was reported in waitresses (Bruynzell and De Boer, 1997).

Sertoli and co-workers investigated an epidemic of dermatitis from glass fibers which occurred within a workshop of the *Ferrovie dello Stato* (Italian Railways) (Sertoli et al. 1982). Skin lesions were present in about 20% of examined subjects, but also in those personnel who worked in buildings, which were far from it and were not directly exposed to the specific hazard (for example, clerks).

The same author (Sertoli, personal communication) reports on two other episodes concerning fiberglass dermatitis epidemics. The first took place on one of the floors of a new building, built for a daily newspaper and reserved for the administration.

This dermatitis was caused by a malfunctioning air-conditioning filter system, which allowed glass fibers to be released into the environment. The second episode took place in a factory producing fabrics for interior decoration. About 50% of the inside workers complained of itching. Four months earlier, drilled boards of phonosorbent aluminum, containing 60-mm thick wads of glass wool treated with thermohardener resins wrapped up in polyvinyl chloride (PVC), were installed in order to reduce the noise level in the weaving department. One or more wraps had broken, maybe because of a manufacturing defect or when they were

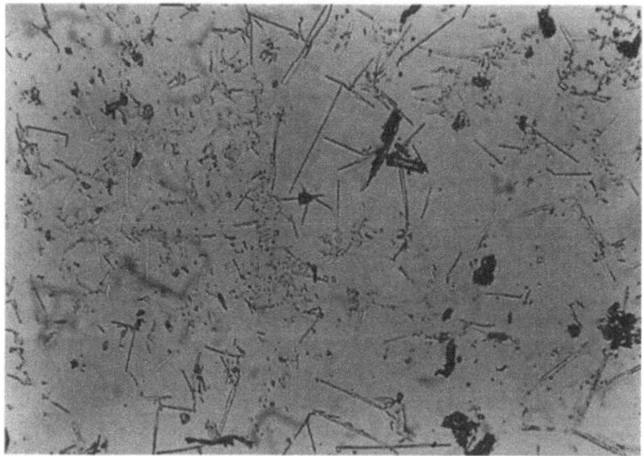

Fig. 2. Microphotography (×100): dust sample coming from the surface of a loom of the same textile industry. Note the presence of fiberglass spicules mixed with dust fluff

Table 2. Nonoccupational hazards of fiberglass contact

Home environment: thermal and acoustic insulation systems, upholstery, curtains, cloths
for furniture in general, clothing, overalls
School environment: desks
Hobbies

inserted into the boards, and, as a result, induced by vibration, glass wool fibers
were discharged through the holes into the environment, falling on the looms and
other surfaces (cylinders, pieces, tables, etc.; Fig. 2).

Familial fiberglass dermatitis micro-epidemics (Table 2) requiring a careful differential diagnosis with scabies – above all where clothing was washed together
with curtains containing these kind of fibers – were also observed ("pseudoclothing dermatitis").

Histopathology

Histopathological lesions observed in fiberglass dermatitis are almost equal to
those produced by the contact eczema presenting spongiosis, sometimes diastasis
at the level of the basal layer, and lymphocytic perivascular and perifollicular infiltrate (Cuypers et al. 1975 a). The persistence of lesions, and their possible evolution towards nodules, suggests the presence of a continuous stimulus due to the
penetration of fibers into the skin. In this case, the histopathological investigation
presents evidence patterns characteristic of the foreign body granuloma (Siebert
1942, Cuypers et al. 1975 a, Björnberg 1985).

Diagnosis

The diagnosis of fiberglass dermatitis is fundamentally based on the clinical observation and accurate collection of anamnestic data. Though not pathognomonic
skin lesions, these nevertheless, show the characteristic distribution and evolution
previously described, while the subjective itching symptomatology has to be considered with particular care. While collecting anamnestic data, the possible onset
of similar lesions in other subjects of the working and/or the familial environment should be carefully investigated (epidemics or micro-epidemics). The identification of the sources of exposure is relatively easy in those cases in which onset took place in the working environment and can be confirmed by the inspection of the factory and by the knowledge of the technological cycle. The investigation is more difficult in the case of non-professional exposure because it also
involves the collection of detailed information concerning the subject's lifestyle,
including possible changes. Diagnosis can be then confirmed by the detection of
glass fibers on those portions of skin affected by dermatitis. This can be confirmed through the "adhesive tape stripping" technique with a piece of scotch
tape applied repeatedly to the affected area and then directly observed under the
optical microscope or by maceration of the corneous samples taken by scraping
with one or more drops of potassium hydroxide at 20% (Deeken 1978, Cronin
1980).

As previously described, the histological investigation of skin samples from the affected areas does not produce any peculiar alteration; it is however possible, though not easy, to find spicules of glass fibers, especially if the observation is carried out under a polarized light which makes them birefringent (Garcia-Patos and Pujol 1994). Furthermore, when the presence of glass fibers in tissues is suspected, an X-ray should be carried out to confirm the results obtained through the histological investigation.

Differential Diagnosis

Due to its clinical characteristics, fiberglass dermatitis, can be associated with the group of generalized acute prurigo and itching caused by external causes.

Fiberglass dermatitis is subject to differential diagnosis (Table 3) first of all if the itching is suspected to be an expression of epizoonosis (Sertoli et al. 1992). Urticaria papulosa (strophulus, simplex acute prurigo, acute prurigo, lichens urticatus by insect stings and bites – mosquitoes, midges, bugs, fleas, etc.), typical in children, is characterized by the presence of itching papules – gathered together or in rows – showing sometimes a centered blister, on the trunk, upper and lower limbs where insects have bitten. These lesions appear about 12–72 hours after the bite or sting and are accompanied by a strong itching; they regress slowly and completely leaving a spot or a pigmented nodule. The form occurring in adults is usually due to professional causes and rarely has an epidemic character; it

Table 3. Most common simple itching (*sine materia*) or prurigo in differential diagnosis with fiberglass dermatitis

By external cause
Urticaria papulosa[a]
Acariasis[a]
Pediculosis[a]
Swimmers' prurigo[a]
Phytodermatitis by thorns[a]
Prurigo by Thaumatopea pinivora hairs[a]
Prurigo by irritant solid airborne particles[a]
Actinic prurigo
Eczema prurigo
Improper or excessive use of detergents
Side effects of drugs
By internal cause
Pruritus senilis
Psychosomatic pruritus
Delusions of parasitosis
Biliary stasis
Diabetes mellitus
Uremia
Pregnancy
Dysthyroidisms
Cancers
Hodgkin's disease or chronic leukemias
Myeloma

[a] Also in epidemics.

appears in the spring-summer period, and is mainly connected with activities carried out in the agricultural and forest environment; papules, even in the case of adults, prevail over any other possible lesions so that dermatosis is less polymorphous.

In the form typical of scabies, *Sarcoptes scabiei*, var. *hominis*, affected sites have a symmetrical disposition and affect hands – particularly the interdigital spaces – wrists, elbows, ankles, feet, in men the penis and scrotum are involved also, and in women areola mammae, waist and umbilical area, buttocks, thighs and armpits; in adults, back and face are not involved. The fundamental lesion is identified with the burrow dug (not always easily noticeable) by the female mite in the corneum and represented by a grayish straight line ending up, at one of the extremities, with a blister. Erythematous papules both isolated and in groups, can be observed. Dark red nodules at elbows, armpits and genitalia can occur mainly in man but regress spontaneously. Itching, which is the most characteristic symptom, appears mostly at night. The main elements needed to carry out a differential diagnosis are the sites involved and the symmetrical disposition of lesions, the observation of mites under the microscope in scrapings from skin lesions and also by the kind of itching, the disappearance of lesions after specific therapy and the rarity of relapses.

More difficult is the differential diagnosis of professional acariasis by mites from animals, such as: *Sarcoptes scabiei* var. *animalis* (dogs, horses, cows, pigs, sheep etc.); *Cheyletiella parasitovorax* in rabbits (through the cat); *Dermanissus gallinae* o *D. avium* and other professional and environmental acariasis (Sertoli 1991).

Differential diagnosis can be carried out with the rare pediculosis corporis by *Pediculus humanus* var. *corporis*, but in this case, clear erythematous patches together with papules and sometimes wheals are present; petechias, linear parallel excoriations by scraping (caused by an intense pruritus), melanodermias in its most advanced stages and, above all, anamnestic data together with the findings of the insect or the nits contribute to its differentiation from fiberglass dermatitis.

The latter has also to be differentiated from the dermatitis by contact with plant thorns like those of the barberry (*Berberis vulgaris*) or of the cactus (*Opuntia Lingularis, Opuntia Tunia Mills* or prickly pear) families.

Urticaria papulosa-like patterns can also be caused by contact with the chitinous hairs of grubs, e.g. Processionary moth's grubs (*Thaumatopea Pinivora*), sometimes floating in the air (Sertoli et al. 1991).

Also solid particles in the environment (sawdust, small cardboard fragments, wood or metal filings, cement powder causing the so-called "cement scabies" etc.) can come into contact with the skin, irritating it and provoking itching. Other prurigo, in differential diagnosis with fiberglass dermatitis, are listed in Table 3.

In particular accurate personal and familial anamnesis, together with appropriate clinical and instrumental investigations, is necessary in order to eliminate systemic diseases characterized by itching and papulous rashes.

At the beginning – months before its onset – Hodgkin's disease can manifest with nonspecific and polymorphous skin lesions, characterized by itching and excoriated papules. Itching is typically exacerbated by spirits and is accompanied by abundant night sweating. We must keep in mind that a strong and generalized itching can also be the aspecific symptom of chronic leukemia (sometimes papules are also present) and myeloma.

Prevention

To prevent the onset of fiberglass pathologies, a good level of personal hygiene together with accuracy in fiberglass production are fundamental (Sertoli et al. 1992, Chang et al. 1996, Stam-Westerveld 1996).

In particular, the following points have to be kept in mind:

1. In the different stages of production, closed cycles have to be adopted.
2. Storage, packaging and transportation of materials to the place in which they are prepared and applied should be carried out in special sealed containers.
3. Cutting of fiberglass-manufactured products should be carried out in the forms required for use, so that successive operations are not necessary.
4. To cut and apply felts hand tools (special knives) should be used instead of power-driven tools.
5. For insulation using the spray method, a wet technique should be used instead of a dry technique; at the end of the work, the spraying machine should be cleaned in the same place that the operations took place.
6. To clean production and application departments, a vacuum cleaner should be used.
7. Both the containers used for transportation and the processing residues should be stored to avoid any kind of dispersion.

Particular safety regulations should be observed while removing fiberglass insulation (Sertoli et al. 1982).

Removal of non-resined materials is highly risky; every single operation should be preceded by suitable humidification of materials or by adequate ventilation of the rooms and localized aspiration. Special rooms for personal hygiene (showers, bathrooms), secluded from those in which fibers are processed, should be available. Protective clothing must always be worn and they should be changed and washed frequently but always in the working place and not at home to avoid any kind of contamination. Clothing should be warm enough and their weft closely woven. Barrier creams, base, emollient, ointments and silicon sprays have not proved useful in preventing fiberglass dermatitis; on the contrary, in some cases they can exacerbate itching (Bensöe et al. 1987).

Therapy

Fiberglass dermatitis therapy is solely symptomatic so that antihistaminic drugs can be administered p.o. or corticosteroid low power topical drugs can be applied, together with antibiotics in case of bacterial overlapping (Lachapelle et al. 1992). Removal of fibers from the corneum can be attempted through the adhesive scotch tape or plumbers' duct tape (Deeken 1978).

Medicolegal Aspects

Italian legislation and accepted, though limited, practice consider fiberglass dermatitis as an industrial accident, especially given the concentration in time and, in many cases, the unpredictability of the causal event. However, there is some contention about whether this practice is sufficient to warrant this conclusion, particularly since this disease heals rather quickly without any complications or permanent consequence.

Allergic Contact Dermatitis (ACD) from Fiberglass

Regarding the pathogenetic mechanism by allergic contact, we point out the following: 36 workers out of 160, that is to say, 54% of the total workers tested in a fiberglass factory, presented positive reactions, particularly, to the epoxy resins used for the finishing of fibers (Cuypers et al. 1975b). In 1979, Dahlquist and co-workers reported on five glass fiber spinners sensitized to epoxy resin containing low-molecular-weight oligomers.

In 1980, Kalimo and co-workers described a subject sensitized to p-tert-butyl-formaldheyde resin used for the finishing of glass fibers.

In 1985, Conde-Salazar and co-workers announced the case of a worker who had been working for 4 years in a glass fiber factory and presented with eczematous lesions, first on the left forearm and then on hands, trunk and lower limbs. He also presented a sensitization to epoxy resin containing a 628 kD molecular weight oligomer.

In a group composed of 130 workers who were in contact with glass fibers coated with epoxy resins, 6 were sensitized to epoxy resin, and 1 to the cresilglycidyl ether, a diluent used as reagent: lesions covered mainly hands, forehands and, to a lesser extent, face and neck (Holness and Nethercott 1989).

In a PRCB factory, Bruze and Almgren found 6 workers, out of the 19 tested, sensitized to epoxy resin. During the production of manufactured articles, (made of copper sheets and rolled fiberglass soaked with epoxy brominated resins) subjects were exposed mainly to nonpolymerized resins and to powders from fiberglass tissues soaked with resins.

In a factory where skis were produced with fiberglass reinforced plastics, 6 workers of 22 presented with sensitization to an epoxy-resin low-molecular-weight oligomer and three among them were sensitized to diethyleneglycol diglycidyl ether, a new reactive diluent. Three subjects were sensitized to other epoxy and polyamidic reactive diluents used to harden resins. In all the subjects, dermatitis was localized on the back of the hands, but in some it also involved the face, trunk and lower limbs. Furthermore, another worker showed a positive reaction to the cobalt used as an accelerating agent for polyester resin binding in fiberglass-reinforced sheets, whose presence was demonstrated by atomic absorption spectrophotometer (Jolanki et al. 1996). A worker in a manufacture of children's rides developed vesicular dermatitis of the palms. He added fiberglass, unsaturated polyester resin and catalysts (methyl ethyl ketone-mek-peroxide and cobalt) to an automated mixing machine. The patch tests were positive to mek peroxide and cobalt chloride (Bhushan et al. 1997).

Kanerva and coworkers (2000) describe a patient with occupational vesicular hand ACD. He worked in an aircraft plant and was exposed to preimpregnated epoxy fiberglass (prepregs). Patch tests with reactive diluents, demonstrated present in prepregs by gas and liquid chromatographic methods, triglycidyl-p-aminophenol (TGPAP), tetraglycidyl-4,4'-methylene dianiline (TGMDA) and prepregs products provoked positive reactions whereas standard epoxy provoked a weak (?+) reaction.

References

Adams RM (1990) Dermatitis due to fibrous glass. In: Adams RM (ed) occupational skin disease. Saunders, Philadelphia, pp 16–17

Adams RM (1995) Occupational contact dermatitis. In: Guin JD (ed) Practical contact dermatitis. Mc Graw-Hill, New York, pp 585–587

Bensöe N, Björnberg A, Lowhagen GB et al (1987) Glass fibre irritation and protective creams. Contact Dermatitis 17:69–72

Beyer AV, Vossmann D (1996) Glasfaser-induzierte chronische Dermatitis. Dermatosen 44:225–227

Björnberg A (1985) Glass fiber dermatitis. Am J Ind Med 8:395–400

Björnberg A, Lowhagen GB, Tengberg JE (1979a) Does occupational exposure to glass fiber increase the general skin reactivity to irritants? Contact Dermatitis 5:175–177

Björnberg A, Lowhagen GB, Tengberg JE (1979b) Relationship between intensities of skin test reactions to glass fibres and chemical irritants. Contact Dermatitis 5:171–174

Bruynzeel DP, de Boer EM (1997) Waitresses' itch. Contact Dermatitis 36:308

Bruze M, Almgren G (1989) Occupational dermatoses in workers exposed to epoxy-impregnated fiberglass fabric. Dermatosen 37:171–175

Bhushan M, Craven NM, Beck MH (1997) Contact allergy to methyl ethyl ketone peroxide and cobalt in the manufacture of fiberglass-reinforced plastics. Contact Dermatitis 39:203

Camarasa JG, Moreno A (1984) Fiberglass dermatitis. Contact Dermatitis 10:43

Carrino L (1988) Plastici rinforzati con fibre di vetro: tecnologie di produzione, settori di utilizzo e tendenze di sviluppo dei processi e dei sistemi. In: Seminario Nazionale "Strategie per la difesa nel comparto delle vetroresine". Reggio Emilia, Proceedings, pp 167–193

Chang CH, Wang CM, Ho CK et al (1996) Fiberglass dermatitis: a case report. Kaohsiung J Med Sci 12:491–494

Conde-Salazar L, Guimaraens D, Romero VL et al (1985) Occupational dermatitis from glass fiber. Contact Dermatitis 13:195–196

Cronin E (1980) Fibre glass. In: Cronin E (ed) Contact dermatitis. Churchill Livingstone, Edinburgh, pp 78–80

Cuypers JMC, Hoedemaker J, Nater JP et al (1975a) The histopathology of fiber-glass dermatitis in relation to von Hebra's concept of eczema. Contact Dermatitis 1:88–95

Cuypers JMC, Bleumick E, Nater JP (1975b) Dermatologische Aspekte der Glasfarefabrikation. Dermatosen 23:143–154

Dahlquist S, Fregert S, Trulsson L (1979) Allergic contact dermatitis from epoxy resin finished glass fiber. Contact Dermatit:190

Deeken JH (1978) Tape treatment for fiberglass splinters. Arch Dermatol 114:623

Erwin JR (1947) Fiberglass plastics-Industrial medical aspects and experiences. Ind Med 16:439–441

Farkas J (1983) Fiberglass dermatitis in employers of project office in a new building. Contact Dermatitis 9:79

Fisher AA (1982) Fiberglass vs mineral wool (rockwool) dermatitis. Cutis 29:412, 415–416

Fisher AA (1986) Fiberglass and rockwool dermatitis. In: Fisher AA (ed) Contact Dermatitis. Lea & Febiger, Philadelphia, pp 566–569

Fisher BK, Warkentin JD (1969) Fiber glass dermatitis. Arch Dermatol 99:717–719

Fleming MG, Bergfeld WF (1990) The ethiology of irritant contact dermatitis. In: Jackson E, Goldner R (eds). Marcel Dekker, New York, pp 41–66

Garcia-Patos V, Pujol RM (1994) Generalized pruritus with flexural micropapules in a 16-month-old girl. Arch Dermatol 130: 785–788

Grzegorczyk L (1982) Zur Bedeutung physikalischer Faktoren fur die Entsthung von Berufsdermatosen. Dermatosen 30:179–181

Grzegorczyk L (1987) "Glasshände" ein neues berufsbedingtes Syndrom. Dermatosen 35:62–64

Heisel EB, Mitchell JH (1957) Cutaneous reactions to fiberglass. Ind Med Surg 26:547–550

Holness DL, Nethercott JD (1989) Occupational contact dermatitis due to epoxy resin in a fiberglass binder. J Occup Med 31:87–89

International Labour Office (1983) Fibres, man-made glass and mineral. In: Parmeggiani L (ed) Encyclopedia of occupational health and safety. ILO, Geneva, pp 852–855

Jolanki R, Tarvainen K, Tatar T et al (1996) Occupational dermatoses from exposure to epoxy resin compounds in a ski factory. Contact Dermatitis 34:390–396

Kalimo K, Saarni K, Kytta J (1980) Immediate and delayed type reactions to formaldehyde resin in glass wool. Contact Dermatitis 6:496

Kanerva L, Jolanki R, Estlander T, et al (2000) Airborne occupational allergic contact dermatitis from triglycidyl-p-aminophenol and tetraglycidyl-4,4'-methylene dianiline in pre-impregnated epoxy products in the aircraft industry. Dermatology 201:29–33.

Koh D, Khoo NY (1994) Identification of a printed circuit board causing fibreglass irritation among electronics workers. Contact Dermatitis 30:46–47

Koh D, Aw TC, Foulds IS (1992) Fiberglass dermatitis from printed circuit boards. Am J Ind Med 21:193–198

Konzen JL (1987) Fiberglass and the skin. In: Maibach HI (ed) Occupational and industrial dermatology. Year Book Medical Publishers, Chicago, pp 282–285

Lachapelle JM (1986) Industrial airborne irritant or allergic contact dermatitis. Contact Dermatitis 14:137–145

Lachapelle JM, Frimat P, Tennestedt D, et al (1992) Dermatoses aéroportées. In: Lachapelle JM, Frimat P, Tennestedt D, et al G (eds) Dermatologie Professionelle et de l'environment. Masson, Paris, pp 142–143

Lammintausta K, Maibach HI (1990) Contact dermatitis due to irritation. In: Adams RM (ed) Occupational skin disease. WB Saunders, Philadelphia, pp 1–12

Lechner W, Hartmann AA (1979) Glasfaserinduzierte Fremdkorpergranulome. Hautarzt 30:100–101

Marks JG jr, DeLeo VA (1992) Occupations commonly associated with contact dermatitis. In: Marks JG jr, DeLeo VA (eds) Contact and occupational dermatology. Mosby Year Book, St. Louis, pp. 276–278

Meneghini CL (1977) Fiberglass dermatitis. Contact Dermatitis 3:218

Okano M, Kozuka T, Tanigaki et al (1987) Fiberglass dermatitis in Japan: report of four cases. J Dermatol 14:590–593

Patroni M (1989) Fibre di vetro in ambiente di vita. G Ital Ig Ind 15:59–70

Rietschel RL, Fowler JF jr (1995) Textile and shoe dermatitis. In: Rietschel Rl, Fowler JF jr (eds) Fisher's Contact Dermatitis. Williams & Wilkins, Baltimore, pp 366–367

Ruegger M (1996) Are artificial mineral fibers harmful to health and unsuitable for asbestos substitute? Schweiz Rundschau Med Prax 85:961–966

Sertoli A (1991) Dermatosi professionale da artropodi. In: Sertoli A (ed) Dermatologia allergologica professionale ed ambientale. Il Pensiero Scientifico, Roma, pp 7–13

Sertoli A, Farli M (1991) Dermatite da fibre di vetro. In: Sertoli A (ed) Dermatologia allergologica professionale ed ambientale. Il Pensiero Scientifico, Roma, pp 40–41

Sertoli A, Spallanzani P, Cappelli V et al (1982) Patologia dermatologica da fibre di vetro in una officina delle Ferrovie dello Stato. Boll Coll Med Ital Trasport 2:31–38

Sertoli A, Giorgini S, Farli M (1992) Fiberglass dermatitis, Clin Dermatol 10:167–174

Siebert WJ (1942) Fiberglass health hazards investigation. Ind Med 11:6–7

Stam-Westerveld EB (1996) Man-made vitreous fiber: glass fiber and rockwool dermatitis. In: van der Valk GM, Maibach HI (eds) The irritant contact dermatitis syndrome. CRC Press, Boca Raton, pp 121–126

Stam-Westerveld EB, Coenraads PJ, van der Valk PGM et al (1994) Rubbing test responses of the skin to man-made mineral fibres of different diameters. Contact Dermatitis 31:1–4

Sulzberger MB, Baer RL (1942) The effects of fiber glass on animal and human skin. Ind Med Surg 11:482–484

Tarvainen K, Jolanki R, Forsman-Gronholm L et al (1993) Exposure, skin protection and occupational skin disease in the glass-fibre-reinforced plastics industry. Contact Dermatitis 29:119–127

Tarvainen K, Estlander T, Jolanki R et al (1994) Occupational dermatoses caused by man-made mineral fibers. Am J Contact Dermat 5:22–29

Tarvainen K, Kanerva L, Jolanki R et al (1995) Occupational dermatoses from the manufacture of plastic composite products. Am J Contact Dermat 6:95–104

TIMA (1991) Man-made vitreous fibres: nomenclature, chemical and physical properties by the Nomenclature Committee of TIMA. TIMA, Stamford

Verbeck SJA, Bluise-Van Unnik EMM, Malten KE (1981) Itching in office workers from glass fibres. Contact Dermatitis 7:354

Wang BJ, Lee JY, Wang RC (1993) Fiberglass dermatitis: report of two cases. J Formos Med Assoc 92:755– 758

CHAPTER 6

Occupational Skin Granulomas   **6**

P. D. Pigatto, A. S. Bigardi, P. Persichini

Granuloma is a chronic proliferative inflammatory reaction surrounded and delimited by healthy tissue (Rabinowitz 1996). Histology distinguishes two granuloma types: the more frequent foreign-body granuloma and a second so-called allergic granuloma. This type of reaction may "transform itself" into an allergic skin granuloma when the etiologic agent remains in the lesion for some time and, in the final analysis, behaves as an allergen. Occupational granuloma is a well-known and well-defined nosographic entity. Silica occupational granulomas of the skin are described in mineworkers (Mesquita-Guimaraes et al. 1987) and stonemasons (Mowry et al. 1991).

At an industrial level beryllium (mainly in the form of beryllium fluoride) is used in the production of fluorescent lamps, light copper, nickel, and iron alloys. After penetrating the skin beryllium causes allergic rather than foreign-body granulomas. Beryllium allergic granulomas may therefore occur not only in mineworkers, but also in people working in the production of metals, fluorescent lamps, and X-ray screens. Zirconium-contact occupational skin granulomas in workers who handle steel frequently or alloys with a high steel content, have been reported as having a particular clinical presentation: multiple, rather than individual lesions with a lupoid appearance (Palmer and Walton 1967). Cadmium is a bivalent metal that is used as an anticorrosive and in the production of conducting alloys, in association with nickel, copper, and silver. One of its salts (cadmium sulfide) is used as a colorant for paints and rubber; cadmium acetate is used in the production of craftware. There are reports in the literature of cadmium granulomas with a sarcoid-like appearance. Occupational exposure to rare metals has been well reviewed (McFadden et al. 1989; Kusaka 1993). Interdigital trichogranuloma is a common disorder among those who cut men's hair but is much less common among those who cut women's hair; perhaps because of the particular characteristic of men's hair or the type of hair cutting involved. A case of subungual trichogranuloma has been described in a hairdresser for both men and women (Abdel-Aziz 1981). Interdigital trichogranulomas or interdigital sinuses are the result of penetration of the skin by short, sharp, hair clippings. This form is described historically (Currie et al. 1953) and well clinically (Zerboni et al. 1990). Among the hypotheses concerning the pathogenesis of this condition, the most accredited is that which considers the interdigital space as a *locus minoris resistentiae*, resulting from occupational contact with detergents, constant steeping in water, and repeated traumas from cutting instruments. Subungual hair penetration appears to be much less common; onycholysis may be both a risk factor for and a consequence of cut hairs becoming imbedded subungually (Hogan et al. 1988).

This form is very similar to that which occurs in people working with animals. Work-related and histological granulomas are the lesions described on the hand of a milkman by Beer et al. (1992). Skin granulomas caused by sheep wool are reported and well known (Lambert et al. 1995).

Another cause of occupational skin granuloma is the starch found in surgical gloves (Ellis 1997). Once it penetrates the skin, the starch can give rise to a foreign body granuloma and develops when microinjuries of the skin are present. The intradermal penetration of the oils used in high-pressure air-compressed lubrication can cause oleomas or oleogranulomas, which appear as yellow-ish, rarely phlegmatic nodules (Macaulay 1986). Important granulomas include those caused by atypical mycobacteria, in particular *Mycobacterium marinum*. This micro-organism seems to find its ideal habitat in aquariums and manifests locally on the hands of people who, for work or pleasure, come into contact with such (Fischer 1988; Ang et al. 2000).

Still now, several authors (Gillingham 1989) reported several cases of accidental self-injection in the poultry service people of oil-based vaccines for chickens.

The oil-based vaccines induce severe local inflammation at the injection site and within a few minutes the area become red, swollen and painful. If the emulsion is not removed early the most severe reactions occur in fingers and hands, where granuloma eventually appear. Moreover a compression of the digital vessels may occur with the subsequent death of the bone and finger tissue.

References

Abdel-Aziz AH (1981) Pilonidal sinus caused by cutting trauma. Cutis 28:455–457

Ang P, Rattana-Apiromyakij N, Goh CL (2000) Retrospective study of Mycobacterium marinum skin infections. Int J Dermatol 39:343–347

Beer WE, Wayte DM, Morgan GW (1992) Knobbly granuloma annulare(GA) of the fingers of a milkman – a possible relationship to his work. Clin Exp Dermatol 17:63–64

Currie AR, Gibson R, Goodall AL (1953) Interdigital sinuses of barber's hands. Br J Surg 41:278–286

Ellis H (1997) Hazards from surgical gloves. Ann R Coll Surg Engl 79:161–163

Fischer AA (1988) Swimming pool granulomas due to Mycobacterium Marinum: an occupational hazard of lifeguards. Cutis 41:397–398

Gillingham S (1989) Accidental selfinjection. Canada Poultryman April 1989:17–18

Haustein UF (1975) Occupationally induced foreign body granulomas of the skin. Dermatol Monatsschr 161:807–816

Hogan DJ (1988) subungual trichogranuloma in hairdresser. Cutis 42:105–106

Hollander A (1976) Recent progress in American dermatology. Hautarzt 27:8–11

Jones DP (1996) Accidental self-inoculation with oil based veterinary vaccines. NZ Med J 109:363–365

Kusaka Y (1993) Occupational disease caused by exposure to sensitising metals. Jpn J Ind Health 35:75–87

Lambert D, Terrussot MC, Dalac S, Boulitrop-Morvan C (1995) Granulome à la laine de brebis. Ann Dermatol Venereol 122:534–535

Macaulay JC (1986) Occupational high-pressure injection injury. Br J Dermatol 115: 379–381

McFadden N, Lyberg T, Hensten-Pettersen A (1989) Aluminium induced granulomas in a tattoo. J Am Acad Dermatol 20:903–908

Mesquita-Guimaraes J, Azevedo F, Aguiar S (1987) Silica granulomas secondary to the explosion of a land mine. Cutis 40:41–43

Mowry RG, Sams WM Jr, Caulfield JB (1991) Cutaneous silica granulomas: a rare entity or rarely diagnosed? Report of two cases with review of the literature. Arch Dermatol 127:692–694

Palmer L, Walton W (1967) Lupus miliaris disseminata faciei: zirconium hypersensivity as possible cause. Cutis 7:744–748

Rabinowitz LO, Zain MT (1996) A clinicopathologic approach to granulomatous disease. J Am Acad Dermatol 35:15–33

Zerboni R, Moroni P, Cannavò SP, et al (1990) Sinus pilonidale interdigitale dei parrucchieri. Med Lav 81:138–141

CHAPTER 7

Occupational Dermatitis Artefacta

7

G. ANGELINI

Introduction

The classification of self-inflicted dermatoses is still very vague. They come under the heading of simulated or artefactual diseases (Table 1), the best-known example of which is Münchhausen's syndrome. In their turn, self-inflicted skin conditions can be subdivided into various clinical forms (Table 2). Dermatitis artefacta is one of the most important of these pictures.

Table 1. Simulated diseases

Münchhausen's syndrome
Self-inflicted dermatoses
Self-mutilations
Vulvodinia
Glossodinia
Factitious pyrexia

Table 2. Self-inflicted dermatoses

Dermatitis artefacta
Pathomimic artefacts
Heteropathomimic artefacts
True simulation
True heterosimulation ("witchcraft syndrome")
Behavioural disorders
Neurotic excoriations
Acne excoriée
Trichotillomania
Onychotillomania
Factious cheilitis
Callosities of the hands
Dermatological pathomimicry
Painful bruising syndrome
Psychogenic purpura
Religious stigmata

Definition

Dermatitis artefacta is a self-inflicted complaint provoked by the patient for various purposes and by various means. Disease can be simulated with illegal intent: to gain advantage from situations of a professional nature (to obtain prolongation of a disease or its recognition as a professional affliction, to attain a higher class of disability pension) or to escape various duties, e.g. military, especially in the case of compulsory military service, or a prison sentence. In all these cases, the simulators are fully conscious of what they are doing and why (Meneghini and Rantuccio 1962; Lyell 1979; Meneghini and Angelini 1979; Petruzzellis et al. 1988); there are no psychic disturbances underlying these particular forms of behaviour.

In contrast, in other subjects, the simulated disease is due to psychiatric problems such as psychoses, mental retardation and personality disorders. In these cases, the intrinsic reason for the lesions is different, as the subject generally hopes to attract the attention of the people he is surrounded by and of the doctor, or else he is reacting to difficult or unfavourable environmental conditions with involuntary somatisation at the skin level. These unconscious simulators are prevalently female.

Artefact skin diseases for illicit purposes, aiming to gain some advantage, are true *simulations*. Lesions provoked by subjects with psychological disturbances, i.e. irresponsibly and without a venal interest, are described as *pathomimic*. In this chapter, only true simulations for professional purposes will be examined.

Diagnostic Criteria

Site

The lesions are usually localised in areas exposed to the possible action of occupational risks and of easy access, such as the left arm (or the right if the simulator is left handed), the lower limbs, the anterior region of the chest, the abdomen and, rarely, the face (but almost exclusively in cases of pathomimic, psychologically-induced simulations) and the neck. The back is usually left alone, unless the simulator can persuade a friend to collaborate, so as to prove the spontaneous nature of the clinical form.

Morphology

Unlike spontaneous lesions, those of dermatitis artefacta do not usually present a rounded or oval appearance, conforming with the skin irritation cones. They are generally irregular, occasionally even having a bizarre, decorative appearance, with clearly defined margins, broken lines and acute angles. They are sometimes noticeably linear, or monomorphous, with little involvement of the surrounding skin. Often, particularly in cases of ulcerous or ulcero-escharotic lesions, there is a distinct pattern visible, which reproduces the shape and size of the object used to inflict the lesions. In oedema from interrupted blood flow, signs of arrest at the ligature point are often evident together with an identical, hard consistency along the whole length of the region involved (Angelini et al 1982; Angelini et al. 1990; Angelini and Bonamonte 2002).

Lesions

Virtually all elementary lesions can be observed, perhaps excluding nodules, gummata, atrophy and sclerosis. Erythematous lesions are usually livid or cyanotic with clear-cut margins; purpuric lesions, usually due to suction or stricture from bandaging, and excoriations are also frequently observed. Vesicular lesions are rare, whereas irregular bullous lesions are quite common, caused using vegetable extracts or chemical substances (Fig. 1). Ecchymoses are often observed, procured by repeated trauma from pinching or beating with various objects (wooden sticks, sand bags).

Subcutaneous introduction of various substances (paraffin, milk) gives rise to infiltrating lesions, which can later take on a wooden consistency (paraffinomas) and may evolve into ulcers. Ulcerous or ulcero-escharotic lesions are very commonly observed (Fig. 2).

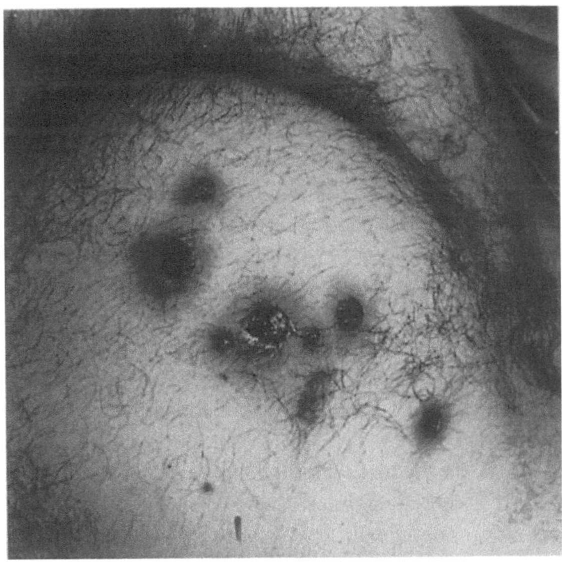

Fig. 1. Bullous and escharotic lesions from chromic mixture. Similar lesions were present at other sites

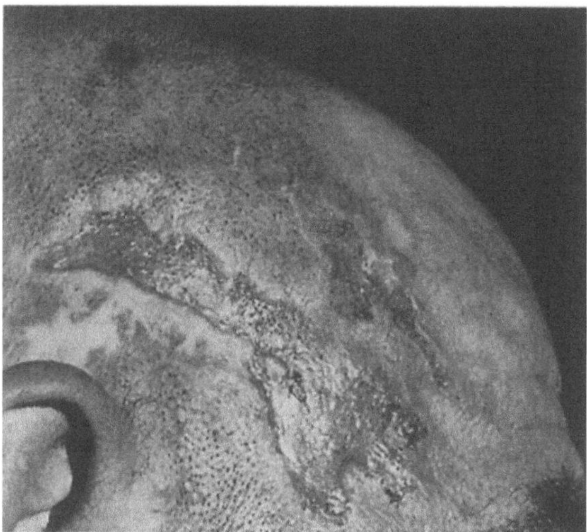

Fig. 2. Ulcerative lesion from chromic mixture at unusual site

Complementary Investigations

In all cases of primitive occupational dermatitis artefacta, rather than secondary forms due to worsening of the existing condition, the various laboratory tests give normal results, apart from inflammatory-type findings in acute pictures. Instrumental tests will also be negative in cases of artefactual arterial or venous afflictions.

Extraneous material on the surface of suspicious lesions can be elicited by means of surface biopsy, performed by stripping with a polyethylene polyester plaster with a drop of cyanoacrylate glue placed in the centre. The plaster is held against the skin surface for 30–60 s and then detached. The layer of corneum cells obtained can be used for histological examination or cultures. In cases of ulcerous lesions, brushing the base of the ulcer can lead to an approximate identification of the foreign material. Determination of the pH may be helpful to demonstrate the use of acid or alkaline substances applied shortly before and not rinsed away.

In all cases, histopathological examination is clearly necessary to make a definite differential diagnosis with respect to spontaneous clinical forms presenting the same appearance.

Clinical Course

The most common artefact lesions have a sudden acute onset and rapidly resolve; exceptions to this rule are constituted by pictures associated with severe trophic damage to the dermal–hypodermal tissues (ulcers, gangrene, paraffinomas). For

Table 3. Most common etiological agents of occupational dermatitis artefacta

Physical agents	Metal objects, paper knives, scissors, tweezers, pincers, forks, various tools, fingernails, small sand-bags, haemostatic ligatures, pumice stone, incandescent needles, lighted cigarettes
Chemical agents	
Acids	Hydrochloric, acetic, formic, trichloroacetic, chromic acids
Alkalis	Sodium and potassium salts, caustic potash, chlorinated lime and calcium oxide
Solvents	Trementin oil, boiling oils and liquids, propane gas, liquid paraffin, petrol, salt
Biological agents	
Plants	Nettle, cactus, agave, ferula, primula, fig latex
Animals	Jellyfish, sea-anemones, caterpillars, sardines, biological secretions (urine, faeces)

rapid healing, it is essential that the topical medication be applied under occlusive bandaging and constant medical and paramedical supervision.

Etiological Agents

The etiological agents may be physical, chemical or biotic in nature (Table 3), although those in the first two categories are more commonly used. Amongst physical-type agents, fingernails should also be taken into account. Chemical substances most commonly belong to the class of strong acids and alkalis. Strong acids have a corroding action, while weak acids have an astringent effect. Hydrochloric acid provokes deep burns and blisters may form; sulphuric acid carbonises the skin, forming ulcers that are slow to heal; nitric acid has a marked oxidising effect and induces deep burns of an intense, yellowish colour. Strong alkaline substances destroy wide areas of skin, solubilising the tissues and causing hard eschars to form.

The many different, complex mechanisms of action of the numerous biotic agents can essentially be summarised under the heading 'pharmacological', due to the freeing of proteolytic biochemical mediators and enzymes.

In reality, identifying the etiologic agent is often very difficult, owing to the obstinate reticence of most simulators. In these cases, some general assumptions can be made: blisters are more commonly induced by vegetable substances, ecchymoses by mechanical agents and ulcers by chemical substances.

Occupational Dermatitis Artefacta

From a pathogenetic viewpoint, occupational dermatitis artefacta can be subdivided into two subgroups: (1) dermatitis provoked directly on healthy skin and (2) aggravation of a pre-existing contact dermatitis. Diagnosis of the latter forms can be fairly simple when the simulator intends to reproduce a picture of eczema on healthy non-sensitised skin. In fact, it is difficult to provoke erythemato-vesicular spongiotic lesions in different phases of evolution, so that self-inflicted lesions tend to manifest as groups of gross blisters.

If the patient aggravates a pre-existing spontaneous eczematous dermatitis, it should be remembered that the simulator may be perfectly well aware of what substance provokes his dermatitis and may make use of it during convalescent periods. In addition to the above-two classical types of occupational dermatitis artefacta, provoked on healthy or on damaged skin, there is another aspect to the problem. This is constituted by attempts to produce positive results to skin tests that would otherwise give negative results. As these methods of diagnostic investigation have grown more common, simulators' concern has shifted from the clinical disease picture towards the results of such tests, knowing that recognition of his condition as a professional complaint largely depends on the latter (Meneghini and Rantuccio 1962; Meigel and Koops 1978; Lyell 1986; Maurice et al. 1987). Clearly, in suspicious cases, the patch tests must be applied without allowing the patient to identify the site of the individual substances and the results must be interpreted with some caution.

Diagnosis, Differential Diagnosis and Complications

Among the various assessment criteria, clinico-morphological examination is undoubtedly the most important. The types of lesions and especially their arrangement and configuration are all elements of considerable diagnostic value. Nevertheless, this criterion must not be overemphasised because spontaneous dermatitis can sometimes assume equally bizarre shapes. A diagnosis of simulated dermatitis should only be made after all the other possible extraneous causes have been diligently and impartially excluded on the basis of anamnestic and clinical data. In short, a diagnosis of dermatitis artefacta should not be the result of a process of elimination but should be regarded as a possible diagnosis among others. Even when the diagnosis of simulation is almost certain it is always best to request a neuropsychiatric consultation to exclude concomitant or prevalent psychiatric disturbances.

Owing to its variable aspects, differential diagnosis of dermatitis artefacta is made in the presence of different dermatological conditions. In the case of fairly superficial ulcerative lesions, extending centrifugally, pyoderma gangrenosum must be excluded. Ulcerative lesions of the legs in a young subject, in the absence of vascular conditions, call for investigations aiming to exclude some rare conditions, such as haematological diseases, thrombocytaemia, lymphoproliferative syndromes, collagenases, Wegener's disease and cryoglobulinaemia, before thinking of dermatitis artefacta.

Bullous lesions from suction or chemical agents should be differentiated from pemphigoid. Porphyria cutanea tarda lesions on the hands and arms may look like artefacta, as may bizarre forms of skin necrosis occasionally observed in polyarteritis nodosa.

Among the complications of dermatitis artefacta we must include the risk of sepsis, the possible but rare thickening of a bone cortex after persistent constric-

Table 4. Differential diagnosis between occupational dermatitis artefacta (ODA) and pathomimic artefacta (PA)

Criteria	ODA	PA
Gender	Generally male	Generally female
Age	Young and adult	Young and adult
History	Episodic affliction with acute onset	Chronic history of complaint
Cutaneous sites	Hands, arms, and unusual sites	Generally face and arms
Morphology	More bizarre lesions	Less bizarre lesions
Causal agents	Highly varied, strange and unimaginable	Common mechanical objects or chemical agents

tion of a limb with ties or bandages, and the equally rare observation of subcutaneous fibrosis after chronic lymph oedema. Naturally, deep destructive lesions leave ugly scars, keloids and retractions.

Criteria for differential diagnosis between occupational dermatitis artefacta and pathomimic artefacta, (apart, of course, from the psychiatric problems underlying the latter), are reported in Table 4. These criteria are based on our experience of many cases of unconscious simulators, in addition to 46 cases of deliberate simulation (Meneghini and Angelini 1979; Angelini and Bonamonte 1998).

Conclusions

To conclude, the diagnostic criteria for professional dermatitis artefacta can be summarised as follows:

Presumptive Criteria

The presumptive criteria raise a suspicion of fraud and are based particularly on detailed history of the development of the lesions and of working conditions (loss of job, reduced hours and hence salary, disagreements with the employer).

Probability Criteria

The probability criteria serve to confirm the suspicion and are based on clinico-morphological findings, observation of the lesions over time and the results of occlusive bandaging. In many cases, the morphology of the lesions alone is enough to justify the diagnosis.

This is supported by the fact that the simulator often tries to reproduce a clinical picture of professional contact dermatitis on healthy skin without considering the difficulties inherent in the lack of pre-existing sensitisation to the relevant chemical agents. Diagnosis is more difficult if the self-inflictor aims to aggravate and prolong a pre-existing eczematous dermatitis, when continual hospital supervision may be necessary to solve the problem.

Certainty Criteria

The certainty criteria are constituted by the identification of residues of the causal agent (chemical or biological) on the damaged site or by a partial or complete confession.

Measures

In cases of true simulated dermatitis, the dermatologist must unmask the situation and explain his/her conclusions in clear terms to the individual involved, once sufficient evidence has been achieved to prove that diagnosis. The professional and legal consequences are usually fairly serious and the dermatologist may be of considerable help to the legal doctor. It must be remembered that, although there is no specific law regulating this act, conscious simulation comes under the general heading of fraudulent acts.

References

Angelini G, Meneghini CL, Vena GA (1982) Secrétan's syndrome: an artefact oedema of the hand. Contact Dermatitis 8:345–346

Angelini G, Vena GA, Meneghini CL (1990) Occupational traumatic lymphedema of the hands. Dermatol Clin 8:205–208

Angelini G, Bonamonte D (1998) Occupational dermatitis artefacta. Proceedings of the 19th World Congress of Dermatology, Sydney, 15–20 June

Angelini G, Bonamonte D (2002) Aquatic dermatology. Springer, Milano

Lyell A (1979) Cutaneous artifactual disease. A review, amplified by personal experience. J Am Acad Dermatol 1:391–407

Lyell A (1986) Dermatitis artefacta in relation to the syndrome of contrived disease. Clin Exp Dermatol 11:109–126

Maurice PDL, Rivers JK, Jones C, Cronin E (1987) Dermatitis artefacta with artefact of patch tests. Clin Exp Dermatol 12:204–206

Meigel WN, Koops DH (1978) Skarifikationsartefakte der Testreaktion bei einer berufsdermatologischen Begutachtung. Hautartz 27:349–351

Meneghini CL, Rantuccio F (1962) Patomimie cutanee professionali. Giorn It Dermatol 103:143–155

Meneghini CL, Angelini G (1979) Occupational dermatitis artefacta. Berufsdermatosen 27:163–165

Petruzzellis V, Angelini G, Vena GA (1988) La dermatite artefatta. Boll Dermatol Allerg Profes 3:23–40

CHAPTER 8

Physical Causes: Heat, Cold, and Other Atmospheric Factors

8

W. Uter

This chapter is based on the corresponding paper by W. Uter and L. Kanerva in the *Handbook of Occupational Dermatology* and on Kanerva (1999). It is dedicated to Lasse Kanerva, one of the most profound experts in this field, with whom I was lucky enough to co-operate – and hopefully will be again.

Heat

Thermal Burns

The lowest temperature at which a burn can occur has been estimated to be 44°C (111°F) (Moritz and Henriques 1947). Burns may be of environmental, domestic or industrial origin, the latter often having characteristic occupational patterns. They may be caused by direct contact with hot objects or flames (e.g., heat torch), infrared radiation (IR) heat or accidental exposure to laser energy absorbed by skin chromophores. The well-known classification of burns is based on the depth of the burn as first, second, or third degree (Burke and Bondoc 1993).

After successful treatment of the acute-phase, impairment due to burn scars may result. Pigmentation, vascularity, pliability, scar height and – in more severe cases – joint mobility and muscle strength are the main parameters for dermatological evaluation (Jonsson et al. 1997, Sullivan et al. 1990). Especially in black persons, disfigurement due to pigmentary changes must additionally be considered, with final evaluation of permanency not until 18–24 months after complete healing. Squamous cell carcinoma arising from burn scars was described by Marjolin in 1828; the criteria established by Ewing (1935) for associating a carcinoma with a previous burn are still considered valid.

Electrical Burns

Electrical burns are due to heat and direct injury by electricity, the severity depending, for example, on current voltage, thickness and wetness of the skin, and duration of contact (Kennedy 1992). High-voltage burns are severe; low-voltage (even with 24 V) burns are milder but penetrate more deeply than is apparent by following nerves and vessels, and extending some distance away from the edge of the visible wound, with delayed (up to 2 weeks) rupture of blood vessels as late complication (Kennedy 1992). Magnetic resonance imaging (MRI) is a new aid in the diagnostic evaluation of high-voltage electrical burns (Nettelblad et al. 1996).

Burns from lightning cause a bizarre, superficial macular erythema arranged in a streaked feather- or fern-like pattern, without blanching on diascopy and fading within 24–48 h. Lightning injuries are obviously an occupational risk of outdoor workers.

Erythema *Ab igne*

Chronic exposure to heat – directly or via IR – insufficient to produce burn, can cause erythema *ab igne* and skin cancer. Erythema *ab igne* is characterized by a mottled, reticulate hyperemia with melanoderma and teleangiectases and sometimes superficial epidermal atrophy and subepidermal blistering. It is still observed in people who sit in front of wood fires or apply heater cushions (Kennedy 1992). Workers at risk of developing erythema ab include stokers, blacksmiths, glassblowers, bakers (especially those using old-fashioned brick-lined ovens), cooks and others working over a heat source. After an interval of 30 years or more, thermal skin injury and erythema *ab igne* may proceed to cancer (Kaplan 1987).

Erythermalgia

Erythermalgia is a syndrome of bilateral symmetric burning sensation and redness of the lower, or sometimes upper, extremities initiated by exercise or exposure to heat (Heller Page and Shear 1993; Drenth and Michiels 1994). Thus, occupational factors may aggravate symptoms (Table 1). Primary erythermalgia usually arises in childhood; secondary erythermalgia develops in adults in association with or without an apparent underlying disorder or as side effect of drugs (Drenth and Michiels 1994).

Table 1. Occupations with potential exposure to excessive heat

Furnace work (animal rendering workers, boiler heaters, coke oven operators, foundry workers, glass manufacturing workers, kiln workers, rubber (tire) manufacturing workers, smelter workers, steel and metal forges)
Plant operators working *near* hot containers or furnaces
Road construction (asphalt, bitumen)
Food preparation (bakers, cannery workers, cooks and other kitchen workers)
Service work (cleaners, firemen, shipyard workers when cleaning cargo holds
Outdoor work during hot weather (e.g., sailors passing hot climatic zones, soldiers)
Hot and humid indoor work (miners in deep mines, greenhouse workers, maintenance workers in nuclear plants and others with tight protective clothing)

Miliaria

Miliaria is caused by sweat retention leading to swelling of the keratin within sweat ducts, resulting in pore closure and rupture of the ducts immediately beneath the obstruction. If the obstruction occurs within the stratum corneum, miliaria crystallina (sudamina) results, producing small, clear vesicles that soon rupture, resulting in desquamation, which may be the only concern of patients in this otherwise asymptomatic condition.

When closure occurs deeper in the granular layer, firm vesicles are formed accompanied by marked, often paroxysmal pruritus and burning. Called miliaria rubra, the small erythematous macules and vesicles unassociated with follicular openings are easily confused with contact dermatitis. This condition may appear as early as a few days after exposure to a hot, humid environment, but most commonly after one to several months (Lillywhite 1992), especially at the trunk and intertriginous. In extensive involvement hyperpyrexia and heat exhaustion or subsequent miliaria profunda (see below) may occur. Successive lesions may be pustular from infiltration of inflammatory cells and complicated by secondary bacterial infection.

If obstruction is even deeper, i.e., in the dermo-epidermal junction zone, miliaria profunda results (Kirk et al. 1996). The deep-seated, asymptomatic vesicles appear much like gooseflesh, but close examination shows that they spare the follicles. The pale white papules (1–3 mm in diameter) are most prominent on the trunk. Erythema and pruritus are mild or absent. Heat exhaustion and collapse are common sequelae; a particularly severe variant has been termed tropical anhidrotic asthenia (Cage et al. 1987).

Occupations associated with excessive heat exposure are listed in Table 1; in addition, work in the tropics may be inadvisable for very susceptible persons.

Miscellaneous Conditions

Intertrigo can occur from excessive sweating, especially in obese persons, not infrequently accompanied by secondary bacterial or candidal infection. The interdigital space between the third and fourth fingers is a common site among cannery workers, bartenders, medical and dental personnel, and others performing wet work for prolonged periods. Cooks, swimming instructors, nurses and others exposed to moisture are also disposed to this condition. Acne vulgaris and rosacea can be aggravated by prolonged chronic exposure to heat, especially intense heat from ovens, steam, open furnaces or heat torches. Herpes simplex may be triggered by sudden blasts of heat.

Cold

The effect of cold is the result of a complex interaction of climatic factors (air temperature, mean radiant temperature, humidity and wind), protection (clothing) and metabolic heat production (activity). Cooling the brain leads to confusion and later to lack of coordination, while cooling the limbs results in numbness and clumsiness. Local cooling usually produces discomfort and local harmful effects before more significant whole-body cooling develops. As local (e.g., digit) cooling conversely depends on whole-body heat balance, it is important to control body cooling by appropriate protective clothing (Holmer 1993). In addition to physiologic responses to "abnormal" cold, abnormal reactions to "normal" cold may occur in some individuals.

Frostbite

The degree of cellular injury depends on: (1) the minimum temperature, (2) the duration of time at that temperature, (3) the cooling rate, with rapid cooling causing more destructive intracellular ice crystal formation and, hence, more destruction, (4) rewarming rate (in slow rewarming, intracellular ice crystals become larger and more lethal for the cell) and, finally, (5) repeated freeze-thaw cycles lead to greater injury. Different cell types vary in their susceptibility to cold, melanocytes being particularly sensitive.

High wind speeds ("wind chill") increase the risk of freezing of the exposed skin. As the skin surface temperature falls from $-4.8\,°C$ to $-7.8\,°C$, the risk of frostbite increases from 5% to 95% (Danielsson 1996). Exposed parts, i.e., toes, feet, fingers, ears, nose and cheeks are most often affected. Today, many cases of frostbite occur in those taking part in winter sports; other occupations at risk are listed in Table 2.

As tissue temperature falls, the area becomes and remains deceptively numb, and the initial redness is gradually replaced by a white, waxy appearance with blistering and, later, necrosis and gangrene in the more severe cases. In early stages MRI and magnetic resonance angiography (MRA) provide for early recognition of the depth of damage (Barker et al. 1997). Long-term effects may include telangiectasias, vasomotor instability with Raynaud-like changes, paresthesia and hyperhidrosis. Squamous cell carcinoma may arise in the old scars (Rossis et al. 1982).

Treatment entails rapidly rewarming the part; a whirlpool or waterbath, or warm air for 20 min (until the most distal part is flushed) is useful for this purpose, with a recommended temperature no higher than blood temperature (Daniels 1987) or $42\,°C$ (Heller Page and Shear 1993). Rewarming is painful and causes an increase in erythema and blistering. The popular old idea of rubbing the affected part with snow has a disastrous effect.

Table 2. Workers potentially exposed to excessive cold

Cooling room workers, e.g., packing and commissioning deep-frozen goods
(Dry-) ice and liquefied gas workers
Firefighters, divers, sailors (especially on ice-breakers) and fishermen, rescue workers
Outdoor workers during cold weather, including winter-sports instructors
Researchers in cold laboratories and polar areas

Immersion Foot: Nonfreezing Cold Injury

Formerly called trench foot, immersion foot results from exposure to cold temperatures above freezing for several days. Under moist conditions and if aggravated by constrictive clothing, continuous exposure for as little as 19 h may be sufficient (Rietschel and Allen 1976). Immersion foot is less severe than frostbite and develops in three stages: initial erythema, edema and tenderness (stage I); followed within 24 h by paresthesia, marked edema, numbness and sometimes bullae (stage II). Gangrene (stage III) does not develop unless there is infection. Convalescence may be prolonged; treatment is similar to frostbite.

In industries where workers are required to stand for long periods in cold, wet mud or water, immersion-type injuries may be frequent (Chow et al. 1980). Interestingly, immersion foot can also develop in warm water (Humphrey and Ellyson 1997), including the tropics (tropical immersion foot).

Chilblains (Perniosis)

The mildest form of cold injury, chilblains or perniosis, occurs as an abnormal reaction to cold in the temperate humid climate of northwestern Europe. The lesions are reddish blue discolorations that become swollen and boggy, with tense bullae and prutitus or burning. Ulcerations and subsequent scarring may occur. The dorsa of the proximal phalanges of the fingers and toes, heels, lower legs, thighs, nose and ears are particularly affected. While in children an incidence peak at the beginning of winter is observed, chilblains in outdoor workers often start in the spring months (Champion 1992). Prophylaxis with warm housing, warm clothing and regular exercise is most important.

Pulling-Boat Hands

This dermatosis has been described from coastal New England (Toback et al. 1985). Erythematous macules and plaques, followed by small vesicles and an itching and burning sensation developed on the dorsa of the hands and fingers of instructors and students after 3–14 days aboard a pulling boat. High humidity, cool air and wind, were considered triggers of this nonfreezing type dermatosis.

Other Atmospheric Factors

Low humidity of the air is believed to cause dehydration of the horny layer and impairment of the epidermal barrier function (Agner and Serup 1989), i.e., increased irritability of the skin. Subclinical xerotic changes may occur within hours of exposure and are more pronounced in atopics (Eberlein-König et al. 1996). According to clinical experience (Kavli and Förde 1984), epidemiological results (Uter et al. 1998) and experimental data (Agner and Serup 1989) low ambient absolute humidity (which coincides with low indoor relative humidity, except when air conditioning is employed) is a risk factor for irritant dermatitis. As the hands in particular may additionally be exposed to a variety of occupational irritants, this fairly inalterable environmental condition puts extra emphasis on the necessity of adequate skin protection, be it domestic or occupational.

Windspeed has been found to be a significant risk factor in the occurrence of "dry flaking" facial skin (Cooper et al. 1992). Parish (1992), who exposed the hands of volunteers to "a cold dry wind" for 3 h daily, found visible alteration (roughness, desquamation) and impaired lipid and enzyme composition of the epidermis after a few days.

In addition to natural environmental conditions, anthropogenic factors may lead to occupational (skin) disease, like exposure to high levels of ultrahigh frequency radiofrequency radiation (UHF, 785 MHz mean frequency) during work on a television mast, causing an immediate sensation of intense heating and later transient erythema, malaise, numbness and pain (Schilling 1997), or Microwave radiation (1–30 GHz) causing burns, sometimes with subsequent paraesthesia (Kennedy 1992).

Low Indoor Humidity

The water content of the horny layer remains below a critical value of 10% when the relative humidity is less than 50% at room temperature (Rycroft 1985), aggravated by high temperature and convection. Such conditions may occur in an open-plan office, next to or under the ventilation system, or in special production halls, e.g., for soft contact lenses (Rycroft 1985) or clean rooms in the electronics industry. Some of the occupations in which low-humidity dermatoses have been reported are listed in Table 3.

Low humidity dermatoses are far more distressing, with intense pruritus and burning, than their comparative paucity of physical signs might suggest (Rycroft 1985). Skin lesions may eventually evolve through dryness of the skin to erythema and round or oval patches of eczema. Fair-skinned individuals apparently are at higher risk. Both atopics and nonatopics have been affected. Differential diagnoses include irritant or allergic airborne contact dermatitis, psychological causes, menopausal hot flashes, rosacea and seborrheic eczema.

Table 3. Reported low-humidity risk occupations

Cabin crew of long distance airplanes
Office work
Silicon-chip and soft contact lens manufacturing
Resident staff in hospitals and hotels
Traveling salesmen (from automobile heaters)

Visual Display Units

In some countries, patients often complain of skin symptoms from work with visual display units (VDU). However, organizational conditions such as high workload and inability to take rest breaks, rather than electromagnetic emissions, were found to be associated with the reported skin symptoms (Bergqvist and Wahlberg 1994). Possibly independent from an initial cause of skin problems, psychological conditioning may lead to a perpetuation of symptoms even without exposure, as illustrated by experiments with affected office workers (Swanbeck and Bleeker 1989).

References

Agner T, Serup J (1989) Seasonal variation of skin resistance to irritants. Br J Dermatol 121:323–328

Barker JR, Haws MJ, Brown RE, Kucan JO, Moore WD (1997) Magnetic resonance imaging of severe frostbite injuries. Ann Plast Surg 38:275–279

Bergqvist U, Wahlberg JE (1994) Skin symptoms during work with visual display terminals. Contact Dermatitis 30:193–196

Burke JF, Bondoc CC (1993) Burns: the management and evaluation of the thermally injured patient. In: Fitzpatrick TB, Eisen AZ, Wolff K, et al. (eds) Dermatology in general medicine, 4th edn. McGraw-Hill, New York, pp 1592–1598

Cage GW, Sato K, Schwachman H (1987) Eccrine glands. The management and evaluation of the thermally injured patient. In: Fitzpatrick TB, Eisen AZ, Wolff K, et al. (eds) Dermatology in general medicine, 3rd edn. McGraw-Hill, New York, pp 691–704

Champion RH (1992) Reactions to cold. In: Rook A, Wilkinson DS, Ebling FJG, et al. (eds) Textbook of dermatology, 5th edn. Blackwell, Oxford, pp 833–847

Chow S, Westfried M, Lynfield Y (1980) Immersion foot: an occupational disease. Cutis 25:662

Cooper MD, Jardine H, Ferguson J (1992) Seasonal influence on the occurrence of dry flaking facial skin. In: Marks RG, Plewig G (eds) The environmental threat to the skin. M. Dunitz, London, pp 159–164

Daniels F (1987) Physiologic factors in the skin's reactions to heat and cold. In: Fitzpatrick TB, Eisen AZ, Wolff K, et al. (eds) Dermatology in general medicine, 3rd edn. McGraw-Hill, New York, pp 1412–1424

Danielsson U (1996) Windchill and the risk of tissue freezing. J Appl Physiol 81:2666–2673

Drenth JPH, Michiels JJ (1994) Erythromelalgia and erythermalgia: diagnostic differentiation. Int J Dermatol 33:393–397

Eberlein-König B, Spiegl A, Przybilla B (1996) Change of skin roughness due to lowering air humidity in climate chamber. Acta Dermatol Venerol 76:447–449

Ewing J (1935) Modern attitude toward traumatic cancer. Arch Pathol 19:690–728

Heller Page E, Shear NH (1993) Disorders due to physical factors. In: Fitzpatrick TB, Eisen AZ, Wolff K, et al (eds) Dermatology in general medicine, 4th edn. McGraw-Hill, New York, pp 1581–1592

Holmer I (1993) Work in the cold. Review of methods for assessment of cold exposure. Int Arch Occup Environ Health 65:147–155

Humphrey W, Ellyson R (1997) Warm water immersion foot: still a threat to the soldier. Mil Med 162:610–611

Jonsson CE, Schuldt K, Linder J, Bjornhagen V, Ekholm J (1997) Rehabilitative, psychiatric, functional and aesthetic problems in patients treated for burn injuries – a preliminary follow-up study. Acta Chir Plast 39:3–8

Kanerva L (1999) Physical causes of occupational skin disease. In: Adams RM (ed) Occupational skin disease, 3rd edn. Saunders, Philadelphia, pp 35–58

Kaplan RP (1987) Cancer complicating chronic ulcerative and scarifying mucocutaneous disorders. Adv Dermatol 2:19–46

Kavli G, Förde OH (1984) Hand dermatoses in Tromsö. Contact Dermatitis 10:174–177

Kennedy CTC (1992) Reactions to mechanical and thermal injury. In: Rook A, Wilkinson DS, Ebling FJG, et al. (eds) Textbook of dermatology, 5th edn. Blackwell, Oxford, pp 777–832

Kirk JF, Wilson BB, Chun W, Cooper PH (1996) Miliaria profunda. J Am Acad Dermatol 35:854–856

Lillywhite LP (1992) Investigation into the environmental factors associated with the incidence of skin disease following an outbreak of Miliaria rubra at a coal mine. Occup Med (Oxf) 42:183–187

Moritz AR, Henriques FC Jr (1947) Studies in thermal injuries. II. The relative importance of time and surface temperature in the causation of cutaneous burns. Am J Pathol 23:695–720

Nettelblad H, Thuomas KA, Sjöberg F (1996) Magnetic resonance imaging: a new diagnostic aid in the care of high-voltage burns. Burns 22:117–119

Parish WE (1992) Chemical irritation and predisposing environmental stress (cold wind and hard water). In: Marks RG, Plewig G (eds) The environmental threat to the skin. M. Dunitz, London, pp 185–193

Rietschel RL, Allen AM (1976) Immersion foot: a method for studying the effects of protracted water exposure on human skin. Mil Med 141:778–780

Rossis CG, Yiacoumettis AM, Elemenoglou J (1982) Squamous cell carcinoma of the heel developing at site of previous frostbite. J R Soc Med 75:715–718

Rycroft RJG (1985) Low humidity and microtrauma. Am J Ind Med 8:371–373

Schilling CJ (1997) Effects of acute exposure to ultrahigh radiofrequency radiation on three antenna engineers. Occup Environ Med 54:281–284

Swanbeck G, Bleeker T (1989) Skin problems from visual display units – provocation of skin symptoms under experimental conditions. Acta Derm Venereol Suppl (Stockh) 69:46–51

Sullivan T, Smith J, Kermode J, McIver E, Courtemanche DJ (1990) Rating the burn scar. J Burn Care Rehabil 11:256–260

Toback AC, Korson R, Krusinski PA (1985) Pulling boat hands: a unique dermatosis from coastal New England. J Am Acad Dermatol 12:649–655

Uter W, Gefeller O, Schwanitz HJ (1998) An epidemiological study of the influence of season (cold and dry air) on the occurrence of irritant skin changes of the hands. Br J Dermatol 138:266–272

CHAPTER 9

Occupational Contact Urticaria

9

I. ALE, H. I. MAIBACH

Nomenclature and Clinical Manifestations

The contact urticaria syndrome (Maibach 1975; Von Krogh 1982; Von Krogh 1981) comprises a variegate group of inflammatory reactions that usually appear in minutes after cutaneous or mucosal contact with the eliciting substance and disappear within a few hours. The clinical manifestations can be classified according to morphology and severity and may be localized or generalized and may also involve organs other than the skin. Wheal-and-flare at the contact site is the prototype of contact urticaria, while generalized urticaria following a local contact is uncommon. In the invisible contact urticaria, only subjective symptoms (itching, tingling, burning) without objective changes or only a mild transient erythema occur. In some patients lesions may evolve to dermatitis (Maibach 1976). Extracutaneous symptoms may occur as a part of a more severe reaction including rhinoconjunctivitis, asthma attack, gastrointestinal symptoms and anaphylaxis.

Occupational contact urticaria (OCU) refers to immediate contact reactions that appear after exposure to urticariogenic agents in the work environment. OCU is believed to be common in occupational settings (Von Krogh 1982; Von Krogh 1981; Amin 1997) and its prevalence should be expected to rise as a result of the worker's exposure to an ever-increasing number of industrial materials.

Classification

Contact urticaria can be classified on the basis of pathogenesis as nonimmunologic, immunologic and of uncertain mechanism

Nonimmunologic Contact Urticaria

Nonimmunologic contact urticaria (NICU) is the most frequent form and may occur in most or almost all exposed individuals. The mechanism of action is the result of a direct nonallergic release of vasoactive substances, which causes a localized response (Laithi 1980). Clinical manifestations depend mainly on the concentration of the contactant, the duration of exposure, and aggravating factors, such as rubbing and scratching. The reaction, often redness without edema rather than a real wheal and flare, characteristically remains localized. Systemic reactions are probably not evoked. Occupational agents capable of inducing NICU include many substances used as preservatives, flavoring and fragrances in the food, cosmetic and pharmaceutical industries.

Immunologic Contact Urticaria

Immunologic contact urticaria (ICU) seems to be mediated by an immediate IgE-mediated hypersensitivity, although the role of other immunoglobulin classes has been postulated in certain cases. In skin challenge, the molecules of the agent readily penetrate the epidermis and react with specific IgE molecules attached to mast cells membranes causing release of histamine and other vasoactive substances and inflammatory mediators, such as prostaglandins, leukotrienes, chemotactic factors and kinins. Not only do mast cells and basophils have receptors for IgE molecules, but also Langerhans cells, eosinophils, B and T lymphocytes, monocytes, and other cell types. Hence, ICU may have a more complicated mechanism than previously thought. It can be hypothesized that protein allergens for type I immediate reactions bind to specific IgE molecules in the surface of Langerhans cells, which are capable of processing and presenting the allergen to the T helper 2 (Th2) lymphocytes inducing a delayed-type hypersensitivity response. This may be the mechanism whereby repeated immediate contact reactions lead to more persistent eczematous skin lesions (Bruynzeel-Koomen 1986). ICU reactions may extend beyond the contact area and generalized urticaria or anaphylaxis may occur. Food allergens are the most common cause of immediate allergic contact reactions, although a wide variety of occupational agents have been implicated in the cause of these reactions. The international epidemic of ICU to latex proteins has led to awareness chiefly in the health care professions.

Contact Urticaria of Uncertain Mechanism

The pathogenetic mechanism in these cases is unclear. The clinical reaction may resemble that of ICU, but no specific IgE can be demonstrated in the patient's serum or in the tissues.

A classical example is provided by ammonium persulphate. This agent produces a heterogeneous clinical picture, which may include generalized urticaria, respiratory symptoms and even anaphylactoid reactions (Von Krogh 1982; Von Krogh 1981). The small prevalence of these reactions suggests individual reactivity. Although the symptoms correspond to an immunologic reaction, IgE antibodies against ammonium persulphate could not been demonstrated and passive transfer was negative. In addition, some individuals react in the first exposure, as in NICU.

Etiologic Agents

To determine prevalence or incidence of OCU with certainty is difficult, since data from epidemiological studies, with the exception of OCU caused by natural rubber latex, remain limited.

Food Products

Workers in the diverse areas of the food industry are exposed to a variety of food-derived and food-associated substances, which are capable of inducing immediate contact reactions, with urticarial lesions and flares of dermatitis at the contact areas (Veien 1983; Hafner 1992; Niinimäki 1995). Etiologic agents include substances such as preservatives, flavorings, stabilizers, emulsifiers, antioxidants, etc. In addition, agents other than food-derived materials, such as grain storage mites, fungus, antibiotics, latex, etc., are capable of inducing immediate contact reactions in exposed workers (Maibach 1995). However, most of the responsible substances for immediate-type reactions in the food industry are food-derived protein allergens (Taylor 1987) (Table 1). The primary route of exposure for food allergens is through ingestion, since food proteins can permeate the gut mucosal membranes. Skin is relatively impermeable to macromolecules such as protein allergens; however, exposure through skin contact can produce immediate and delayed contact allergy in food workers. The existence of a work-related dermatitis may impair the skin barrier function and predispose to the development of immediate contact reactions. Conversely, immediate contact reactions may lead to dermatitis. Contact urticaria and vesicular-immediate reactions as causal factors of hand eczema were described by Maibach (1976) and Maibach and Johnson (1975). Hannuksela (1980) used the term "atopic contact dermatitis" to designate ICU in atopic subjects. Hjorth and Roed-Petersen (1976), described a particular form of chronic dermatitis in kitchen workers. Most of the affected workers had chronic hand dermatitis, sometimes associated with urticarial or vesicular exacerbations a few minutes after contact with protein allergens. Patch tests were often negative, but prick or scratch tests with the responsible foods were positive. Specific IgE antibodies to the responsible substances were detected in some cases. They coined the term "protein contact dermatitis" (PCD) to designate this composite reactions.

Work-associated dermatitis and immediate reactions are well known in bakers. Several proteins were identified as allergenic in wheat flour (Sutton 1984), and there is extensive cross-reactivity between cereals, such as wheat, rye, barley, oat, corn and rice. In addition, flour additives and flavoring agents are also capable of inducing allergic reactions. Enzymes, such as amylases, proteases, cellulases, lipoxygenases, etc., can cause immediate hypersensitivity reactions, such as ICU, rhinoconjunctivitis and asthma, as well as dermatitis (Morren 1993; Vanhanen 1996; Kanerva 1998; Kanerva 1997) (Table 2). Positive prick tests, scratch chamber tests and RAST (radioallergosorbent tests) to the responsible enzymes were observed in affected workers. Although bakers probably represent the most ex-

Table 1. Foods and food additives causing contact urticaria

Animal Products	Fruits (I)
Meat (I)	Apple[a]
Beef[a]	Apricot
Chicken[a]	Apricot stone[a]
Lamb	Banana
Pork[a]	Kiwi
Sausage	Litchi
Turkey	Lemon[a]
Liver[a]	Lemon peel[a]
Calf[a]	Lime[a]
Pork[a]	Mango
Fish[a] (I) (NI)	Orange
Frog[a]	Peach
Seafood[a] (I)	Plum
Cod[a]	Strawberry[a] (I?)
Crab	Watermelon[a]
Herring[a]	Nuts
Lobster[a]	Almond
Oysters[a]	Peanuts
Plaice[a]	Peanut butter
Shrimp[a]	Seeds (I)
Scallops[a]	Sesame seeds
Cheese[a] (I)	Sunflower seeds
Eggs[a] (I)	Grains (I)
Honey (I)	Buckwheat
Milk[a] (I)	Flour
Vegetables (I)	Maize
Asparagus[a]	Malt
Beans[a]	Rice
Cabbage[a]	Wheat
Carrots[a]	Wheat bran
Castor bean[a]	Flavorings and fragrances
Celery[a]	Balsam of Peru (I) (NI)
Chives	Benzaldehyde[a] (NI)
Coffee been (green)[a]	Benzoic acid (NI)
Cucumber pickle[a] (I?)	Cassian (cinnamon) oil
Endive[a]	Cinnamic acid (NI)
Garlic[a]	Cinnamic aldehyde (NI)
Lettuce[a]	Condiments and spices
Mustard[a]	Cayenne pepper (NI)
Onion[a]	Caraway
Parsley[a]	Coriander
Parsnip[a]	Curry (U)
Potato[a]	Paprika (I)
Rocket	Thyme (NI)
Rutabaga (Swede)	Other food-related materials
Soybean[a]	Fungi
Stock	Mushrooms[a] (I)
Tomato[a] (I) (NI)	Salami casing molds[a] (I)
Winged bean[a]	

I, Immunologic contact urticaria; NI, non-immunologic contact urticaria; U, uncertain mechanism.

[a] Occupational contact urticaria.

Table 2. Enzymes causing contact urticaria

α Amylase[a] (I)
Cellulase[a] (I)
Papain[a] (I)
Xylanase[a] (I)

I, Immunologic contact urticaria.
[a] Occupational contact urticaria.

posed occupational group, enzymes may affect workers in several industries, such as paper, textile and pharmaceutical industries, starch, wine and sugar production, farming, etc. (Kanerva 1998; Kanerva 1997).

Immediate contact reactions to fruits and vegetables are fairly common among food industry workers (Alonso 1993; Krook 1977). These reactions are more common in atopic patients and frequently are associated with pollen allergy (Hannuksela 1977). The allergen characterization in fruits, vegetables and pollens has been conducted to identify profilins, a group of actin-binding proteins, as common antigenic determinants (Valenta 1977). Specific IgE antibodies from patients' serum have been found to react with profilins isolated from fruits, vegetables and spices as well as with birch, timothy and mugwort pollens (Halmepuro 1984; Ebner 1995).

Animal derived foods have been found to cause OCU and PCD in food industry workers. Responsible agents are not only raw meat from different animals, such as cow (Fisher 1982; Jovanovic 1992), chicken (Harrington 1981), lamb (Maibach 1976) pork (Kanerva 1996) and fish (Melino 1987); but also any part of the animal handled, such as skin, gut, liver and blood (Beck 1982; Fisher 1977; Moseng 1982). Animal derivatives, such as eggs (Valero 1996; Smith 1990; Rudzki 1977) and milk products (Nestle 1997) have also produced immediate contact reactions in food industry workers. Occupational egg allergy with respiratory symptoms and immediate contact reactions have been described in bakers, confectionary and factory workers (Valero 1996; Smith 1990). According to skin and nasal provocation tests and specific IgE RAST results, many different allergenic fractions may be involved, namely, ovoalbumin, ovomucoid, lysozyme, etc (Valero 1996; Rudzki 1977). Nestle and Elsner (1997) reported occupational hand dermatitis and immediate contact reactions in cheese makers, with immediate skin-test reactions to various milk products.

Animals and Animal-Derived Products

OCU and PCD following contact with animals or animal derived products have been widely reported in different occupations. In 1978 Hjorth applied the term "fat eczema" to describe an itchy vesicular hand dermatitis with the characteristics of PCD in workers in contact with viscera and mesenteric fat from pigs. Since then many cases of OCU and PCD to animal products have been described in slaughterhouse workers, butchers, cooks, etc (Hansen 1989; Zenarola 1991; Göran-

Table 3. Animals, plants and derivatives (natural products) causing contact urticaria

Animals and their derivatives	Plants and their derivatives
Ammniotic fluid[a] (I)	Abietic acid (U)
Anisakis simplex (worm)	Algae (I)
Blood[a] (I)	Aloe
Brucella abortus (I)	Birch (leaves, sap) (I)
Calf[a]	Bougainvillea (U)
Caterpillars (NI)	Camomille[a]
Cephalopods (Loligo vulgaris)[a]	Chrysanthemum[a] (I)
Chironomus (I)	Cinchona[a] (U)
Cockroaches[a] (I)	Colophony[a] (I)
Corals (NI)	Cornstarch[a] (I)
Cow[a]	Cotoneaster
Dander[a] (I)	Crataegus (I)
Dog	Dandelion[a] (I)
Gut (pig)[a] (I)	Elm tree (U)
Guinea pig[a]	Eruca sativa (I)
Hair (rat, mice)[a] (I)	Eucalyptus (I)
Hair (Human)	Ficus benjamina[a] (I)
Hedgehogs	Gerbera[a] (I)
Horse	Grevillea juniperina (NI) (I?)
Jellyfish (I) (NI)	Golden rod[a] (I)
Liver (mice)[a] (I?)	Hakea suaveolens
Locust[a] (I)	Larch
Lumbrinereis impatiens (worm)	Latex rubber[a] (I)
Mites[a] (I)	Lichens
Moths (NI)	Lilies[a] (I)
Nereis diversicolor	Lime
Placenta (cow)[a] (I)	Limonium trataricum (dried flowers)[a] (I)
Pig[a]	Mahogany[a]
Rat[a]	Mulberry
Saliva[a] (I)	Obeche[a] (I)
Sea anemona (NI)	Phaseolus multiflorus (U)
Seminal fluid (I)	Poppy flowers (Papaver rhoeas) (I)
Serum (amphibian)[a] (I)	Spathe flower[a] (I)
Silk[a] (I)	Semecarpus anacardium (U)
Spider mite[a] (I)	Teak (I)
Pearl oysters[a]	Tobacco[a] (I)
Rat tail[a] (I)	Tropical woods[a] (I?)
Urine (mice, rat)[a] (I)	Tulips[a] (I)
	Turpentine (NI)
	Verbena (V. hybrida & elegans)[a] (I)
	Yucca aloifolia[a]

I, Immunologic contact urticaria; NI, non-immunologic contact urticaria; U, uncertain mechanism.
[a] Occupational contact urticaria.

son 1981). Veterinary surgeons, especially those who perform obstetric work with cows, are also exposed. Contact with obstetric fluids is the most frequent cause of these reactions (Rudzki 1982; Hjorth 1980; Prahl 1979; Degreff 1984) (Table 3). Animal hair, blood and saliva have also been reported as causative agents (Prahl 1979; Degreff 1984). Hjorth (1980) studied 36 veterinary surgeons with incapacitating hand dermatitis. Sixteen of them stated that vaginal or rectal examinations caused a flare of dermatitis. Scratch tests with obstetric fluid from cows were performed on 15 of them and 5 reacted positively. Prick tests with animal hair were positive in 18 subjects, and 4 had a positive RAST to cow hair. Cow dander was reported as a cause of occupational immediate and delayed allergy in farmers. In Finland, allergy to cow dander represents 25% of reported occupational dermatitis in farmers and it is the most frequent cause of OCU (Kanerva 1996). Susitaival et al. (1995) prick- and patch-tested 104 farmers with hand dermatitis; 41 were positive to cow dander; one-third had an immediate positive reaction; one-third had a delayed reaction and one-third had both immediate and delayed reactions.

Animals used in biological research, such as rats, mice, guinea pigs, hamsters, rabbits, frogs, toads, etc., have been reported to produce respiratory and cutaneous immediate allergic reactions in people working with them (Davies 1983; Burrows 1979; Hunskaar 1990; Karches 1993; Wong 1984; Thomsen 1987). The main allergens in rat and mice are urinary proteins (Gordon 1993). Allergens are also present in saliva, fur and feces (Walls 1985).

Plants and Plant-Derived Products

Contact urticaria and immediate respiratory symptoms from flowers, flower pollen and plants have been reported in florists, floriculturists and gardeners (Lahti 1986; Estlander 1998; Paulsen 1997) (Table 3). De Jong et al. (1998) studied 14 Dutch subjects with occupationally related rhinoconjunctivitis, asthma and contact urticaria from handling flowers. Skin prick testing with home made pollen extracts from 17 different flowers growing in The Netherlands was positive in most cases. Since all patients were allergic to mugwort pollen, it was concluded that it could be used as a screening test for a possible flower allergy.

Wood can also cause immediate contact reactions in exposed workers. OCU and respiratory symptoms from tropical woods (Lauan, Philippine, Red Mahogany) (Göransson 1980) and obeche wood (Kanerva 1998) have been reported in wood workers and carpenters.

Immediate allergic reactions to natural rubber latex (NRL), a plant-derived product, are a major occupational problem for health care workers. Since the first description in 1979 (Nuter 1979) the reports of immediate reactions to NRL have greatly increased. Not only an increased incidence but, also, greater awareness and better diagnostic techniques explain the rising number of diagnosed cases (Beaudouin 1990; Hesse 1996; Turjanmaa 1995). Prevalence of latex allergy in health care personnel in different countries has been shown to vary between 3% and 16% (Turjanmaa 1995), but comparison of different materials is not easy because of dissimilar diagnostic methods and inclusion criteria. The principal source of latex exposure is surgical gloves. Contaminated glove powder may act as carrier of latex proteins and spread them into the air (Turjanmaa 1997). Allergen content varies widely between different brands, thus, use of low-allergen non-powdered gloves is crucial in the primary prevention of latex allergy (Turjanmaa 1988). In secondary prevention, when even low-allergen non-powdered gloves are not tolerated, latex free gloves should be used.

Medicaments and Cosmetics

Immediate contact reactions to medicaments have been described in heath care and pharmaceutical industry workers, veterinarians and other exposed workers (Fisher 1982; Sherertz 19994). Antibiotics, such as penicillin (Boonk 1981), mezlocillin (Keller 1992a), streptomycin (Levene 1969) and cephalosporins (Tuft 1975; Miyahara 1993); antineoplasic agents (Schena 1996); analgesics (Sertoli 1980), antiseptics (Freitas 1986) etc., have been reported to induce respiratory symptoms and OCU, mostly of the immunologic type (Table 4). Cosmetic prod-

Table 4. Topical drugs and cosmetics causing contact urticaria

Medicaments	Chlorhexidine (I)
Acetylsalicylic acid	Chlorocresol[a] (NI) (I?)
Aescin (saponine from dried seeds) (I?)	Formaldehyde[a] (NI) (I)
Antibiotics (I)	Gentian violet (I)
Ampicillin	Imidazolidinyl urea (NI)
Bacitracin	Kathon CG (NI)
Cephalosporins[a]	Mercurochrome (I)
Chloramphenicol	o-Phenylphenate (I)
Gentamycin	Parabens (I?)
Iodochlorhydroxyquin	Phenylmercuric acetate[a] (I)
Mezlocillin[a]	Phenylmercuric propionate (I)
Neomycin	Sodium benzoate[a] (NI)
Penicillin[a]	Sodium hypochlorite (I)
Rifamycin	Sorbic acid (NI)
Streptomycin[a]	Cosmetics, fragrances and emulsifiers
Virginiamycin	Hair care products
Antineoplastic agents	Ammonium, potassium and sodium persulphate[a] (U)
Cisplatin[a] (I)	Basic blue 99 (amino ketone dye)[a] (I)
Mechlorethamine (I)	Henna[a] (I)
Benzocaine (U)	Protein hydrolysate[a] (I?)
Benzoyl peroxide (I)	Paraphenylenediamine[a] (I)
Capsaicin (NI)	Emulsifiers
Carboxymethylcellulose sodium (I)	Cetyl alcohol (U)
Chloroform (NI)	Stearyl alcohol (U)
Dinitrochlorobenzene	Polysorbate (I?)
Diphenylcyclopropenone (I)	Sorbitan monolaurate (I?)
Dimethylsulfoxide (NI)	Sorbitan monostearate (I?)
Lindane (I)	Sorbitan sesquioleate (I?)
Nicotinic acid esters (NI)	Fragrances
Pentamidine isethionate[a] (I)	α-Amyl cinnamic aldehyde (NI)
Phenothiazines (I)	Anisyl alcohol (NI)
Chlorpromazine	Balsam of Peru[a] (NI) (I?)
Levopromazine (I)	Cassia oil (NI)
Promethazine	Cinnamic aldehyde (NI)
Pilocarpine (U)	Cinnamic alcohol (NI)
Pyrazolones (I)	Cinnamic acid (NI)
Aminophenazone	Coumarin (NI)
Methamizole[a]	Eugenol (NI)
Prophylphenazone	Fragrance mix (NI)

Table 4 (continued)

Steroids	Geraniol (NI)
Tar extracts (NI)	Hydroxycitronellal (NI)
Tincture of benzoin (NI)	Other substances
Preservatives and disinfectants	Allantoin (I?)
Acetic acid	Aloe gel (I?)
Alcohols (NI) (I)	Benzophenone (NI)
Amyl-Ethyl-Butyl-Isopropyl-Benzyl	Chamomile extract (I?)
Ammonia (I)	Lecithin (I?)
Benzoic acid (NI) (I?)	Melissa extract (I?)
Bronopol (NI)	Pyrrolidone carboxylate (NI)
Butilated hydroxytoluene (I?)	Propylene glycol (NI)
Camphor (NI)	Resorcinol (NI)
Chloramine (I)	Wool alcohols (I)

I, Immunologic CU; NI, non-immunologic CU; U, uncertain mechanism.
[a] Occupational CU.

ucts also have been reported to induce immediate reactions. Ammonium persulphate and other persulphates used in hair bleaches represent the most common cause of OCU in hairdressers (Fisher 1985). The pathogenic mechanism of these reactions remains uncertain. Other potential agents of OCU in hair bleaches are sodium silicate (filler material) ammonia and colorants such as henna (Majoie 1992). Natural products, such as protein hydrolysates in shampoos, hair conditioners and other cosmetic products have been reported as a cause of immunological OCU.

Miscellaneous Agents

Plastics, metals, solvents, rubber, and various chemical agents have been reported to produce immediate contact reactions in workers in the chemical and oil industry, rubber industry, plastic manufacturing industry, metallurgy, etc. (Table 5).

Diagnosis

In addition to a detailed clinical history concerning any occurrence of immediate reactions – whether limited to the skin or not – and their association with occupational exposure, diagnostic tests should be performed. Guidelines for evaluating immediate-type responses have been recommended by von Krogh and Maibach (Von Krogh 1982; Von Krogh 1981). The initial tests should be performed on healthy skin, preferably in an open application, and the area should be examined after 20–30 min (preferably the area should be examined again after 1 h). In case of a negative result, the open test should be repeated on a slightly effected (or previously dermatitic) area. If this is also negative, a patch test should be done, first on healthy and then on lesional or previously affected skin. Finally, invasive tests, such as scratch or prick tests can be performed with caution.

Table 5. Miscellaneous chemicals causing contact urticaria

Acetyl acetone (I)	Cobalt[a] (I)
Acid anhydrides[a] (I)	Cooper
Methylhexahydrophtalic anhydride	Gold
Methyltetrahydrophtalic anhydride	Iridium[a] (I)
Phtalic anhydride	Mercury (I?)
Acrylic acid (I?)	Nickel[a] (I)
Acrylic monomers[a] (I)	Palladium
Aliphatic polyamide[a] (I)	Platinum salts[a] (I)
Aminodiphenylamine[a] (I)	Rhodium[a]
Aminothiazole	Ruthenium
Aziridine[a] (I?)	Tin
Butylhidroxytoluol	Zinc
Calcium hypochloride	Methyl ethyl ketone (I)
Carbamates[a] (I)	Monoamylamine (I)
Carbonless copy paper[a] (I)	Naphta[a] (NI)
Chlorotalonil[a] (I)	Naphthylacetic acid
Citraconic anhydride	Nylon (I)
Denatonium benzoate[a] (I?)	Oleylamide
Dicyanidiamide	Phosphorous sesquisulfide
Diethylfumarate	Polypropylene[a]
Diethyltoluamide (I)	Potassium ferricyanide
Diglycidyl ether of bisphenol A[a] (I)	Sodium fluoride
Formaldehyde resin[a] (I)	Sodium silicate
Fumaric acid	Sodium sulfide
Maleic anhydride[a] (I)	Sulfur (NI)
Metals	Trichloroethanol (U)
Aluminum	Vinyl pyridine[a]
Chromium[a] (I)	Xylene[a]

I, Immonologic contact urticaria; NI, non-immunologic contact urticaria; U, uncertain mechanism.
[a] Occupational contact urticaria.

Occlusive application, as in the scratch-chamber test, is convenient when testing non-standardized materials, especially when a delayed reading is needed (PCD). The rationale behind this step-by-step procedure is to minimize the risk of adverse extracutaneous reactions. Life-threatening reactions when performing tests have been documented, especially when testing with occupational materials (Von Krogh 1982; Haustein 1976).

Conclusion

OCU represents an increasing problem in occupational dermatology. Current industrial processes involving new chemicals, oblige practitioners, researchers and medical authorities to join their efforts to investigate the capacity of occupational materials to induce immediate contact reactions, as has been the case for delayed-type contact sensitizers. Studies on the mechanism of immediate contact reactions and standardization of human and animal models constitute a challenge for future research.

References

Alonso MD, Martin JA, Cuevas M, et al (1993) Occupational protein contact dermatitis from lettuce. Contact Dermatitis 29:109–110

Amin S, Tanglertsampan C, Maibach HI (1997) Contact urticaria syndrome (1997) Am J Contact Dermatitis 8:15–19

Beaudouin E, Pupil P, Jacson F, et al (1990) Allergie professionelle au latex. Enquete prospective sur 907 sujets du milieu hospitalier. Rev Fr Allergol 30:157–161

Beck H, Knudsen N (1982) Type I and type IV allergy to specific chicken organs. Contact Dermatitis 3:217–218

Boonk WR (1981) Dermatologic hazards from hidden contact with penicillin. Dermatosen 29:131–135

Bruynzeel-Koomen C (1986) IgE on Langerhans cells: new insights into the pathogenesis of atopic dermatitis. Dermatologica 172:181–183

Burrows D (1979) Urticaria from rats. Contact Dermatitis 5:122

Davies GE, Thompson AV, Niewola Z, et al (1983) Allergy to laboratory animals: a retrospective and a prospective study. Br J Ind Med 40:442–449

Degreff H, Bourgeois M, Naert C, et al (1984) Protein contact dermatitis with positive RAST caused by bovine blood and amniotic fluid. Contact Dermatitis 11:129–130

De Jong NW, Vermeulen AM, Gerth van Wijk R, de Grrot H (1998) Occupational allergy caused by flowers. Allergy 53:204–209

Ebner C, Hirschwehr R, Bauer L, et al (1995) Identification of allergens in fruits and vegetables: IgE cross reactivities with the important birch pollen allergens Bet v1 and Bet v2 (birch profiling). J Allergy Clin Immunol 95:962–969

Estlander T, Kanerva L, Tupasela O, Jolanki R (1998) Occupational contact urticaria and type I sensitization caused by gerbera. Contact Dermatitis 38:118–120

Fisher AA, Stengel F (1977) Allergic occupational hand dermatitis due to calf's liver. An urticarial "immediate" type hypersensitivity. Cutis 19:561–565

Fisher AA (1982) Contact urticaria due to medicaments, chemicals and food. Cutis 30:168–172

Fisher A (1982) Contact urticaria from handling meats and fowl. Cutis 30:726–729

Fisher AA (1985) The persulphates – a triple threat. Cutis 35:520–525

Freitas JP, Brandao FM (1986) Contact urticaria to chlorocresol. Contact Dermatitis 15:252

Göransson K (1980) Contact urticaria and rhinoconjunctivitis from tropical woods (Lauan, Philippine, Red Mahogany). Contact Dermatitis 6:223–224

Göranson K (1981) Occupational contact urticaria to fresh cow and pig blood in slaughtermen. Contact Dermatitis 7:281–282

Gordon S, Tee RD, Newman Taylor AJ (1993) Analysis of rat urine proteins and allergens by sodium dodecyl sulfate polyacrylamide gel electrophoresis and immunoblotting. J Allergy Clin Immunol 92:298–305

Hafner J, Riess CE, Wüthrich B (1992) Protein contact dermatitis from paprika and curry in a cook. Contact Dermatitis 26:51–52

Halmepuro L, Vuontela K, Kalimo K, et al (1984) Cross-reactivity of IgE antibodies with allergens in birch pollen, fruits and vegetables. Int Arch Allergy Appl Immunol 74:235–240

Hannuksela M, Lahti A (1977) Immediate reactions to fruits and vegetables. Contact Dermatitis 3:70–84

Hannuksela M (1980) Atopic contact dermatitis. Contact Dermatitis 6:30–32

Hansen KS, Petersen HO (1989) Protein contact dermatitis in slaughterhouse workers. Contact Dermatitis 21:221–224

Harrington CI (1981) Chicken sensitivity. Contact Dermatitis 7:126

Haustein UF (1976) Anaphylactic shock and contact urticaria after the patch test with professional allergens. Allergie Immunol 22:349–352

Hesse A, Lacher U, Koch HU, et al (1996) Update on the latex allergy topic. Hautarzt 47:817–824

Hjorth N, Roed Petersen J (1976) Occupational protein contact dermatitis in food handlers. Contact Dermatitis 2:28–42

Hjorth N (1978) Gut eczema in slaughterhouse workers. Contact Dermatitis 21:221–224

Hjorth N, Roed-Petersen J (1980) Allergic contact dermatitis in veterinary surgeons. Contact Dermatitis 6:27–29

Hunskaar S, Fose RT (1990) Allergy to laboratory mice and rats: a review of the pathophysiology, epidemiology and clinical aspects. Lab Animals 24:358–374

Jovanovic M, Oliwiecki S, Beck M (1992) Occupational contact urticaria from beef associated with hand eczema. Contact Dermatitis 27:188–189

Kanerva L (1996) Occupational IgE-mediated protein contact dermatitis from pork in a slaughterman. Contact Dermatitis 34:301–302

Kanerva L, Susitaival P (1996) Cow dander – the most common cause of occupational contact urticaria in Finland. Contact Dermatitis 35:309–310

Kanerva L, Brisman J (1997) Contact urticaria, dermatitis and respiratory allergy caused by enzymes. In: Amin S, Lahti A, Maibach HI (eds) Contact urticaria syndrome. CRC Press, Boca Raton, pp 129–142

Kanerva L, Vanhanen M, Tupasela O (1998) Occupational contact urticaria from cellulase enzyme. Contact Dermatitis 38:176–177

Kanerva L, Tuppurainen M, Keskinen H (1998) Contact urticaria caused by obeche wood (*Triplochiton Scleroxylon*). Contact Dermatitis 38:170–171

Karches F, Fuchs T (1993) A strange manifestation of occupational contact urticaria due to mouse hair. Contact Dermatitis 28:200

Keller K, Schwanitz HJ (1992) Combined immediate and delayed hypersensitivity to mezlocillin. Contact Dermatitis 27:348–349

Krook G (1977) Occupational dermatitis from Lactuca Sativa (lettuce) and Cichorium (Endive). Simultaneous occurrence of immediate and delayed allergy as a cause of contact dermatitis. Contact Dermatitis 3:27–36

Lathi A (1980) Nonimmunologic contact urticaria. Acta Derm Venereol Suppl (Stockh) 60 [Suppl 1]:1–50

Lahti A (1986) Contact urticaria and respiratory symptoms from tulips and lilies. Contact Dermatitis 14:317–319

Levene GM, Withers AFD (1969) Anaphylaxis to streptomycin and hyposensitization (parasensitization). Trans St John's Hosp Dermatol Soc 55:184

Maibach HI (1976) Immediate hypersensitivity in hand dermatitis. Arch Dermatol 112:1289–1291

Maibach HI (1995) Contact urticaria from mold on salami casing. Contact Dermatitis 32:120–121

Majoie ML, Bruynzeel DP (1992) Occupational immediate-type hypersensitivity to henna in a hairdresser. Am J Contact Dermatitis 7:38–40

Melino M, Toni F, Rigguzzi G (1987) Immunologic contact urticaria to fish. Contact Dermatitis 31:55–57

Miyahara H, Koga T, Imayama S, Hori Y (1993) Occupational contact urticaria syndrome from cefotiam hydrochloride. Contact Dermatitis 29:210–211

Morren MA, Janssen V, Dooms-Goossens A, et al (1993) Alfa-amylase, a flour additive: an important cause of protein contact dermatitis in bakers. J Am Acad Dermatol 29:723–728

Moseng D (1982) Urticaria from pig's gut. Contact Dermatitis 8:1235–136

Nestle FO, Elsner P (1997) Occupational dermatoses in cheese makers: frequent association of irritant, allergic and protein contact dermatitis. Dermatology 194:243–246

Niinimäki A, Hannuksela M, Makinen-Kiljunen S (1995) Skin prick tests and in vitro immunoassays with native spices and spice extracts. Ann Allergy Asthma Immunol 75:280–286

Nuter AF (1979) Contact urticaria to rubber. Br J Dermatol 101:597–598

Paulsen E, Søgaard J, Andersen KE (1997) Occupational dermatitis in Danish gardeners and greenhouse workers (I). Prevalence and possible risk factors. Contact Dermatitis 37:263–270

Prahl P, Roed-Petersen J (1979) Type I allergy from cows in veterinary surgeons. Contact Dermatitis 5:33–38

Rudzki E, Grzywa Z (1977) Contact urticaria from egg. Contact Dermatitis 3:103–104

Rudzki E, Rebandel P, Grzywa Z, et al (1982) Occupational dermatitis in veterinarians. Contact Dermatitis 8:72–73

Schena D, Barba A, Costa G (1996) Occupational contact dermatitis due to cisplatin. Contact Dermatitis 34:2320–2321

Sertoli A, Marliani A, Lmobardi P, Panconesi E (1980) Immediate sensitization to methamizole verified by patch tests. Contact Dermatitis 6:294

Sherertz E (1994) Occupational skin disease in the pharmaceutical industry. Dermatol Clin 12:533–536

Smith AB, Bernstein DI, London M et al (1990) Evaluation of occupational asthma from airborne egg protein exposure in multiple settings. Chest 98:398–404

Susitaival P, Husman L, Hollmen A, et al (1995) Hand eczema in Finnish farmers. A questionnaire-based clinical study. Contact Dermatitis 32:150–155

Sutton R, Skerritt JH, Baldo BA, Wrigley CW (1984) The diversity of allergens involved in bakers asthma. Clin Allergy 14:93–107

Taylor SL, Lemanski RF, Bush RK, Busse WW (1987) Food allergens: structure and immunological properties. Ann Allergy 59:93–99

Thomsen RJ, Honsinger RW (1987) Immediate hypersensitivity reaction to amphibian serum manifesting as eczema. Arch Dermatol 123:1436–1437

Tuft L (1975) Contact urticaria from cephalosporins. Arch Dermatol 111:1609

Turjanmaa K, Laurila K, Mäkinen-Kiljunen S, Reunala T (1988) Rubber contact urticaria. Allergenic properties of 19 brands of latex gloves. Contact Dermatitis 19:362–367

Turjanmaa K, Mäkinen-Kiljunen S, Reunala T, et al (1995) Natural rubber latex allergy, the European experience. Immunol Allergy Clin N Am 15:71–88

Turjanmaa K (1997) Contact urticaria from latex gloves. In: Amin S, Lahti A, Maibach HI (eds) Contact urticaria syndrome. CRC press, Boca Raton pp 173–187

Valenta R, Duchêne M, Ebner C, et al (1992) Profilins constitute a novel family of functional plant pan-allergens. J Exp Med 175:377–385

Valero A, Lluch M, Amat P, et al (1996) Occupational egg allergy in confectionary workers. Allergy 51:588–592

Vanhanen M, Tuomi T, Hokkane H, et al (1996) Enzyme exposure and enzyme sensitization in the baking industry. Occup Environ Med 53:670–676

Veien N, Hattel T, Justesen O, Norholm A (1983) Causes of eczema in the food industry. Dermatosen 31:84–86

Von Krogh G, Maibach HI (1982) The contact urticaria syndrome. Semin Dermatol 1:59–66

Von Krogh G, Maibach HI (1981) The contact urticaria syndrome – an update review. J Am Acad Dermatol 5:328–342

Walls AF, Longbottom JL (1985) Comparison of rat fur, urine, saliva and other rat allergen extracts by skin testing, RAST and RAST inhibition. J Allergy Clin Immunol 75:242–251

Wong AV, Shih-Wen H, Burnett JW (1984) Hypersensitivity to rat saliva. J Am Acad Dermatol 11:606–608

Zenarola P, Lomuto M (1991) Protein contact dermatitis with positive RAST in slaughterman. Contact Dermatitis 24:134–135

CHAPTER 10

Occupational and Environmental Acne   10

J.S. Taylor, J.K. McDonnell

Introduction

Occupational and environmental acne results from various chemical exposures and from a variety of environmental, physical and mechanical factors. The eruption may be mild, involving localized exposed or covered areas of the body, or severe, explosive and disseminated with the involvement of almost every follicular orifice. Occupational and environmental acne is separated into oil acne, coal-tar acne, acne cosmetica, acne mechanica, tropical acne and chloracne. Chloracne almost always represents a cutaneous sign of systemic exposure to highly toxic chemicals.

Oil Acne

Oil acne is the most common form of occupational acne and is most commonly observed in workers employed in the machine tooling trades. Others affected may include auto, airplane and truck mechanics, petroleum refiners, and rubber workers. The incidence of oil acne has declined in recent years because of decreased use of pure cutting oils and improved industrial and personal hygiene practices (Kokelj 1992).

Cutting oils, especially insoluble (straight) oils, and semi-synthetic coolants have been the most commonly incriminated oil acnegens (Taylor 1987). In mechanics, prolonged exposure to grease, lubricating oils and kerosene may induce oil acne (Upreti et al. 1989).

Prolonged oil exposure produces a reactive follicular hyperkeratosis and results in sebum retention. This manifests clinically as multiple open comedones, inflammatory folliculitis and microcystic lesions caused by the oil itself. Lesions are distributed primarily over exposed areas, such as the dorsal hands and extensor forearms. Oil-soaked clothing may produce lesions on the thighs, lower abdomen and buttocks (Kokelj 1992). The face may be involved from wiping the brow with an oil-contaminated sleeve. Although the lesions are commonly referred to as oil boils, they usually do not develop from bacteria present in the oils (Taylor 1987). The inflammatory lesions are more prominent than in chloracne and may mimic conglobate cystic acne.

Oil acne is treated with the usual acne vulgaris modalities, such as topical benzoyl peroxide and retinoic acid. Systemic treatment is often needed with tetracycline, erythromycin or minocycline, or with isotretinoin in severe cases. The key factor is avoiding contact with oils and grease. Work clothes should be changed daily and frequent cleansing of the skin with soap and water is advised.

Coal-Tar Acne

Coal-tar oils, creosote and pitch can produce a comedonal type of acne, which shows a predilection for exposed areas, particularly the malar regions (Bertolini 1989; Adams et. al., 2000). Coal-tar plant workers, roofers, road maintenance workers and construction workers are among those at risk. Coal-tar acne may be complicated by phototoxic reactions affecting both the skin and the eyes and resulting in hyperpigmentation known as coal-tar melanosis. Late complications include the development of pitch and tar papillomas, keratoses and acanthomas (Taylor 1987).

Acne Cosmetica

Acne cosmetica may develop in actors and models who are often required to wear heavy, greasy make-up; cosmetologists may also be affected (Kligman and Mills 1972). Acne cosmetica consists of essentially non-inflammatory, small, closed comedones and a few intermittent papules and pustules.

Cosmetic ingredients found experimentally to be comedogenic include lanolin, petrolatum, certain vegetable oils and pure chemicals such as butyl stearate, lauryl alcohol and oleic acid. Many of these substances are now avoided or modified by cosmetic manufacturers and cosmetics are frequently advertised as non-comedogenic.

Acne Mechanica

Repeated or prolonged physical insults to the skin, such as rubbing, pressure, friction, pinching or pulling, may produce an acneiform eruption that can be strikingly inflammatory in nature. An example is the local pressure and rubbing against seat covers which occurs in truck drivers. Other occupational causes of acne mechanica include the use of face masks (as in hospital workers or cleanroom workers in the semiconductor industry), belts, straps, tight-fitting work clothing, football shoulder pads, football helmets, hats, and telephones (Mills and Kligman 1975). Violinist's neck is also a variant of acne mechanica (Omohundro and Taylor 1998).

Clinically, crops of inflammatory papules and pustules appear in affected areas of skin. Deep, inflammatory nodules may result from prolonged pressure. It has been emphasized that acne mechanica is a complication of acne vulgaris and that external physical forces merely exacerbate the underlying disease focally (Mills and Kligman 1975). We have seen it as a complication of friction and sweating in chloracne.

Tropical Acne

Tropical acne may result from exposure to excessively hot or humid environments. Tropical acne has been observed most commonly in soldiers stationed in tropical climates, but variants may result from chronic exposure to other hot and/or humid environments as can be found in foundries (Mathias 1994).

Onset is explosive in nature and typically occurs several months after entering the hot, humid environment. This is a severely inflammatory condition, with the development of papules, pustules, nodules, and draining sinuses as in acne conglobata. Patients often feel quite ill, and acute-phase reactants may be elevated. There is characteristic involvement of the buttocks and upper thighs, but lesions may be extensive, with the neck, arms, and trunk being affected. The face is usually spared (Sperling 1994).

Cultures have not identified a consistent pathogen, and the role of bacterial infection is felt to be unimportant. Antibiotic therapy is without significant benefit. The only effective therapeutic measure is to remove the patient from the precipitating environment (Sperling 1994).

Chloracne

Chloracne results from environmental exposure to certain halogenated aromatic hydrocarbons. Chloracne is considered one of the most sensitive indicators of biological response to these chemicals and it occurs regardless of whether chemical exposure has occurred via skin contact – the usual route – inhalation or ingestion (Crow and Puhvel 1991).

Chloronapthalenes and polychlorinated biphenyls (PCBs) were the causative agents in the pre-World-War-II era. Since then, trace contaminants formed during the manufacture of PCBs and other polyhalogenated compounds, especially herbicides, have been the major causes of chloracne. These include polyhalogenated dibenzofurans, polychlorinated dibenzo-p-dioxins and chlorinated azo- and azoxy benzenes.

Chloracnegenic compounds are structurally similar, sharing relative molecular planarity and containing two benzene rings with halogen atoms occupying at least three of the lateral ring positions. The position of halogen substitution appears to be critical, as reduced biological activity results from substitution into positions that lead to molecular non-planarity (Kokelj 1992).

Chloracne-Producing Chemicals and Sources of Exposure

Table 1 provides a partial list of past and present sources of the various chloracnegens. The majority of chloracne cases have resulted from occupational exposure during chemical manufacturing or rarely from end product use.

Occupational Exposure

Selected outbreaks will be discussed as classified by chemical cause.

Table 1. Partial list of past and present sources of chloracnegens

Chloracnegen	Source
Polychloronaphthalenes	Electrical insulators; fire-resistant materials; wood preservatives; boat hull coatings (anti-magnetic properties); high-pressure additives for lubricants
Polychlorobiphenyls (PCBs)	Hydraulic fluids; plastics; adhesives; fire retardants in transformers; sealants
Polychlorodibenzofurans (PCDFs), especially tri-, tetra-, penta- and hexachlorodibenzofuran	Contaminants of PCBs and various chlorinated phenols
Polychlorinated phenols	Wood preservatives; leather; paper industry applications; herbicides; fungicides; algicides; insecticides; disinfectants
Dioxins	Contaminant of agent orange, formed during production of chlorinated organic solvents (hexachlorophene and the herbicide 2,4,5,-T); products of combustion
3,4,3′,4′ tetrachloro azo- and azoxy-benzenes	3, 4-dichloroaniline herbicide intermediates
Trifluoromethyl – pyrazole derivative	Pharmaceutical drug development (Scerri et al. 1995)

Polyhalogenated Naphthalenes

Industrial use of the polyhalogenated naphthalenes (PCNs), occupational chloracne outbreaks and experimental human and animal studies have been reviewed (Taylor 1979). No occupational cases of PCN chloracne have been reported since 1972. Trace contamination of PCBs with hexachloronaphthalenes and of polybromodiphenyls (PBBs) with polybromonaphthalenes are potential current, but unlikely, sources of exposure (Taylor 1979).

Polychlorinated Biphenyls/Polyhalogenated Dibenzofurans

PCBs are chloracnegens as has been demonstrated in reports in capacitor workers (Taylor et al. 1979) and in other workers (Longnecker et al. 1997). Cutaneous hyperpigmentation eye discharge and palpebral edema have also been reported (Taylor et al. 1979). Since polyhalogenated dibenzofuans (PHDFs) contaminate PCBs and polyhalogenated phenols, their cutaneous effects are discussed under those headings.

Dioxins

Dioxin, specifically TCDD, is the paradigm for chemicals causing chloracne and also for the biological importance of trace industrial contaminants. Dioxins contaminate polychlorophenols, especially the herbicides 2,4,5-T and pentachlorophenol (PCP) and herbicide intermediates (2,4,5-trichlorophenol). TCDD is one of the most toxic small molecules and is also one of the best-studied toxic chemicals, largely after intense scrutiny over its use in the Vietnam war.

More than 20 outbreaks of dioxin chloracne, as well as its other health effects, have been reviewed (Taylor et al. 1979; Mukerjee 1998).

Chloracne is the hallmark of dioxin exposure in humans; however, its absence does not exclude dioxin exposure. There is no apparent dose-response model for chloracne in exposed human populations. It may develop weeks or months after exposures. In Germany, six workers who developed chloracne after an industrial accident had an estimated mean TCDD body burden shortly after the accident of 44 µg (range 9.7–124 µg). Thus, a body burden of 9.7 µg, as measured in adipose tissue, may be the lowest observable effect level for TCDD-related chloracne in humans. Thirty-two years after exposure, the German workers still had detectable levels of TCDD in adipose tissue, and one still had chloracne (Agency for Toxic Effects of Chemical Substances 1993).

A case of palmoplantar keratoderma, scleroderma and chloracne was reported in an agricultural worker who had been a weed sprayer for 5 years. He had used 2,4,5-trichlorophenoxyacetic acid and/or 2,4-dichlorophenoxyacetic acid, both of which may contain chlorinated dibenzodioxins as impurities. He also had been chronically exposed to multiple other, non-chloracne associated herbicides, some of which have been associated with scleroderma. Safety equipment was not utilized (Poskitt et al. 1994). Punctate keratoderma of the palms and soles has also been reported (Geusau et.al. 2000).

PCP is frequently used as a wood preservative, herbicide and fungicide, as well as in the leather and paper industry (O'Malley et al. 1990). A retrospective review of 648 medical and personnel records from individuals manufacturing PCP between 1938 and 1978 demonstrated 47 cases of chloracne occurring in a 25-year period. These workers were exposed only to PCP for 2 years prior to their diagnosis. During the commercial synthesis of PCP, varying amounts of polychlorinated aromatic by-products, including dioxins, are produced (O'Malley et al. 1990).

Cole et al. (1986) reported an unusual case of occupational chloracne that developed in a carpenter who assembled piers for small boat marinas using PCP-treated lumber. Samples of treated lumber contained 10–40 times the amount of octachlorodibenzodioxin (OCD) than untreated wood. The yellow residue from treated wood contained 400 ppm OCD compared with technical grade PCP which contained 1600 ppm OCD. This case is unusual because the only source of PCP exposure was pressure-treated lumber. Coenrads et.al. (1999) determined threshold levels of dibenzodioxins and dibenzofurans in blood lipids which caused chloracne in a PCP production facility in China.

Azo and Azoxybenzenes

We first documented cases of chloracne from tetrachloroazoxybenzene (TCAOB) in 1977. Tetrachlorozobenzene (TCAB) was also produced during the synthesis of 3,4-dichloroaniline or during its further conversion to herbicides. More than 90%

of 41 workers in a small chemical plant developed chloracne. Family members of four workers, none of whom had been in the plant, also developed chloracne, probably from exposure at home to contaminated tools or work clothes (Taylor et al. 1977). Eight years later, three of five workers with chloracne still had some evidence of chloracne and scarring. Similar episodes of chloracne have been reported from the production of the pesticide-herbicide Proponil in Arkansas in 1977. We are aware of other reports of TCAB and TCAOB chloracne in the United States and England in the 1970s and 1980s (Taylor and Lloyd 1982).

An outbreak of chloracne in 17 workers from a British plant manufacturing dichloroaniline-derived herbicides was reported in 1993. TCAB and TCAOB were the acnegens. Comedones evolved 6–12 weeks after exposure to these chloracnegenic contaminants. Cutaneous xerosis and folliculitis, on the trunk, limbs, thighs and buttocks, previously uncommonly described, was present in 50% of exposed workers. A direct toxic effect on epidermal keratinocytes or a secondary effect due to a perifollicular inflammatory reaction has been theorized (McDonough et al. 1993). They suggested that folliculitis and xerosis should be included in the clinical spectrum of chloracne.

In 1996, nine workers from a Mexican chemical plant were evaluated for the effects of chronic exposure to mono-, ortho- and paradichlorobenzenes. They had a mean exposure of 24 working years and worked in all stages of chemical production. Safety equipment was not used, and direct contact with the chlorobenzenes occurred via the skin and respiratory tract. The nine workers had a polymorphic acneiform eruption consisting mainly of comedones and cysts. Hyperpigmentation of the face and oral cavity was also observed. All workers reported chronic conjunctivitis with thick secretions from meibomian glands. Hepatic involvement including elevated serum alkaline phosphatase and lower extremity peripheral neuropathy were also evident (Vazquez et al. 1996).

Non-Occupational Exposure

Non-occupational chloracne has resulted from industrial accidents, contaminated industrial waste and poisoned food products. Extensive environmental contamination with TCDD, occurred in July, 1976, at a chemical plant near Seveso, Italy. An explosion occurred during the manufacturing of trichlorophenol that resulted in the formation and ultimate discharge into the atmosphere of an estimated 2 kg of TCDD. The contaminated area encompassed more than 200 acres of land, and 135 cases of chloracne, mostly in children, were confirmed among the 2000 area inhabitants. The toxic cloud caused the death of hundreds of fowl in the first days after the explosion; the development of chloracne occurred after different time periods.

Ingestion alone of PCBs and their thermally degraded polychlorinated dibenzofurans (PCDFs) played a major role in two mass "oil-poisoning" episodes – Yusho in Japan (1968) and in Taiwan in (1979), the largest epidemics of chloracne to date. In both countries, several thousand persons were affected after eating rice-based cooking oil that had been accidentally contaminated with large amounts of tetrachlorobiphenyl. Dermatologic manifestations included chloracne, hyperpigmentation and hypersecretion of conjunctival meibomian glands. Most clinical manifestations were observed in patients who had directly ingested the oil. PCBs and PCDFs can persist in human tissues (similar dioxins have half-lives in humans of about 7 years) in the offspring of exposed females, described as cola babies because of their dark color. Generalized hyperpigmentation, meibomian gland enlargement with eye discharge and nail deformities occurred in congenitally exposed individuals. Severe chloracne scars were observed 11 years post-congenital exposure in some affected individuals in Taiwan (Hsu et al. 1995).

We studied 128 children who were transplacentally exposed to PCBs and dibenzofurans in Taiwan, their parents and siblings who were directly exposed, and 115 control children. Direct exposure of the mothers stopped in 1979 and the children were born as late as 1985. On cutaneous examination in 1985, key findings were of a much higher rate of dystrophic fingernails and pigmented or dystrophic toe nails than in controls. Increased rates of hyperpigmentation and acne were also seen in the exposed groups. The cutaneous findings were part of a transplacental neuroectodermal dysplasia, with dental abnormalities, a growth deficit, developmental delay, and a behavior disorder. The findings in transplacentally exposed children differ from those seen in people directly exposed, particularly the higher prevalence of acne in the latter group (Gladen et al. 1990; Hsu et al. 1995). A recent 14-year follow-up study (Guo, et.al. 1999) identified increased chloracne, "skin allergy", goiter, arthritis and anemia in a cohort of 795 PCB exposed Taiwanese.

In 1982, eight members of a Spanish family were poisoned by consumption of olive oil contaminated with PCDDs and PCDFs. The entire family had varying degrees of acneform lesions. Hyperpigmentation of the face was also reported. These lesions are comparable in severity to those described in the Yusho incident. The olive oil consumed was stored in a 50-l plastic container, which had presumably stored hexachlorobenzene and pentachlorophenol prior to the oil. There were high serum levels of PCDDs and PCDFs, which returned to normal when measured 5 years after oil consumption ceased (Rodriguez-Pichardo et al. 1991).

Mechanism

The mechanism for development is still unclear. TCDD is known to have an effect on in vitro keratinocyte differentiation, which may include changes in the epithelium of the pilosebaceous unit. Contrary to data from animal experiments, changes in epidermal retinal have not been observed in epidermal tissue from humans with chloracne (Coenraads 1999)

Histology

Histologic changes in the skin may begin within 5 days of severe exposure to chloracnegenic chemicals (Hambrick 1957). Lesions demonstrate squamous metaplasia and plugging of infundibular ducts in addition to atrophy of sebaceous glands. The specificity of these findings is unclear. A characteristic of chloracne is the rapid transformation of sebaceous glands into comedones. Biopsies from Seveso showed eccrine duct metaplasia with possible acrosyringeal cyst formation. Foreign body granulomas around detached walls of eccrine gland excretory ducts may also be present (Omohundro and Taylor 1998).

Diagnosis

Chloracne is diagnosed by a compatible clinical picture with distribution of comedones and non-inflammatory cysts beyond the typical locations of acne vulgaris. Documentation of significant exposure to known chloracnegens and the absence of other external causes is also required. Based on cutaneous findings alone, it may be very difficult to differentiate chloracne from early acne vulgaris (Table 2) and senile (solar) comedones of the Favre-Racouchot syndrome. Dowling-Degos' disease also can be considered in the clinical differential diagnosis (Kersevovich et al. 1992). Differentiation of chloracne from other types of environmental acne – oil folliculitis, pitch acne and tropical acne – is listed in Table 3.

Table 2. Clinical features of acne vulgaris compared with chloracne (after Peter Pochi)

Clinical features	Acne vulgaris	Chloracne
Usual age	Teenage	Any
Comedones	Present	Many (if absent, not chloracne)
Straw-coloured cysts	Rare	Pathognomonic
Temporal comedones	Rare	Diagnostic
Inflammatory papules and cysts	Common	Uncommon
Retroauricular involvement	Uncommon	Common
Nose involvement	Often spared	Often spared
Associated systemic findings	Rare	Common

Table 3. Differential diagnosis of various forms of occupational and environmental acne

	Etiology	Location	Lesion
Chloracne	Halogenated aromatics	Malar; retroauricular; mandibular	Comedones; straw-colored cysts (0.1–1.0 cm)
Oil folliculitis	Oil	Arms; thighs; buttocks	Erythematous; papules; pustules
Pitch acne	Tar/pitch	Exposed facial areas, especially malar	Open comedones
Tropical acne	Heat/humidity	Back; neck; buttocks; proximal extremities	Nodules, cysts

Cutaneous Manifestations

Clinical features of chloracne include multiple closed comedones and straw-colored cysts distributed primarily over the malar crescents and retroauricular folds, typically sparing the nose. This pattern of distribution is of significant diagnostic importance. Inflammatory lesions occur but are less frequent than in other forms of acne. As toxicity increases, the posterior neck, trunk and extremities, buttocks, scrotum and penis may become involved. Dermatologic observations associated with chloracne, which may lead to identification of specific exposures, include hyperpigmentation of the skin (PCBs, TCDD), mucous membrane and nail hyperpigmentation (PCBs), follicular hyperkeratosis (PCBs, TCDD [Seveso]), conjunctivitis and meibomian gland changes (PCBs), facial erythema and edema (trichlorophenol, hypertrichosis (TCDD), hyperhidrosis of the palms and soles (TCDD, PCBs) folliculitis and xerosis (TCAB, TCAOB) and actinic elastosis (TCDD). Erythema and edema of the exposed face and extremities associated with trichlorophenol production was also seen in the Seveso cases. These "pre-chloracne" lesions were also accompanied by vesiculobullous and necrotic lesions on finger tips and palms, and papulonodular lesions, all of which resolved within a few weeks. Hyperkeratotic, infiltrative erythematous granuloma annulare (Geusault et. al. 2000) or erythema elevatum diutinum-like lesions were also seen in association with chloracne 2 months after the explosion. Axillary involvement and follicular hyperkeratosis are linked with inhalation or ingestion of chloracnegens (Taylor 1979).

Hypertrichosis in association with chloracne has been mainly confined to the temples and may rarely be a sign of hepatic porphyria. However, hypertrichosis has also been described in chloracne patients with normal uroporphyrin levels (Jirasek et al. 1973 and Crow and Puhvel 1991).

Non-Cutaneous Manifestations

Patients with chloracne should have complete physical and laboratory evaluations to exclude systemic poisoning.

Epidemiologic data suggesting that high-level dioxin exposure causes liver function abnormalities and chloracne are incontrovertible (Longnecker et al. 1997). Crow and Puhvel (1991) suggested that the degree of hepatic injury is dependent on the specificity of the toxicant involved, rather than a consistent consequence of all forms of chloracnegen exposure.

Porphyria cutanea tarda (PCT) has been reported in humans following TCDD exposure (Bleiberg et al. 1964). TCDD is a porphyrinogen in animal models and inhibits uroporphyrinogen decarboxylase, the enzyme precipitating PCT in some patients (Mukerjee 1998).

Other systemic disorders reported with chloracne include peripheral neuropathy, hypertriglyceridemia, hypercholesterolemia, bronchitis, renal and pancreatic involvement (Taylor 1987).

Populations occupationally or accidentally exposed to chemicals contaminated with dioxin may have an increased incidence of soft-tissue sarcomas and non-

Hodgkin's lymphoma. Non-cancer health effects have been reviewed (Sweeney 2000). To date, no comprehensive studies have been conducted to determine any health impact to the general population from environmental exposure to PCDDs (Mukerjee 1998).

Treatment

Chloracne tends to resolve slowly upon cessation of chemical exposure. Its duration correlates with the severity of the disease, which usually reflects the degree and extent of exposure. The severely exposed victims of Yusho in 1968 had characteristic chloracne lesions that continued to develop for as long as 14 years postexposure.

Treatment has been difficult as the modalities that are useful in acne vulgaris are often ineffective in chloracne. Topical application of retinoic acid (0.005–0.3% concentration) or of tretinoin (Retin-A) gel or cream is of some benefit in controlling comedones, but other topical agents are of little use (Caputo et al. 1988). A combination of tetracycline and short courses of orally administered prednisone help with severe inflammatory cases. A trial regimen of methotrexate, 25 mg every 10 days for several months was unsuccessful (Taylor et al. 1977).

There are anecdotal reports of the efficacious use of oral 13-cis retinoic acid (isotretinoin) which, if instituted early, may prevent cyst formation. Isotretenoin 0.3–1 mg/kg/day may be indicated in severe cases for a course of 20 weeks. The drug should be administered only by those experienced in its use and in strict accordance with current prescribing instructions. The hepatotoxicity and lipid abnormalities sometimes associated with chloracne are theoretical reasons to avoid isotretinoin.

Isotretinoin is a potent teratogen with other potentially significant side effects and requires close monitoring (Gawkrodger 1991). Isotretinoin has been less effective in other reports (Scerri, et.al 1995).

Light cautery following topical anesthesia with EMLA (eutectic mixture of local anesthetic) cream has been used successfully in six patients with resistant chloracne lesions (Yip et al. 1993). Other therapies include acne surgery and dermabrasion. Olestra, a non-digestible and non-absorbable dietary fat substitute increased fecal excretion of TCDD in 2 individuals exposed to an unknown source of TCDD. This is sufficient to reduce the elimination half-life of TCDD from about 7 years to 1–2 years (Geusau et al., 1999).

References

Adams BB, ChettyVB, Mutasim DF (2000) Periorbital comedones and their relationship to pitch tar: a cross-sectional analysis and a review of the literature, J Am Acad Dermatol 42:624–7

Agency for Toxic Substances and Disease Registry (1993) Dioxin toxicity. Am Fam Physician 47:855–861

Bertolini R (1989) Acne. A summary of the occupational health concern. Canadian Centre for Occupational Health and Safety. Hamilton, Ontario. Report No. F89–1E:1–7

Bleiberg J, Wallen M, Brodken R et al (1964) Industrial acquired prophyria. Arch Dermatol 89:793–797

Caputo R, Monti M, Ermacora E, et al (1988) Cutaneous manifestations of tetrachlorodibenzo-and I;p and D;-dioxin in children and adolescents. J Am Acad Dermatol 19:812–819

Coenraads PJ, Olick, Tang NJ (1999) Blood lipid concentrations of dioxins and dibenzofurans causing chloracne. Br J Dermatol 141:694–7

Cole GW, Stone O, Gates D, Culver D (1986) Chloracne from pentachlorphenol – preserved wood. Contact Dermatitis 15:164–168

Crow KD, Puhvel MS (1991) Chloracne (halogen acne). In: Marzulli FN, Maibach HI (eds) Dermatoxicology. Hemisphere, New York, pp 647–667

Gawkrodger DJ (1991) Chloracne: causation, diagnosis and treatment. J Dermatol Treatment 2:73–76

Geusau A, Tschachler E, Meixner M et al (1999) Olestra increases fecal excretion of 2, 3, 7, 8-tetrachlorodibenzo-p-dioxin. Lancet 354:1266–7

Geusau A, Jurecka W, Nahavandi H, et al (2000) Punctate keratoderma-like lesions on the palms and soles in a patient with chloracne. A new clinical manifestation of dioxin intoxication. Br J Dermatol 143:1067–71

Gladen BC, Taylor JS, Wu YC, Ragan NB, Rogan WJ, Hsu CC (1990) Dermatologic findings in children exposed transplacentally to heat-degraded polychlorinated biphenyls in Taiwan. Br J Dermatol 122:799–808

Guo YL, Yu M-L, Hsu C-C, Rogan WJ (1999). Chloracne, goiter, arthritis and anemia after poly-chlorinated biphenyl poisoning: 14 year follow-up of the Taiwan Yucheng Cohort. Environ Health Perspect 107:715–719

Hambrick GS (1957) The effects of substituted napthalenes on the pilosebacious apparatus of rabbit and man. J Invest Dermatol 28:29–103

Hsu MM-L, Mak C-P, Hsu C-C (1995) Follow up of skin manifestations in Yu-Cheng children. Br J Dermatol 122:799–808

Jirasek L, Kalensky J, Kubec K (1973) Acne chlorina and porphyria cutanea tarda during the manufacturing of herbicides Part I. Cesk Dermatol 48:306–317

Kersevovich J, Langenberg A, Odom RB, et al (1992) Dowling-Degos' disease mimicking chloracne. J Am Acad Dermatol 27:345–348

Kligman AM, Mills OH (1972) Acne Cosmetica. Arch Dermatol 106:843–850

Kokelj F (1992) Occupational Acne. Clin Dermatol 10:213–217

Longnecker MP, Rogan WJ, Lucier G (1997) The human health effects of DDT (dichlorodiphenyltrichloroethane) and PCBs (polychlorinated biphenyls) and overview of organochlorines in public health. Ann Rev Public Health 18:211–44

Mathias CGT (1994) Occupational Dermatoses. In: Zenz C, Dickerson OB, Horvath EP (eds) Occupational medicine, 3rd edn. Mosby, St. Louis, pp 93–131

McDonough AJ, Gawkrodger DJ, Walker AE (1993) Chloracne-study of an outbreak with new clinical observations. Clin Exp Dermatol 18:523–525

Mills OH, Kligman A (1975) Acne Mechanica. Arch Dermatol 111:481–483

Mukerjee D (1998) Health impact of polychlorinated dibenzo-p-dioxins: a critical review. J Air Waste Manag Assoc 48:157–165

O'Malley MS, Carpenter AV, Sweeney MH, Fingerhut MA, et al (1990) Chloracne associated with employment in the
production of pentachlorophenol. Am J Ind Med 17:411–421

Omohundro C, Taylor JS (1998) Occupational acne. In: English JSC (ed) A colour handbook of occupational dermatology. Manson, London, pp 121–134

Poskitt LB, Duffill MB, Rademaker M (1994) Chloracne, palmoplantar keratoderma and localized scleroderma in a weed sprayer. Clin Exp Dermatol 19:264–267

Rodriguez-Pichardo A, Camacho F, Rappe C, Hansson M, Smith AG, Greig JB (1991) Chloracne caused by ingestion of olive oil contaminated with PCDDs and PCDFs. Hum Exp Toxicol 10:311–322

Scerri L, Zaki I, Millard LG (1995) Severe halogen acne due to a trifluoromethylpyrazole derivative and its resistance to isotretinoin. Br J Dermatol 132:144–148

Sperling L (1994) Skin disease associated with excessive heat, humidity, and sunlight. In: Zajtchuk R (eds) Textbook of military medicine, part III. Sergent General, Department of the Army, Washington DC, pp 44–45

Sweeney MH, Mocarelli P (2000) Human health effects after exposure to 2, 3, 7, 8 TCDD. Food Addit Contam 17:303–316

Taylor JS (1979) Environmental chloracne: update and overview. Am NY Acad Sci 320:295–307

Taylor JS (1987) Pilosebaceous unit. In: Maibach HI (ed) Occupational and industrial dermatology. Year Book Medical Publishers, Chicago, pp 105–120

Taylor JS, Lloyd KM (1982) Chloracne from 3, 3' and 4,4'-tetrachloroazoxybenzene and 3,3' and 4,4'-tetrachloroazobenzene: update and review. In: Hutzinger O (ed) Chlorinated dioxins and related compounds. Pergamon, Oxford, pp 535–544

Taylor JS, Wuthrich RC, Lloyd KM, Poland A (1977) Chloracne from manufacture of a new herbicide. Arch Dermatol 113:616–619

Upreti RK, Das M, Shanker R (1989) Dermal exposure to kerosene. Vet Hum Toxicol 31:16–20

Vazquez ER, Macias PC, Tirado JG, Solana CG, Casanova A, Moncada JF (1996) Chloracne in the 1990s. Int J Dermatol 35:643–645

Yip J, Peppall L, Gawkrodger DJ, Cunliff WJ (1993) Light cautery and EMLA in the treatment of chloracne lesions. Br J Dermatol 128:313–316

CHAPTER 11

Occupational Nail Disorders 11

R. BARAN

Anatomy

The nail plate emerges from beneath the proximal nail fold, which adheres closely to the nail for a short distance and forms a transverse strip of desquamating tissue, the cuticle (first area of weakness), which seals the nail cul-de-sac. The matrix from which the nail is derived extends approximately 6 mm under the proximal nail fold, but its most distal part is visible as the white semicircular lunula. For most of its length, the nail plate, which has a loose attachment to the matrix, lies distally on a firmly adherent nail bed of highly vascular connective tissue containing glomus organs. It is colorless but translucent, transmitting the pink color of the underlying nail bed. The nail bed epithelium presents with parallel longitudinal rete ridges.

The hyponychium (second area of weakness of the nail apparatus) marks the point at which the nail plate separates from the underlying tissue.

The functions of the nail are multiple 1/ to protect the normal nail bed, 2/ to act as a weapon or as a tool for scraping or gripping small objects, 3/ to provide counter-pressure for the pulp, which is essential to the tactile sensation involving the fingers.

Fingernails grow at a rate of 0.1 mm a day; toenails grow much more slowly.

Definition

Occupational nail diseases are abnormalities of one or more of the tissues of the nail apparatus, produced or aggravated by the working environment. But you should:
1. Rule out nail involvement produced by dermatoses which may present with an isolated symptom and lead to a "false positive" diagnosis (Bennet 1975).
2. Determine if it may be exacerbated, precipitated or revealed by occupational trauma (Baran 1992).
3. Visualize what the hands do at work (Fisher 1992).
4. Look for functional distribution of the lesions, for example, commonly first three fingers of the dominant hand are involved in occupational disease (Ronchese 1962 b).
5. Look for occupational stigmata on the nails.
6. Examine the whole skin surface and mucous membranes.

Table 1. Physical hazards

Burns (onycholysis, pterygium)
Cold (Beau's line, nail shedding, koilonychia) (Dolma 1990)
Dishwashers using heavy rubber gloves (subungual hemorrhages) (Long 1958)
Foreign bodies
Ionizing radiation (Dulanto 1979)
Trauma
Vibrating power tools (discoloration, ridging, nail shedding, carpal tunnel syndrome and Raynaud's phenomenon, also observed in typists, violonists and pianists) (Boyle 1988)

Table 2. Acute injuries (Baran 1994)

Acute injuries may be associated with:
  Partial or total hematoma
  Lacerating wounds
  Fractures of the terminal phalanx
  Denudation of the terminal phalanx

Table 3. Delayed post acute traumatic deformities (Baran 1994)

Onycholysis
Split nail deformity
Pterygium
Various nail dystrophies
Hooked nail

Table 4. Workers affected by repeated micro trauma associated with koilonychia. In time, nail changes may become irreversible

Automotive workers (Dawber 1974)
Cabinet makers
Cement workers
Chimney sweeps
Coil winders (Smith 1980)
Glass workers
Hairdressers (thioglycolates) (Alanko 1997)
Homemakers
Mushroom growers (Schubert 1977)
Oil burner repairers (Meyer-Hamme 1983)
Organic chemist (organic solvents) (Ancona-Alayon 1975)
Pin threaders
Rickshaw puller (feet) (Bentley-Philips 1971)
Slaughterhouse workers (Forck 1971)

Table 5. Workers/work tasks affected by repeated microtrauma associated with fingernail fragility. This leads to a gradual destruction of the nail plate, which becomes brittle and atrophic. Nail fragility may occur in isolation or be associated with paronychia and/or onycholysis

Bean shellers and potatoes peelers *(paronychia)*
Butchers
Cement workers
Chemists and laboratory workers *(paronychia)*
Dentist *(onycholysis, subungual hyperkeratosis, dermatitis)*
Engravers *(paronychia)*
Etchers *(paronychia)*
File-makers
Glaziers *(paronychia)*
Hat cleaners *(paronychia)*
Nurses
Optical glass handlers
Packers
Painters *(paronychia)*
Photographers *(paronychia, discoloration)*
Plasterers *(corroded nails)*
Porcelain workers *(serrated nails)*
Pottery workers
Radio workers *(paronychia and nail loss)*
Rope workers
Shoe-shiners
Shoemakers *(onycholysis and paronychia)*
Silk weavers (Ronchese 1955)
Wet work *(paronychia)*
Wood workers *(paronychia and stains)*
Workers exposed to microwave radiation *(onycholysis)*
Workers handling small instruments
Workers lifting repeatedly heavy plastic bags (Schubert 1977)

Table 6. Workers/athletes/performers affected by repeated microtrauma associated with toenail dystrophy

Dancers (exostosis) (Sebastian 1977)
Rickshaw pullers (koilonychia) (Bentley-Philips)
Miners (onychomycosis) Gugnani 1989)
Sportsmen (hematoma; nail shedding)
 Athletes
 Joggers
 Walkers
 Squash players
 Soccer players
 Tennis players

Table 7. Workers/work tasks affected by repeated microtrauma associated with onycholysis of mechanical origin (Forck 1967; Ronchese 1962; Somov 1976)

Chicken-processing plant workers
Cropping
Fur workers
Milking
Nut cracking
Poultry plucking
Separating meat from bone
Scraping
Shell casing
Destalking mushrooms

Table 8. Foreign bodies that cause onycholyisis associated with repeated microtrauma. This may be associated with an acute trauma (metal) or repeated microtrauma (in hair dressers, for example)

Animal (bristles, sea urchin, oyster shell)	
Metal, glass, fiber glass (Rogailin 1975), plastic	They may also produce paronychia and bacterial infection.
Splinters of hair (Buendia-Eisman 1997)	
Vegetable (thorn, splinter, hyacinth and narcissus bulbs raphide cells with crystals of calcium oxalate) (Hjorth 1968)	

Occupational onycholysis is most frequently due to chemical irritants or sensitizers. In addition, there are infective causes, which tend to be limited to medical personnel and occupations, which entail prolonged soaking of the hands (*Candida* and *Pseudomonas*)

Occupational traumatic abnormalities in the nail area represent one of the most important chapters in this field. This includes major trauma, repeated microtrauma and foreign body injury. Tables 1–9 presents an overview of these areas and the occupations associated with them.

Variations in Color

The term chromonychia indicates an abnormality in color of the substance and surface of the nail plate and/or subungual tissues.

Abnormalities of color depend on the transparency of the nail, its attachment to the underlying tissues and the character of the latter (Tables 10–12).

Bacterial Infections

The usual microorganisms which may develop in abrasions or lacerations of the nail area are coagulase-positive staphylococci and various streptococci (Barnham

Table 9. Workers/work tasks affected by paronychia

Agricultural workers
Automotive workers (sulphuric acid exposure from batteries)
Bakers and pastry cooks
Barbers and hairdresser (onycholysis)
Bartenders
Bean shellers
Book binders (paste)
Bricklayers (limes, cement, mortar)
Builders and carpenters (including glass fibre)
Button makers
Cement workers
Chemists and laboratory workers
Chicken factory workers
Cooks
Cosmetic workers
Dentists (Kanerva 1997)
Dyers (aniline dyes, producing stains and necrosis)
Engravers, glass etchers (brittle nail)
Fishermen
Fishmongers
Florist and gardeners (onycholysis) (hyacinth, narcissus bulbs, tulip fingers)
(fungal infection)
Glaziers (brittle nail)
Ground keepers
Hair dresser
Janitorial and domestic workers
Meat handlers
Mechanics
Milkers (onycholysis from bristle)
Oil-rig workers
Painters
Photographic developers (brittle nail, discoloration)
Pianists
Physicians, dentists' nurses
Potato peelers
Radio workers (methanol, causing pigmentation and nail loss)
Salt plant workers (ulcers)
Shoes workers (brittle nails)
Tanners (whitlow)
Textile workers (threads of fabric)
Violonists (nail dystrophy)
Wood workers (brittle nails, stains)
Wool workers (wool thread)

Table 10. Variations in color of the nail plate

Sign	Workers affected
Leuconychia	Arsenic workers
	Butchers
	Keypunchers (Roberts 1984)
	Salt plant workers and those in contact with salted intestines (Honda 1976; Ferreira Marques 1939)
	Weedkillers (paraquat) (Frenk 1966; Botella 1985)
	Workers manufacturing thallium rodenticides
	Fly tier's finger (apparent leuconychia) (Dobbelaere 1974)
Blue	Anodizers (aluminum)
	Local argyria (MacAulay 1990; Bergfeld 1987)
	Auto mechanics (oxalic acid in radiators)
	Cyanosis from methaemoglobinemia or sulphhaemoglobinemia
	Dye makers
	Electroplaters
	Gold plasters
	Metal cleaners, metal patina solution
	Ink makers
	Paints removers
	Photographers
	Rust removers
	Silver workers (presenting generalized argyria) (Sarsfield 1992)
	Textile workers
Brown/Black	Cigar makers
	Cobblers
	Coffee bean workers
	Cooks and bakers (burnt sugar)
	Electric bulb cleaners (hydrochloric acid)
	Gunsmith
	Hairdressers
	Photographers
	Roadway pavers
	Shoe-shiners
	Vintners (red wine)
	Walnut pickers (pecans)
	Woodworkers (varnish)
	Woodworkers (ebony, mahogany) (Harris 1989)
Green (usually caused by *Pseudomonas* infection)	Bartenders
	Dish-washers
	Electricians
	Fruit handlers
	Laundry workers
	Metallurgists
	Restaurant workers
	Sugar factory workers

Table 10 (continued)

Sign	Workers affected

Yellow	Epoxy system handlers
	  Metaphenylenediamine (Cohen 1985)
	  4,4'-Methylenedianiline (Cohen 1985)
	Flower handlers
	Pesticide workers
	  Diquat (Samman 1961; Clark 1970)
	  Paraquat (Hearn 1971)
	  Dinitro-orthocresol (Baran 1974)
	  Dinobuton (Wahlberg 1974)
	Workers handling chromium salts
	Workers handling dyestuffs
	  Dinitrosalicylic acid (Fregert 1980)
	  Dinitrobenzene
	  Dinitrotoluene
	  Trinitrotoluene

Table 11. Chemical sensitizers. (Contact sensitization occurring through the nail plate is probably rare. Usually sensitizers alter the distal sub- and periungual tissue)

Flowers and plants	Alstroemeria (onycholysis) (Rycroft 1981; Marks 1988) Hydrangea (paronychia) (Bruynzeel 1986) Nasturtium (finger tip dermatitis) (Derrick 1997) Tabernaemontana coronaria (finger tip dermatitis) (Bajaj 1996) Tulip fingers (painful onycholysis and fissured keratotic eczema) (Gette 1990) Rhus dermatitis from poison ivy, oak and sumac (onycholysis, yellowish discoloration of the nail) (Fulghum 1972)
Chemicals	Acrylic resins[a] (Kanerva 1997; Kanerva 1997) "Cain" (local anesthetics) and propanidid (Castalain 1980) Cement dermatitis from dichromate content (koilonychia, fissures) Codein (onycholysis, subungual hyperkeratosis, nail atrophy) (Romaguera 1983) Ethyl cyanoacrylate (Shelley 1988) Epoxy resin (Castelain) Hydroxylamine (onycholysis, paronychia) (Baran 1991) 1-methylquinoxalinium-p-toluen sulphonate (periungual dermatitis) (English 1986) Mydriatic agents containing tropicamid and phenylephrin hydrochloride (nurses) (Okamoto 1991) Nonoxynol-6 (transverse nail dystrophy) (Nethercott 1984) Quaternium 15 (subungual hyperkeratosis, onycholysis) (Marren 1991) p-Tertiary butyl phenol formaldehyde (onycholysis subungual hyperkeratosis, nail atrophy, periungual dermatitis) (Rycroft 1980) Thiourea (Dooms-Goossens 1988) Turpentine (periungal dermatitis, subungual hyperkeratosis)
Protein contact dermatitis	Baits (onycholysis, paronychia) (Montel 1957) Food animal origin (food handlers) (Tosti 1992) Vegetable origin

Table 12. Chemical irritants

Alkalis
Alkaline chlorine-containing compounds (Coskey 1974)
Aminoethyletanolamine-containing soldering flux (onycholysis, periungual dermatitis)
(Goh 1985)
Detergents (onycholysis, subungual bleeding ulcerations) (Göthe 1972)
Formaldehyde
Gold potassium cyanide (purplish-brown discoloration, onycholysis) in electroplaters,
electronic workers (Budden 1978)
Hydrofluoric acid (excruciating pain, onycholysis) (Shewmake 1979; Baran 1980)
Organic solvents and motor oils (onycholysis, subungal hyperkeratosis, nail softening)
Oxalic acid (bluish discoloration, brittle nails)

Table 13. Viral infections

Herpes simplex (Rames 1984; Kanaar 1967; Rosato 1970; Hsedicke 1989; Amichai 1993)
Human orf (Groves 1991)
Milker's nodule
Viral warts (Jablonska 1987; Aloi 1988; Keefe 1994; Moragon 1987; Rülinger 1984)

Table 14. Fungal infections

Fungal agent	Occupational realm
Candida spp (onycholysis paronychia)[a]	Dishwashers, poultry and fish handlers
Dermatophytic toenail infection	Increased prevalence in ore miners
T. rubrum is the most common dermatophyte,	(Tappeiner 1966) and others who work
sometimes responsible for the one hand-two	in hot, humid environment
foot tinea syndrome	
T. mentagrophytes var. *interdigitale*	Washing facilities
Molds, especially *scytalidium* spp. involves	Miners
the toenails	

[a] *Candida* fungal infection of the nail area is a common condition involving occupations which require the hands to be wet for prolonged periods.

Table 15. Individuals at risk of fungal infections (Baran 1997)

Athletes
Dustmen
Employees of indoor swimming pools
Excavation workers
Mine workers
Rubber-industry workers
Sewage workers
Soldiers
Steel and furnace workers
Wood-cutters

Table 16. Occupational systemic conditions

Condition	Exposure to
Clubbing (resulting from pneumoconiotic lung diseases)	Asbestos (Petry 1966) Talc Berryllium (Kern 1990) Silica Cobalt (Desoille 1962) Tungsten (Desoille 1962)
Pseudoclubbing (systemic sclerosis with acroosteolysis)	Vinyl chloride monomer
Cutaneous hemangioendothelioma	Polyvinyl chloride (Davis 1990)
Collagen diseases Systemic sclerosis	Vinyl chloride monomer Epoxy resin (vapors) Trichlorethylene, trichlorethane Silica (Rustin 1989)
Sclerodactyly (nail fold capillary changes, Raynaud's phenomenon, acroosteolysis) (Bachurzewska 1989; Flindt-Hansen 1987)	
Lupus eythematosus-like erythema and periungual telangiectasia	Substances on coffee plantations (Narahari 1990) (workers)

1984; Barnham 1980) (Tables 13–16). *Pseudomonas* infection is responsible for the green nail syndrome. Such infected nails, in health care personnel, may then be a source of nosocomial infections especially from nurses with artificial nails in whom Serratia, Acinobacter and *Pseudomonas* have been found.

Acute paronychia is frequent enough in meat handlers (Barnham 1984). Erysipeloid infection is rare and can be observed in meat and fish handlers. Prosector's wart [tuberculosis verruca cutis (Goette 1978)] has its source in a tuberculous infected cadaver. It may be seen in pathologists, morgue attendants and other hospital personnel.

In mycobacterium marinum infection (Califano 1998), called fish-tank granuloma or swimming-pool granuloma, the association of skin infection with aquariums and tropical fish has been noted. A prick from a rose thorn might also cause the infection. This is characterized by the presence of one papule, nodule, or erythematous plaque with a verrucous surface on the dorsum of the distal phalanx of the finger.

Pasteurella tularensis is transmitted to man by direct contact with infected wildlife (rabbits are the principal reservoirs of tularemia in nature). Over half the patients with any cutaneous ulcers, present with multiple lesions including shallow erosions into the subungual tissues (Young 1969).

References

Alanko K, Kanerva L, Estlander T et al (1997) Hairdresser's koilonychia. Am J Contact Derm 8:177–178

Aloi FG, Molinero A, Passera A et al (1988) Viral warts in butchers. Clinical and statistical study. G Ital Dermatol Venereol 123:341–344

Amichai B, Grunwald MH, Abraham A et al (1993) Tense bullous lesions on fingers. Arch Dermatol 129:1043–1048

Ancona-Alayon A (1975) Occupational koilonychia from organic solvents. Contact Derm. 1:367–369

Bachurzewska B, Boruka I (1986) Dermatosen in Beruf und Umwelt. Occup Environm Derm 34:77–79

Bajaj AK, Pasricha JS, Gupta S et al (1996) Tabernaemontana coronaria causing fingertip dermatitis. Contact Derm 35:104–105

Baran R, Dawber RPR (1994) Nail diseases and their management. Blackwell Science. Oxford

Baran R, Levy JL (1992) Onychopathies et travail. Rev Med Travail 19:47–49

Baran R (1974) Nail damage caused by weed killers and insecticides. Arch Dermatol 110:467

Baran R (1991) Onycholysis from hydroxylamine. Contact Derm 24:158

Baran R (1997) Epidemiology and prevention of onycholysis. In Grob JJ, Stern RS, Mackie RM, Weinstock WA (eds) Epidemiology, causes and prevention of skin diseases. Blackwell Science, Oxford, pp 276–278

Barnham M, Kerby J (1984) A profile of skin sepsis in meat handlers. J Infect 9:43–50

Barnham M, Kerby J, Skillin J (1980) An outbreak of streptococcal infection in a chicken factory. J Hyg Camb 84:71–75

Bennet JH (1975) The "false positive" diagnosis: skin disorders that mimic an occupational dermatitis. Cutis 15:410–411

Bentley-Philips B, Bayles MAH (1971) Occupational koilonychia in toenails. Br J Dermatol (85) 140–144

Bergfeld WF, McMahon JT (1987) Cutaneous metalloid hyperpigmentation. In: Callen JP, Dahl MV, Golitz LE, Stegman SJ (eds) Advances in dermatology, vol 1, Yearbook, Chicago, pp 123–124

Botella R, Sastre A, Castells A (1985) Contact dermatitis to paraquat. Contact Derm 13:123–124

Boyle JC, Smith NJ, Burke FD (1988) Vibration white finger. Hand Surg 13B:171–175

Bruynzeel DP (1986) Allergic contact dermatitis to hydrangea. Contact Derm 14: 128

Budden MG, Wilkinson DS (1978) Skin and nail lesions from gold potassium cyanide. Contact Derm 4:172–173

Buendia-Eisman A, Serrano-Ortegas, Ortega del Olmo RM (1997) Hair fragments as a subungual foreign body. Eur J Dermatol 7:517–518

Califano L, Cannavo SP, Malara G et al (1998) Verrucous nodule of the finger. Arch Dermatol. 134:365–366

Castelain PY and Piriou A (1980) Contact dermatitis due to propanidid in an anesthetist. Contact Derm 6:360

Castelain PY, Com J and Castelain M (1992) Occupational dermatitis in the aircraft industry: 35 years of progress. Contact Derm 27:311–316

Clark DG and Hurst EW (1970) The toxicity of diquat. Br J Indust Med 27:51–55

Cohen SR (1985) Yellow staining caused by 4,4′-methylenedianiline exposure. Arch Dermatol 121:1022–1027

Coskey RJ (1974) Onycholysis from sodium hypochlorite. Arch Dermatol 109:96

Davis MFP, Curtis M, Howat JMT (1990) Cutaneous hemangioendothelioma: possible link with chronic exposure to vinyl chloride. Br J Indust Med 47:65–67

Dawber R (1974) Occupational koilonychia. Br J Dermatol. 91 [Suppl 10]:11

De Berker D, Dawber R, Wojnarowska F (1994) Subungual hair implantation in hairdressers. Br J Dermatol 130:400–401

Derrick E, Darley C (1997) Contact dermatitis to nasturtium.Br J Dermatol 136:287–299

Desoille H, Brouet G, Assouly M et al (1962) Fibrose pulmonaire diffuse chez un sujet exposé aux poussières de cobalt et de carbure de tungstène. Arch Mal Prof 23:570–578

Dobbelaere F and Bouffioux J (1974) Leuconychia en bandes due au paraquat. Arch Dermatol 30:283–384

Dolma T, Norboo T, Yayha M et al (1990). Seasonal koilonychia in Ladakh. Contact Derm 22:78–80

Dooms-Goossens A, Dubusschère K, Morren M et al (1988) Silver polish: another source of contact dermatitis reactions to thiourea. Contact Derm 19:133–135

Dulanto (De) F, Camacho F (1979) Radiodermatitis. Acta Derm Sif 70:67–94

English JSC, White IR, Rycroft RJC (1986) Sensitization by 1-methylquinoxalinium-*p*-toluene sulfonate. Contact Derm 14:261–262

Ferreira Marques J (1939) Une forme particulière de leuconychie, la leuconychie en large bande longitudinale (stigmate professionel). Ann Dermatol 10:688–691

Fisher AA, Baran R (1992) Occupational nail disorders with a reference to Koebner's phenomenon. Am J Contact Derm 3:404–406

Flindt-Hansen H, Isager H (1987) Scleroderma after occupational exposure to trichlorethylen et trichloretane. Acta Derm Venereol 67:263–264

Forck G, Kästner H (1967) Charakteristische onycholysis traumatica bei Fleissbandarbeiter in Geflügelschlachterei. Hautarzt 18:85–87

Fregert S, Trulson L (1980) Yellow stained skin from dinitrosalicylic acid. Contact Derm 6:362

Frenk F, Leu F (1966) Leukonychie durch beruflichn Kontakt mit gesalzenen Därmen. Hautarzt 17:233–235

Fulghum DD (1972) Allergic contact onycholysis due to poison ivy oleoresin. Contact Derm Newsletter 11:266

Gette MT, Marks JE (1990) Tulip fingers. Arch Dermatol. 126:203–205

Goette DK, Jacobson KW, Doty RD (1978) Primary inoculation tuberculosis of the skin. Prosector's paronychia. Arch Dermatol 114:567

Goh CI (1985) Occupational dermatitis from soldering flux among workers in electronic industry. Contact Derm 13:85–90

Göthe CJ, Nilzen A, Holmgren A et al (1972) Medical problems in the detergent industry caused by proteolytic enzymes from bacillus subtiles. Acta Allerg 27:63

Groves RW, Wilson-Jones E, MacDonald DM (1991) Human orf and milkers nodules: a clinico pathologic study. J Am Acad Dermatol 25:706–711

Gugnani HC, Oyeka CA (1989) Foot infections due to Hendersonula toruloidea and Scytalidium hyalinun in coal miners. J Med Vet Mycol. 27:169–179

Haedicke GJ, Crossman JAI, Fisher AE (1989) Herpetic whitlow of the digits. J Hand Surg 14B:443–446

Harris AO, Rosen T (1989) Nail discoloration due to mahogany. Cutis 43:55–56

Hearn CED, Keir W (1971) Nail damage in spray operators exposed to paraquat. Br J Indust Med 28:399

Hjorth N, Wilkinson DS (1968) Contact dermititis. 4. Tulip fingers, hyacinth itch and lily rash. Br J Dermatol 80:696

Honda M, Hattori S, Koyama L et al (1976) Leukonychia striae. Arch Dermatol 112:1147

Jablonska S, Obalek S, Favre M et al (1987). The morphology of butcher's warts as related to papilloma-virus types. Arch Dermatol Res 279:566–572

Kanaar P (1967) Primary herpes simplex infection of fingers in nurses. Dermatologica 134:346

Kanerva L, Estlander T, Jolanki R (1997) Occupational allergic contact dermatitis caused by acrylic tri-cure glass ionomer. Contact Derm 37:49–50

Kanerva L, Henricks-Eckerman ML, Jolanki R et al (1997) Plastics/acrylics: material safety data sheets need to be improved. Clin Dermatol 15:533–546

Kanerva L, Henriks-Eckerman ML, Estlander T et al (1997) Dentists's occupational allergic paronychia and contact dermatitis caused by acrylics. Eur J Dermatol 7:177–180

Kanerva L, Jolanki R, Estlander T (1997) 10 years of patch testing with the (meth)acrylate series. Contact Derm 37: 255–258.

Kanerva L, Mikola H, Henriks-Eckerman ML et al (1998) Fingertip paresthesia and occupational allergic contact dermatitis caused by acrylics in a dental nurse. Contact Derm 38:114–116

Keefe M, al Ghamdi A, Coggon D et al (1994) Cutaneous warts in butchers. Br J Dermatol 130:9–14

Kern DG (1990) Occupational disease. In: Scher R, Daniel C (eds). Nails: therapy, diagnosis, surgery. Saunders, Philadelphia, pp 224–243

Long PI (1958) Subungual hemorrhage in pan washer. JAMA 168:1226

MacAulay JC (1990) Fly tiers finger. Can J Dermatol 2:67

Marks JG (1988) Allergic contact dermatitis to alstroemeria. Arch Dermatol 124:914–916

Marren P, de Berker D, Dawber R et al (1991) Occupational contact dermatitis due to quaternium 15 presenting as nail dystrophy. Contact Derm 25:253–255

Meyer-Hamme S, Quadripur SA (1983) Berufsbedingte koilonychia. Hautarzt 34:577–579

Montel MI, Gouyer E (1957) L'Escavenite. Bull Soc Fr Dermatol Syphil 64:672

Moragon M, Ibanez MD, San Juan L et al (1987) L'incidence des verrues vulgaireschez les travailleurs d'abattoirs industriels de volaille de la province de Valence. Arch Mal Prof 48:41–43

Narahari SR, Skiniva CR, Kelkar SK (1990) LE-like erythema and periungual telangiectasia among coffee plantations workers. Contact Derm 22:296–297

Nethercott JR, Lawrence MJ (1984) Allergic contact dermatitis due to nonoxylphenol ethoxylate. Contact Derm 10:235–239

Okamoto H, Kawai S (1991) Allergic contact sensitivity to mydriatic agents on a nurse's fingers. Cutis 47:357–358

Petry H (1966) Uhrglasnägel und Trommelschlegelfinger bei Asbestose. Int Arch Geweberpath Gewerberghyg 22:55–59

Rames S, Folkmar Tand Roed-Petersen B (1984) Herpes simplex as a possible occupational disease in dentists of the county of Aarhus, Denmark. Acta Derm Venereol 64:163–165

Roberts AHN (1984) Subungual melanoma following a single injury. J Hand Surg 9B:328–330

Rogaïlin VI, Selisski GD, Zakharov GA (1975) Clinical characteristic of skin disease in production of glass fibre. Sovietsk Med 9:154

Romaguera C, Grimalt F (1983) Dermatitis de contacto profesional por codeina. Bol Inform G.E.I.D.C. 5:21–2.

Ronchese F (1955) Peculiar silk weavers nails. A new type of artefact. Arch Dermatol. 71:525–526

Ronchese F (1962) Nail defect and occupational trauma. Arch Dermatol 85:404

Ronchese F (1962 b) Nails: injuries and disease in traumatic medicine and surgery for the attorney, vol 6. Butterworth, Washington, pp 626–639

Rosato FE, Rosato EF, Plotkin SA (1970) Herpetic paronychia, an occupational hazard of medical personnel. New Engl J Med 282:804–805

Rosenthal EA (1983) Treatment of fingertip and nail bed injuries. Orthop Clin N Am 14:675–697

Rüdlinger R, Bunney MH, Grab R et al (1984) Warts in fish handlers. Br J Dermatol 120:375–381

Rustin MHA, Bull HA, Ziegler V et al. (1989) Silica exposure and silica-associated systemic sclerosis. Br J Dermatol 121 [Suppl 34]:29–30

Rycroft RJG, Calnan CD (1981) Alstroemeria dermatitis. Contact Derm 7:284

Rycroft RJG, Wilkinson JD, Homes R et al (1980) Contact sensitization to p-tertiary butylphenol (PTBP) resin in plastic nail adhesive. Contact Derm 5:441–445

Samman PD (1961) Onychia due to synthetic nail coverings. Experimental studies. Trans St Johns Hosp Dermatol Soc 46:68–73

Sarsfield P, White JE, Theaker JM (1992) Silverworker's finger: an unusual occupational hazard mimicking a melanocytic lesion. Histopathology 20:73–75

Schubert B, Minard JJ, Baran R et al (1977) Onychopathie des champignonnistes. Ann Dermatol Venereol (Paris) 104:627–630

Sebastian G (1977) Subungual Exostose der Grosszehe: Berufsstigma bei Tänzern. Derm Monatsschr 163:998–1000

Shelley DE, Shelley WB (1988) Nail dystrophy and periungual dermatitis due to cyanoacrylate glue sensitivity. J Am Acad Dermatol 19:574–575

Shewmake SW, Anderson BG (1979) Hydrofluoric acid burns. Arch Dermatol 115:593–596

Smith SJ, Yoder FW, Know DW (1980) Occupational koilonychia. Arch Dermatol 116:861

Somov BA, Lipets ME, Ivanov VV et al (1976) Occupational onycholysis. Vestn Derm Venereol 2:51–55

Tappeiner J, Male O (1966) Nagelveränderungen durch Schimmelpilze. Derm Int 5:145

Tosti A, Guerra L, Morelli R et al (1992) Role of foods in the pathogenesis of chronic paronychia. J Am Acad Dermatol. 27:706–710

Wahlberg JE (1974) Yellow staining of hair and nails and contact sensitivity to dinobuton. Contact Derm Newsl 16:481

Young IS, Bicknell DS, Archer BG et al (1969) Tularemia epidermic: Vermont, 1968. Forty-seven cases linked to contact with muskrats. New Engl J Med 280:1253

CHAPTER 12

Non-Eczematous Occupational Contact Reactions 12

C.L. GOH

Introduction

Contact reactions may present as non-eczematous lesions. The following non-eczematous contact reactions have been described:
1. Erythema multiforme-like eruption [urticarial papules and plaque eruptions (UPPE)]
2. Purpuric eruption
3. Lichen planus-like eruption
4. Papular and nodular eruption
5. Granulomatous reaction
6. Pustular eruption
7. Erythema and exfoliation
8. Pseudoscleroderma

Erythema Multiforme-Like Reaction (UPPEs)

Several contact allergens, e.g., metal, topical medicaments, wood and industrial chemicals have been reported to cause "erythema multiforme-like" eruptions. These allergic contact reactions can be confirmed by positive patch-test reactions. The morphology of these reactions includes target-like erythemacular, and urticarial lesions. Such eruptions have been described as UPPE to distinguish them from the erythema-multiforme (Goh 1989).

Clinical Features

The characteristic presentation is usually an eczematous lesion on the primary contact site followed shortly with urticarial, papular and plaque lesions on the primary contact site, spreading to adjacent skin and occasionally distant sites.

Patch Test

In all cases, a positive patch test to the contact allergen can be elicited. The patch-test reaction is always eczematous.

Histology

The epidermis is normal or shows mild spongiosis with upper dermal edema and perivascular lymphohistiocytic infiltrate. Vacuolar degeneration of the basal cells is occasionally present. Goh postulated that the allergen is absorbed percutaneously and evokes an allergic contact dermatitis at the primary site, while concurrently forming immune complexes with a circulating antibody (Goh 1989).

Woods and Plants

Holst et al. (1976) described three carpenters who developed erythema multiforme-like eruption from contact allergy to three different tropical woods – Rio rosewood (Dalbergia nigra), pao ferro (Mackerium scleroxylon) and Euculyptus saligna. The antigen in pao ferro was R-3,4-dimethoxy-dalbergione. A wooden bracelet (Fisher 1986) and pendant (Fisher and Bikowski 1981) made from Dalbergia nigra were also reported to cause erythema multiforme-like eruption. The specific chemical antigen was identified as quinone R-4-methoxy-dalbergione (Hausen 1981). Non-occupational causes have also been reported. Irvine et al. (1988) reported reaction to pao ferro (Machaerium scleroxylon) in a hobbyist handling the wood. Plants reported to cause erythema multiforme-like eruption include poison ivy (Toxicodendron) (Schwartz and Downham 1981; Mallory et al. 1982), primula (Primula obconica) (Hjorth 1966) and mugwort (Artemesia vulgaris) (Kurz and Rapaport 1979). Mallory et al. (1982) reported urticarial eruptions with black deposits on the skin of four patients with Toxidocendron radicansdermatitis. Urticaria, erythema multiforme-like eruptions, in a patient with Rhus dermatitis was reported by Schwartz and Downham (1981). They recommended that patients with such reactions should be screened for systemic involvement as previous reports have shown that nephritis can be an associated feature (Meneghini and Angelini 1981; Fisher 1986).

Metals and Chemicals

Non-occupational UPPE from nickel was first described by Calnan (1956). Cook reported UPPE in a 13-year-old girl due to allergic contact dermatitis from nickel and cobalt from the metal studs in jeans (Cook 1982). Friedman and Perry (1985) described a garment worker who developed UPPE on her hands from nickel dermatitis from her scissors.

Laboratory Chemicals

9-bromofluorene has been reported to cause UPPE (De Feo 1966). A phenyl sulfone derivative was incriminated as a cause of UPPE (Roed-Petersen 1975).

Industrial Chemicals

Nethercott et al. (1982) reported of four men working with printed circuit boards who developed erythema multiforme. Formaldehyde was suspected to be the cause of the eruption since two of the workers gave a positive reaction to formaldehyde. Trichloroethylene was suspected to cause erythema multiforme in five workers in an electronic factory in Singapore (Phoon et al. 1984).

Goh (1988) reported erythema multiforme-like eruption in a worker with contact allergy to trinitrotoluene in an ammunitions factory. Patch test to trinitrotoluene was strongly positive.

Recently, contact dermatitis to natural rubber latex was also reported to cause UPPE (Bourrain et al. 1996). Airborne erythema multiforme-like eruptions were also reported in individuals exposed to pyrethrum (Garcia-Bravo et al. 1995).

Pigmented Purpuric Reaction

Occupational contact allergy occasionally presents as purpuric eruption. The eruption may or may not be preceded by erythema or itch. Percutaneous absorption of contact allergens appears to form immune complexes with a circulating antibody that becomes deposited in the microvasculature, producing the vasculitic lesions. However, such immune complexes cannot be identified (Calnan and Peachey 1971). Purpuric eruption associated with allergic contact dermatitis to rubber chemical phenyl-nisopropyl PPD (IPPD) in clothing was described by Batschvarov and Minkov in 1968. Allergic contact dermatitis to IPPD, in rubber boots, was also reported to cause a purpuric eruption (Calnan and Peachey 1971). Fisher (1974) reported similar eruptions in three patients caused by a rubber diving suit, elasticized shorts and a rubberized support bandage. Romaguera and Grimalt (1977) reported similar eruption from IPPD in a rubberized brassiere. Shmunes (1978) reported purpuric allergic contact dermatitis to paraphenylenediamine from black hats.

Lichen Planus-Like and Lichenoid Reaction

Occupational allergic contact dermatitis to some color developers may manifest as lichen planus-like eruptions. Such eruptions often present as itchy, dusky or violaceous papules or plaques on areas of skin exposed to the allergen. The eruptions clear when the allergen is removed. The histological features of patients with lichen planus-like eruptions from color developer pose interesting features. Buckley (1958), Canizares (1959) and Hyman and Berger (1959) reported the histology as compatible with lichen planus in a number of instances, but some authors reported nonspecific chronic dermatitis changes. Fry reported that only two of five patients' biopsies showed histology suggestive of lichen planus (Fry 1965). Kodak CD2 (4-diethyl-2-methylphenylenediamine), Kodak CD3 (4-ethyl-2-methanesulfonylaminoethyl-2-methyl-phenylenediamine sesquisulfate monohydrate), Agfa TSS (4-amino-diethylanilinesulfate), Ilford MI 210 (ethyl-[5-hydroxy-amyl] paraphenylenediamine hydrogen sulfate), and Kodak CD4 (2-amino-5-ethyl- [beta hydroxyethyl] amino toluene sulfate) are reported allergens (Goh et al. 1984).

Recently, lichen planus-like eruptions have been reported from contact with methacrylic acids esters used in the car industry. Histologically, the lesions showed all the features of classical lichen planus. Patch testing revealed positive reactions to methacrylic acid esters (Kawamura et al. 1996).

Nodular and Papular Reactions

Contact allergy to gold has been reported to cause papular and nodular eruptions (Shelly 1963). These occurred peculiarly on the earlobes after ear piercing with gold earrings. Similar eruptions have been observed on the hands and forearms of gold electroplaters who develop contact allergy to gold salts. The eruptions characteristically persist for months after the patients have avoided contact with metallic gold (Petros and Macmillan 1973). In some patients, the patch test also evokes an unusual reaction; the reaction is infiltrative and tends to persist for months (Monti et al. 1983). The reaction to gold in these individuals appeared to provoke lymphoplasia. Histology of such eruptions or its patch test reaction may show dense lympho-monocytic infiltrate in the dermis (Iwatsuki et al. 1982).

Granulomatous Reaction

Contact reactions to metals and metallic salts can manifest as granulomatous lesions. Skin injury from zirconium, silica, magnesium, beryllium may cause granulomas (Rubin 1956). Some reactions are due to delayed-type allergic reaction and some are nonallergic reactions. Clinically, the granulomatous eruptions appear as inflamed papules. Eczema is usually present but pruritus is usually minimal. The histology shows epithelioid cells and may be indistinguishable from sarcoid.

Contact with sheep wool has been reported to cause granulomatous eruptions. Each diseased skin area was closely related to the tight contact with the sheep's wool and, on histological slides, each granuloma was centered by a tiny ply of wool (Lambert et al. 1995).

Pustular Reaction

Pustular reaction to contactant was first observed in patch-test reaction. The pustules are sterile and are transient. Fisher et al. (1959) reported that metallic salts, e.g., nickel, copper, arsenic and mercurial salts, may produce pustular reaction. Stone and Johnson explained that such reactions may represent an enhanced reaction of prior inflammation, rather than an irritant or allergic reaction, because such a reaction can be elicited in non-nickel-sensitive patients (Stone and Johnson 1967). Hjorth reported that atopics are more predisposed to such reactions (Hjorth 1977). Wahlberg and Maibach believed that such pustular reactions are usually irritant in nature but may also be a manifestation of allergic reactions (Wahlberg and Maibach 1981).

Conde-Salazar reported a subcorneal pustular eruption in a patient with trichloroethylene exposure (Conde-Salazar et al. 1983). The patient reacted systemically upon cutaneous challenge test made by exposing only the right leg to an environment saturated with trichloroethylene (to avoid inhalation) with reappearance of erythema on the exposed area within a few hours and fleeting exanthema on the trunk and in the flexures.

Erythema and Exfoliation

Exposure to trichloroethylene, appears to cause localized or generalized erythema with or without papular and/or vesicular eruption to be followed by skin exfoliation. The skin reaction is believed to be a toxic or allergic reaction from percutaneous or mucosal absorption of the chemicals.

Trichloroethylene

Generalized erythema followed by exfoliation after exposure to trichloroethylene was reported by Schwartz et al. (1947). It was believed to be due to systemic sensitization to trichloroethylene. Similar eruption was also documented by Bauer and Rabens (1977).

Nakayama et al. (1988) also reported a generalized erythema and exfoliation with mucous membrane involvement in a patient exposed to trichloroethylene. The patient had a positive patch-test reaction to trichloroethylene and trichloroethanol (its metabolite). Goh and Ng (1988) reported of a patient with recurrent localized erythematous xerotic plaques, which became parched and fissured on the arms and trunk of a patient with trichloroethylene. The route of entry of trichloroethylene was from the respiratory tract and it was believed to be a form of systemic trichloroethylene toxicity in a sensitized individual.

Methyl Bromide

Exposure to methyl bromide caused sharply demarcated erythema with vesiculation in six workers during fumigation work (Hezemans-Boer et al. 1988). Plasma bromide levels after exposure strongly suggested percutaneous absorption of methyl bromide. The lesions were especially more prominent on skin that was relatively moist or subject to mechanical pressure, such as axillae, groin and abdomen. Microscopically, early skin lesions revealed necrosis of keratinocytes, severe edema of the upper dermis, subepidermal blistering and diffuse infiltration of neutrophils.

Scleroderma-Like Reaction

Solvents have been reported as predisposing or eliciting factors in some patients with scleroderma-like reaction. The reaction is suspected to result from repeated cutaneous contact with the solvent. The pathogenic mechanism is unknown. Walder (1983) reported six scleroderma patients who had close contact with aromatic hydrocarbon solvents, such as benzene, toluene and white spirit. The associated scleroderma is limited to the skin of hands and feet where the direct contact took place.

Yamakage and Ishikawa (1982) also reported that various aliphatic hydrocarbons, such as naphtha,-hexane, and hexachloroethane, can induce a generalized morphea-like sclerosis either by vapor exposure or by direct contact.

In a recent report of an analysis of 28 men suffering from systemic sclerosis collated over a 25-year period, 21 (75%) were suspected to be associated with occupational scleroderma. The most frequent chemical was organic solvents which were found in 13 of the patients (46%) (Zachariae et al. 1997).

References

Batschvaros B, Minkow DM (1968) Dermatitis and purpura from rubber in clothing. Trans St John's Hospit Derm Soc 54:73–78

Bauer M, Rabens SF (1977) Trichloroethylene toxicity. Int J Dermatol 16:113–116

Bourrain JL, Woodward C, Dumas V, Caperan D, Beani JC, Amblard P (1996) Natural rubber latex contact dermatitis with features of erythema multiforme. Contact Dermatitis 35:55–56

Buckley WR (1958) Lichenoid eruptions following contact dermatitis. Arch Dermatol 78:454–457

Calnan CD (1956) Nickel dermatitis. Br J Dermatol 68:229–232

Calnan CD, Peachey RDG (1971) Allergic contact purpura. Clin Allergy 1:287–290

Canizares O (1959) Lichen planus-like eruption caused by color developer. Arch Dermatol 80:81–86

Conde-Salazar L, Guimaraens D, Romero LV, Yus ES (1983) Subcorneal pustular eruption and erythema from occupational exposure to trichloroethylene. Contact Dermatitis 9:235–237

Cook LJ (1982) Associated nickel and cobalt contact dermatitis presenting as erythema multiforme. Contact Dermatitis 8:280–281

De Feo CP (1966) Erythema multiforme bullosum caused by 9-bromofluorene. Arch Dermatol 94:545–551

Fisher AA (1974) Allergic petechial and purpuric rubber dermatitis. The PPPP syndrome. Cutis 14:25–27

Fisher AA (1986) Erythema multiforme-like eruptions due to exotic woods and ordinary plants: part I. Cutis 37:101–104

Fisher AA (1986) Erythema multiforme-like eruptions due to topical medications: part II. Cutis 37:158–161

Fisher AA, Bikowski J (1981) Allergic contact dermatitis due to wooden cross made of Dalbergia nigra. Contact Dermatitis 7:45–46

Fisher AA, Chargrin L, Fleischmayer R, et al. (1959) Pustular patch test reactions. Arch Dermatol 80:742–752

Friedman SF, Perry HO (1985) Erythema multiforme associated with contact dermatitis. Contact Dermatitis 12:21–23

Fry L (1965) Skin disease from color developers. Br J Dermatol 77:456–461

Garcia-Bravo B, Rodriguez-Pichardo A, de-Pierola SF, Camacho F (1995) Airborne erythema-multiforme-like eruption due to pyrethrum. Contact Dermatitis 33:433

Goh CL (1988) Erythema multiforme-like eruption from trinitrotoluene allergy. Int J Dermatol 27:650–651

Goh CL (1989) Urticarial papular and plaque eruption. A manifestation of allergic contact dermatitis. Int J Dermatol 28:172–176

Goh CL, Kwok SF, Rajan VS (1984) Cross sensitivity in color developers. Contact Dermatitis 10:280–285

Goh CL, Ng SK (1988) A cutaneous manifestation of trichloroethylene toxicity. Contact Dermatitis 18:59–60

Hausen BM (1981) Woods injurious to human health. Walter de Gruyter, Berlin, p 59

Hezemans-Boer M, Toonstra J, Meulenbelt J, Zwaveling JH, Sangster B, van Vloten WA (1988) Skin lesions due to exposure to methylbromide. Arch Dermatol 124:917–921

Hjorth N (1966) Primula dermatitis. Trans St John's Hospit Derm Soc 52:207–219

Hjorth N (1977) Diagnostic patch testing. In: Marzulli F, Maibach HI Dermatoxicology and pharmacology. John Wiley, New York, p 344

Holst R, Kirby J, Magnusson B (1976) Sensitization to tropical woods giving erythema multiforme-like eruptions. Contact Dermatitis 2:295–296

Hyman AB, Berger RA (1959) Lichenoid eruption due to color developer. Arch Dermatol 80:243–244

Irvine C, Reynolds A, Finlay AY (1988) Erythema multiforme-like reaction to "rosewood". Contact Dermatitis 19:224–225

Iwatsuki K, Tagami H, Moriguchi T, Yamada M (1982) Lymphoadenoid structure induced by gold hypersensitivity. Arch Dermatol 118:608–611

Kawamura T, Fukuda S, Ohtake N, Furue M, Tamaki K (1996) Lichen planus-like contact dermatitis due to methacrylic acid esters. Br J Dermatol 134:358–360

Kurz G, Rapaport MJ (1979) External/internal allergy to plants (Artemesia). Contact Dermatitis 5:407–417

Lambert D, Terrussot MC, Dalac S, Boulitrop-Morvan C (1995) Granulome a la laine de brebis. Ann Dermatol Venereol 122:534–535

Mallory SB, Miller OF, Tyler WB (1982) Toxicodendron radicans dermatitis with black lacquer deposit on the skin. J Am Acad Dermatol 6:363–368

Meneghini CL, Angelini G (1981) Secondary polymorphic eruptions in allergic contact dermatitis. Dermatologica 163:63–70

Monti M, Berti E, Cavicchini S, Sala F (1983) Unusual cutaneous reaction after gold chloride patch test. Contact Dermatitis 9:150–151

Nakayama H, Bobayashi M, Takahashi M, Ageishi Y, Takano T (1988) Generalized eruption with severe liver dysfunction associated with occupational exposure to trichloroethylene. Contact Dermatitis 19:48–51

Nethercott JR, Albers J, Gurguis S, et al (1982) Erythema multiforme exudativum linked to the manufacture of printed circuit boards. Contact Dermatitis 3:314–322

Petros H, Macmillan AL (1973) Allergic contact sensitivity to gold with unusual features. Br J Dermatol 88:505–508

Phoon WH, Chan MOY, Rajan VS, et al (1984) Stevens-Johnson syndrome associated with occupational exposure to trichloroethylene. Contact Dermatitis 10:270–276

Roed-Petersen J (1975) Erythema multiforme as an expression of contact dermatitis. Contact Dermatitis 1:270–271

Romaguera C, Grimalt F (1977) PPPP syndrome. Contact Dermatitis 3:103–3

Rubin L (1956) Granulomas of axillae caused by deodorants. JAMA 162:953–955

Schwartz RS, Downham TF (1981) Erythema multiforme associated with Rhus contact dermatitis. Contact Dermatitis 27:85–86

Schwartz L, Tulipan L, Birmingham A (1947) Occupational disease of the skin, 3rd edn. Lea Febiger, Philadelphia, p 771

Shelly WB, Epstein E (1963) Contact-sensitivity to gold as a chronic papular eruption. Arch Dermatol 87:388–391

Shmunes E (1978) Purpuric allergic contact dermatitis to paraphenylenediamine. Contact Dermatitis 4:225–229

Stone OJ, Johnson DA (1967) Pustular patch test – experimentally induced. Arch Dermatol 95:618–619

Wahlberg JE, Maibach HI (1981) Sterile cutaneous pustules – a manifestation of primary irritancy? J Invest Dermatol 76:381–383

Walder BK (1983) Do solvents cause scleroderma? Int J Dermatol 22:157–158

Yamakage A, Ishikawa H (1982) Generalized morphea-like scleroderma occurring in people exposed to organic solvents. Dermatologica 165:186–193

Zachariae H, Bjerring P, Sondergaard KH, Halkier-Sorensen L (1997) Occupational systemic sclerosis in men. Ugeskr-Laeger 28:2687–2689

CHAPTER 13

Occupational Connective Tissue Disorders 13

U. F. Haustein, B. Lietzberg

Connective tissue disorders involving occupational factors are, first of all, systemic sclerosis (SSc), probably also lupus erythematosus (LE) and very rarely dermatomyositis, mixed connective tissue disease (MCTD), rheumatoid arthritis (RA) and Sjögren's syndrome (Zschunke et al. 1990; Koeger et al. 1991).

Systemic Sclerosis

Introduction

SSc, characterized by fibrosis of the skin and internal organs, is a disease of unknown etiology with a pathogenesis that is still vague. The prevalence in a Caucasian population is estimated at 0.3–1.9 per 100,000 (Haustein and Albrecht 1993). Women are affected three to six times more frequently (Medsger and Masi 1971; Sluis-Cremer et al. 1985). In recent years, some environmental substances have been reported as inducing factors in SSc and in so-called scleroderma-like diseases (SLD) (Table 1).

Table 1. Factors inducing systemic sclerosis (SSc) or scleroderma-like diseases (SLD), respectively

SSc	SLD
Mineral	Chemical compounds
Silica	Plastics
Solvents	Vinyl chloride
Chlorinated hydrocarbons	Epoxy resins (bis(4-amino-3-methylcyclohexyl)-methane)
Aromatic hydrocarbons	Solvents
	Chlorinated hydrocarbons
	Aromatic hydrocarbons
	Aliphatic hydrocarbons
	Pesticides
	Drugs (e.g. bleomycin, pentazocine)
	Others
	Aniline and fatty acid anilides (oleylanilides)
	Paraffin, silicon

Silica (Quartz)

Next to oxygen, silicon is the most common substance in our environment. Silicon has never been found in its elementary state. In nature it exclusively occurs in compounds derived from silicon dioxide (silica = SiO_2). Silica is a regular constituent part in about 92% of all rock.

The three important crystalline structures of silica are quartz, tridymite, and cristobalite. These compounds are also called "free silica" to distinguish them from the silicates, minerals containing silica bound to one or more metallic cations (American Thoracic Society 1997).

From the chemical point of view, quartz is an extremely inert material. It cannot be destroyed by water or solvents. Only hydrofluoric acid is capable of dissolving quartz. It may easily be detected by crystallographic methods, for example X-ray diffractometry and polarization microscopy, but it is difficult to trace by chemical analysis.

Epidemiological and Clinical Aspects

In 1914, the Scottish physician Bramwell reported a coincidence between "sclerodermia" and occupations involving exposure to silica dust. Five of the nine patients who reported diffuse SSc worked as stonemasons. Bramwell supposed that holding the chisel and working under cold-weather outdoor conditions might be work-associated causative factors.

Erasmus (1957) observed 17 cases of SSc among 8,000 underground miners in South Africa, 6 of them with silicosis. In order to get an impression about the morbidity of SSc, he examined 25,000 male and 27,000 female infirmary patients. He found one male patient (also a miner) and nine female patients with SSc and suggested a greater incidence among miners than among non-miners. In the following years (from 1960 until 1969), 29 additional cases of SSc were registered in miners who had been working in the South African gold mines. That corresponds to an incidence of 7.7 cases per 100,000 miners per year in contrast with an incidence of 0.33 in 100,000 in a control group consisting of railway and harbor workers. From 1955 to 1984, a total of 79 definite or probable cases of SSc in miners were registered. These investigations were related exclusively to Caucasian individuals (Sluis-Cremer et al. 1985). Cowie (1987) analyzed the occurrence of SSc in a native South African male population. Among miners he found an incidence of 8.2 per 100,000 versus merely 0.3 per 100,000 among inhabitants serving as a control group. In the Republic of South Africa, SSc has been acknowledged since 1974 as an occupational disease in miners that has to be compensated by law (Sluis-Cremer et al. 1985).

In the United States, Rodnan and colleagues (1967) analyzed the occupations of 60 male patients with SSc. They reported that 26 of them had been coal miners and 10 of them had been foundry workers exposed to quartz sand. In eight of the patients, SSc was associated with silicosis of the lungs. This association between SSc and silicosis has been confirmed by other groups (Beck et al. 1976; Ziegler et al. 1982).

One report on the increased prevalence of SSc in workers exposed to silica dust, mainly in the mining of ores in the former German Democratic Republic, was published in 1976 by Zschunke, whose findings initiated a study that appears to be the most extensive evaluation until now. A first analysis, which included all SSc patients from the whole country, was performed by our group in 1981 and revealed that 77% of all male patients with SSc had been exposed to silica dust in the workplace. In addition, half of the patients showed simultaneous silicosis of the lungs (Ziegler et al. 1981, 1982, 1986; Haustein and Ziegler 1985). Continuing this evaluation, records are currently available on 137 male patients with SSc. Silica dust exposure was established in 111 of these patients, and silicosis was found in 57 of them (Haustein and Herrmann 1994). The comparable occupational silica exposure in the general population of an industrial area is estimated as being 10% or less. Utilizing epidemiological tools, the following risk was calculated: the likelihood (odds ratio) that SSc will develop in men with silicosis who are older than 40 years of age is 12 times higher than in workers who are the same age but not exposed to silica dust. Ten female patients with SSc were also exposed to silica dust in the workplace. One of them had also developed silicosis. In contrast to the male patients, the epidemiologic research concerning females lacks evidence, probably due to their small numbers.

All our patients fulfilled the criteria of the American College of Rheumatology (ACR). The average time of exposure was 13.6 years. The delay in symptomatic disease (from beginning of exposure to onset of SSc) was 24.3 years on average. In some cases, the silica exposure lasted until the onset of SSc. The majority of pulmonary silicosis started before SSc in 41 of 57 (72%); the reverse was true in a minor fraction (19%). In 9%, both diseases were detected at the same time. From the remaining 54 SSc patients without silicosis, 25 (46%) developed lung fibrosis within 2 years. Raynaud's phenomenon was observed as a preceding or concurrent symptom in 107 of the 111 silica-dust-exposed SSc patients (96%). Skin involvement occurred before pulmonary symptoms in 36 of 111 (32%), at the same time in 5 of 111 (5%), after silicosis in 41 of 111 (37%), and in 29 of 111 (26%) patients no respiratory disorders were observed.

The occupations of our silica-exposed SSc patients are listed in Table 2. Fifty-seven of the 77 miners were exclusively exposed through uranium mining, 8 through coal mining, and 12 through both. Forty-two of the 111 patients had

Table 2. Occupations of our systemic sclerosis patients with verified silica-dust exposure ($n = 111$)

Occupation	Number of patients
Miner	77
Foundry worker	10
Quarryman	6
Sand-blaster	5
Dental mechanic	4
Sandstone sculptor	3
Glass grinder	3
Cast polisher	3

never worked in uranium mines. Twelve of these 42 suffered from silicosis. The odds ratio of the 42 patients who never worked in uranium mines to develop SSc was still 3.9. Since uranium mines were shut down between 1980 and 1989, we could follow up only the sequelae of this exposure. Today, only a few patients are still alive or have been recently diagnosed.

It is possible that sclerosis of the lungs, fibrosis due to nonspecific dust impact, and genuine silicosis might be confused in several cases; however, fibrosis of the lungs accompanied by SSc obviously occurs in subjects exposed to silica dust rather than in those who have not been exposed in such a way. The rate of silicosis in the male patients with SSc presented by our group is higher than the number reported by Erasmus (1957) and Rodnan et al. (1967). This difference might be explained by regional variations in defining silicosis in the past, by differences in the composition of the rocks, and at least in several cases by the radioactivity of the uranium. Progress in the differential diagnosis has been achieved by high-resolution computer tomography.

Sluis-Cremer et al. (1985) suggested that a brief exposure to dust with high silica content causes SSc without simultaneous silicosis. This would imply that the mode of exposure determines whether SSc with or without silicosis might develop. We do not share the opinion that SSc in these patients is not idiopathic SSc, but rather should be labeled as SLD (Siegel 1977). The symptomatic criteria for diagnosing SSc (compiled by the ACR; Masi 1980) have been fulfilled by almost all patients investigated (Table 3). According to our view, Rodnan et al. (1967), Rustin et al. (1990), and Gabay and Kahn (1992) emphasized the lack of differences between so-called idiopathic SSc and SSc in patients with silicosis.

Typical workplaces in which exposure to silica dust must be taken into account are listed in Table 4. However, numerous hidden sources of silica exposure exist, e.g., cleansers used in housekeeping (Mehlhorn et al. 1990; Koeger et al. 1992) and polishes used in various jobs. Even fondant powders contained quartz in the

Table 3. Clinical features and laboratory findings of systemic sclerosis patients associated with silicosis (n=37), limited:diffuse form = 22:15

Symptoms/laboratory findings	Number of patients	Limited form	Diffuse form
Raynaud's phenomenon	36	21	15
Finger-tip ulcers	28	15	13
Arthralgia	28	13	12
Lung involvement	37	22	15
Esophagus involvement	29	16	13
Heart involvement	11	3	8
Muscle involvement	9	2	7
Kidney involvement	5	0	5
Anti-nuclear antibodies (ANA)	35	20	15
Anti-topoisomerase antibodies (ATA)	13	1	12
Anti-centromere antibodies (ACA)	9	8	1
Platelet factor 4	27	14	13
β-Thromboglobulin	27	15	12
Endothelin	17	7	10

Table 4. Workplaces associated with silica-dust exposure (according to Zschunke et al. 1990)

Mining industry	Underground workers
Extracting and processing of stones (sandstone, granite, slate, fluor-spar, mica)	Quarrymen, crushers, sculptors, stone masons, workers producing slate pencils, workers handling slate powder, e.g. as a carrier for hexachlorocyclohexane insecticides, workers producing roof paper
Producing and processing of chamotte	Grinders, mixers, stove fitters, blast furnace-lining bricklayers
Foundry industry	Moulders, coremakers, casters, cast dressers
Tire industry and industries producing other products made from natural or synthetic rubber, e.g., cables	Workers handling talc that is sometimes heavily contaminated by silica
Industries producing pottery including glassware	Workers handling raw material, in particular sand and kaolin; the latter also regularly contains considerable quantities of silica
Dental technical laboratories (polishing and embedding materials)	Dental technicians

past and were found to be a cause of silicosis (Beck and Irmscher 1974). Silicosis was also observed in female laundry workers washing dust-contaminated clothes (Evans and Posner 1971). One anecdote refers to a husband and his wife who both developed SSc, the husband after silica exposure and his wife probably by inhaling dust from his clothes (Christy and Rodnan 1984). Koeger et al. (1992) reported of two patients who developed edematous scleroderma and subluxing arthropathy, respectively, after applying aerosole silicon glaze on cables over a 20-year period.

Yamamoto et al. (1994) described an SSc patient with high levels of serum immunoglobulin E who developed nodular scleroderma. He had been working on polishing watches with an abrasive agent composed mainly of aluminum, chromium dioxide, and silica.

It is also known that dental technicians are exposed to various particulate matters including silica, alloys, and acrylic plastics which may induce pneumoconiosis and probably other occupational lung diseases (Choudat 1994). The prevalence of pneumoconiosis is 1/0 or greater of about 15% in technicians with 20 or more years of exposure. Compensation should be paid to those suffering from this work-related disease (Choudat 1994).

Yánez-Díaz et al. (1992) presented two male patients with SSc and pulmonary silicosis after occupational exposure to silica, and one of them to trichloroethylene as a degreasing agent.

Gabay and Kahn (1992) have analyzed 202 SSc patients diagnosed at the Rheumatology Department, University Bichat (Paris) since 1976. Among them were 39 male patients (women/men = 4.2/1). Eleven of them had been exposed to silica dust for between 4 years and 33 years (mean ± SD 14.5 ± 11.4 years) (as miners, foundry workers, or bricklayers), one to solvents (as a painter), and two to both.

The mean age at onset of disease was 50.4±10.19 years (range 31–72 years) with Raynaud's phenomenon before onset of disease (mean duration 6 months). The delay between the beginning of exposure and onset of disease was 24.4±12.2 years (range 4–45 years). There were no significant differences between the two groups (induced SSc versus "primitive" SSc) regarding age at onset of disease, mortality, systemic manifestations except myositis (which occurred only in the "primitive" group), therapy, anti-nuclear antibodies (ANAs) and anti-Scl-70 antibodies [anti-topoisomerase antibodies (ATAs)]. Among the 163 female patients there was no silica-induced case.

Surprisingly, an occupational analysis of 56 men with SSc in the United Kingdom showed no evidence of silica exposure implicated in the onset of the disease (Silman and Jones 1992).

Englert et al. (2000) performed a case-control study in Australia with 160 male SSc patients having both the diffuse and limited disease subtypes and 83 controls. This study's findings demonstrate higher crude and socioeconomically-adjusted frequencies of silica exposure in cases than controls (37.5% vs 13.3%) indicating an estimated relative risk magnitude two to fourfold.

Among 139 patients occupationally exposed to silica dust (examined between 1981 and 1984), Ebihara and Kawami (2000) found 3 with SSc and one with polyarteritis nodosa. Another patient with SSc had been exposed to asbestos dust.

Case reports and epidemiological studies reporting on patients suffering from SSc and silicosis are summarized in Table 5.

Silica and Other Autoimmune Diseases

Evaluating 764 patients with connective tissue disease (CTD) hospitalized in the clinic of the University Pitié-Salpêtrière/Paris, Koeger et al. (1995) found 24 (3%) patients with silica-associated CTD. Eight of them had SSc, in four cases in association with Sjögren's syndrome and in three cases in association with silicosis. RA has been found in five patients (four in association with Sjögren's syndrome), systemic LE in four patients (three with silicosis), discoid LE in one patient, and dermatomyositis in association with Sjögren's syndrome in three patients. The last three patients had erosive polyarthritis and Sjögren's syndrome, Grave disease, and inflammatory polyarthralgia. Three additional cases of autoimmune diseases, after unusual exposure to silica (abrasive cleansing powder) or silicon glaze, have been reported by the same authors (Koeger et al. 1992).

Steenland and Brown (1995) updated a study of 3,328 gold miners who worked underground for at least 1 year between 1940 and 1965 in South Dakota. Multiple-cause analysis revealed significant excesses of arthritis, musculoskeletal diseases, and various cutaneous disorders (including SSc and systemic LE).

Evidence that occupational exposure to silica is also associated with autoimmunity was reinforced by the observation that workers from a factory that produced scouring powder with a higher than usual silica content (70–90% powdered quartz) exhibited a high prevalence of clinical and biological autoimmune manifestations (Table 6). Among a group of 50 workers, Sanchez-Roman et al.

Table 5. Published cases of systemic sclerosis (SSc) in association with silica exposure and silicosis, respectively

	Author	Cases	Diagnosis	Occupation	Exposure
1914	Bramwell	5	Diffuse scleroderma	Stone masons	Silica dust
1957	Erasmus	17	SSc, 6 with silicosis	Underground miners	Silica dust
1959	Francia et al.	6	SSc and silicosis		
1967	Rodnan et al.	36	SSc, 8 with silicosis	26 Coal miners, 10 foundry workers	Silica dust (coal miners), quartz sand (foundry workers)
1955–1984	Sluis-Cremer et al. (including the cases of Erasmus 1957)	79	SSc	Gold miners	Silica dust
1987	Cowie	10	SSc, 6 with silicosis	Gold miners	Silica dust
1981–1997	Haustein and Herrmann (1994) (some of these patients were also reported by Ziegler et al. 1986, Baur 1994, Mehlhorn 1994)	111	SSc, 57 with silicosis	Uranium mining (57), coal mining (8), both (12)	Silica dust (uranium)
1984	Christy and Rodnan	2	SSc	The husband developed SSc after silica exposure and his wife probably by inhaling dust from his clothes	Silica dust
1990	Mehlhorn et al.	1	SSc	Cleaning woman	Scouring powder containing crystalline silica
1992	Koeger et al.	1	Edematous scleroderma	Sprayed silicon-glaze on cables	Silicon-glaze
1992	Yánez-Díaz et al.	1	SSc, silicosis	Lead mine	Silica dust
1992	Yánez-Díaz et al.	1	SSc, silicosis	Lead mine	Fiberglass, (trichloroethylene)
1992	Gabay and Kahn	11	SSc	Miner, foundry worker, bricklayer	Silica dust
1992	Gabay and Kahn	2	SSc	Miner, foundry worker, bricklayer	Silica and solvents

Table 5 (continued)

	Author	Cases	Diagnosis	Occupation	Exposure
1994	Yamamoto et al.	1	Multiple papules in an area of non-sclerotic skin in SSc	Polishing watches	Abrasive agent (aluminum, chromium dioxide, silica)
1995	Koeger et al.	8	SSc, 3 with silicosis	Underground worker, sand molder, dental prosthetist, foundry engineer, marble sculptor, miner, sandblaster, mason, sandstone cutter	Silica dust
1996	Wichmann et al. (including the patients reported by Sanchez-Roman et al. 1993)	12	SSc	Scouring powder	Silica content: 70–90% powdered quartz
2000	Englert et al.	60		13 Construction 5 mining 8 manufacturing 1 rock-driller	
2000	Ebihara and Kawami	3 Total = 350	SSc		silica dust

Table 6. Autoimmune diseases in association with silica exposure (according to Sanchez-Roman et al. 1993 and Wichmann et al. 1996)

	Sanchez-Roman et al. (1993), 50 workers; number (%)	Wichmann et al. (1996), 52 workers, same factory; number (%)
Systemic sclerosis (SSc)	5 (10)	12 (23)
Systemic lupus erythematosus (SLE)	3 (6)	16 (31)
Polymyositis (PM)		1 (2)
Overlap syndrome (SLE/SSc)	5 (10)	7 (14) (included in SLE, SSc, PM and undefined collagen disease)
Secondary Sjögren's syndrome	6 (12) (included in the three first clinical diagnosis)	
Undefined collagen disease	19 (38) (including three cases of primary Sjögren's syndrome)	15 (29)
Asymptomatic subjects	19 (38)	15 (29)

(1993) demonstrated symptoms of systemic illness in 32 (64%) and ANA in 36 (72%) of them.

Wichmann et al. (1996) showed that individuals chronically exposed to silica, independent of whether they are suffering from CTD, have antibodies to myeloperoxidase (MPO).

In 9 of 11 patients with silica exposure and renal involvement with systemic vasculitis, Chevalier et al. (working in Angers) found various antibodies indicative of autoimmunity, such as MPO-anti-neutrophil cytoplasmic antibodies (ANCA) and ANA at low titers, with anti-RO/Sjögren's syndrome-A in two patients, but without anti-double-stranded DNA (dsDNA) (Conrad et al. 1997).

According to our data, Conrad et al. (1997) demonstrated that uranium miners with heavy exposure to silica run a higher risk of developing SSc and systemic LE than miners with slight or no exposure, because they showed a higher frequency of SSc-specific autoantibodies [anti-centromere antibodies (ACAs), ATAs, anti-nucleolar antibodies] related to the intensity of the silica exposure and to preceding symptoms of SSc (Raynaud's phenomenon, diffuse interstitial lung fibrosis).

By summarizing various studies and case reports, Gregorini (working in Brescia) showed that extrapulmonary silicotic lesions and/or autoimmune processes may play a role in kidney diseases after silica exposure, more specifically MPO-ANCA-positive microscopic polyangiitis and its renal-limited form of "idiopathic", rapidly progressive glomerulonephritis (Conrad et al. 1997).

In conclusion, silica may induce systemic diseases with various clinical and serological manifestations: systemic sclerosis with ACA, ATA or anti-nucleolar antibodies, systemic LE and systemic LE (SLE)-like diseases with anti-dsDNA and/or anti-RO/SS-A and anti-cardiolipin antibodies, and necrotizing systemic vasculitis with renal involvement and MPO-ANCA (Conrad et al. 1997).

Pathogenesis

Silica-associated SSc is clinically, serologically, and immunologically indistinguishable from idiopathic SSc (Haustein and Ziegler 1985; Rustin et al. 1990; Gabay and Kahn 1992).

Quartz is absorbed both via inhalation and percutaneously. Silicosis of the lung is caused by particles with a diameter of less than 5 µm. The orifice of the sebaceous glands in healthy individuals is approximately 24 times wider than the particle size relevant for silicosis. At the extremities, there are up to 50 follicles per square centimeter (Plewig and Kligman 1978). Miners experience microinjuries of their hands and forearms quite frequently. Therefore, it is not surprising that about 150 particles of quartz between 1 µm and 20 µm could be traced in a single biopsy specimen (Ziegler et al. 1988).

In several patients we determined the silica content in skin specimens obtained from fingers, dorsum of the hand, and lower arms by polarization and phase-contrast microscopy, and in two cases by electron spectroscopy for chemical analysis. As shown in Table 7, silica crystals can be found in a high percentage of silica-exposed subjects. In the majority of occupations, the mechanical forces (e.g. in air or compressed air, drilling or hewing) are substantial and may promote the penetration of silica crystals by micro-wounding. However, these data do not distinguish patients from silica-exposed miners without skin and lung diseases.

This mechanism of penetration might serve as an explanation for the observation that symptoms start at the distal portions of extremities in the majority of cases.

Silica particles are ingested by macrophages (Fig. 1), e.g., in the lung or skin, and can be transported to extrapulmonary sites (Holt 1981). Subsequently, activated macrophages release enhanced amounts of interleukin (IL)-1α and -β (Oghiso and Kubota 1986). Similarly, silica-stimulated monocytes can release fibroblast-proliferation-inducing factors (Schmidt et al. 1984), leading to stimulation of collagen production by fibroblasts, too. The spontaneous secretion of IL-1 from silicotic rat alveolar macrophages can be inhibited by anti-Ia antibodies (Struhar and Harbeck 1989). Furthermore, silica added to antigen- or mitogen-stimulated lymphocyte cultures increases the number of immunoglobulin-secreting cells (Moseley et al. 1988). IL-1α and -β also affect T-helper lymphocytes promoting production and release of IL-2. IL-2 may stimulate B lymphocytes synthesizing immunoglobulins and (auto)antibodies. Activated T lymphocytes also produce other lymphokines (e.g., macrophage-activating factors) which are capable of stimulating macrophages and fibroblasts.

Table 7. Silica in exposed skin areas

Subjects	Positive/total
Silica-induced SSc	24/26
Silicosis	4/5
Silica-exposed miners (without SSc/silicosis)	3/5
Non-exposed controls	1/6

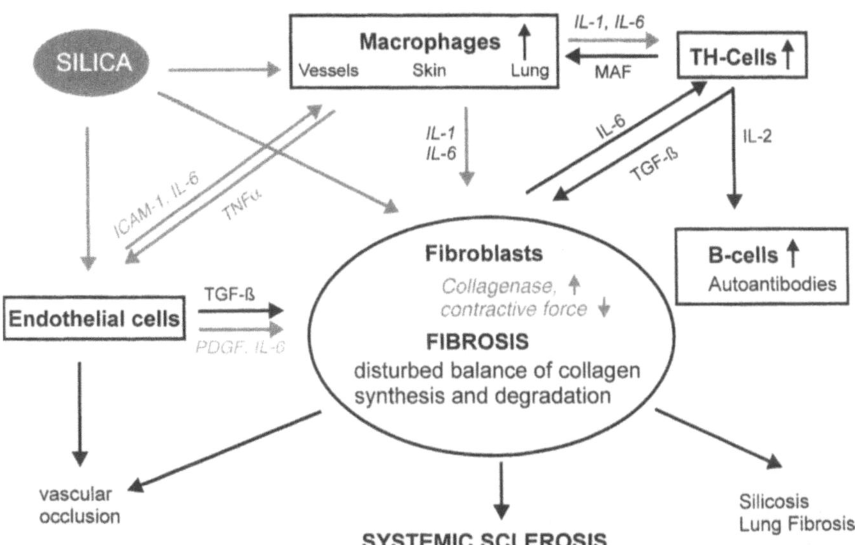

Fig. 1. Silica can activate various cell types involved in the pathophysiology of systemic sclerosis (SSc). Macrophages activated by silica in vitro liberate the same cytokines and growth factors known to be active in the pathophysiology of idiopathic SSc. Microvascular endothelium is involved in silica-induced as well as idiopathic SSc with similar activation patterns in vitro and in vivo. Dermal fibroblasts are affected by silica in vitro, and fibroblasts are the cells producing large amounts of extracellular matrix in vivo. In vitro, the synthesizing capacity of fibroblasts depends greatly on culture conditions. All these effects are based on our in vitro experiments with silica shown in italic. These effects are similar to pathophysiological events known from idiopathic SSc

These mechanisms are continuously triggered by silica, which is not chemically reactive and remains in the tissue over an extended period. Nevertheless, it has toxic effects on macrophages in a dose-dependent manner. After phagocytosis and destruction of these cells, silica is set free in the tissue, and the process of ingestion through phagocytosis might start again. In this way, a vicious cycle of a dysfunctional inflammatory response is established (Haustein and Herrmann 1994).

However, Adamson et al. (1989) have shown that silica and irradiation are each able to enhance the number of interstitial cells in the lung. In addition, the content of cells, protein, and hydroxyproline is increased in bronchoalveolar lavage fluids. Taken together, irradiation plus silica exposure might lead to a synergistic enhancement of their effects.

Obviously, the endothelial cell damage occurs early, before systemic symptoms appear. This is suggested by the observation that Raynaud's phenomenon often precedes SSc and by elevated levels of von Willebrand factor and circulating immune complexes not only in silica-induced SSc, but also in healthy silica-exposed miners.

Concerning the involvement of blood vessels, Dowd and Ziegler (1987) demonstrated decreased formation of prostacyclin, a vasodilating lipid mediator originating from endothelial cells. The lack of prostacyclin formation was shown in patients with Raynaud's phenomenon as well in patients with SSc who had been exposed to silica. Furthermore, there are certain patterns of ultrastructural changes of the endothelial layer, which seem to be characteristic of SSc (Haustein and Klug 1975; Haustein et al. 1986). Accordingly, subintimal fibrosis of small arteries has been described by Fleischmajer et al. (1983).

Silica seems to be a potent activator of endothelial cells in vitro, too. Incubation of human dermal microvascular endothelial cells (HDMEC) with silica at non-toxic concentrations increased the steady-state levels of the messenger RNA (mRNA) for intercellular adhesion molecule 1 (ICAM-1), and also increased the corresponding levels of this cell-surface protein as shown by fluorescence-activated cell-sorter (FACS) analysis; the incubation also increased the level of soluble protein in the culture fluid, as shown by means of ELISA, in a dose- and time-dependent manner. Additionally, increased levels of IL-6 in the culture supernatants have been found and a significant increase in collagenase I mRNA in HDMEC has been demonstrated (Anderegg et al. 1997).

The intratracheal instillation of silica crystals (a quartz) into the lungs of C57BI/6 mice resulted in a significant increase in levels of ICAM-1 in lung tissue and bronchoalveolar lavage fluids (Nario and Hubbard 1996).

In patients with SSc, Frank et al. (1993) found a slight decrease of IL-1 basal secretion from monocytes in comparison with healthy volunteers, and no changes in IL-6 and tumor necrosis factor a (TNFa) production. In monocyte-enriched cultures from healthy donors, a dose-dependent modulation of the cytokine pattern (IL-1a, IL-1β, IL-6, TNFa) could be demonstrated after silica phagocytosis. Using titanium dioxide for phagocytosis, no comparable effects were observed. The impact of silica on cytokine secretion of monocytes might explain inflammatory tissue reactions and increased collagen synthesis in silica-associated SSc.

The incubation of fibroblasts in culture with silica demonstrated the induction of interstitial collagenase I mRNA and protein in the monolayer and a decreased ability to contract collagen fibers in a three-dimensional gel. Unexpectedly, we could not find an increase in the expression of collagen I or III mRNA (Anderegg et al. 1996).

Taken together, the enhanced expression of ICAM-1 by endothelial cells might cause enhanced adhesion of activated (and activating) mononuclear cells to the microvascular wall. Together with increased collagenase activities originating from endothelial cells and the neighboring dermal fibroblasts, the extravasation of monocytes into the surrounding tissue could be realized. The resulting perivascular infiltrate may take part again in the activation of fibroblasts to produce more collagen and matrix proteins in skin or lung tissue. The mechanism of SSc due to silica is summarized in Fig. 1.

Vibration

Vibrations caused by pneumatic tools are known to induce Raynaud's phenomenon, which regresses after cessation of the exposure. To what extent vibration hammers, which are often used in mining and treating stones, take part in promotion of SSc is still vague (Blair et al. 1974). However, it is extremely unlikely that some of the patients, such as sandblasters, glass grinders, cast polishers, and stove fitters, have ever worked with pneumatic tools. Increased incidences of Raynaud's phenomenon, sclerodactyly and edema of the hands were observed in chain-saw workers and in individuals operating jack-hammers (Nagata et al. 1993).

Human Lymphocyte Antigen Association

The association of immunological disorders with certain human lymphocyte antigen (HLA) alleles emphasizes the role of genetic factors in determining susceptibility to environmental factors (Table 8). Rihs et al. (1994) analyzed the association of circulating autoantibodies and HLA alleles in 71 uranium miners and 1 cleaning woman. They showed a positive correlation of anti-Scl-70 to DR3 (1*0300) and DQ2 (1*0201) as well as of ACA to DR1 (1*0101–1*0103), DR8 (1*0801–1*0804), and DQ4 (1*0400). Significant differences between affected and unaffected miners have not been observed.

In addition, Rihs et al. (1996) studied the genetic association of HLA-DPB1 alleles in 54 patients with idiopathic SSc, 26 uranium miners with SSc, and 70 unrelated, healthy control subjects. The data show that anti-Scl-70 expression in idiopathic SSc patients is linked with DPB1*1301, whereas anti-Scl-70-positive miners do not exhibit such a DPB1 association. Furthermore, the data indicate that glutamate at position 69 of DPB1 might be involved in the susceptibility to idiopathic anti-Scl-70 expression.

Additionally, DRB1*0301 and DQB1*0201 were significantly increased in ATA-positive, silica-associated SSc patients, and DRB1*0800 and DQB1*0402 were ele-

Table 8. Association between human lymphocyte antigen (HLA) alleles and several subgroups of systemic sclerosis (SSc) patients according to Rihs et al. (1994, 1996), Baur et al. (1996) and Conrad et al. (1997)

Circulating autoantibody	SSc patient subgroup	HLA alleles
Anti-Scl-70/anti-topoisomerase antibodies	Uranium miner	DR 3 (DRB 1*0300), DQ2 (DQB 1*0201)
	Silica-associated SSc	DRB 1*0301, DQB 1*0201
	Idiopathic SSc	DPB 1 (1*1301, *0601, *1701)
Anti-centromere	Uranium miners	DR 1 (1*0100, *0101-*0103), DR 8 (1*0800, *0801-*0804), DQ (1*0400)
	Silica-associated SSc	DRB 1*0800, DQB 1*0402

vated in ACA-positive, silica-associated SSc patients compared with unrelated controls and the idiopathic SSc group studied (Conrad et al. 1997). Conrad et al. (1998) tested sera of 1795 uranium miners for autoantibodies typical for systemic autoimmune diseases. The autoantibody prevalence in uranium miners without SSc, SLE and other autoimmune diseases was significantly higher than in a control group. In general, it was associated with intensity of exposure as well as clinical symptoms of SSc or SLE, but not with silicosis. The autoantibody prevalences and specificities in uranium miners with SSc and SLE were similar to those in "idiopathic" diseases, however, miners with SSc had more topoisomerase I-antibodies and miners with SLE had no Sm-antibodies. DRB*0301, DQB1*0201, TNFa2 and TNF2 alleles were significantly more prevalent in uranium miners with SSc compared to idiopathic SSc, blood donors, miners without SSc. This indicates the capacity of silica to induce the production of TNFa and reactive oxygen species by macrophages.

One TNFa2 allele (associated with an increased TNF production capacity) was only increased in silica-associated SSc, independently of any DRB alleles. The results of this study reinforce the idea that not only structural conditions of antigen binding encoded by major histocompatibility class-II genes, but also an association to a certain TNF region, may be important for the generation of an immune response through regulation of TNF production, which is modified in silica-associated SSc patients due to continuous ingestion of silica by macrophages (Conrad et al. 1997).

Conclusion

As silica cannot be removed from the body once it is incorporated, its deleterious precipitating effect is unavoidable. This indicates that the clinical course of silica-induced disorders is quite similar to classical autoimmune diseases or SSc, characterized by progressions and remissions. The subsequent therapy should take these findings into account and has to be adjusted according to the criteria for the extent, organ involvement, and clinical activity of the disease. The best way to prevent this type of SSc is to minimize the exposure to silica.

However, continuous efforts are still required to encourage acknowledgment of SSc as an occupational disease after long-term silica exposure. Individual decisions by clinical experts should provide the basis enabling social and financial support to reduce the harm caused by silica-induced SSc.

Scleroderma-Like Diseases

In contrast to silica and several solvents, a whole variety of substances are reported to induce SLD, which can be distinguished from SSc using the following criteria:
- Type of skin manifestation, in particular acrosclerosis, circumscribed and generalized morphea, fibrotic nodules, or joint contractures.

- Visceral involvement due to toxic damage of liver, kidney, nervous system and muscles, or angiosarcoma of the liver.
- Laboratory findings, discrete thrombocytopenia, and absence of autoantibodies.
- Cessation or reversal of the disease process after early discontinuation of exposure.
- Female preponderance for idiopathic SSc is often not observed in occupationally induced SLD.

Vinyl Chloride

Individuals cleaning or inspecting autoclaves for polymerization of vinyl chloride (VC) to polyvinyl chloride (PVC) are in danger of developing SLD with high incidence (Lelbach and Marsteller 1981; Ostlere et al. 1992). Cleaning is usually performed by scraping and water splashing. In this way, workers are exposed to the remnants of the monomer.

The first large study was conducted in Rumania in 1963, where 168 PVC workers had been observed over 4 years (Suciu et al. 1963). The symptoms included pruritus of the arms and face, and scleroderma-like lesions, which mostly disappeared after the worker left the workplace. Later on, the disease was described in detail and labeled as occupational acro-osteolysis (OAOL) in England, France, and the United States (Cordier et al. 1966; Harris and Adams 1967; Wilson et al. 1967; Dinman et al. 1971; Markowitz et al. 1972). The disease is characterized by Raynaud's phenomenon, papular-fibrotic skin lesions on the wrist and dorsa of the hands, and osteolysis in the middle of the distal phalanges (bullet holes), mainly of the first three fingers, which became shortened and shapeless. OAOL occurred only in those workers who had been exposed to the VC monomer and was most common in reactor cleaners (Lelbach and Marsteller 1981).

Histopathological examination of scleroderma-like lesions showed distended collagen fibers, shrinkage of elastic fibers, interstitial edema, sometimes perivascular lymphocytic infiltrates, swollen endothelial cells of the enlarged capillaries, and marked acanthosis in the epidermal layer (Czernielewski et al. 1979).

In 1974, Lange et al. reported of a systemic form of VC disease. Changes included skin sclerosis, pulmonary fibrosis, fibrosis of the liver and spleen, and disturbances in the capillary vascular system, joints, and musculature. Further manifestations are paresthesia, thrombocytopenia, leukopenia, and splenomegaly (Bachner et al. 1974). Capillary microscopy reveals that abnormalities of the nailfold in VC workers are similar but less pronounced than those found in SSc (Maricq et al. 1976). Distal pitting scars, esophageal dysmotility, renal disease, and cardiac disease are generally absent.

Leukopenia, as well as angiosarcoma of the liver, drew attention to the carcinogenic and mutagenic properties of VC. The relationship between VC disease and SSc is shown in Table 9.

Finally, common symptoms of VC-related diseases such as fatigue, cold, burning pain, emotional instability, loss of libido, and impotence should be mentioned (Penin et al. 1975; Veltman 1980). After discontinued exposure, skin lesions, capillary abnormalities and acro-osteolytic lesions will revert to an almost normal

Table 9. Relationship between vinyl chloride (VC) disease and systemic sclerosis (SSc) (according to Veltman 1980, Haustein and Ziegler 1985)

	Percentage (%)
Features of VC disease resembling SSc	
Raynaud's phenomenon	33–74
Fibrotic skin, sclerodactyly	10
Resorption of bone at the distal phalanges	11
Pulmonary fibrosis	13
Esophageal variation	23
Skin capillary abnormalities	23
Arthralgia	82
Myalgia	16
Features of VC disease different from SSc	
Paresthesia	80
Thrombocytopenia	76
Splenomegaly	48
Reticulocytosis	35
Central nervous system symptoms	17
Leukopenia	8
Angiosarcoma of the liver	6
No calcinosis	

status (Veltman 1980). VC is a volatile gas. It is not quite clear to what extent inhalation of VC might induce skin lesions; however, remnants of the gaseous monomer VC have been demonstrated in the polymer PVC. VC is stored and metabolized by the organism. One of its metabolites, thiodiglycolic acid, can easily be detected in urine samples, even when levels of VC in the atmosphere are considerably lower (Mueller et al. 1978). So-called activated metabolites of VC (Fig. 2) may participate in the pathogenesis. Other mechanisms might affect the individual's cellular immune response, especially in workers exposed to the small molecules of VC (Kohanka 1982). Circulating immune complexes were found to be increased (Milford 1976). However, autoantibodies – particularly ANA, ATA, and ACA – could not be traced (Black et al. 1983). HLAs of the pattern HLA DR5, HLA DR3, HLA A1, HLA B8, and HLA B3 prevail in patients with VC disease. The genetic background, together with the impairment of cellular immune functions, might lead to an increased susceptibility to the disorder (Black et al. 1983). One of the main targets of VC-inducible effects seems to be microvascular tissues. Fibrosis of the vessel wall results in fibrosis of other organ systems. Patients with VC disease have fewer capillary abnormalities of their fingers than patients with SSc, but they have more than healthy controls (Maricq 1981).

In rats fed for 2 years with 30 mg VC per kilogram of body weight, thickening of the skin with collagen deposition as well as an increase in glycosylated lysine and hydroxylysine have been described, indicating an increased collagen synthesis (Knight and Gibbons 1987).

Reducing maximum concentrations in the work place from 500 ppm to negligible levels (ppm) by automation and contact-free technology will subsequently decrease the number of reported cases.

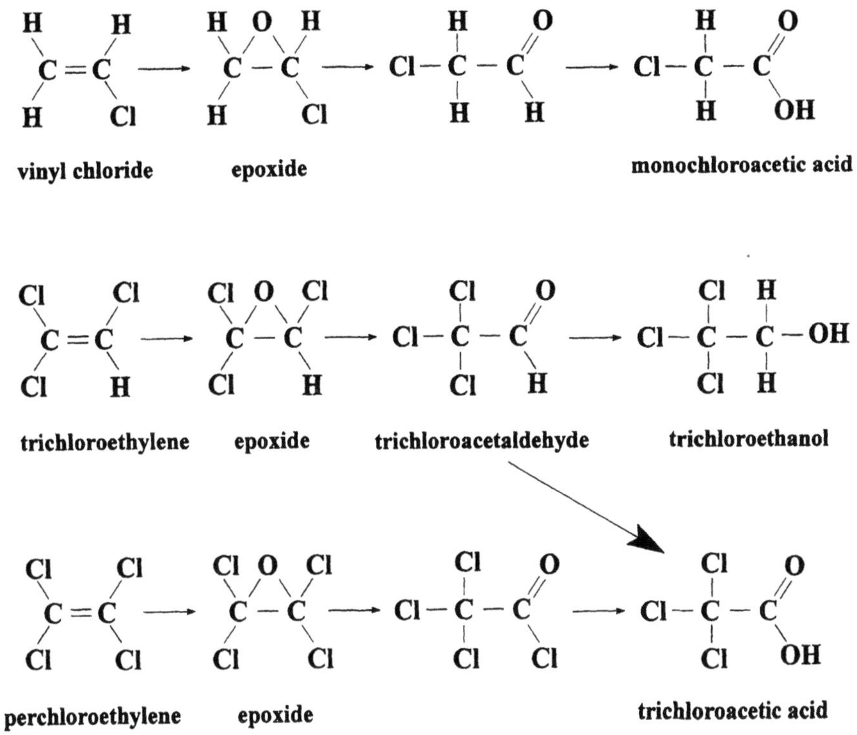

vinyl chloride   epoxide   monochloroacetic acid

trichloroethylene   epoxide   trichloroacetaldehyde   trichloroethanol

perchloroethylene   epoxide   trichloroacetic acid

Fig. 2. Metabolism of chlorinated ethylenes (reprinted from Bolt et al 1982, with permission from Elsevier)

PVC Dust

Recently, a case of MCTD in a male patient occupationally exposed to PVC and other toxic agents was presented. Clinical symptoms consisted of typical signs of SLE, rheumatoid arthritis, and lupoid hepatitis. MCTD diagnosis was confirmed serologically by the presence of μ_1-ribonucleoprotein-autoantibodies. Prednisone, 60 mg daily, produced remission (Panaszek et al. 1993). Studnicka et al. (1995) presented a 58-year-old patient exposed to thermoplastic dusts, mainly PVC, for 10 years. He developed pneumoconiosis and secondary SSc.

Bis(4-Amino-3-Methylcyclohexyl)Methane (Polymerization of Epoxy Resins)

Two male patients (of 233 workers) with a newly diagnosed SLD induced by epoxy resins were reported from Japan in 1980 (Yamakage et al. 1980). Ishikawa et al. (1995) described the clinical and laboratory findings of these patients after a 17-year follow-up from 1976 to 1993. Both patients had been employed by a chemical factory since May 1975, and were continuously exposed to a polymerization process of epoxy resins. First symptoms appeared after 1 month (patient 1)

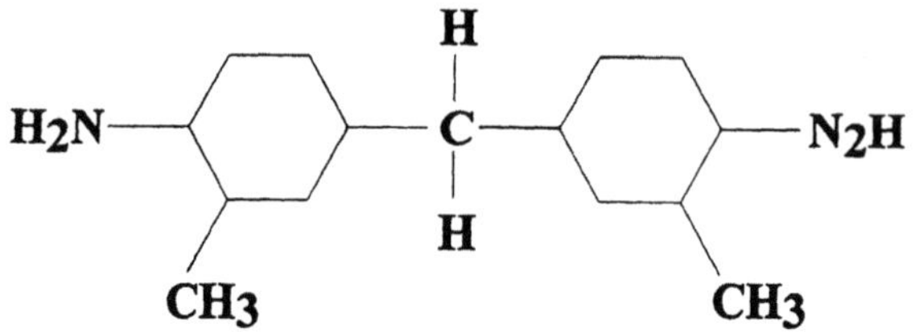

Fig. 3. Bis(4-amino-3-methylcyclohexyl)methane

and 1.5 months (patient 2). After this brief exposure, the patients developed erythema and edema, which evolved to generalized dermal sclerosis and alopecia, weakness, and muscle atrophy, but no Raynaud's phenomenon or ANA. Treatment was started with a small dose of prednisolone and discontinued in 1980. The hair loss recovered in 1977, the sclerotic skin changes disappeared by 1980, and the sclerodactyly recovered in 1993. Bis(4-amino-3-methylcyclohexyl)methane (BAMM), a new type of plasticizer belonging to the cyclohexamines (Fig. 3), was suspected as the causative agent from the list of chemical substances used.

BAMM may interfere with the amine metabolism, which has been suggested to be disturbed in SSc patients (Stachow et al. 1979). In addition, oligomers of epoxy resins, being strong sensitizers, might induce dysfunctional immune responses (Thorgeirsson et al. 1978). Using SSc-inducing glycosaminoglycans in lymphocyte transformation tests, splenocytes of mice experimentally treated with BAMM showed a positive response (Ishikawa et al. 1982). Intraperitoneal injections of one compound produced skin sclerosis in a murine model (Yamakage et al. 1980).

A 33-year-old man developed SSc without scleroderma while working after being exposed from 20 to 30 years of age to epoxy resin polymerization during surfboard manufacturing (Inachi et al. 1996). The symptoms included a shortening of the frenulum linguae, diffuse hyperpigmentation and facial telangiectasia, positive ANA, and pulmonary dysfunction, but no acrosclerosis or sclerodactyly. Modest dermal collagen proliferation in the forearm skin confirmed SSc without scleroderma.

Chlorinated Hydrocarbons, Aliphatic Hydrocarbons

The chlorinated hydrocarbons trichloroethylene and perchloroethylene (Fig. 2) are widely used as solvents and cleaners. They may be considered closely related to VC because of the clinical similarity of the disorders caused by these compounds to VC disease. Trichloroethylene is more volatile (boiling point 87.2 °C) and much more toxic than perchloroethylene (boiling point 121.1 °C). It penetrates the skin and, in its vaporous state, is also absorbed by the alveolar capillaries. Prolonged contact with the skin will induce irritative dermatitis (Schirren 1971; Bauer and Rabens 1977). Besides the well-described toxic effects in the nervous system, liver, kidney, and bone marrow, several reports on SLD resembling VC disease have been published (Reinl 1957; Saihan et al. 1978). Sparrow (1977) observed an SLD similar to VC disease, probably caused by perchloroethylene.

Recently, Flindt-Hansen and Isager (1987) reported three cases of SSc after occupational, prolonged (4–12 years), and intensive exposure to trichloroethane and/or trichloroethylene during metal-cleaning procedures. According to the ACR-criteria, all three cases could be classified as definite SSc.

Another case of SSc (with pos. ANA) after working with trichloroethylene (Czirják et al. 1993) was observed in a female patient after inhalation for 2 years (beginning at the age of 40 years).

Lockey et al. (1987) described a 47-year-old woman with previously excellent health who developed fatal SSc after a single 2.5-h predominantly dermal exposure to trichloroethylene. An additional case of SSc in a 51-year-old female worker has been presented, who developed SSc after 15 years of exposure to perchloroethylene (Szeimies et al. 1992).

A 26-year-old woman with localized scleroderma after 1 year of exposure to various organic solvents, including trichloroethylene, tetrachloroethylene, acetone, benzene, isopropyl alcohol, dimethyl phthalate, methoxyethanol, polyethylene glycol, polyvinyl alcohol, polyvinyl acetate, xylene and phenol, has been presented by Czirják et al. (1994). Disseminated circumscribed scleroderma (morphea) has been described in a painter exposed to perchloroethylene (Hinnen et al. 1995).

Recently, two cases of fasciitis (no scleroderma) with eosinophilia associated with prolonged exposure to trichloroethylene were reported: the first case (a 63-year-old woman) by drinking contaminated water from a residential well, and the second (a 65-year-old man) through occupational exposure (Waller et al. 1994).

Czirják et al. (1987) analyzed 21 female patients with SSc. In eight of them, occupationally hazardous agents were considered: trichloroethylene in one, organic solvents in six, and polyethylene and possibly its derivatives in the last. Another patient had been heavily exposed to trichloromethane during 13 years of work renovating carburetors in Israel (Tibon-Fisher et al. 1992).

The analysis of 61 patients with SSc (Czirják et al. 1989) revealed a female-to-male ratio of 60:1. Prior occupational exposure to chemicals (mainly organic solvents) was found in 17 (28%) of the patients, with a mean age of 49 ± 8 years. The exposure preceded the onset of disease by 9 ± 7 years. The mode of exposure was mainly through inhalation, with a duration of 6.3 ± 6.5 years. Features from patients with exposure to organic solvents were clinically indistinguishable from the other cases studied.

As mentioned by Yamakage and Ishikawa (1982), various aliphatic hydrocarbons, such as naphtha and h-hexane, are able to induce generalized morphea-like sclerosis, either by exposure to vapor or by direct skin contact with the liquid substance. Further features of the induced disorder are sclerodactyly, Raynaud's phenomenon, esophageal dysfunction, and fibrosis of the lung. The disease could be reproduced by chronic intraperitoneal injection of these organic compounds in animal experiments.

A 41-year-old male foundry worker with exposure to trichloroethane, xylene, trimethylbenzene, and naphthalene for 15 years developed the following symptoms: sclerodactyly, digital pitting scars, Raynaud's phenomenon, impotence, reflux esophagitis and ANA titers of 1:320 (Brasington and Thorpe-Swenson 1991).

Trichloroethylene elicits acute pulmonary cytotoxicity in mice, which involves Clara cells of bronchioles. Forkert and Forkert (1994) examined the effects of a single dose of trichloroethylene in lungs of mice and showed that structural and functional abnormalities progress for at least 3 months. Pulmonary fibrosis was first detected at 15 days and was ongoing and diffuse in the alveolar zone, resulting in thickening of alveolar septa and destruction of lung structure. The fibrosis was most pronounced at 90 days. Levels of total lung hydroxyproline content were not significantly different in control and treated mice at days 30 and 60, but were significantly increased at day 90, while the proline content remained unchanged. The increase in collagen deposition at 90 days coincided with a significant increase in lung elastic recoil (Forkert and Forkert 1994).

As shown in Fig. 2, chlorinated hydrocarbons such as VC, perchloroethylene and trichloroethylene are metabolized via similar pathways (Lockey et al. 1987). However, the significance of the P 450 system for metabolization and in the detoxification of putative SSc-inducing environmental toxins has not been studied so far.

Aromatic Hydrocarbons

In 1983, Walder reported of six patients with limited scleroderma who were exposed to aromatic hydrocarbon solvents, such as benzene, toluene, xylene, white spirit, and diesel oil. Unlike chlorinated hydrocarbons, these aromatic hydrocarbons do not cause systemic disorders. The scleroderma-like lesions were limited to hands and feet, and directly exposed body parts.

Recently, however, a sclerodermatous syndrome with unusual features and visceral involvement has been reported following prolonged occupational exposure (32 years) to a wide variety of organic solvents (including benzene in various forms, toluenes, toluidines, xylenes, xylidenes, aniline compounds, and ethanolamine and its derivatives) (Bottomley et al. 1993). Associated functional changes include cold sensitivity, restrictive pulmonary disease, peripheral neuropathy, esophageal dysfunction, labile hypertension, and a monoclonal paraproteinemia.

Garcia-Zamalloa et al. (1994) described a 56-year-old patient who developed SSc with skin, lung, and pericardial affections after he had worked in a rubber transformation section of a tire factory for 23 years. He had been exposed to toluene (an aromatic hydrocarbon), heptane (an aliphatic hydrocarbon), dimethylbuthylphenyldiamine (an aromatic amine), and octhyphenol formaldehyde (a formaldehyde derivative), cutaneously and by inhalation. Exposure to nonchlorinated hydrocarbon and sulfated substances was also assessed. Two male patients developed SLD after occupational exposure to various chemicals (respectively, meta-phenylenediamine, VC, and silicon tetrachloride) in the same building. The most attractive candidate for a potential causative agent in this SLD is meta-phenylenediamine (Owens and Medsger 1988).

In our own clinical practice, we examined a 58-year-old painter who had been exposed to a wide variety of organic solvents for 30 years. He developed an SLD of the skin, esophagus and lung, with polyneuropathy and chronic hepatosis and elevated titers of ANA and Scl-70-antibodies. The second patient was a 49-year-old woman who had sewn leather in an oil bath containing various oils and organic solvents for 12 years. She suffered from an acrosclerosis of the hands, lung fibrosis and kidney involvement, chronic hepatitis, and peripheral neuropathy including positive ANA and ACA titers (Haustein and Albrecht 1996).

Bovenzi et al. (1995) examined 21 patients (16 women, 5 men) with SSc or localized variants of scleroderma. A significant association was found between exposure to organic solvents (aromatic hydro-carbons) and SSc (3 men, 1 woman).

Finally, SLD has also been reported in a 53-year-old man after exposure to LOC, a domestic detergent widely used in Japan. Its constituents are polyoxyethylene alkyl ether and fatty acid alkanol amide (Tanaka et al. 1993).

In a recently performed occupational analysis of 56 men with SSc in the United Kingdom showing no evidence of silica exposure implicated in the onset of the disease, only exposure to organic solvents were reported to any extent. No significant increase in exposure to organic solvents was found in a case control analysis (Silman and Jones 1992).

Table 10 summarizes data on patients with SSc or SLD in association with exposure to organic solvents.

Pesticides/Herbicides

Dunnill and Black (1994) reported a case of generalized cutaneous sclerosis associated with prominent myositis and esophageal involvement in a patient exposed to herbicides containing bromocil, diuron, and aminotriazole. There was no evidence of lung involvement, and antibody titers were in the normal range. Treatment with oral prednisolone resulted in modest improvement of the cutaneous changes, particularly of the face, trunk, and proximal limbs.

Another case of sclerodermiform lesions after use of various herbicides has been described by Poskitt et al. (1994). A 53-year-old man developed chloracne, palmoplantar keratoderma and scleroderma after many years of exposure to a variety of chloracnegens.

Dermatohistopathological changes, selected as an example of highly organized connective tissue, were studied by eight different staining and histochemical techniques in 896 biopsies of macroscopically uninvolved skin from the gluteal region of 56 patients with acute phospho-organic pesticide intoxication between days 2 and 15 after intoxication (Tashev and Tsonev 1990). Nonspecific changes affecting mainly the elastic and collagen components were found. The reticular net, vessels, matrix and cell elements were far less affected, indicating their relative stability to the pesticides' toxicity.

Mixed Connective Tissue Disease

Vincent et al. (1996) reported a 25-year-old woman who developed Sharp's syndrome 5 years after diagnosis of acute silicosis due to inhalation of the scouring powder Ajax (Colgate Palmolive Co.), containing 95% silica, 2% alkylbenzosulphonate, and 3% trichlorocyanuric acid. MCTD due to PVC dust is mentioned above (Panaszek et al. 1993).

Table 10. Cases of systemic sclerosis (SSc) and scleroderma-like diseases (SLD) in association with exposure to solvents

Author	Number	Clinical symptoms	Exposure
Sparrow 1977	1	SLD	Perchloroethylene
Walder 1983	6	SLD	Benzene, toluene, xylene, white spirits, diesel oil
Czirják et al. 1987	8	SSc	Trichloroethylene (1), organic solvents (6), polyethylene (1)
Lockey et al. 1987	1	SSc	Trichloroethylene
Flindt-Hansen and Isager 1987	3	SSc	Trichloroethylene, trichloroethane
Owens and Medsger 1988	2	SLD	Meta-phenylenediamine, silicon tetrachloride (hydrochloric acid and free silica), meta-phenylenediamine, vinyl chloride and silicon tetrachloride
Czirják et al. 1989	17	SSc	Benzene and petroleum-derived crude solvents (3), organic solvents (isopropyl alcohol, terpene derivatives) (4), ethyl acetate and other solvents (3), organic solvents (not well defined) (4), silica dust, paints and solvents (1), ethylene derivatives (1), trichloroethylene (1)
Szeimies et al. 1990	1	SSc	Perchloroethylene
Brasington and Thorpe-Swenson 1991	1	SSc	Trichloroethane, xylene, naphthalene, trimethylbenzene
Yánez-Díaz et al. 1992	1	SSc, silicosis	Trichloroethylene, fiberglass
Tibon-Fisher et al. 1992	1	SSc	Trichloromethane
Gabay and Kahn 1992	3	SSc	Solvents (1), solvents and silica dust (2)
Czirják et al. 1993	1	SSc	Trichloroethylene
Tanaka et al. 1993	1	SLD	LOC (domestic detergent, constituents: polyoxyethylene alkyl ether, fatty acid alkanol amide)
Bottomley et al. 1993	1	SLD	Organic solvents (including benzene in various forms, toluenes, toluidines, xylenes, xylidenes, aniline compounds, and ethanolamine and its derivatives)
Waller et al. 1994	2	Fasciitis, eosinophilia	Trichloroethylene
Czirják et al. 1994	1	Localized scleroderma	Trichloroethylene, tetrachloroethylene, acetone, benzene, isopropyl alcohol, dimethyl phthalate, methoxyethanol, polyethylene glycol, polyvinyl alcohol, polyvinyl acetate, xylene, phenol
Garcia-Zamalloa et al. 1994	1	SSc	Toluene, heptane, dimethylbutylphenyldiamine and octyphenol formaldehyde, exposure to nonchlorinated hydrocarbon and sulphated substances was also assessed
Hinnen et al. 1995	1	Disseminated morphea	Perchloroethylene
Bovenzi et al. 1995	4	Scleroderma	Organic solvents (aromatic hydrocarbons)
Haustein and Albrecht 1996	2	SLD	Wide variety of organic solvents (for 30 years), various oils and organic solvents (for 12 years)

Sjögren's Syndrome

Three cases of primary Sjögren's syndrome were described by Puisieux et al. (1994) in silicotic coal miners. One patient had cryoglobulinemia and polyneuritis. Another had Raynaud's phenomenon, arthralgia, purpura and polyneuritis. Capillary microscopy revealed normal findings in all three patients. ANA were detected only in one patient, who also had anti-SS-A (RO) and anti-SS-B (LA) antibodies. Although the prevalence of SSc, RA, and probably SLE is significantly higher after long-standing occupational exposure to silica, so far no case of Sjögren's syndrome has been described in the course of pulmonary silicosis.

Lupus Erythematosus

Silica-induced LE is a chronic multiorgan system autoimmune disease with frequent exacerbations and remissions similar to the natural course of mixed connective tissue disease. The pathomechanism of LE is not yet completely understood. Based on a genetic background, a major role seems to be played by disturbances of immune regulation, such as T-cell abnormalities, including T-cell cytokine network, polyclonal B-cell stimulation, immune complex formation, defects in the clearance of immune complexes, and dysregulation of apoptosis. Various environmental factors have been discussed, such as drugs, solvents, and silica.

There is only scant knowledge with reference to occupational influences on LE. Exposure to heat, cold, and wind were cited in the past (Warde 1903). Sunlight was frequently considered an eliciting factor for the primary manifestations, and the exacerbations as well (Baer and Harber 1965; Epstein et al. 1965; Diezel et al. 1977). However, among 236 patients examined, only six showed an improvement after the patients moved from an outdoor job to an indoor workplace. In this study, no relationship between occupation and LE could be confirmed (Nebe and Lenz 1971). In terms of association with silicosis of the lung in the former German Democratic Republic, 193 male infirmary patients were examined, with three cases of coincidental silicosis among them (Ziegler et al. 1987).

Further reports exist about the association of LE with silicosis (Hatron et al. 1982) or with occupational silica exposure (Ebihara and Kawami 1985). In addition, Mehlhorn and Gerlach (1990) and our group (Ziegler et al. 1991) demonstrated several cases in the uranium-mining industry in East Germany. The former author observed 37 patients with LE who had been exposed to quartz over many years (Mehlhorn and Gerlach 1990). Thirty of them suffered from silicosis. In a survey of 877 male LE patients (592 systemic LE, 279 discoid LE), we only found seven patients with silicosis out of 428 systemic LE patients over 40 years of age (Ziegler et al. 1991). Recently, we reported of four additional male SLE patients with long-term silica exposure (12–23 years) and silicosis (Haustein 1998). In 1996, Wichmann et al. published a study of 16 systemic LE patients among a group of 52 workers occupationally exposed to silica.

Siebels et al. (1993) presented case histories of five patients with silicosis who had developed SLE and microscopic polyarteritis in two cases each, and rapidly progressive glomerulonephritis (limited Wegener's granulomatosis) in one case.

Recently, a male patient who had worked as a stone cutter and had developed silicosis and systemic LE was also reported by Siebels et al. (1995).

Koeger et al. (1995) observed four patients with SLE (three with silicosis) and one with discoid LE among 24 cases of silica-associated CTD.

Conrad et al. (1996) described 28 definite and 15 likely SLE patients among 15,000 heavily silica-exposed miners, probably part of the same group analyzed by Mehlhorn and Gerlach (1990). Therefore, the prevalence of SLE in the population of highly quartz-dust-exposed uranium miners may be estimated as up to 93 of 100,000. ANA could be detected in all definite and in 72.9% of probable patients having SLE. Middle-to-high-titred ANA were present in 94.4% of definite and in 54.7% of probable patients having SLE. In patients exhibiting definite SLE, clear positive results were obtained for anti-dsDNA in 38.9%, anti-RO/SSA in 38.9%, and anti-LA/SSB in 11.1%. In uranium miners without SLE, the prevalence of ANA was significantly higher than the age- and gender-related control group. Furthermore, an increase in ANA titers in heavily rather than slightly exposed uranium miners could be detected. Table 11 comprises data of patients with LE in association with silica exposure.

An ANA profile suggestive of Sjögren's syndrome or SLE without symptoms of either disease occurred in a patient with chronic obstructive pulmonary disease. He worked for less than 5 years as a maintenance mechanic in a plant in South Carolina manufacturing silica flour and industrial sand (Johnson and Busnardo 1993). Excessive occupational exposure to free silica by inhalation was documented. An open-lung biopsy revealed an early stage of silicosis characterized by perivascular and peribronchial accumulation of macrophages, as well as early granuloma formation.

Dermatomyositis

Few reports are available on dermatomyositis after occupational exposure. Koeger et al. (1991) described dermatopolymyositis in two men and one woman after 5, 16 and 21 years of occupational exposure to silica. Pulmonary involvement was present as diffuse interstitial fibrosis in two patients whose lung biopsies revealed high particulate silica contents. Another patient with polymyositis among 52 workers from a factory producing scouring powder with a higher than usual silica content (70–90% powdered quartz) was described by Wichmann et al. (1996). Among 24 patients with silica-associated CTD, three patients have been diagnosed with dermatomyositis and Sjögren's syndrome (Koeger et al. 1995).

Rheumatoid Arthritis

Rosenman and Zhu (1995) found an association between silicosis and RA using hospital discharge data from Michigan between the years 1990 and 1991, examining potential associations between pneumoconiosis and pulmonary hypertension, lung cancer, obstructive lung disease, and connective tissue disease among both male and female patients. In an updated multivariate analysis of 3328 gold miners

Table 11. Lupus erythematosus (LE) in association with silica exposure

Author	Cases	Diagnosis	Exposure (occupation)
Ziegler et al. 1987	3	SLE and silicosis	Silica
Mehlhorn and Gerlach 1990	37	25 SLE and silicosis, 5 discoid LE and silicosis, 4 SLE, 3 discoid LE	Silica (36 ore miners, 1 foundry worker)
Ziegler et al. 1991	30	LE, 5 with silicosis	Silica (16 ore miners, 3 foundry workers, 2 underground workers, 2 enamellers, 1 sandblaster, quarry worker, stove bricklayer, grindstone maker, well driller, glass industry worker)
Siebels et al. 1993	2	SLE and silicosis	Silica
Siebels et al. 1995	1	SLE and silicosis	Silica (stone cutter)
Koeger et al. 1995	5	4 SLE (3 with silicosis), 1 discoid LE	Silica (mason, miner, dental prothetist, scouring and tooth powder worker)
Wichmann et al. 1996	16	SLE	Silica (scouring powder factory)
Haustein and Albrecht 1996	1	SLE and silicosis	Silica (uranium hewer)
Conrad et al. 1996 (partially the same group as analyzed by Mehlhorn and Gerlach 1990)	43	28 SLE, 15 probable SLE	Silica (uranium miners)
Haustein 1998	4	SLE and silicosis	Silica (uranium hewer, cast polisher, stone mason, uranium driller)

who worked underground for at least 1 year in South Dakota between 1940 and 1965, an extended follow-up from 1977 to 1990 revealed significant excesses of arthritis, musculoskeletal diseases, and skin conditions including SLE and SSc, in addition to silicosis and tuberculosis, but without lung cancer (Steenland and Brown 1995). The study of Koeger et al. (1995) presented five patients with RA (four in association with Sjögren's syndrome).

Conclusion

Connective tissue disorders such as SSc, LE, Sjögren's syndrome, dermatomyositis and RA can be induced by occupational exposure to silica, solvents, and other chemical offenders. An enhanced genetic susceptibility seems to favor these disorders. SSc is the most frequent and best-studied disease. While silica precipitates SSc, the other offenders induce scleroderma-like diseases with different clinical and laboratory findings than with SSc. Taking a careful case history of patients with SSc will help to identify the occupational causes. The best way to prevent this type of connective tissue disease is to minimize the exposure to occupational substances. However, efforts in the form of individual expert decisions have to be made in order to acknowledge these disorders as occupational diseases and provide some social and financial support to patients and reduce the harm caused by these disorders.

Acknowledgment. We gratefully acknowledge Ulf Anderegg (PhD) for helpful discussions and Jörg Kleine-Tebbe (MD) for editorial assistance.

References

Adamson IYR, Letourneau HL, Bowden DH (1989) Enhanced macrophage fibroblast interactions in the pulmonary interstitium increases fibrosis after silica injection to monocyte-depleted mice. Am J Pathol 134:411–418

American Thoracic Society (1997) Adverse effects of crystalline silica exposure. Am J Respir Crit Care Med 155:761–765

Anderegg U, Vorberg S, Herrmann K, Haustein UF (1996) Increased expression of interstitial collagenase in silica-treated fibroblasts. Eur J Dermatol 6:51–55

Anderegg U, Vorberg S, Herrmann K, Haustein UF (1997) Silica directly induces intercellular adhesion molecule 1 (ICAM-1) expression in cultured endothelial cells. Eur J Dermatol 7:27–31

Bachner U, Etzel F, Lange CE, Marsteller HJ, Veltman G (1974) Haemostaseologische Aspekte bei der Vinylchlorid-Krankheit. Dtsch Med Wochenschr 99:2409–2410

Baer RL, Harber LC (1965) Photobiology of lupus erythematosus. Arch Dermatol 92:124–128

Bauer M, Rabens SF (1977) Trichloroethylene toxicity. Int J Dermatol 16:113–116

Baur X (1994) Systemische Sklerodermie im Uranerzbergbau der ehemaligen SDAG Wismut. Arbeitsmed Sozialmed Umweltmed Sonderheft 22:5–7

Baur X, Rihs HP, Altmeyer P, Degens P, Conrad K, Mehlhorn J, Weber K, Wiebe V (1996) Systemic sclerosis in German uranium miners under special consideration of autoantibody subsets and HLA class II alleles. Respiration 63:368–375

Beck B, Irmscher G (1974) Silikosen durch weniger bekannte Expositionsarten. Z Erkr Atmungsorgane 140:282–293

Beck B, Irmscher G, Zschunke E (1976) Sklerodermie und Silikose – Versuch einer Synopsis. Z Gesamte Inn Med 31:493–496

Black CM, Welsh KI, Walker AE, Bernstein RM, Catoggio LJ, McGregor AR, Jones JK (1983) Genetic susceptibility to scleroderma-like syndrome induced by vinyl chloride. Lancet 1:53–55

Blair HM, Headington JT, Lynch PJ (1974) Occupational trauma, Raynaud's phenomenon and sclerodactylia. Arch Environ Health 28:80–81

Bolt HM, Laib RJ, Filser JG (1982) Reactive metabolites and carcinogenicity of halogenated ethylenes. Biochem Pharmacol 31:1–4

Bottomley WW, Sheehan-Dare RA, Hughes P, Cuncliffe WJ (1993) A sclerodermatous syndrome with unusual features following prolonged occupational exposure to organic solvents. Br J Dermatol 128:203–206

Bovenzi M, Barbone F, Betta A, Tommasini M, Versini W (1995) Scleroderma and occupational exposure. Scand J Work Environ Health 21:289–292

Bramwell B (1914) Diffuse sclerodermia: its frequency; its occurrence in stone-masons; its treatment by fibrolysin injections – elevations of temperature due to fibrolysin. Edinburgh J Med 12:387–401

Brasington RD, Thorpe-Swenson AJ (1991) Systemic sclerosis associated with cutaneous exposure to solvent: case report and review of the literature. Arthritis Rheum 34:631–633

Choudat D (1994) Occupational lung diseases among dental technicians. Tuber Lung Dis 75:99–104

Christy WC, Rodnan GP (1984) Conjugal progressive systemic sclerosis (scleroderma): report of the disease in husband and wife. Arthritis Rheum 27:1180–1182

Conrad K, Mehlhorn J, Lüthke K, Dörner T, Frank KH (1996) Systemic lupus erythematosus after heavy exposure to quartz dust in uranium mines: clinical and serological characteristics. Lupus 5:62–69

Conrad K, Humbel RL, Tan EM, Shoenfeld Y (1997) Autoantibodies – diagnostic, pathogenetic and prognostic relevance. Clin Exp Rheumatol 15:457–465

Conrad K, Mehlhorn J, Frank KH (1998) Markers of systemic autoimmune disease in uranium miners. In: Conrad K, Humbel RL, Meurer M, Shoenfeld Y, Tan EM (eds) Pathogenic and diagnostic relevance of autoantibodies. Pabst Science Publishers, Volume 9, pp 151–152

Cordier JH, Fieviez C, Lefevre MJ, Sevrin A (1966) Acroosteolyse et lesions cutanees chez deux ouvriers affectees au nettoyage d'autoclaves. Can Med Travail 4:3

Cowie RL (1987) Silica-dust-exposed mine workers with scleroderma (systemic sclerosis). Chest 92:260–262

Czernielewski A, Swierczynska-Kiec M, Gluszcz M (1979) Dermatological aspects of so called vinyl chloride monomer disease. Derm Beruf Umwelt 27:108–112

Czirják L, Dankó K, Schlammadinger J, Surányi P, Tamási L, Szegedi GY (1987) Progressive systemic sclerosis occurring in patients exposed to chemicals. Int J Dermatol 26:374–378

Czirják L, Bokk Á, Csontos G, Lörincz G, Szegedi G (1989) Clinical findings in 61 patients with progressive systemic sclerosis. Acta Derm Venereol 69:533–536

Czirják L, Schlammadinger J, Szegedi G (1993) Systemic sclerosis and exposure to trichloroethylene. Dermatology 186:236–7

Czirják L, Pocs E, Szegedi G (1994) Localized scleroderma after exposure to organic solvents. Dermatology 189:399–401

Diezel W, Meffert H, Günther W, Huse K, Sönnichsen N (1977) Exazerbation des Lupus erythematodes visceralis infolge UV-Bestrahlung. Dermatol Monatsschr 163:290–295

Dinman BD, Cook WA, Whitehouse WM, Magnuson HJ, Ditcheck T (1971) Occupational acroosteolysis: an epidemiological study. Arch Environ Health 22:61–65

Dowd PM, Ziegler V (1987) Endothelial cell cultures in silica induced systemic sclerosis. Abstr Sympos Aktuel Probl Arbeitsderm Leipzig, p 51

Dunnill MG, Black MM (1994) Sclerodermatous syndrome after occupational exposure to herbicides-response to systemic steroids. Clin Exp Dermatol 19:518–520

Ebihara I, Kawami M (1985) Health hazards of mineral dust with special reference to the causation of immuno-pathologic systemic diseases. J Sci Labour 61:1–31

Ebihara I, Kawami M (2000) Mineral Dust Exposure and Systemic Diseases. JEPTO 19:109–127

Englert H, O'Connor H, Small-McMahon J, Chambers P, Davis K, Brooks P (2000) Male systemic sclerosis and occupational silica exposure – a population-based study. Aust NZ J Med 30:215–220

Epstein IH, Tuffanelli DL, Dubois EL (1965) Light sensitivity and lupus erythematosus. Arch Dermatol 91:483–485

Erasmus LD (1957) Scleroderma in gold-miners on the Witwatersrand with particular reference to pulmonary manifestations. South Afr Lab Clin Med 3:209–231

Evans DJ, Posner E (1971) Pneumoconiosis in laundry workers. Environ Res 4:127–128

Fleischmajer R, Perlish IS, Duncan M (1983) Scleroderma: a model for fibrosis. Arch Dermatol 119:957–962

Flindt-Hansen H, Isager H (1987) Scleroderma after occupational exposure to trichlorethylene and trichlorethane. Acta Derm Venereol 67:263–264

Forkert PG, Forkert L (1994) Trichloroethylene induces pulmonary fibrosis in mice. Can J Physiol Pharmacol 72:205–10

Francia A, Monarca A, Cavallot A (1959) Osservazioni clinico-roentgenologiche sollàssociazione silicosi-sclerodermia. Med Lav 50:523

Frank R, Giese T, Dummer R, Walther T, Rytter M, Ziegler V, Haustein UF (1993) Silica-induced cytokine release in human monocyte cultures and its possible involvement in the pathophysiology of silica-associated scleroderma. Eur J Dermatol 3:304–309

Gabay C, Kahn MF (1992) Les sclérodermies masculines; rôle de l'exposition professionelle. Schweiz Med Wochenschr 122:1746–1752

Garcia-Zamalloa AM, Ojeda E, Gonzalez-Beneitez C, Goni J, Garrido A (1994) Systemic sclerosis and organic solvents: early diagnosis in industry. Ann Rheum Dis 53:618

Harris DK, Adams WGF (1967) Acroosteolysis occurring in men engaged in the polymerisation of vinyl chloride. BMJ 3:712–714

Hatron PY, Plouvier B, Francois M (1982) Assoziation von systemischem Lupus erythematodes und Silikose. Kasuistik (5 Pat.). Rev Med Intern 3:245–246

Haustein UF (1998) Silica-induced Lupus erythematosus. Acta Derm Venereol 78:73–74

Haustein UF, Albrecht M (1993) Zur Epidemiologie und Klinik der systemischen Sklerodermie. Z Hautkr Geschlechtskr 68:651–658

Haustein UF, Albrecht M (1996) Berufsbedingte progressive Sklerodermie, Pseudosklerodermie und systemischer Lupus erythematodes. Derm Beruf Umwelt 44:77–80

Haustein UF, Herrmann K (1994) Environmental scleroderma. Clin Dermatol 12:467–473

Haustein UF, Klug H (1975) Zur Ultrastruktur der Hautkapillaren bei Lupus eythematodes, Dermatomyositis und progressiver Sklerodermie. Dermatol Monatsschr 161:353–363

Haustein UF, Ziegler V (1985) Environmentally induced systemic sclerosis-like disorders. Int J Dermatol 24:147–151

Haustein UF, Herrmann K, Boehme HJ (1986) Pathogenesis of progressive systemic sclerosis. Int J Derm 25:286–293

Hinnen U, Schmid-Grendelmeier P, Muller E, Elsner P (1995) Exposure to solvents in scleroderma: disseminated circumscribed scleroderma (morphea) in a painter exposed to perchloroethylene (in German). Schweiz Med Wochenschr 125:2433–2437

Holt PF (1981) Transport of inhaled dust to extrapulmonary sites. J Pathol 133:123–129

Inachi S, Mizutani H, Ando Y, Shimizu M (1996) Progressive systemic sclerosis sine scleroderma which developed after exposure to epoxy resin polymerization. J Dermatol 23:344–346

Ishikawa H, Yamakage A, Tamura T, et al (1982) Scleroderma induced by epoxy resins with special reference to experimental scleroderma with Bis(4-amino-3-methylcyclohexyl)-methane as the probable causative agent. J UOEH 4:225–235

Ishikawa O, Warita S, Tamura A, Miyachi Y (1995) Occupational scleroderma. A 17-year follow-up study. Br J Dermatol 133:786–789

Johnson WM, Busnardo MS (1993) Silicosis following employment in the manufacture of silica flour and industrial sand. J Occup Med 35:716–719

Kilburn KH, Warshaw RH (1992) Prevalence of symptoms of systemic lupus erythematosus (SLE) and of fluorescent antinuclear antibodies associated with chronic exposure to trichloroethylene and other chemicals in well water. Environ Res 57:1–9

Knight KR, Gibbons R (1987) Increased collagen synthesis and cross-link formation in the skin of rats exposed to vinyl chloride monomer. Clin Sci (Colch) 72:673–678

Koeger AC, Alcaix D, Rozenberg S, Bourgeois P (1991) Occupational exposure to silicon and dermatopolymyositis. 3 cases (in French). Ann Med Interne 142:409–413

Koeger AC, Marre JP, Rozenberg S, Gutmann L, Bourgeois P (1992) Autoimmune diseases after unusual exposure to silica or silicones. 3 cases. (in French). Ann Med Interne 143:165–70

Koeger AC, Lang T, Alcaix D, Milleron B, Rozenberg S, Chaibi P, Arnaud J, Mayaud C, Camus JP, Bourgeois P (1995) Silica-associated connective tissue disease. A study of 24 cases. Medicine (Baltimore) 74:221–237

Kohanka V (1982) Epidemiologic studies of the delayed-type immunity in workers exposed to vinyl chloride monomers (in German). Boerg Vener Szemle 58:145–149

Lange GE, Juehe S, Veltman G (1974) Ueber das Auftreten von Angiosarkomen der Leber bei zwei Arbeitern der PVC-herstellenden Industrie. Dtsch Med Wochenschr 99:1598–1599

Lelbach WK, Marsteller HJ (1981) Vinyl chloride-associated disease. Ergeb Inn Med Kinderheilkd 47:1–110

Lockey JE, Kelly CR, Cannon GW, Colby TV, Aldrich V, Livingston GK (1987) Progressive systemic sclerosis associated with exposure to trichloroethylene. J Occup Med 29:493–496

Maricq HR (1981) Vinyl chloride disease. International Conference on Progressive Systemic Sclerosis. Austin, 9 October 1981

Maricq HR, Johnson MN, Whetstone CL, LeRoy EC (1976) Capillary abnormalities in polyvinyl chloride production workers. Examination by in vivo microscopy. JAMA 236:1368–1371

Markowitz SS, McDonald CJ, Fethiere W (1972) Occupational acroosteolysis. Arch Dermatol 106:219–233

Masi AT (1980) Preliminary criteria for the classification of systemic sclerosis. Arthritis Rheum 23:581–590

Medsger TA, Masi AT (1971) Epidemiology of systemic sclerosis. Ann Intern Med 74:714–721

Mehlhorn J (1994) "Quarzinduzierte" Progressive Systemische Sklerodermie – Exposition, Klinische Beobachtungen, Lungenfunktion. Arbeitsmed Sozialmed Umweltmed Sonderheft 22:8–11

Mehlhorn J, Gerlach C (1990) Gemeinsames Auftreten von Silikose und Lupus erythematodes. Z Erkr Atmungsorgane 175:38–41

Mehlhorn J, Gerlach C, Ziegler V (1990) Berufsbedingte progressive systemische Sklerodermie durch ein quarzhaltiges Scheuermittel. Derm Beruf Umwelt 38:180–184

Milford WA (1976) Evidence of an immune complex disorder in vinyl chloride workers. Proc R Soc Med 69:289–291

Moseley PL, Monick M, Hunninghake GW (1988) Divergent effects of silica on lymphocyte proliferation and immunoglobulin production. J Appl Physiol 65:350–357

Mueller G, Norpoth K, Kusters E (1978) Determination of thiodiglycolic acid in urine specimens of vinyl chloride exposed workers. Int Arch Occup Environ Health 41:199–205

Nagata C, Yoshida H, Mirbod SM, Komura Y, Fujita S, Inaba R, Iwata H, Maeda M, Shikano Y, Ichiki Y, et al (1993) Cutaneous signs (Raynaud's phenomenon, sclerodactylia and edema of the hands) and hand-arm vibration exposure. Int Arch Occup Environ Health 64:587–591

Nario RC, Hubbard AK (1996) Silica exposure increases expression of pulmonary intercellular adhesion molecule-1 (ICAM-1) in C57Bl/6 mice. J Toxicol Environ Health 49:599–617

Nebe H, Lenz U (1971) Untersuchungen ueber berufliche Noxen beim Lupus erythematodes. Dermatol Monatsschr 157:500–504

Oghiso Y, Kubota Y (1986) Enhanced interleukin 1 production by alveolar macrophages and increase in Ia-positive lung cells in silica-exposed rats. Microbiol Immunol 30:1189–1198

Ostlere LS, Harris D, Buckley C, Black C, Rustin MH (1992) Atypical systemic sclerosis following exposure to vinyl chloride monomer. A case report and review of the cutaneous aspects of vinyl chloride disease. Clin Exp Dermatol 17:208–210

Owens GR, Medsger TA (1988) Systemic sclerosis secondary to occupational exposure. Am J Med 85:114–116

Panaszek B, Malolepszy J, Wrzyszcz M, Jutel M, Machaj Z (1993) Mixed connective tissue disease in a male patient chronically exposed to toxic chemicals (in Polish). Pol Tyg Lek 48:430–432

Penin H, Sager G, Lange GE, et al (1975) Neurologisch-psychiatrische und elektroenzephalographische Befunde bei Patienten mit Vinylchlorid-Krankheit. Proc. 15. Jahrestagung Dt Gesellschaft Arb Med, Gentner, Stuttgart, pp 299–304

Plewig G, Kligman A (1978) Acne. Springer, Berlin Heidelberg New York

Poskitt LB, Duffill MB, Rademaker M (1994) Chloracne, palmoplantar keratoderma and localized scleroderma in a weed sprayer. Clin Exp Dermatol 19:264–267

Puisieux F, Hachulla E, Brouillard M, Hatron PY, Devulder B (1994) Silicosis and primary Gougerot-Sjogren syndrome (in French). Rev Med Intern 15:575–579

Reinl W (1957) Sklerodermie durch Trichloraethyleneinwirkung? Zentralbl Arbeitsmed 7:58–60

Rihs HP, Conrad K, Mehlhorn J, May-Taube K, Welticke B, Frank KH, Baur X (1994) Association between HLA-D alleles and scleroderma-specific autoantibodies in quartz dust exposed persons (in German). Z Arztl Fortbild (Jena) 88:513–518

Rihs HP, Conrad K, Mehlhorn J, May-Taube K, Welticke B, Frank KH, Baur X (1996) Molecular analysis of HLA-DPB1 alleles in idiopathic systemic sclerosis patients and uranium miners with systemic sclerosis. Int Arch Allergy Immunol 109:216–222

Rodnan GP, Benedek TG, Medsger TA, Cammarata RJ (1967) The association of progressive systemic sclerosis (scleroderma) with coal miners pneumoconiosis and other forms of silicosis. Ann Intern Med 66:323–334

Rosenman KD, Zhu Z (1995) Pneumoconiosis and associated medical conditions. Am J Ind Med 27:107–113

Rustin MHA, Bull HA, Ziegler V, Mehlhorn J, Haustein UF, Maddison PJ, James J, Dowd PM (1990) Silica-associated systemic sclerosis is clinically, serologically indistinguishable from idiopathic systemic sclerosis. Br J Dermatol 123:725–34

Saihan EM, Burton JL, Heaton KW (1978) A new syndrome with pigmentation scleroderma, gynaecomastia, Raynaud's phenomenon and neuropathy. Br J Dermatol 99:437–441

Sanchez-Roman J, Wichmann I, Salaberri J, Varela JM, Nunez-Roldan A (1993) Multiple clinical and biological autoimmune manifestations in 50 workers after occupational exposure to silica. Ann Rheum Dis 52:534–538

Schirren SM (1971) Skin lesions caused by trichloroethylene in a metal working plant. Berufsdermatosen 19:240–245

Schmidt JA, Oliver CN, Lepe-Zuniga JL, Green I, Gery I (1984) Silica-stimulated monocytes release fibroblast proliferation factors identical to interleukin 1. J Clin Invest 73:1462–1472

Siebels M, Schulz V, Andrassy K (1993) Silicosis and systemic diseases (in German). Immun Infekt 21:53–54

Siebels M, Schulz V, Andrassy K (1995) Systemic lupus erythematosus and silicosis (in German). Dtsch Med Wochenschr 120:214–218

Siegel RC (1977) Scleroderma. Med Clin North Am 61:283–296

Silman AJ, Jones S (1992) What is the contribution of occupational environmental factors to the occurrence of scleroderma in men? Ann Rheum Dis 51:1322–1324

Silver RM, Sahn EE, Allen JA, Sahn S, Greene W, Maize JC, Garen PD (1993) Demonstration of silicon in sites of connective tissue disease in patients with silicone-gel breast implants. Arch Dermatol 129:63–68

Sluis-Cremer GK, Hessel PA, Hnizdo E, Churchill AR, Zeiss EA (1985) Silica, silicosis and progressive systemic sclerosis. Br J Ind Med 42:838–843

Sparrow GP (1977) A connective tissue disorder similar to vinyl chloride disease in a patient exposed to perchloroethylene. Clin Dermatol 2:17–22

Stachów A, Jablonska S, Skiendzielewska A (1979) Biogenic amines derived from tryptophan in systemic and cutaneous scleroderma. Acta Derm Venereol 59:1–5

Steenland K, Brown D (1995) Mortality study of gold miners exposed to silica and nonasbestiform amphibole minerals: an update with 14 more years of follow-up. Am J Ind Med 27:217–229

Struhar D, Harbeck RJ (1989) Anti-Ia antibodies inhibit the spontaneous secretion of IL-1 from silicotic rat alveolar macrophages. Immunol Lett 23:31–33

Studnicka MJ, Menzinger G, Drlicek M, Maruna H, Neumann MG (1995) Pneumoconiosis and systemic sclerosis following 10 years of exposure to polyvinyl chloride dust. Thorax 50:583–5

Suciu I, Drejman I, Valaskai M (1963) Contributii la studiul imbolnavirilor produse de clorina de vinil. Med Int 15:967–978

Szeimies RM, Lissner A, Meurer M (1992) Perchlorethylen-induzierte systemische Sklerodermie. Derm Beruf Umwelt 40:66–69

Tanaka M, Niizeki H, Shimizu S, Miyakawa S (1993) Scleroderma after exposure to domestic detergent LOC. J Rheumatol 20:1993–1994

Tashev TS, Tsonev I (1990) The connective tissue changes in patients with acute poisonings by organophosphate pesticides (in Bulgarian). Vutr Boles 29:83–87

Thorgeirsson A, Fregert S, Ramnaes O (1978) Sensitization capacity of epoxy resin oligomers in the guinea pig. Acta Derm Venereol 58:17–21

Tibon-Fisher O, Heller E, Ribak J (1992) Occupational scleroderma due to organic solvent exposure. Harefuah 122:530–532, 551

Varga J, Schumacher R, Jimenez SA (1989) Systemic sclerosis after augmentation mammoplasty with silicone implants. Ann Intern Med 111:377–383

Veltman G (1980) Klinische Befunde und arbeitsmedizinische Aspekte der Vinylchlorid-Krankheit. Dermatol Monatsschr 166:705–712

Vincent M, Pouchelle C, Martinon S, Gerard F, Arthaud Y (1996) Connective tissue disease due to intentional inhalation of scouring powder. Eur Respir J 9:2688–2690

Walder WB (1983) Do solvents cause scleroderma? Int J Dermatol 22:157–158

Waller PA, Clauw D, Cupps T, Metcalf JS, Silver RM, Leroy EC (1994) Fasciitis (not scleroderma) following prolonged exposure to an organic solvent. J Rheumatol 21:1567–1570

Warde WB (1903) Lupus erythematosus: some illustrative cases. Br J Dermatol 15:161–168

Wichmann I, Sanchez-Roman J, Morales J, Castillo MJ, Ocana C, Nunez-Roldan A (1996) Antimyeloperoxidase antibodies in individuals with occupational exposure to silica. Ann Rheum Dis 55:205–207

Wilson RH, McCormick WE, Tatum CF, Greech JL (1967) Occupational acroosteolysis: report of 31 cases. JAMA 201:577–580

Yamakage A, Ishikawa H (1982) Generalized morphea-like scleroderma occurring in people exposed to organic solvents. Dermatologica 165:186–193

Yamakage A, Ishikawa H, Saito Y, Hattori A (1980) Occupational scleroderma-like disorder in men engaged in the polymerization of epoxy resins. Dermatologica 161:33–44

Yamamoto T, Furuse Y, Katayama I, Nishioka K (1994) Nodular scleroderma in a worker using a silica-containing abrasive. J Dermatol 21:751–754

Yánez-Diaz S, Moran M, Unamuno P, Armijo M (1992) Silica and trichloroethylene-induced progressive systemic sclerosis. Dermatology 184:98–102

Yoshida S, Gershwin ME (1993) Autoimmunity and selected environmental factors of disease induction. Semin Arthritis Rheum 22:399–419

Ziegler V, Koepping H, Münzberger H, Haustein UF, Löschke K (1981) Arbeitsmedizinische Aspekte der progressiven Sklerodermie. Wiss Z Karl-Marx-Univ Leipzig 30:478–482

Ziegler V, Pampel W, Zschunke E, Münzberger H, Mährlein W, Koepping H (1982) Kristalliner Quarz – (eine) Ursache der progressiven Sklerodermie? Dermatol Monatsschr 168:398–401

Ziegler V, Haustein UF, Mehlhorn J, Münzberger H, Rennau H (1986) Quarzinduzierte Sklerodermie, sklerodermie-aehnliches Syndrom oder echte Sklerodermie? Dermatol Monatsschr 172:86–90

Ziegler V, Kipping D, Herrmann K, Haustein UF, Löschke K (1987) Quarz – seine Relevanz für die Dermatologie. Derm Beruf Umwelt 35:199–204

Ziegler V, Keyn J, Mehlhorn J, Kipping D, Haustein UF (1988) Qarznachweis in Sklerodermiehaut. Dermatol Monatsschr 174:688–689

Ziegler V, Pfeil B, Haustein UF (1991) Berufliche Quarzstaubexposition – Progressive Sklerodermie und Lupus erythematodes. Z Hautkr Geschlechtskr 66:968–970

Zschunke E (1976) Dermatologische Probleme in der Arbeitsmedizin. Dermatol Monatsschr 162:454–458

Zschunke E, Ziegler V, Haustein UF (1990) Occupationally induced connective tissue disorders. In: Adams RM (ed) Occupational skin disease. Saunders, Philadelphia

CHAPTER 14

Operational Definition of Occupational Allergic Contact Dermatitis

14

S. I. ALE, H. I. MAIBACH

Introduction

When establishing the diagnosis of Occupational Allergic Contact Dermatitis (OACD), two prerequisites should be fulfilled: recognizing the existence of an occupational exposure; and demonstrating that this exposure represents a cause or substantial aggravating factor in the patient's dermatitis. To accomplish this goal, the physician relies on a detailed history, a complete physical examination and comprehensive skin testing.

Diagnosis of OACD

The assessment starts with a thorough dermatological history (Table 1). The physician should investigate all probable sources of allergenic exposure in the patient's workplace, and determine whether or not this exposure may be responsible for the patient's dermatitis. In addition, history should provide insights in differentiating OACD from other exogenous or endogenous dermatoses. This is crucial when dealing with multifactorial dermatitis. Previous episodes of dermatitis, presence of other skin diseases and personal or family atopy must also be recorded.

Exposure Assessment in OACD

Assessment of exposure must include all suspicious occupational and non-occupational agents. A workplace visit usually proves valuable. When assessing exposure, many quantitative and qualitative parameters have to be considered (Table 2). The environmental evaluation involves the determination of the intrinsic hazardous potential and other physicochemical characteristics of the suspected agent. Assessment of the hazardous potential of the substance or product comprises data from predictive toxicological assays, including mathematical models (Hostynek 1998), in vitro-in vivo methods (Basketter 1996) and in vivo testing in animals and in humans (Andersen 1985; Rietschel 1995). Besides, the physicochemical properties of the substance, i.e., pH, solvent properties, hygroscopicity, volatility, oxidizing capacity, substantivity, binding capacity, wash-and-rub resistance to removal, etc., should always be considered.

Table 1. Clinical data for the assessment of OACD

1. History of exposure to the sensitizer (present or past)
Occupational exposure
  Complete job description and materials
  Other materials present in the working environment
  Other workers similarly affected
  Process change before the onset of the dermatitis
Non-occupational exposure
  Homework, hobbies
  Skin care products, pharmaceutical products, jewelry and clothing
Indirect contact (contaminated objects, connubial dermatitis, etc.)
Seasonal related contact (plants and other environmental agents)
Photoexposure
Type of exposure: dose, frequency, cutaneous site, total area of contact
Environmental conditions: humidity, temperature, occlusion, vapors, powders, mechanical
trauma, friction, etc.

2. Clinical characteristics of the present dermatitis
Time of onset (onset after the patient began work)
Characteristics of the initial lesions
Effect of holidays and time-off work
Dermatitis site and distribution of the lesions (patient exposed to the suspicious agent at
work and distribution of the dermatitis consistent with occupational exposure)
Some morphologies suggest specific allergens
Time relationship between exposure and the development or aggravation of the lesions

3. History of previous dermatitis and other clinical events
Past exogenous dermatitis with similar or different characteristics
Previous patch testing
Other endogenous skin diseases (psoriasis, atopic dermatitis, stasis, etc.)

4. Personal and family atopy and history of other family skin diseases

Table 2. Parameters of exposure

Hazardous potency of the substance/product
Other intrinsic (physicochemical) properties of the substance
Concentration of the substance
Duration of exposure
Frequency of exposure
Route of exposure
Skin site and total area of exposure
Specific exposure mechanisms
Simultaneous exposure factors (occlusion, temperature, humidity, mechanical trauma, etc.)

Skin contact with hazardous agents is a sine qua non condition, but whether
or not this contact will result in the development of OACD depends on a combination of exposure characteristics and individual susceptibility. Quantitative data
regarding exposure (i.e., dose, duration, frequency and total area of exposure)
should also be determined. Delayed sensitivity is a dose-related phenomenon and
there is a threshold surface concentration of the allergen required to induce sensi-

tization and/or elicitation of the response (Marzulli 1976; Upadhye 1992). Finally, we have to consider concomitant exposure factors that might enhance the percutaneous penetration of the hazardous substance and are unique to the workplace or task, i.e., wet work, irritation, occlusion, temperature, humidity and mechanical trauma (Andersen 1994; Meneghini 1985; Shmunes 1988).

Sometimes, even when a meticulous clinical history and thorough exposure evaluation is carried out, the source of exposure remains unidentified. This can be due to multiple causes; the exposure may be indirect (produced through a contaminated item), infrequent or occasional. We also have to consider substances of personal hygiene, measures of skin protection (such as gloves, glasses, barrier creams, etc.) and medicaments used by the patient (Table 1). All other potential causes of contact dermatitis from non-occupational exposure should be excluded by a thorough history and comprehensive patch testing.

Relationship Between Exposure and Clinical Dermatitis

To ascertain whether the exposure is relevant to the patient's dermatitis, the following factors should be taken into account: existence of a temporal relationship between the exposure and the evolution of the dermatitis and appropriate morphology (correspondence between the exposure and the clinical pattern of the dermatitis).

Time Relationship Between Dermatitis and Exposure

Time relationship between the occupational exposure and the clinical course of the dermatitis varies depending on many different factors related to the exposure, individual susceptibility and type of dermatitis. Usually, occupational contact dermatitis improves when the patient is off work and relapses when work is resumed. Allergic contact dermatitis improves more slowly than irritant contact dermatitis when exposure is discontinued and recurs faster (in a few days) after returning to work. The elicitation time depends on the characteristics of the sensitizer, intensity of exposure and degree of sensitivity. Lesions usually appear 24–72 h after the last exposure to the causative agent, but they may develop as early as 5 hours or as late as 7 days after exposure. A clinical course characterized by iterative, sudden flares of dermatitis, usually indicates allergic sensitization. Nevertheless, confounding factors should always be considered. Sometimes, exposure may continue even when the patient is off work, due to the existence of non-occupational sources; therefore, failure to improve does not necessarily invalidate a causal relationship. Besides, severe chronic dermatitis may require 3–4 weeks away from work before apparent improvement occurs.

Clinical Morphology of the Dermatitis

The pattern of distribution of OACD is usually the single most important diagnostic clue and should be consistent with the exposure, correlating with occupational gestures and activities. Usually the most affected areas are those of maximum contact with the offending allergen, but sometimes, the most severe dermatitis appears in an area distant to the apparent site of contact. This can be due to the transfer of the antigen to other body sites by the hands, which spreads the allergen to different areas of the body, such as the face, neck and genitalia. Sometimes, clinical examination reveals a distinct occupational "mark" that points out the causative agent. However, most of the time the clinical situation is intricate and the diagnostic approach needs to be systematic and critical. Dermatitis is often the joint outcome of endogenous, irritant and allergic factors. Previous irritant dermatitis produced by an irritant working environment may predispose to allergic contact dermatitis [9]. In some dermatitis – especially hand dermatitis – constitutional, irritant and allergic factors frequently coexist.

Visiting the Workplace

The accurate diagnosis of OACD often requires a workplace visit. This activity – although time consuming – enables the physician to obtain a whole picture of the real situation at the working milieu and then, many details acquire clinical significance. It also allows the identification of putative sources of exposure, as well as establishing the actual degree of skin contact. It makes it possible to reconstruct the occupational gestures, to appreciate the working conditions (space, temperature, ventilation) and the existence of adequate protective measures. Visiting the workplace also enables the detection of allergens missed from patch testing as well as the assessment of relevance of previously unexplained positive reactions.

Patch Testing in OACD

In the diagnostic study of OACD, extensive patch testing including the screening standard tray, additional series of allergens according to the occupation, and substances used by the patient in the workplace is often required. Four particular substantial aspects have to be considered when performing patch tests in the assessment of OACD: interpreting results, especially evaluating false-positive and false-negative reactions; deciding when to re-test; deciding when to perform special tests; and assessing clinical relevance of positive reactions. The most significant aspect in evaluating a positive patch test reaction is ascertaining whether the response represents a true positive allergic or a false-positive reaction. Irritant reactions are the principal cause of false-positive responses and are frequently observed when testing with industrial chemicals. Testing with industrial substances should always be undertaken with caution. It is imperative to follow the established guidelines; materials of unknown composition are never to be used under occlusion and open tests with diluted substances should be preferred as an initial approach, progressively increasing the concentration as far as no response – either allergic or irritant – appears. When a new compound gives a positive reaction, testing in control subjects is required. Information about the materials to be tested should be procured from labels of ingredients, product databases or the material safety data sheets. When not enough information is available, the product's manufacturer can be consulted. Specialized textbooks regarding test's concentration for many non-standardized materials are currently available (De Groot 1986.

False-negative reactions represents a further complication of patch testing. Many causes of false-negative reactions exist, however, in occupational dermatology, the most significant causes of false-negative reactions are: failure of the patch test to reproduce the conditions of exposure, for example, sweating and friction experienced at work may not be adequately reproduced in patch testing; inadequate penetration of the allergen: the allergens are applied on normal skin in patch testing, whilst the clinical lesions results from an allergen contacting compromised skin; and insufficient concentration of allergen in the samples acquired from the workplace; the concentration of the allergen in the product may be too low to elicit a positive patch test reaction, but enough to produce a dermatitis through multiple exposures. When patch testing results are negative, but strong suspicion of contact allergy from an occupational substance persists, performing some additional tests can be helpful: (a) patch test with the suspicious product's extracts, (b) patch test on a previous dermatitic site, or close to a dermatitis area (careful interpretation is needed); and (c) special tests, i.e., Provocative Use Test (PUT) or a Repeated Open Application Test (ROAT), etc. (Hannuksela 1997).

Assessment of Clinical Relevance

In assessing the clinical relevance of a positive patch test reaction, we must establish whether the responsible allergen either represents the primary cause or an aggravating factor of the patient's dermatitis. An allergen is clinically relevant if: 1) we can establish the existence of an exposure and, 2) the patient's dermatitis is explainable with regard to that exposure (Ale 1995). It must also be determined, whether the positive reaction represents the cause of the current dermatitis ("current" or "present" relevance) or a previous one ("past" relevance). In addition, current or past relevance can be scored according to the degree of clinical certainty, using terms such as: "relevance doubtful", "relevance possible" and "relevance likely" (Lachapelle 1997). Finally, if the source of the positive response is not traced, we consider the response as being of "unknown" relevance. A judgment of unknown relevance often reflects physicians' ignorance of the chemical environment and the pattern of cross-sensitivity rather than actual irrelevancy. In some circumstances, it may be difficult to substantiate the presence of the allergen in the patient's environment. This may be due to the difficulty in detecting certain allergens or to our restricted knowledge about the composition of many products. Industrial products are often not labeled with ingredient content and

Table 3. Suggested guidelines for the assessment of relevance. Modified from Ale (1995)

Re-interrogate the patient in light of the test results
Perform a workplace visit
Look for all probable sources of allergen exposure (including indirect, infrequent and concealed)
Seek cross-reacting substances
Obtain information from "lists" of allergens, databases, material safety data sheets, manufacturers, etc.
Perform physicochemical analysis of products
Perform additional testing procedures with the suspected allergen(s), products presumably containing the suspected allergen and product's extracts
Use open tests and serial dilution if necessary
Perform PUT and ROAT

substances added to raw materials or used in the manufacturing process may be not declared. Physicochemical analysis of the suspected item(s) is useful but difficult to perform in complex products. Additional skin tests are frequently necessary for relevance assessment. Testing with products that may contain the causative allergen and to which the patient refers being exposed can be helpful. However, patch testing with the unmodified product may give false-negative results, usually because of insufficient concentration of the allergen in the product. This may be partially overcome by performing the test with the product's extracts or performing use tests, such as the PUT or ROAT (Table 3).

Operational Definition of OACD

As seen above, diagnosis in occupational contact dermatitis is complex. Nine steps in the assessment of OACD can be considered as follows:

1. History of occupational exposure
2. Existence of time relationship between occupational exposure and onset of dermatitis
3. Morphology of the dermatitis consistent with occupational exposure
4. Positive diagnostic patch test with appropriate vehicle and concentration
5. Repeat patch test – when appropriate – to exclude ESS (excited skin syndrome) and "rogue" reactions
6. Perform serial dilution of the chemical tested
7. Review controls for non-irritating concentrations and performing special tests for not commonly utilized allergens
8. Perform PUT or ROAT to define clinical relevance
9. Clearing of the dermatitis when allergen is removed, or exposure is significantly decreased

No single criterion provides sufficient evidence for probable occupational origin of allergic contact dermatitis. The above guidelines can provide a simplified rational approach for an operational definition of OACD that may represent a useful tool until more information becomes available.

References

Andersen E, Maibach HI (1985) Guinea pig sensitization assays: an overview. In: Andersen E, Maibach HI (eds) Contact allergy, predictive tests in guinea pigs (Current problems in dermatology, vol 14). Karger, Basel, pp 263–290

Andersen KE (1994) Mechanical trauma and hand eczema. In: Menné T, Maibach HI (eds) Hand eczema, CRC Press, Boca Raton, FL, pp 31–34

Ale SI, Maibach HI (1995) Clinical relevance in allergic contact dermatitis. An algorithmic approach. Dermatosen 43:119–121

De Groot AC (1986) Patch testing concentrations and vehicles for 2800 allergens. Elsevier, Amsterdam

Basketter DA, Gerberick GF, Kimber I, Loveless SE (1996) The local lymph node assay: A viable alternative to currently accepted skin sensitization tests. Food Chem Toxicol 34: 985–990

Hannuksela M. (1997) The repeated open application test (ROAT). Contact Dermatitis 36: 39–43

Hostýnek JJ (1998) Structure-activity relationship in contact sensitization: classification and ranking of allergens. In: Marzulli FN, Maibach HI (eds) Dermatotoxicology methods: the laboratory worker's vademecum. Taylor and Francis, Washington DC, pp 115–120

Lachapelle J-M (1997) A proposed relevance scoring system for positive allergic patch test reactions: practical implications and limitations. Contact Dermatitis 36:39–43

Marzulli FN, Maibach HI (1976) Effects of vehicles and elicitation concentration in contact dermatitis testing. 1. Experimental contact sensitization in humans. Contact Dermatitis 2:325–329

Meneghini CL (1985) Sensitization in traumatized skin. Am J Ind Med 8:319–321

Rietschel RL, Fowler JF Jr (1995) Predictive testing for human contact dermatitis. In: Rietschel RL, Fowler JF Jr (eds) Fischer's contact dermatitis, 4th edn. Williams and Wilkins, Baltimore, pp 33–37

Shmunes E (1988) Predisposing factors in occupational skin diseases. Dermatol Clin 6:7–13

Upadhye MR, Maibach HI (1992) Influence of area of application of allergen on sensitization in contact dermatitis. Contact Dermatitis 27:281–286

CHAPTER 15

The Role of Atopy in Working Life   15

K. KALIMO, K. LAMMINTAUSTA

Atopy

The definition of atopy includes atopic dermatitis (AD), established by Hanifin and Rajka (1980), with suggested major and minor criteria, including other atopic diseases such as allergic rhinitis (AR), conjunctivitis (AC) or asthma (A). Atopic skin diathesis (ASD) (Lamintausta and Kalimo 1981; Diepgen et al. 1991; Diepgen and Fartasch 1992) includes dry skin, history of low threshold for pruritus in contact with dust or rough materials, pruritus when sweating and white dermographism.

In recent epidemiological studies, the occurrence of AD has shown variable, although, in the majority, increasing frequencies varying from 10% to 16% of the general population (Varjonen et al. 1992; Williams 1992; Schultz-Larsen et al. 1996).

Hand Eczema and AD

According to epidemiological studies the reported point prevalence of hand eczema has changed, with figures from 2% to about 22% (Agrup 1969; Peltonen 1979; Lantinga et al. 1984; Meding and Swanbeck 1989; Menné et al. 1992; Susitaival et al. 1994).

A previous history of AD, or ASD, during childhood has been reported in 20–90% of hand eczema patients (Lammintausta and Kalimo 1981; Shmunes and Keil 1984; Baurle et al. 1985; Nilsson et al. 1985; Rystedt 1985a,b, 1986; Meding and Swanbeck 1990a; Funke et al. 1995). Simultaneously, AD is present in the hands of about 40% of patients (Rystedt 1985c; Lammintausta et al. 1991); thus, the prevalence of atopic hand eczema follows the prevalence of AD, both with high figures.

Certain features of atopy are associated with the development of hand eczema (Lammintausta and Kalimo 1981; Lammintausta 1982; Nilsson et al. 1985; Rystedt 1985a,b, 1986; Meding and Swanbeck 1990a; Diepgen et al. 1991; Diepgen and Fartasch 1992; Funke et al. 1995). The major risk factor is a history of severe AD during childhood, especially if dermatitis was localized in the hands, 60–90% of these patients and 40% of patients with moderate AD develop hand eczema later in working life. Episodes of hand eczema can occur even if the patients are just doing clean, dry office work.

A significant association between atopy and hand dermatitis has also been found in patients who present only with ASD especially when they are exposed to skin irritation. A history of AR or A was reported to suggest an increased risk for hand eczema by Meding and Swanbeck (1990a), while no risk was found in atopics who had AR, AC or A without any signs of ASD, by other investigators (Lammintausta and Kalimo 1981; Rystedt 1986; Diepgen and Fartasch 1992). The frequency of hand dermatitis is highest among the younger workers; with age, all atopic symptoms show a tendency to decline. Concerning gender differences, women are likely to suffer almost twice as often from hand dermatitis as men (Meding and Swanbeck 1990a). This can partly depend on different duties at work and at home and working manners, as well as on constitutional factors.

Allergy and AD

Atopic patients have an increased risk of developing immunoglobulin E (IgE) antibodies against common allergens. Thus, they often suffer from allergy to pollens, epithelia and different foods. This can lead to manifestation of symptoms when working in contact with food (e.g., in a bakery or kitchen) or with animals (Kanerva and Susitaival 1996). In such positions, it is common to suffer from rhinitis, asthma and conjunctivitis. Natural rubber latex allergy has become a significant health problem, causing symptoms from local reactions to severe anaphylactic shock. AD patients possessing the risk of developing IgE antibodies are also at risk of developing latex allergy (Turjanmaa 1994).

Several allergens that give rise to IgE production may also lead to the development of local contact eczema (protein contact dermatitis), if continuous exposure to the skin takes place (Hjort and Roed-Petersen 1976). It seems evident that both animal epithelia and food products may give rise to contact sensitisation, although many of these substances are simultaneously strong irritants (Kanerva and Susitaival 1996).

With regard to contact allergy, it seems that AD patients develop contact allergy, but the positive reactions include topical treatments they have used. The most common contact allergens include nickel, fragrances, neomycin, balsam of Peru, cobalt, colophony, chromate, propyleneglycol, formaldehyde and wool alcohols (Rystedt 1985d, 1986; Lammintausta et al. 1992).

Skin Irritation

An irritant contact eczema is frequently seen to develop in AD patients and in workers with ASD. The decreased capacity of atopic skin to resist external irritation is poorly understood. Depending on the different methods used, reports from experimental studies on the irritability of the atopic skin are contradictory (Gallacher and Maibach 1998). The interindividual variation in the irritation reactivity of the skin in atopic and non-atopic subjects is extensive. Increased transepidermal water loss has been reported in atopics (Hannuksela and Hannuksela

1995; Goh 1997). Epidemiologic data strongly suggest that AD is a dose-dependent risk factor for skin irritation since 90% of atopic patients developed hand dermatitis if heavy wet-work exposure lasted for 2 h compared with 50% hand eczema cases in non-exposed workers (Lammintausta and Kalimo 1993).

Occupational Hand Eczema and AD

According to long-term follow-up studies, it appears that young atopic subjects who belong to the risk groups often develop skin problems when they enter working life (Lammintausta and Kalimo 1981; Shmunes and Keil 1984; Baurle et al. 1985; Nilsson et al. 1985; Rystedt 1985 a, b, c, 1986; Meding and Swanbeck 1989, 1990 a; Lammintausta et al. 1991; Funke et al. 1995). Increased exposure to wet work, foods and chemicals, dirt and mechanical friction seems to be especially hazardous for them. Some of the workers cannot manage to continue in their chosen occupation and have to plan job changes, whereas others are able to continue even in the same position in which the eczema started. In some cases "hardening" may also develop. Intensive patient education and treatment programs have improved the prognosis (Coenraads et al. 2001). The principal reason behind the better prognosis may be the improved protection and skin care and adequate rationalisation of working methods. Although the individual prognosis is highly variable, hand eczema in atopic workers is generally more persistent (Meding and Swanbeck 1990 a, b; Lammintausta and Kalimo 1993; Shum KW et al. 2000).

The distinction between endogenous AD and dermatitis caused by external factors is often difficult. In the case of an AD patient, the diagnosis of an occupational hand eczema requires that AD has been symptom free and hand eczema is seen to develop or deteriorate significantly in the working environment. Sometimes the dermatitis flares up so that the association is evident and the diagnosis of an occupational skin disease may be made. However, the practice of compensatory principles is variable in different countries (Bruze 1994).

Risk Occupations

The increased risk of hand eczema seems to depend on multiple factors. Exposure to common irritating factors, wet work, detergents, chemicals, dirt and mechanical friction are the most common causes for the development of hand eczema at work. Exposure to airborne allergens or irritants can also lead to dermatitis. In addition, jobs with changes in temperature and humidity or with extensive sweating increase the risk of dermatitis. The prevalence of hand eczema is high in hairdressing, food handling, cleaning and nursing and also in domestic work. The frequency of sick leave taken by atopic patients is comparable with that of non-atopics, although some of the sick-leave periods were of longer duration (Rystedt 1985 c; Lammintausta et al. 1991; Lammintausta and Kalimo 1993; Holm and Veierod 1994; Meding 1996; Uter et al. 1999 a, b).

Counselling

Working life will never be risk free and, therefore, it is important that AD patients are aware of the specific character of their skin. Working conditions may develop and change continuously, and risks can be decreased by, for example, automatisation. The prognosis in AD is highly variable (Rystedt 1985c; Meding and Swanbeck 1990b; Lammintausta and Kalimo 1993). It is evident that good motivation and thorough understanding of the risks will result in a better prognosis in working life. Therefore, it is important that the AD patients get information as early as at school age regarding the risks and treatment alternatives associated with atopy (Lammintausta and Kalimo 1993; Diepgen 1996; Shum et al. 2000; Coenraads et al. 2001). It is also evident that not all AD patients are willing or able to move to those positions in which the exposure to skin irritation can be eliminated. There may also be other factors involved since approximately 10% of patients with severe AD did not develop hand dermatitis during wet-work exposure (Lammintausta et al. 1991; Diepgen and Fartasch 1992).

Summary

The prevalence of atopic patients is remarkable. Both AD and ASD patients have an increased risk of hand dermatitis in working life, especially if the dermatitis was severe in early childhood and if there is involvement of the hands. This risk is increased in women and in occupations with exposure to skin-irritating factors, wet work, detergents, other chemicals, friction, food and animals. However, many workers are able to work successfully when they are provided with information concerning the risks and how to treat and protect. If they are well motivated to perform the work, their ability to manage in working life is good. Thus, no absolute restrictions for atopic subjects should be given.

References

Agrup G (1969) Hand eczema and other hand dermatoses in South Sweden (thesis). Acta Derm Venereol Suppl (Stockh) 61:49

Baurle von G, Homstein OP, Diepgen T (1985) Professionelle Handekzeme und Atopie. Dermatosen 5:161–165

Bruze M (1994) Principles of occupational hand eczema. In: Menn and Eacute; T, Maibach HI (eds) Hand eczema. CRC Press, Boca Raton, pp 166–178

Coenraads PJ, Span L, Jaspers JP, Fidler V (2001) Intensive patient education and treatment program for young adults with atopic eczema. Hautarzt 5(5):428–433

Diepgen T (1996) Epidemiological studies on the prevention of occupational contact dermatitis. Curr Probl Dermatol 25:1–9

Diepgen TL, Fartasch M (1992) Recent epidemiological and genetic studies in atopic dermatitis. Acta Derm Venereol Suppl (Stockh) 176:13–18

Diepgen TL, Fartasch M, Hornstein OP (1991) Criteria of atopic skin diathesis. Dermatosen 39:79

Funke U, Diepgen T, Fartasch M (1995) Identification of high risk groups for irritant contact dermatitis by occupational physicians. Curr Probl Dermatol 23:64–72

Gallacher G, Maibach HI (1998) Is atopic dermatitis a predisposing factor for experimental acute irritant contact dermatitis? Contact Dermatitis 38:1–4

Goh CL (1997) Comparing skin irritancy in atopics and nonatopics to sodium lauryl sulphate and benzalkonium chloride using TEWL measurements. Environ Dermatol 4:30–32

Hanifin JM, Rajka G (1980) Diagnostic features of atopic dermatitis. Acta Derm Venereol Suppl (Stockh) 92:44–47

Hannuksela A, Hannuksela M (1995) Irritant effects of a detergent in a wash and chamber tests. Contact Dermatitis 32:163–166

Hjort N, Roed-Petersen J (1976) Occupational protein contact dermatitis in food handlers. Contact Dermatitis 2:28–42

Holm JO, Veierod MB (1994) An epidemiological study of hand eczema. III. Characterization of hairdressers with and without hand eczema, regarding demographic factors and medical histories. Acta Derm Venereol Suppl (Stockh) 187:15–17

Kanerva L, Susitaival P (1996) Cow dander, the most common cause of occupational contact urticaria in Finland. Contact Dermatitis 35:309–310

Lammintausta K, Kalimo K (1981) Atopy and hand dermatitis in hospital wet work. Contact Dermatitis 7:301–308

Lammintausta K, Kalimo K (1993) Does a patient's occupation influence the course of atopic dermatitis? Acta Derm Venereol 73:124–128

Lammintausta K, Kalimo K, Raitala K, Forsten Y (1991) Prognosis of atopic dermatitis. A prospective study in early adulthood. Int J Dermatol 30:563–568

Lammintausta K, Kalimo K, Fagerlund V-L (1992) Patch test reactions in atopic patients. Contact Dermatitis 26:234–240

Lantinga H, Nater JP, Coenraads PJ (1984) Prevalence, incidence and course of eczema on the hands and forearms in a sample of general population. Contact Dermatitis 10:135–139

Meding B (1996) Prevention of hand eczema in atopics. Curr Probl Dermatol 25:116–122

Meding B, Swanbeck G (1989) Epidemiology of different types of hand eczema in an industrial city. Acta Derm Venereol Suppl (Stockh) 69:227–233

Meding B, Swanbeck G (1990a) Predictive factors for hand eczema. Contact Dermatitis 23:154

Meding B, Swanbeck G (1990b) Consequences of having hand eczema. Contact Dermatitis 23:6–14

Menné T, Borgen O, Green A (1992) Nickel allergy and hand dermatitis in a stratified sample of the Danish female population; an epidemiological study including a statistic appendix. Acta Derm Venereol Suppl (Stockh) 62:35–41

Nilsson E, Mikaelsson B, Andersson S (1985) Atopy, occupation and domestic work as risk factors for hand eczema in hospital workers. Contact Dermatitis 13:216–223

Peltonen L (1979) Nickel sensitivity in the general population. Contact Dermatitis 5:27–32

Rystedt I (1985a) Atopic background in patients with occupational hand eczema. Contact Dermatitis 12:247–254

Rystedt I (1985b) Factors influencing the occurrence of hand eczema in adults with a history of atopic dermatitis in childhood. Contact Dermatitis 12:185–191

Rystedt I (1985c) Hand eczema and long term prognosis in atopic dermatitis. Acta Derm Venereol Suppl (Stockh) 117:1–59

Rystedt I (1985d) Contact sensitivity in adults with atopic dermatitis in childhood. Contact Dermatitis 12:185–191

Rystedt I (1986) Atopy, hand eczema, and contact dermatitis: summary of recent large scale studies. Semin Dermatol 5:290–300

Schultz-Larsen F, Diepgen T, Svensson A (1996) The occurrence of atopic dermatitis in north Europe: an international questionnaire study. J Am Acad Dermatol 34:760–764

Shmunes E, Keil J (1984) The role of atopy in occupational dermatoses in South Carolina. Contact Dermatitis 11:174–178

Shum KW, Lawton S, Williams HC, Docherty G, Jones J (2000) The British Association of Dermatologists audit of atopic eczema management in secondary care. Phase 3: audit of service outcome. Br J Dermatol 142(4):721–727

Susitaival P, Husman L, Horsmanheimo M, Notkola V, Husman K (1994) Prevalence of hand dermatoses among Finnish farmers. Scand J Environ Health 20:206–212

Turjanmaa K (1994) Update on occupational natural rubber latex allergy. Dermatol Clin 12:561–567

Uter W, Pfahlberg A, Gefeller O, Schwanitz HJ (1999a) Hand dermatitis in a prospectively-followed cohort of hairdressing apprentices: final results of the POSH study. Prevention of occupational skin disease in hairdressers. Contact Dermatitis 41:280–286

Uter W, Pfahlberg A, Gefeller O, Schwanitz HJ (1999b) Risk of hand dermatitis among hairdressers versus office workers. Scand J Work Environ Health 25:450–456

Varjonen E, Kalimo K, Lammintausta K, Terho P (1992) Prevalence of atopic disorders among adolescents in Turku, Finland. Allergy 47:243–248

Williams HC (1992) Is the prevalence of atopic dermatitis increasing? Clin Exp Dermatol 17:385–391

CHAPTER 16

Diagnostic Patch Testing   **16**

J. E. WAHLBERG

Patch testing is a well-established method of diagnosing contact allergy and allergic contact dermatitis, a delayed type of hypersensitivity (type-IV reaction). Patients with a history and clinical picture of contact dermatitis are exposed to the suspected allergens, materials or products under controlled conditions to verify the diagnosis. Besides testing patients with hand, arm, face or leg eczema, testing of other types of eczema (atopic, seborrhoic dermatitis, nummular eczema) is sometimes indicated, especially when the dermatologist suspects contact allergy to prescribed topical medicaments and their vehicles. The procedure can also be used before recommending alternative protective gloves, skin care products, corticosteroids, etc. in a particular patient. If the patient does not react to the alternatives tested, it is very unlikely that the same individual will react to the products in ordinary use. Patch testing is usually required in medicolegal cases of compensation. Much effort has been put into standardization of allergens, vehicles, concentrations, patch test materials, tapes and the scoring of test reactions; the procedure is today considered accurate and reliable. Standardization has facilitated comparisons of contact allergy frequency in selected industrial populations and between clinics and geographical areas.

Patch testing with standard allergens can be carried out by any dermatologist after adequate training, while testing with materials and products brought by the patient requires special resources and facilities.

Test Systems

One can distinguish two test systems – the original, in which the allergens, patches and tapes are supplied separately (Finn chamber, Al-test, van der Bend square chambers and others) and the modern ready-to-use system, in which only a covering material has to be removed before the test is applied (true test system). At present, the latter test system is available for 23 standard allergens. Testing with screening series and with materials brought by the patient is therefore carried out according to the original system.

Allergens

The standard patch test allergens sold by Chemotechnique Diagnostics (2001) and Hermal (2001) can, according to these suppliers' product catalogues, be considered chemically defined and pure. The catalogues contain lists of approximately 300 allergens in alphabetical order, allergens in the European standard series, as well as tables of mixes and lists of screening series (Table 1). They also contain information on the occurrence of allergens, cross-reactivity patterns and additional practical advice on the patch test procedure.

Standard Series

The present European standard series contains 23 items, but six of them are mixes; so in fact, at least 24 additional allergens are applied. The basic idea of using mixes instead of single allergens is to save time and space, and the screening capacity is thereby greatly increased.

Screening Series

To evaluate the significance of special exposures, mainly occupational, a number of screening series are available (Table 1). They are compiled from the experience

Table 1. Commercially available screening series and number of allergens in each series

Chemotechnique (2001)	Number	Hermal (2001)	Number
Bakery	19	Antimicrobials, preservatives, antioxidants	32
Corticosteroid	08	Cosmetics	13
Cosmetics	48	Dental materials	20
Dental	30	Hairdressing	07
Epoxy	09	Medicaments	36
Fragrance	24	Metal compounds	07
Hairdressing	26	Metal working/technical oils	24
Isocyanate	06	Miscellaneous	24
Medicament	13	Perfumes, flavors	14
(Meth)acrylate: adhesives, dental and other	15	Photoallergens	18
Nails-artificial	13	Photographic chemicals	10
Printing	24	Plants	07
Oil and cooling fluid	35	Plastic, glues	28
Photographic chemicals	16	Rubber chemicals	10
Plant	13	Sunscreen agents	09
Plastic and glues	25	Textile and leather dyes	13
Rubber additives	25	Vehicles, emulsifiers	08
Scandinavian photopatch	20		
Shoe	22		
Sunscreen	10		
Textile colors and finish	32		
Various allergens	57		

gathered at departments of occupational dermatology and from the literature. Newly defined allergens are added regularly and these series can be considered to cover the present exposure situation in the occupational setting. However, the allergens are pure chemicals and, if the original offending agent was an impurity, a degradation product, etc., the cause will be missed. A supplementary test with the patient's own working material is therefore highly recommended.

Tests with Substances or Products Brought by the Patient

When patients bring suspected products or materials from their work environment, it is recommended that material safety data sheets, lists of ingredients and other such information be requested from the manufacturer so that a general impression of the product, ingredients, concentrations, intended use, etc. can be formed. There are usually one or two ingredients that are of interest as suspected allergens, while the rest are well-known substances of proven innocuousness, for which detailed information is available.

Based on the list of ingredients the next step is to look for suspected allergens. If these are available from suppliers of patch-test allergens, one can rely on the choice of vehicle and concentration. If one suspects that impurities or contaminants have caused the dermatitis, this can only be discovered through samples of the ingredient from the manufacturer. It is essential to use samples from the actual batch to which the patient has been exposed; but, when testing cutting fluids, for example, unused products must be tested for comparison.

Identification of New Contact Allergens

When testing with products and materials brought by patients, previously unknown allergens are sometimes discovered. A scheme for identification of new allergens is presented in Table 2. If the test is positive in a particular patient, one

Table 2. Scheme for identification of new contact allergens

Clinical
Positive patch-test reaction to a product
Test with ingredients of the product
Serial dilution test to define a threshold of sensitivity
Control test for irritancy
Cross-reactivity – equimolar concentrations
ROAT (repeated open application test)
Experimental
Structural formula
Chemical analysis
Purity
Animal testing
Allergenic potential
Cross-reactivity pattern

has to demonstrate in at least 10–20 unexposed controls that the actual test preparation is nonirritant; otherwise the observed reaction in the patient does not prove allergenicity (Wahlberg 2001).

Vehicles

White petrolatum is the most widely used vehicle and the majority of commercial test preparations are delivered in this vehicle. However, each allergen almost certainly has its own optimal vehicle, and it is improbable that just one vehicle, e.g., petrolatum, could be optimal for all allergens. Liquid vehicles, such as water and solvents (acetone, ethanol, methyl ethyl ketone), are recommended since they facilitate penetration into the skin; but they also have some drawbacks.

Practical Information

For practical information on concentrations, tapes, test sites, application of test preparations to patches, exposure time, reading, recording of test reactions, artifacts, effect of medicaments and irradiation, excited-skin syndrome, compound allergy, cross-sensitivity, false-positive and false-negative test reactions, patch test sensitization and other complications, standard textbooks are recommended (Rietschel and Fowler 1995; Wahlberg 2001).

Relevance

Evaluating the relevance of a reaction is the most difficult and intricate part of the patch-test procedure, and it is a challenge to both dermatologist and patient. The dermatologist's skill, experience and curiosity are crucial factors.

For standard allergens, detailed lists are available that present the occurrence of each in the environment. The patient and the dermatologist should study the lists together, in order to judge the relevance of a positive patch-test reaction in relation to the exposure, site, course and relapse of the patient's current dermatitis. A positive test reaction can also be explained by a previous, unrelated episode of contact dermatitis (past relevance). Sometimes, the relevance of a positive reaction remains unexplained until the patient brings a package or bottle with the allergen in question named on the label. In other cases, chemical analyses demonstrate the presence of the allergen, or the manufacturer finally, after many inquiries, admits that the offending substance is present in the product.

In paints, cutting fluids, glues, skin care products, detergents, etc., it is common that new ingredients are added or replace previous ones, but the product keeps its original trade name. Alternatively, well-known allergens are included in new products, but with other fields of application than the original. To discover the cause of the patient's dermatitis the dermatologist must sometimes be obstinately determined!

Open Tests

Open testing usually means that a product "as is" or dissolved in water or some solvent, e.g., ethanol, acetone or ether, is dropped onto the skin and allowed to spread freely. No occlusion is used. An open test is recommended as the first step when testing poorly defined substances or products, such as those brought by a patient (paints, glues, oils, detergents, cleansing agents based on solvents, etc.). The test site should be checked at regular intervals during the first 30–60 min after application, especially when the history indicates immediate reactions or contact urticaria. A second reading should be done at 3–4 days.

Use Tests

Use tests and open tests are sometimes used as synonyms. The original (provocative) use (or usage) tests were intended to mimic the actual use situation (repeated open applications) of a formulated product, such as an oil, shampoo or a topical medicament. A positive result supported the suspicion that the product had caused the patient's dermatitis. Nowadays, these tests are increasingly used to evaluate the clinical significance of one or more ingredients of a formulated product previously found reactive by ordinary patch testing. The concentration of the particular ingredient can be so low that one may wonder whether the positive patch-test reaction can explain the patient's dermatitis.

Details of the performance of the repeated open application test (ROAT) and its relevance are given in textbooks (Rietschel and Fowler 1995; Wahlberg 2001).

Recommendations

In occupational dermatology patch testing is of great importance in order to obtain an accurate diagnosis. If the offending allergen(s) can be found at comprehensive patch testing (standard allergens plus own materials) it is of the utmost value in order to avoid relapses (secondary prevention). The tests should be carried out by dermatologists with interest in the field and with sufficient experience of patch testing, and using materials and products from the patient's work environment. This knowledge is crucial in medicolegal cases of compensation. As stated, the evaluation of the relevance of a positive test reaction is the most intricate part of the patch-test procedure.

References

Chemotechnique Diagnostics (2001) Patch test products, catalogue. Malmö, Sweden
Hermal (2001) Patch test allergen. Trolab, Reinbeck, Germany
Rietschel RL, Fowler JF Jr (1995) Fisher's contact dermatitis, 4th edn. Williams and Wilkins, Baltimore, pp 11–32
Wahlberg JE (2001) Patch testing. In: Rycroft RJG, Menné T, Frosch PJ, Lepoittevin J-P (eds) Textbook of contact dermatitis, 3rd edn. Springer, Berlin, Heidelberg, New York, pp 435–468

CHAPTER 17

Patch Testing With the Patient's Own Work Materials

17

R. Jolanki, T. Estlander, K. Alanko, L. Kanerva

Introduction

Patch testing the patient's own work materials is important, but it entails many problems. The evaluation of test reactions to the materials in question may be difficult. In many cases, patch testing with the patient-supplied products has been the main clue in revealing the causative agent for allergic contact dermatitis. An allergic reaction produced by the patient's own material may also help to convince the patient and the insurance companies of the causative substances of allergic contact dermatitis.

Patch testing with the patient's materials from the workplace is a screening test. In subsequent testing, it is reasonable to confirm the previous reactions by repeating the investigation and by testing individual constituents of strongly suspected materials. A positive test result to a patient's own material and a simultaneous negative result to the corresponding commercial test substance may reveal that there is something wrong with the commercial test substance (Leisvaara et al. 1998). Unfortunately, a positive test result to separate ingredients, and a negative one to the whole product, may also be possible. The test substances made of individual chemicals often contain the allergen in an optimal concentration and vehicle, whereas the test substance made of a product may include some allergenic ingredients, such as preservatives and fragrances, in too low concentrations or rarely in an inadequate vehicle to induce an allergic test reaction.

Patient-Supplied Materials

Specimens

The selection of patient-supplied materials for patch testing should be based on careful exposure anamnesis. The clinic must have a list of the chemicals handled at the workplace, as well as samples of each chemical corresponding to the situation in which the patient's skin exposure occurs and that is suspected of causing his/her skin problems. Special attention should be paid to materials that are strongly suspected of causing allergic contact dermatitis. Hand creams and cleansers, and protective gloves should also be included in the patient's own materials. The name and address of the manufacturer or the supplier is necessary for further contacts. Sometimes a visit to the patient's workplace is necessary.

If industrial chemicals, such as metal-working fluids, are used diluted, undiluted products must also be supplied to the clinic. If the patient handles chemical mixtures or two-component products in mixture form, the individual chemicals or components should be packed separately. Even solid materials, such as parts of plants should be packed separately to avoid contamination.

Liquid chemicals should be packed separately in tightly closed containers made of some inert material that does not interfere with the chemical product or influence its properties, e.g., polypropylene or glass. Evaporation or hardening of the chemical is not allowed during storage, because the chemical may be needed later for repeat or control tests, or for chemical analyses. The wrapping of the patient's own industrial chemicals should be provided with a label including at least the trade name of the chemical. It is important to confirm that the container really does contain the product named in the label.

Information Regarding the Products

The precise composition of chemical preparations is often unknown (Dooms-Goossens 1995). In the clinic performing patch tests with patient-supplied products, enough information regarding the products must be available to those who conduct the tests. A review of the safety data sheet (SDS) for any given industrial chemical preparation is important because this often reveals enough information for patch testing with the chemical. However, the SDS often does not give detailed information on the exact chemicals present, and most of the harmful chemicals present in a concentrations of less than 1% are not required to be listed (Adams 1995). In the European Union, if a skin-sensitizing chemical is present at a concentration of 0.1% or more in a chemical preparation, it should be listed in the preparation's SDS. More detailed information on the composition may nevertheless be needed, especially for the evaluation of the positive patch-test reaction produced by the chemical. It is also important to determine the degree of acidity or alkalinity of a product, especially if the product is not labeled properly. Sometimes even a chemical analysis is necessary.

Determination of Patch-Test Substances

Most industrial chemicals are not suitable for testing as such, but have to be diluted prior to patch testing. Too low a test concentration may lead to a false-negative or too weak and therefore doubtful reactions. Too high a test concentration may lead to a false test reaction that is difficult to interpret, and which may be very inconvenient or even harmful to the patient. Testing should, if possible, be performed only at specialized clinics, where substances brought in by the patients are routinely used for patch testing, and clinicians who are familiar with the patient's specific problems should perform the readings personally (Beck 1995).

Concentration

Furthermore, chemicals having the potential allergens in high concentrations have to be tested in the proper vehicle and at the right concentration to avoid a false-positive or irritant reaction, active sensitization, a chemical burn or an extremely strong bullous allergic reaction. The proper test concentration and the best vehicle for all the chemical substances should be estimated carefully on the basis of the information on toxicity and the composition of the material available. In addition, one should check which of the individual chemical components are available from the suppliers as patch-test substances, because one may rely on their choice of vehicle and concentration, and these substances, if available, should be included in the test battery of the patient. Sometimes the reported concentrations or a supplier's test concentrations are not appropriate (Jolanki et al. 2000; Kanerva et al. 1998). It is helpful to use selected test series related to a specific type of product aimed to be tested, e.g., metal-working series for metal-working fluids. Several reports provide useful information on the concentrations and vehicles to be used (Fregert 1981; De Groot 1994; Guin 1995; Niklasson 1995; Rietschel and Fowler 1995). The test concentration for the chemical substance should not exceed the previously recommended test concentration for any of the components. This may, however, lead to the risk of over dilution of potential allergens, especially when the responsible ingredient is present at a low concentration or appears as a contaminant in the product.

To avoid complications, patch testing should never be performed with materials of which the composition or skin effects are not known, or are known to be extremely hazardous, such as strong acids or alkalis, or highly toxic chemicals. If the exact nature of the substance is not known, but the group to which it belongs or the purpose for which it is used can be determined, one may proceed with the testing as recommended for that particular group of chemicals (Table 1).

Acrylics are difficult compounds to use in patch testing. Too high a test concentration may sensitize the patient, whereas too low a concentration may cause false-negative patch-test results (Jolanki et al. 2000; Kanerva et al. 1996). Patch testing should be performed with the commercially available (meth)acrylates, and the patient's own acrylics at a low concentration (Table 1). Other highly reactive chemicals such as those used as intermediates in chemical syntheses should also be patch tested (including control tests) with extreme caution due to the risk of active sensitization. Patch-test preparations should match published concentrations and should not exceed 0.1% in concentration of the reactive component.

When a solid non-irritant product is suspected (rubber, wood, paper, etc.), these can usually be supplied as is, with a drop of vehicle in the test chamber or using extracts. Many plants, in particular, are highly irritant (Hausen 1988; Lamminpää et al. 1996), and are preferably to be tested in diluted form after an ultrasonic bath extraction.

In order to find the most suitable test concentration, it is a good idea to use a few different concentrations. Testing with a dilution series helps in the reading and interpretation of the test results; this is especially valuable when one has no previous experience of the products to be tested. A dilution series, e.g., 10–3.2–1%, or 10–5–2.5% is suitable (Fregert 1985).

Table 1. Recommended vehicles and concentrations in dilution series for patch testing industrial chemicals

Chemical	Patch test concentration and vehicle
Acrylics	
Epoxy diacrylates	0.5% pet.
Epoxy dimethacrylates, e.g., dental composite materials	1–2% pet.
Instant glues (cyanoacrylate-based)	1–10% pet. or allow to dry
Methacrylates (prosthesis materials, floor coatings)	2% pet.
Ultraviolet-curable inks and lacquers (acrylate-based)	0.01–0.1% pet.
Adhesive tapes	As such
Alkyd resins	1–10% pet.
Brake fluids	1–5% pet.
Detergents and soaps (without solvents)	
pH < 2	1–10% alkaline buffer (make sure that the pH is 4–9)
pH 2–4	1–10% pet. or aq.
pH 4–9	10–100% pet. or aq.
pH 9–10	1–10% pet. or aq.
pH >10	1–10% acid buffer (make sure that the pH is 4–9)
Epoxy products	
Adduct hardeners	1–10% pet.
DGEBA epoxy resins, liquid	1–2% pet.
DGEBA epoxy resins, solid	10% pet.
Non-DGEBA epoxy resins	0.25–0.5% pet.
Paints, lacquers, glues, etc., solvent-based	1–10% pet. or ac
Paints, lacquers, glues, etc., without solvent	1–2% pet. or ac.
Polyamine hardeners	0.1–1% pet.
Powder paints	5–10 pet. or ac.
Formaldehyde resin products	
Resins, glues, lacquers, etc.	1–10% pet. or acid buffer (make sure that the pH is 4–9)
Glues (excluding epoxy, formaldehyde resin and acrylic)	
Dispersion glues	10–100% pet. or aq.
Solvent-based contact glues	1–10% pet. or allow to dry
Industrial greases	10–100% pet.
Metal-working oils and fluids	
Fluid concentrates	1–10% pet.
Fluid emulsions	As such
Cutting oils	10–100% pet.
Mineral oils	
High-viscosity	10–100% pet.
Low-viscosity	1–10% pet.
Organic solvents	
Aliphatic, cycloaliphatic	1–10% pet.
Aromatic	1–5% pet.
Chlorinated	0.1–1% pet.
Esters	1–10% pet.

Table 1 (continued)

Chemical	Patch test concentration and vehicle
Paints (excluding epoxy, polyester and acrylic)	
Di-isocyanate hardeners of polyurethane paints or lacquers	2–5% pet.
One component, water-based	10–100% pet. or aq.
One component, solvent- or oil-based, e.g., alkyds	1–10% pet.
Powder paints (plastisols)	10–100% pet.
Photographic chemicals	
Developers	0.1–1% alkaline or acid buffer (make sure that the pH is 4–9)
Fixation fluids	0.1–1% aq.
Polyester product	
Cobalt accelerators	0.1–1% pet.
Hardeners of two-component cements	0.1–1% pet.
Lamination resins	1–10% pet.
Powder paints	1–10% pet.
Resins of two-component cements	1–10% pet.
Printing inks (excluding ultraviolet-curable)	1–10% pet.
Reactive intermediates in chemical syntheses	0.01–0.1% pet.
Textile dyes	0.1–1% pet.
Water additives used in offset printing	1–10% aq.

pet., petrolatum; aq., aqua; ac., acetone; DGEBA, diglycidyl ether of bisphenol A.

Vehicles

The selection of the most appropriate vehicle depends on the solubility and other characteristics of the product. White or yellow petrolatum or distilled water are the most recommended vehicles, but also acetone and ethanol of pharmaceutical quality, even olive oil or other vegetable oils and methyl ethyl ketone (MEK) can be used for chemicals that are not water soluble.

For a water-soluble product, the appropriate vehicle is determined on the basis of pH. Water or other vehicles for neutral products, acid buffer for alkaline products (pH above 9), and alkaline buffer for acid products (pH below 4) can be used. One should be especially careful with products that may contain hydrofluoric acid, which can cause chemical burns and should not be tested at all.

Non-irritant solid materials or powders may be tested with a drop of water in a test chamber. Organic solvent vehicles, e.g., acetone, ethanol or methyl ethyl ketone, may be used instead of water, depending on the material or powder to be tested. The use of water or organic solvent improves the extraction of chemicals and their penetration into the skin. Moisturizing also helps the application of a test chamber containing powder or solid material. Water is recommended for textiles and paper, but organic solvents for plastic or rubber materials (Niklasson 1995).

Buffering

The use of buffers greatly widens the range of the possible products that can be used for testing. It also allows the detection of allergy to ingredients (perfumes and preservatives) that otherwise would be missed if the products were diluted to the extent that the pH is within an acceptable range. When using buffer solutions for the dilution of acid or alkaline chemicals, the test concentration may be increased 10-fold or even 1000-fold, and the problem of too low a test concentration can thus be overcome (Bruze 1984). Buffering is used in the testing of washing agents, preservatives, ethanol amines, even phenol formaldehyde resins (Jolanki et al. 2000).

The product should be diluted gradually with buffer until a pH range of 4–9 is reached (Bruze 1984). The buffering does not reduce the irritancy of products by mechanisms other than changes in pH. Products containing hydrofluoric acid (stain removers in the graphic industry, cleaners for metals, etc.) should not be used for testing, even if the pH is adjusted to above 4, as the toxicity of hydrofluoric acid is not mediated only through its acidity. Also, washing agents used for cleaning metal surfaces or the hands in dirty work may contain organic solvents. These products may cause severe irritant reactions if diluted only slightly with acidic buffer solution. The composition of acid and alkaline buffers is described in detail by Bruze 1984.

Recommended Concentrations and Vehicles for Patch Testing the Patients' Own Industrial Chemicals

Table 1 gives some guidelines for recommended test concentrations using dilution series and vehicles for common industrial chemicals, but it is not possible to give precise recommendations for each patient-supplied material.

Preparation of the Patch-Test Substances

It is handy to use disposable containers, syringes, stirrers or sticks to prepare test substances or dose them onto test chambers. If the product is solid (in crystal or powder form), it can be pulverized using a mortar.

The dilutions can be made using disposable syringes for volumetric determination (volume/volume) and electronic scales for the determination of weights (weight/weight).

The test substance should be mixed thoroughly. If the preparation is used to patch test other patients later, it should be protected from heat and light, and preferably be refrigerated. The vehicle should not be allowed to evaporate.

Solid materials, such as paper, textile, plastic products, plant materials and rubber products, can be tested as such, placing scrapings or cut pieces in the test chamber. Nevertheless, tests with such materials often turn out to be falsely negative, because the concentration of the sensitizer in the product is too low or the

Table 2. Materials suitable for extraction and recommended solvents (Jolanki et al. 2000; Niklasson 1995)

Material	Solvent
Paper	Ethanol
Plants and wood dusts	Acetone, ether, ethanol or water
Plastics, e.g., gloves	Acetone
Rubber, e.g., gloves	Acetone or water
Textiles	Ethanol

sensitizer is not released. To overcome this problem, the sensitizer can be extracted with water or organic solvents. The use of an ultrasonic bath makes the extraction process more efficient (Table 2) (Bruze et al. 1992; Niklasson 1995).

Semi-Open Tests in Testing Patient-Supplied Materials

Dooms-Goossens (1995) has suggested the use of a semi-open test for testing patient-supplied products, but it is not yet commonly accepted. All reactions must be verified by means of normal patch testing. One must keep in mind that even a single exposure to a strong allergen may sensitize (Kanerva et al. 1991, 1994; Kanerva and Lauerma 1998).

Evaluation of Test Reactions

An industrial material is usually a mixture of two or more chemicals. To be able to treat the patient's dermatitis and to prevent further cases of sensitization, it is important to find the chemical which was responsible for the positive reaction to his/her own industrial material. It is often possible to discover the allergenic ingredient by comparing concomitant positive reactions to individual test substances in the standard or in additional test series. If this is not possible, even weakly positive (?+) reactions caused by a patient's own substances should be confirmed by repeating the test by using the same test concentration supplemented with a dilution series; in case of a weak reaction, test substances of higher and lower concentrations than that producing the weak reaction should be used. The determination of the particular component to which the patient has been sensitized is sometimes crucial when occupational dermatosis is concerned. The sensitizer can be identified by testing the ingredients of the product separately. Manufacturers or importers are usually willing to supply individual ingredients as such or as ready-made test substances for additional patch testing. The pure components can also be purchased from chemical suppliers. Sometimes the allergen is an impurity or a product of a chemical reaction.

Control Tests

To avoid both false-positive and false-negative reactions, it may be necessary to test a suitable number of control persons with the adopted test substance.

The irritancy of a chemical can be shown by testing at least 20 non-sensitized individuals with a higher test concentration than that to which the patient reacted. Fregert (1985) has suggested that the test concentration for the control test should be ten times higher than the lowest concentration that gave a reaction to the patient. In general, the actual allergen produces a test reaction at a concentration as low as 0.01%. Accordingly, it is possible to consider whether the allergenic component is the main product or an additive. When highly sensitizing chemicals (such as acrylates, intermediates in pharmaceutical syntheses and epoxy compounds) are control-tested, the tenfold concentration may be too high, and the proper test concentration for control tests is usually the same one that gave a clear (2+) reaction in the patient (Jolanki 1991), otherwise there may be risk of active sensitization.

Even when these precautions are taken, weak irritant reactions are still possible. They may be preferable to false-negative reactions that usually are not referred for further examination, and the allergen remains unrecognized.

False-Negative Result

There are some patient-supplied chemicals that are very difficult to test because the concentration of the allergen in the product may be too low to cause a positive response. The allergen release from some solid materials is usually quite low. Moreover, the allergen may not be liberated in sufficient quantity, or the occlusion may be insufficient, so that other testing methods might be required. If there is a clear history of a product inducing a contact allergy reaction, it may be necessary to ask the manufacturer for the ingredients and test them individually at appropriate concentrations in order to detect the allergy. In certain cases, repeated open-application tests (ROAT) (Hannuksela and Salo 1986) can be useful. With the semi-open test method (Dooms-Goossens 1995), it is possible to use undiluted chemicals, but the penetration may be too low to induce test reactions. If a product is under serious suspicion, the different ingredients should be tested individually.

False-Positive Result

One of the problems in the testing of non-commercially available antigens, such as those made from the patient-supplied materials, is the possibility of an irritant reaction causing a false-positive test. The irritant reaction can sometimes be recognized as such, but this requires considerable experience. Serial dilution control tests are helpful in distinguishing between irritant and allergic reactions (Dooms-Goossens 1995; Niklasson 1995).

Active Sensitization

The sensitization risk must be kept in mind especially when performing patch tests with the patients' own substances. Though the patient may handle the chemicals as such, tests with the undiluted chemicals are not recommended (Kanerva et al. 1991). Patch-test preparations should match published concentrations and should not exceed 0.1% in concentration when very reactive components are tested, e.g. intermediates of some chemical syntheses (Sonnex and Rycroft 1986; Niklasson 1995). Active sensitization should also be taken into consideration when control tests are performed.

Compound Allergy

For a review of compound allergy see Bashir et al. (2000).

Need for Chemical Analyses

There are two main reasons for chemical analyses. First, on patch testing, the patient is found to be allergic to a specific chemical, and the causative product(s) are analyzed for the chemical. Second, the patient's own material has caused an allergic test reaction, but SDS or other information from the manufacturer did not reveal the causative chemical. In this case, it may be reasonable to analyze the material of all ingredients, especially if individual ingredients could not be tested separately.

Health Hazards in the Testing Unit

The personnel of the testing unit may be at risk of skin sensitization against the patient's own industrial chemicals. When making the test preparations, protective gloves should be worn, and disposable plastic (polyvinylchloride or polyethylene) or synthetic rubber (nitrile) are the most suitable materials. The use of disposable containers and stirrers, etc. also diminishes exposure to the potential allergenic chemicals. A place for washing the hands and rinsing the eyes should be very near the place where the handling of industrial chemicals takes place, and adequate local exhaust ventilation should be available.

Conclusion

The importance of making a correct diagnosis, especially when patients with a suspected occupational dermatitis are being investigated, is obvious. The outcome has such a great impact on the patient's life that complicated cases with, for example, extensive exposure to several chemicals should be referred to clinics specialized in occupational dermatology, if possible (Niklasson 1995).

Supplementary testing in addition to the standard tray, with selected series, and the patient's own products – plus the suspicious ingredients in those products – gives the best chance of revealing the cause(s) of allergic contact dermatitis. Quality-controlled skin tests with the materials handled by the patient may be the only way to detect contact allergy, especially to the chemical ingredients that are not included in about 500 commercially available patch-test substances. The importance of identifying all contact allergens cannot be overemphasized.

References

Adams RM (1995) Additional sources of information that can be caused in patch testing. Am J Contact Dermatitis 6:40–41

Bashir SJ, Kanerva L, Jolanki R, Maibach HI (2002) Occupational and non-occupational compound allergy. In: Kanerva L, Elsner P, Wahlberg JE, Maibach HI (eds) Handbook of occupational dermatology. Springer, Berlin Heidelberg New York, pp 351–355

Beck MH (1995) The patient with negative patch tests – what now? In: Guin JD (ed) Practical contact dermatitis. A handbook for the practitioner. McGraw-Hill, USA, pp 659–672

Bruze M (1984) Use of buffer solutions for patch testing. Contact Dermatitis 10:267–269

Bruze M, Trulsson L, Bendsöe N (1992) Patch testing with ultrasonic bath extracts. Am J Contact Dermatitis 3:133–137

De Groot AC (1994) Patch testing, 2nd edn. Elsevier, Amsterdam

Dooms-Goossens A (1995) Patch testing without a kit. In: Guin JD (ed) Practical contact dermatitis. A handbook for the practitioner. McGraw-Hill, USA, pp 63–74

Fregert S (1981) Manual of contact dermatitis. Munksgaard, Copenhagen

Fregert S (1985) Publication of allergens. Contact Dermatitis 12:123–124

Guin JD (1995) Practical contact dermatitis. A handbook for the practitioner. McGraw-Hill, USA

Hannuksela M, Salo H (1986) The repeated open application test (ROAT). Contact Dermatitis 14:221–227

Hausen BM (1988) Allergiepflanzen – Pflanzenallergene. Kontaktallergene. Ecomed, Munich

Jolanki R (1991) Occupational skin diseases from epoxy compounds. Epoxy resin compounds, epoxy acrylates and 2,3-epoxypropyl trimethyl ammonium chloride (doctoral dissertation). Acta Derm Venereol Suppl 159:1–80

Jolanki R, Estlander T, Alanko K, Kanerva L (2000) Patch testing with a patient's own materials handled at work. In: Kanerva L, Elsner P, Wahlberg JE, Maibach HI (eds) Handbook of occupational dermatology. Springer, Berlin Heidelberg New York (Ch. 47), 375–383

Kanerva L, Lauerma A (1998) Iatrogenic acrylate allergy complicating amalgam allergy. Contact Dermatitis 38:58–59

Kanerva L, Turjanmaa K, Jolanki R, Estlander T (1991) Occupational allergic contact dermatitis from iatrogenic sensitization by a new acrylate dentin adhesive. Eur J Dermatol 1:25–28

Kanerva L, Tarvainen K, Pinola A, Leino T, Granlund H, Estlander T, Jolanki R, Förström L (1994) A single accidental exposure may result in a chemical burn, primary sensitization and allergic contact dermatitis. Contact Dermatitis 31:229–235

Kanerva L, Estlander T, Jolanki R (1996) False negative patch test reaction caused by testing with dental composite acrylic resin. Int J Dermatol 35:189–192

Kanerva L, Estlander T, Jolanki R (1998) Dental nurse's occupational allergic contact dermatitis from eugenol used as a restorative dental material with polymethylmethacrylate. Contact Dermatitis 38:339–340

Lamminpää A, Kanerva L, Estlander T, Jolanki R (1996) Occupational allergic contact dermatitis caused by decorative plants. Contact Dermatitis 34:330–335

Leisvaara K, Estlander T, Jolanki R (1998) Allergic contact eczema caused by MDI isocyanate in insulation work (in Finnish). In: Kanerva L, Jolanki R, Keskinen H, Savela A, Karjalainen A (eds) Työperäiset allergiat v. 1995–96. Työterveyslaitos, Helsinki, pp 237–240

Niklasson B (1995) Mixing your own antigens. In: Guin JD (ed) Practical contact dermatitis. A handbook for the practitioner. McGraw-Hill, USA, pp 687–695

Rietschel RL, Fowler JJ Jr (1995) Fisher's contact dermatitis, 4th edn. Williams & Wilkins, Philadelphia

Sonnex TS, Rycroft RJG (1986) Allergic contact dermatitis from chloromethyl heterocyclic intermediates in the synthesis of a histamine antagonist. Contact Dermatitis 14:265–267

Wahlberg JE (1998) Identification of new allergens and non-irritant patch test preparations. Contact Dermatitis 39:155–156

CHAPTER 18

Sources of Information on the Occurrence of Chemical Contact Allergens

18

M.-A. FLYVHOLM

Introduction

Information on the occurrence of chemical contact allergens is essential for the prevention and treatment of allergic contact dermatitis. The ideal situation is access to reliable, easy and quick detection and identification of contact allergens in the environment.

Several studies have shown that careful investigation and information on exposure to contact allergens is important for the prognosis of patients with allergic contact eczema (Cronin 1991; Edman 1988; Flyvholm and Menné 1992). Furthermore, early elimination of the exposure to the allergens seems to prevent chronic occurrence of the eczema (Flyvholm and Menné 1992).

Exposure information can be obtained from different sources, such as:

1. Literature
2. Product labelling and declarations
3. Material safety data sheets
4. Inquiries to manufacturers or suppliers
5. Chemical analysis
6. Product databases

The different sources of information have advantages and limitations, and are thus more or less adequate depending on the context in which the information is needed and the nature or the origin of the allergen(s) and product(s) in question (Flyvholm et al. 1995; Flyvholm 1996). This chapter gives a presentation of the different methods used to obtain information on the occurrence of chemical contact allergens with a short discussion on each method followed by a general discussion.

Literature

Textbooks on contact dermatitis frequently include overviews on the occurrence of contact allergens in product categories or occupations based on, for example, published papers, author experience or product databases. These overviews will always be restricted to existing knowledge and the background of the data must be considered when using and evaluating such information. For some substances and product categories, textbook information will be quickly outdated due to changes in technology and lifestyle, but for others it can be expected to last longer. If textbooks are available, they are easy to use.

Scientific journals often publish case reports on new or unrecognised sources of exposure to specific allergens. Due to developments in the field of easy access on-line literature databases, this source of exposure information has become more useful than earlier when literature searches were rather expensive and time consuming.

Product Labelling and Declarations

Product labelling and declarations are the most obvious ways to obtain and provide information on the content of contact allergens in chemical products but, unfortunately, labelling requirements do not cover all product categories. This kind of information on exposure has an advantage in that it is accessible immediately for both patients and doctors, provided that the product package still exists. The labelling or declaration is restricted to the information that the manufacturer, importer or supplier has to or is willing to provide. Furthermore, labelling or declaration is influenced by legislation and regulations concerning what type of product categories to cover, what kind of information to include and how to provide the information. In some cases, compounds added to raw materials may be missing in the declaration. As regards cosmetic products, the fragrances do not have to be included in the declaration, according to the EU rules. For chemical products containing contact allergens, the EU rules require labelling of products (preparations) with Xi (irritating) and Risk Phrase (R43 "may cause contact sensitisation by skin contact"). The default threshold value for labelling the content of contact allergens is 1% (10,000 ppm) although a lower limit has been established for some contact allergens. Another problem in the use of product labelling and declarations is that the names for the allergens are not always easy to read and interpret (De Groot and Weijland 1997).

Product labelling and declarations with sufficient information on specific ingredients, including information on components of less than 1%, is the ideal as regards allergic contact eczema.

Material Safety Data Sheets

Material safety data sheets can, like product declarations, be accessible immediately, provided that they are available and that the user is able to read and understand chemical names. The value of the data is also restricted to the information which the manufacturer, importer or supplier has to or is willing to provide. Material safety data sheets make it possible to include additional information on safe use and precautions in case of accidents. The practical use is dependent on the local management and administration of a workplace system ensuring easy access to the relevant material safety data sheets.

Inquiries to Manufacturers or Suppliers

Inquiries to manufacturers or suppliers in order to obtain information on ingredients in chemical products can, in principle, provide information on ingredients in products used by eczema patients. In practice, this is often very time consuming and sometimes the detailed information may not even be available from a supplier. However, some manufacturers are able to provide detailed information on a specific batch of a product quickly.

Chemical Analysis

Chemical analysis is very suitable for well-defined and known substances if reliable analytical methods are available for the specific allergens. Simple and quick test methods make it possible for clinical departments to analyse products brought in by the patients. Analytical methods requiring specialised laboratory equipment or expertise must be carried out in specialised laboratories, and this may cause time delay or incredibly high expenses for the clinical routine work. For example, nickel and formaldehyde can be detected by simple tests methods, but chromate and epoxy demand methods requiring specialised laboratory equipment and expertise.

Usually, it is necessary to know for which allergens to search before doing chemical analyses, because a thorough chemical identification of all components in complex products is seldom practicable. As only a minor part of the known contact allergens can be detected by routine analytical methods, it is thus only possible to obtain information on exposure to contact allergens by analysing the products in a limited number of cases.

Product Databases

Product databases can, if they are easily accessible and include the relevant product categories, be a quick and easy way to obtain information on contact allergens in chemical products. It should normally be possible to make lists of product categories or single products with the content of specific allergens or lists of allergens occurring in a product category. Depending on the data sources and the degree of specificity, some databases may have restricted access, whereas those with non-confidential data normally can be used without limitations. Databases of relevance in dermatology are reviewed in the *Textbook of Contact Dermatitis* (Dooms-Goossens et al. 1995). The Danish Product Register Database (PROBAS) is an example of a national database established on legal demands and notification rules. This database includes information and evaluations on substances, materials and products used in Denmark; the registered data is focused on use, chemical composition of products, quantities used in Denmark and the adverse effects on health and environment. Further description of PROBAS and registered contact allergens can be found in Flyvholm (2000) and Flyvholm et al. (1992).

Product databases can be used at the single patient level by doctors and patients. On a more general level, the authorities can use databases to survey the use of chemical products and to plan preventive measures. Particularly in the use of administrative databases, the background of the registered data and the product categories included should be considered, see Chap. 26.

Discussion

As indicated in this chapter, different sources of information on the occurrence of contact allergens are suitable for different exposure situations and allergens. Depending on the local facilities and demands, different methods may be preferred, but access to a variety of sources is usually necessary.

Formaldehyde is an example of a contact allergen, which can occur in products from various origins, each of which requires different sources of information (Flyvholm 1997). Thus, formaldehyde is used below to illustrate the advantages and limitations of the different sources of information on the occurrence of chemical contact allergens.

Formaldehyde can occur in chemical products as a component added directly in the manufacturing process or as a component added in raw materials. Some components can release formaldehyde as part of their function in the products, i.e., formaldehyde releasing preservatives (Flyvholm and Andersen 1993). Besides these intentional occurrences of formaldehyde, it can occur as residues from synthesis of other product components and from formation during storage and handling of raw materials or end products. Contamination from packages coated with formaldehyde resins has also been reported.

Textbooks and scientific journals can provide a tremendous amount of data on the occurrence of formaldehyde in chemical products from various sources, which can provide a solid background on potential exposure to formaldehyde. Nevertheless, eczema patients with contact allergy to formaldehyde have previously been able to receive only scanty information on exposure to formaldehyde (Cronin 1991; Flyvholm and Menné 1992). Product labelling and declarations normally give information on components added by the manufacturer. Content derived from raw materials may be missing and content coming from residues, formation in the products or contamination cannot be expected to be covered by labelling and declarations. Material safety data sheets will more or less cover the same formaldehyde sources as labelling and declarations. Inquiries to manufacturers or suppliers could provide, in principle, updated and adequate information on formaldehyde content in the specific products, independently of the origin of formaldehyde, if the products are analysed, or the information obtained may include only added components and eventual content from raw materials. Chemical analysis can provide information on the content of formaldehyde independently of the origin, if analytical methods suitable for the product type are available (Flyvholm et al. 1996). Product databases cannot provide data better than the input data, so databases compiling product labelling and declarations will equal these and so on, which stresses the need to be aware of the background of the product databases.

In conclusion, the best strategy for a dermatological department seems to be a solid background knowledge from the literature combined with routine examination of product labelling, declarations and material safety data sheets for products used by the eczema patients. This may be combined with chemical analysis for detection of allergens originating from raw materials, residues, and formation in the products or contamination. For regulatory purposes and prevention of sensitisation, overviews based on product databases can be of great benefit in the supplying of information which, under other circumstances, could take years to compile from product labelling, declarations, material safety data sheets, inquiries to manufacturers and suppliers, or chemical analysis.

References

Cronin E (1991) Formaldehyde is a significant allergen in women with hand eczema. Contact Dermatitis 25:276–282

De Groot AC, Weijland JW (1997) Conversion of common names of cosmetic allergens to the INCI nomenclature. Contact Dermatitis 37:145–150

Dooms-Goossens A, Dooms M, Drieghe J (1995) Computers and patient information systems. In: Rycroft RJG, Menné T, Frosch PJ (eds) Textbook of contact dermatitis. Springer, Berlin Heidelberg New York, pp 771–784

Edman B (1988) The usefulness of detailed information to patients with contact allergy. Contact Dermatitis 19:43–47

Flyvholm MA (1996) Prevention by exposure assessment. Curr Probl Dermatol 25:97–105

Flyvholm MA (1997) Formaldehyde exposure at the workplace and in the environment. Allergologie 5:225–231

Flyvholm MA (2000) Computerized product database. Registered chemical contact allergens. In: Kanerva L, Elsner P, Wahlberg JE, Maibach HI (eds) Handbook of occupational dermatology. Springer, Berlin Heidelberg New York, pp 451–461

Flyvholm MA, Andersen P (1993) Identification of formaldehyde releasers and occurrence of formaldehyde and formaldehyde releasers in registered chemical products. Am J Ind Med 24:533–552

Flyvholm MA, Menné T (1992) Allergic contact dermatitis from formaldehyde. A case study focussing on sources of formaldehyde exposure. Contact Dermatitis 27:27–36

Flyvholm MA, Andersen P, Beck ID, Brandorff NP (1992) PROBAS: The Danish Product Register Data Base – a national register of chemical substances and products. J Hazardous Mater 30:59–69

Flyvholm MA, Menné T, Maibach HI (1995) Skin allergy: Exposures and dose-response relationships. In: Vos JG, Younes M, Smith E (eds) Allergic hypersensitivities induced by chemicals. Recommendations for prevention. CRC Press, Boca Raton, pp 261–285

Flyvholm MA, Tiedeman E, Menné T (1996) Comparison of 2 tests used for clinical assessment of formaldehyde exposure. Contact Dermatitis 34:35–38

CHAPTER 19

Identification and Assessment in Relation to the Material Safety Data Sheets

19

D. A. Basketter, L. Kanerva

Introduction

The manufacturer's material safety data sheet (MSDS) represents the primary source of information on safety issues related to the material or product to which it is related. It is thus a first point of call for the dermatologist trying to judge whether a particular product/substance might be responsible for a case of occupational skin disease under consideration. Even though current MSDSs are of great help, they may not be exact enough from a dermato-allergist's point of view (Kanerva et al. 1997).

In this chapter, we review how skin irritation/sensitisation information is generated/collated for the MSDS, what it does tell the physician, what it does not tell the physician and how the information given might be refined/improved. We also present recently published data on the quality of currently used MSDS by comparing gas-chromatographic (GC) analyses of acrylate chemicals with MSDS and product declarations (Kanerva et al. 1997). From that study, we can conclude that better MSDS and product declarations should be required from industries before the products are sold; otherwise, many patients/customers could suffer irritation/sensitisation before any preventive measures have been put in place.

What is an MSDS?

An example of a current MSDS is given in Fig. 1. The MSDS is simply a means for a manufacturer to present basic safety information on his product, whether that product is a single substance, a mixture of substances or even a fully finished product. It should contain details of all the known safety hazards presented by the product, both physical and biological, together with details of how these hazards should be managed.

Previously, manufacturers were often unwilling to reveal the chemicals in their products (Kanerva et al. 1996). Examples in Finland were printing plates containing acrylics in the 1970s: hardly any information on the hazardous chemicals was available to the physician. The Finnish Identification and Labelling System for Hazardous Chemicals (286/78) made MSDS mandatory in Finland (Kanerva et al. 1996) in 1978. The EU has also implemented regulations on the preparation of MSDS which have been updated recently (European Community 2001). However, even though current MSDSs are of great help, they may have insufficient detail

1. IDENTIFICATION OF THE SUBSTANCE/PREPARATION AND COMPANY

UNILEVER UK	PRODUCT NAME: **Wonderclean SU**	EMERGENCY TELEPHONE: REF NO: R57166 ISSUE DATE: 14 May 1997
PHYSICAL FORM:	PRODUCT TYPE:	CONTAINER(S):

2. COMPOSITION/INFORMATION ON INGREDIENTS

<u>Occupational Exposure Limit</u>

<u>NAME</u>	<u>RANGE</u>	<u>HAZARD</u>	<u>STEL</u>	<u>TWA</u>
NTA SODIUM SALT		Irritant Harmful		
ALCOHOL C8-18/E6-15		Irritant Harmful		
COCONUT DIETHANOLAMIDE		Irritant		
BENZALKONIUM CHLORIDE		Corrosive Harmful		

STEL - Short Term Exposure Level. TWA - 8hrs Time Weighted Average.
OELs are UK standard, expressed as mg/m³. They are Occupational Exposure Standards, unless marked *, which indicate Maximum Exposure Level

3. HAZARDS IDENTIFICATION: Irritant to skin and eyes

4. FIRST-AID MEASURES

EYE:	Wash immediately with copious amounts of water then obtain medical attention.
SKIN:	Wash thoroughly with water. Remove contaminated clothing.
INGESTION:	Remove material from mouth. Drink 1 or 2 glasses of water (or milk) and obtain medical attention.
INHALATION:	Remove from source of exposure and obtain medical attention.
EQUIPMENT AT WORK PLACE:	Eye and skin washing facilities.

5. FIRE-FIGHTING MEASURES

FLAMMABILITY: Not flammable

SUITABLE EXTINGUISHERS: Any can be used.	EXPLOSIVE HAZARDS: None known.
EXTINGUISHERS NOT TO BE USED: None.	
SPECIAL PROTECTIVE EQUIPMENT: Breathing apparatus should be worn when tackling fires involving this product.	HAZARDOUS COMBUSTION PRODUCTS: Toxic and irritant fumes may be given off when heated to decomposition.

PRODUCT NAME: Quatdet SU321	REF NO: R57166

6. ACCIDENTAL RELEASE MEASURES

PERSONAL PROTECTION	Wear adequate eye protection and gloves.
SPILLAGE CLEAN-UP	Observe local legislation. Absorb large spillage with inert material (e.g. sand) and collect into suitable, labelled containers for disposal at an approved site. Wash residues and small spillages away to drain with water.

7. HANDLING AND STORAGE

HANDLING	Avoid eye and skin contact. Prevent any mist formation.
STORAGE	Store in the original, closed containers under dry conditions. Avoid extremes of temperature.

8. EXPOSURE CONTROLS/ PERSONAL PROTECTION: Protective goggles and gloves.

9. PHYSICAL AND CHEMICAL PROPERTIES

APPEARANCE:

SOLUBILITY IN WATER:	BOILING POINT (°C):
pH:	FLASH POINT (°C):
VISCOSITY AT 20°C:	DENSITY:

10. STABILITY AND REACTIVITY: Stable, no dangerous reactions known.

11. TOXICOLOGICAL INFORMATION

EYE:	Causes irritation.
SKIN:	Causes irritation.
INGESTION:	Causes irritation.
INHALATION:	Causes irritation.

12. ECOLOGICAL INFORMATION: Product should not be discharged directly to the aquatic environment without pretreatment. The cationic component will be efficiently removed in waste water treatment.

13. DISPOSAL CONSIDERATIONS

CONTENTS:	Observe relevant legislation.
EMPTY CONTAINERS:	Observe relevant legislation

14. TRANSPORT INFORMATION

UN NUMBER AND PACKAGING GROUP: Non-dangerous material.

15. REGULATORY INFORMATION

R36	Irritating to eyes and skin.
S26	In case of contact with eyes, rinse immediately with plenty of water and seek medical advice
S37	Wear suitable gloves.

16. OTHER INFORMATION
If the product is used from a spray. Product use instructions must advise against breathing the spray and ensuring that there is adequate ventilation.
Handle and apply only as recommended.

Fig. 1. Material safety data sheet of the product "Wonderclean SU"

Table 1. Possible reasons for material safety data sheets being inaccurate

Low concentrations of chemicals may not be declared
Raw materials may contain hidden impurities
Final product may contain starting materials
Decomposition of components
Contamination of residues
Manufacturing processes may be poorly controlled
Undeclared components may be added intentionally

from a dermato-allergist's point of view (Table 1). We feel that efforts should be taken to achieve more complete MSDSs, and the dermato-allergist also needs to know the components with a lower concentration than the arbitrary 1% cut-off limit; currently, chemicals with a concentration below 1% are usually not declared, even when they are allergenic.

Irritation/Sensitisation Hazard Identification and the MSDS

In this book, we are largely concerned with the threat posed to normal skin by contact with irritant and sensitising substances; it is worth noting that whilst both substances and/or mixtures thereof can be irritating, for skin sensitisation it is the substances themselves that must be allergens (haptens). In this section, approaches to the identification of skin irritants are described briefly, together with a description of how the data may be interpreted in terms of an MSDS. Subsequently, a similar succinct account for skin sensitisers is presented.

Skin Irritation

For many years, the standard approach to the determination of skin-irritation potential has been the Draize rabbit test (Draize 1944, 1959). This simple, 4-h, semi-occluded patch testing, typically using three rabbits, is still the one recommended in regulatory guidelines (Food and Drug Administration 1972; European Community 1988, 1992, 1993; United Nations 1993; Organisation for Economic Cooperation and Development 1993). Generally, the information generated is interpreted against standard criteria, such as those in Europe (European Community 1993), which then serve to convert the continuous erythema/oedema/scaling reaction of skin irritancy into a "yes/no" decision. Thus, in the European Community (EC), and expressed in layman's terms, if a substance induces an average of mild to moderate irritancy in at least two of the rabbits, it is classified as a skin irritant. If it fails to achieve the arbitrary threshold, it is not classified as a skin irritant. Whilst some countries have a slightly different threshold (if they have any at all), the general principle of crude hazard identification using this type of approach is usually followed. It is noteworthy that this test only evaluates the ability of the material in question to give rise to an acute irritant response.

Whilst the test described above is a common way in which an attempt is made at predictive identification of those substances or products with significant skin-irritation potential, other information can also be used. Consideration is given to structure-activity relationships, although it must be said that this subject is in its infancy for skin irritants (Whittle et al. 1996; Barratt 1996). Data may also come from non-standard animal tests, predictive human tests and from human experience. These may cover either acute and/or cumulative irritant responses in skin. It is also possible for manufacturers to use data from in vitro studies. Lastly, where the product is a mixture of two or more substances [a "preparation" in European Union (EU) terminology], the manufacturer may elect to calculate the likely irritancy on the basis of the knowledge of the skin irritancy of the component substances and the concentration at which they occur in the product. For certain types of product, this process has been formalised in the EU as the "conventional method" (European Community 1988).

Whilst the formal classification of skin-irritation potential in the EU for both substances and preparations should lead to a harmonisation of the information applied to the MSDS, this does not in fact occur. The standard rabbit test is highly variable (Weil and Scala 1971). A key problem is that even well defined criteria are still open to differences of interpretation. For most of the types/ sources of information mentioned above, there are no criteria for their interpretation. How much human clinical data and of what type should be sufficient to categorise a product as an irritant? How might in vitro data be interpreted in a meaningful way? In practice, the manufacturer has to make an independent judgement on whether the data are sufficient to cause concern about skin irritancy.

Skin Sensitisation

The generation and interpretation of skin sensitisation data suffers from many of the problems associated with skin irritation data, but has, in addition, special characteristics of its own. As with skin irritation, the protocols commonly used for the predictive identification of skin-sensitising chemicals use a small number of animals to detect the hazard. The most common method employed is the Magnusson and Kligman guinea-pig maximisation test (GPMT) (Magnusson and Kligman 1970), which is very effective at identifying even weak skin sensitisers. The interpretation of the results in terms of classification of a chemical as a skin sensitiser follows a similar process to that for skin irritation, i.e. the continuously variable biological data is converted into a binomial result. Using EU criteria, if at least 30% of the animals are positive in the GPMT, then the chemical is described as a skin sensitiser (European Community 1996). No account is taken of the test concentrations, the intensity of individual reactions or indeed the number of reactions, except to ensure that the latter is above the threshold. Manufacturers use this or similar criteria in an ad hoc way to judge whether their product is a skin sensitiser. Also, in a similar manner to irritancy, it is possible to make use of structure-activity considerations (Barratt et al. 1997). Furthermore, data may also be derived from other animal tests, predictive human tests and from human clinical experience.

Although there appears to be considerable standardisation of test protocols for the predictive identification of skin sensitisers (Organisation for Economic Cooperation and Development 1993), both the use and the interpretation of test data is subject to wide variations (Robinson et al. 1990; Frankild et al. 1996). It is almost impossible to overestimate the variability of the results which can be obtained by different laboratories testing the same substance and using the same protocol.

Recently, the local lymph node assay (LLNA) has been accepted as a valid alternative method for the identification of skin sensitisation (OECD 1993, 2002). Importantly, this method shows real promise in providing a robust and quantitative assessment of the relative sensitising potency of substances (Basketter et al. 2000). Such data would permit classification of allergens into categories (weak/moderate/strong etc.). Use of this approach in an MSDS could be of benefit for risk assessment/management.

MSDS Information – What Does it Tell Me/Not Tell Me?

"Something, but not a lot" is the short answer. What the MSDS does say is that the manufacturer of the product has made a judgement (hopefully on the basis of all the available data) as to whether that product possesses either skin irritating and/or sensitising properties to a "significant" extent. What is significant is generally left to the judgement of the manufacturer although, at least for certain products in the EU, the standard criteria may be applied (European Community 1988, 1993).

However, the information contained on a MSDS is limited in a variety of ways. First, both the derivation of data and its interpretation vary to a considerable degree. For example, lactic acid has been described as corrosive to skin by some manufacturers, yet left unlabeled (i.e. not regarded as significantly irritant) by another (D. Basketter, personal communication). Similar inconsistencies exist for skin sensitisation. One real difficulty can be manufacturers who err wholly on the side of caution and thus label a great many products as irritants; there is a tendency to be more circumspect about the use of the term "sensitising".

Being cautious is not by itself bad. However, it does highlight a further limitation of the MSDS information – that it is binomial, a product is either irritating/sensitising or it is not. This is so far from the truth as to be laughable. The only action that can ensue on the basis of such limited information is to "avoid skin contact". Risk assessment and management activities need to be much more sophisticated to be of real benefit, not least since total avoidance of skin contact is rarely possible.

Most commonly, skin irritation to chemicals occurs clinically as cumulative irritant dermatitis. MSDS data is most often based on evidence of the acute skin-irritation potential of the product. Such data may not always be fully predictive of cumulative irritation potential (Hannuksela and Hannuksela 1995). Furthermore, if the product is a preparation rather than a single substance, MSDS information may be based on the conventional calculation method, in which labelling is only applied if the sum of classified irritants is at least 20% (European Community 1988). To put this in simple terms, it means that 20% aqueous sodium lauryl sulphate would be described as irritant, whilst 19.9% would not be so labelled.

Skin sensitisation can often arise from highly allergenic substances that are present either as impurities or are deliberately added, but at a very low level. Typically, these may not be identified on an MSDS; the manufacturer may not even be aware of their presence. Following EC rules (European Community 1988), a preparation is not normally labelled as skin sensitising if the offending agent is present at a concentration below 1.0%. Yet it is quite obvious that such a judgement of whether a preparation is likely to be sensitising depends not only on the concentration, but also is heavily dependent on the potency of the skin sensitiser as well as on a number of other factors. Skin sensitisation may also arise by oxidation of specific chemicals (Karlberg et al. 1997); an MSDS does not normally address such matters, although this may be changing (Karlberg et al. 1999).

MSDS – Comparison of Data in MSDS
to Chromatographic/Mass Spectrometric Analysis

Identification of allergens can be performed with chromatographic/mass spectrometric (GC/MS) analysis. Here, we review recent data in which GC/MS analysis was compared with data given in MSDSs (Kanerva et al. 1997). Dental acrylics contained up to 37% of undeclared acrylics (triethylene glycol dimethacrylate (TREGDMA). Undeclared 2,2-bis-4-(2-hydroxy-3-methacryloxypropoxy)phenyl-propane (BIS-GMA) was present (at 7.6%) in an adhesive. Many other undeclared methacrylates were present in a concentration greater than 1%, namely ethylene glycol dimethacrylate (EGDMA, 13%), decamethylene dimethacrylate (5.9%) and diethylene glycol dimethacrylate (DEGDMA, 1.5%). A great number of acrylics were present in lower concentrations than 1%. A prosthesis powder contained 3% methyl methacrylate (MMA) and 0.5% I,D-butyl methacrylate, although the MSDS did not declare any acrylics. Acrylic denture-base liquids may contain cross-linking dimethacrylates, and the analysis showed 4.6% EGDMA although it had not been declared in the MSDS.

The analysis of an epoxy acrylate and styrene-based reinforced plastic showed that only styrene was declared as a hazardous compound, although 8.1% of sensitising 2-hydroxypropyl methacrylate (2-HPMA) was present in the plastic.

Acrylic glues used in the construction industry did not contain acrylics (detection limit 0.005%). The main component of the anaerobic glues was TREGDMA. DEGDMA or 2-HPMA were used as reactive diluents. Undeclared 2-HPMA was present (at 7.6%) in one glue. Tetrahydrofurfural methacrylate and isobornyl acrylate were the main components in the analysed two-component glues. Ethyl-hexyl methacrylate and 2-hydroxyethyl methacrylate (2-HEMA) were present as reactive diluents. High concentrations of two sensitisers, HEMA (26%) and isobornyl acrylate (24%), were present, although undeclared. Undeclared epoxy resin (6%) had been added to two glues.

The UV lacquers contained several types of diacrylates, triacrylates and epoxy diacrylates. Up to 46% undeclared diacrylates (tripropylene glycol diacrylates) were analysed. MMA was the main component in two concrete paints. These contained up to 7.3% undeclared butanediol dimethacrylate. UV-light-cured coatings contained up to 13% of undeclared oligotriacrylates and 7.6% undeclared hexanediol diacrylate.

MSDS – Opportunities for Improvement

It must be accepted that there are real practical difficulties in making substantive improvements in the MSDS. That does not mean that they should not be attempted. It is our view that a much greater harmonisation of the current information contained in the MSDS would be helpful. Standardisation of the predictive test methods employed, preferably by adoption of more reliable protocols and the use of suitable benchmarks, would considerably enhance the quality of the information in an MSDS. However, of even greater value would be information on the potency of the sensitisation or irritation hazard present, even if this was seen to be a low risk due, for example, to the presence of a strong sensitiser at a very low concentration. Such information would be of immense practical value in risk assessment/management. In addition, proper attention should be paid to the risk of oxidation of certain materials. Limonene and colophony are not sensitisers, but their oxidation products are (Karlberg et al. 1988). Such knowledge should be encapsulated in the MSDS. Other susceptibilities of the product or other potential impurities should be included.

Conclusion

In summary, the MSDS usually provides only the most basic information on significant intrinsic skin irritation and sensitisation hazards. The quality of any information is highly variable and generally will say nothing about the strength of the hazard presented. Information on sensitising impurities or the risk of their formation, e.g. through oxidation, is normally absent.

Accurate MSDSs are very important when trying to reveal the cause of occupational contact dermatoses. However, most of the analysed acrylate products contained undeclared sensitising acrylics: (meth)acrylates were not declared in 17 of 28 (61%) of the analysed products, and up to 46% of the materials present were undeclared, sensitising acrylics (Kanerva et al. 1997).

Thus, the user of the MSDS has in effect three options: take the information at face value, ignore the information or treat the information as a stimulus to undertake a more detailed search followed by an analysis of the information in the context of the known/expected skin exposure. This last course of action is the one that is recommended if the need for a clinical or safety evaluation is of importance. Information on product ingredients should also be given for sensitising substances present at concentrations lower than 1%. Therefore, better MSDSs and product declarations should be required from industries before their products are put on the market.

References

Barratt MD (1996) Quantitative structure activity relationships for skin irritation and corrosivity of neutral and electrophilic organic chemicals. Toxicol In Vitro 10:247–256

Barratt MD, Basketter DA, Roberts DW (1997) Quantitative structure activity relationships. In: Le Poittevin J-P, Basketter DA, Dooms-Goossens A, Karlberg AT (eds) The molecular basis of allergic contact dermatitis. Springer, Berlin Heidelberg New York, pp 129–154

Basketter DA, Blaikie L, Dearman RJ, Kimber I, Ryan CA, Gerberick GF, Harvey P, Evans P, White IR, Rycroft RJG (2000) Use of the Local Lymph Node Assay for the Estimation of Relative Contact Allergenic Potency. Contact Dermatitis 42:344–348

Consumer Product Safety Commission (1979) Federal Hazardous Substances Act, Code of Federal Regulations. Title 16, part 1500.42. Federal Register

Draize JH, Woodard G, Calvery HO (1944) Methods for the study of imitation and toxicity of substances applied topically to the skin and mucous membranes. J Pharmacol Exp Ther 82:377–390

Draize JH (1959) Dermal toxicity. In: Appraisal of the safety of chemicals in foods, drugs and cosmetics. Association of Foods and Drugs Officials of the United States, Littleton, pp 46–59

European Community (1988) Council Directive of 7 June 1988 on the approximation of the laws, regulations and administrative provisions of the Member States relating to the classification, packaging and labeling of dangerous preparations. Off J Eur Communities L18:14

European Community (1992) Annex to Commission Directive 92/69/EEC of 31 July 1992 adapting to technical progress for the seventeenth time Council Directive 67/548/EEC on the approximation of laws, regulations and administrative provisions relating to the classification, packaging and labelling of dangerous substances. Off J Eur Communities L383A:35

European Community (1993) Council regulation EEC No 793/93 of 23 March 1993 on the evaluation and control of the risks of existing substances. Off J Eur Communities L18:14

European Community (1996) Annex V. Off J Eur Communities L248/226

European Community (2001) Commission Directive 2001/58/EC dated 7/8/2001. Off J Eur Communities L212/24

Food and Drug Administration (1972) United States – Food and Drug Administration. Hazardous substances. Proposed revisions of test for primary skin irritants. Fed Reg 37:27635

Frankild S, Basketter DA, Andersen KE (1996) The value and limitations of rechallenge in the guinea pig maximisation test. Contact Dermatitis 35:135–140

Hannuksela A, Hannuksela M (1995) Irritant effects of a detergent in wash and chamber tests. Contact Dermatitis 32:163–166

Kanerva L, Estlander T, Jolanki R (1996) Allergy caused by acrylics – past, present and prevention. In: Elsner P, Lachapelle JM, Wahlberg J, Maibach HI (eds) Prevention of contact dermatitis (Curr Probl Dermatol, vol 25). Karger, Basel, pp 86–96

Kanerva L, Henriks-Eckerman M-L, Jolanki R, Estlander T (1997) Plastics/acrylics: material safety data sheets need to be improved. Clin Dermatol 15:533–546

Karlberg A-T, Basketter DA, Goossens A, Lepoittevin J-P (1999) Regulatory classification of substances oxidized to skin sensitizers by exposure to the air. Contact Dermatitis 40:183–188

Karlberg A-T, Bohlinder K, Boman A, Hacksell U, Hermansson J, Jacobsson S, Nilsson JLG (1988) Identification of 15-hydroperoxyabietic acid as a contact allergen in Portugese colophony. J Pharm Pharmacol 40:42–47

Karlberg A-T, Goossens A (1997) Contact allergy to oxidized S,D-limonene among contact dermatitis patients. Contact Dermatitis 37:308–309

Organisation for Economic Cooperation and Development (1993) Skin sensitisation test guideline 406

Organisation for Economic Cooperation and Development (2002) Skin sensitisation test guideline 429

Robinson MK, Nusair TL, Fletcher ER, Ritz HL (1990) A review of the Buehler guinea pig skin sensitisation test and its use in a risk assessment process for human skin sensitization. Toxicology 61:91–107

United Nations (1993) Recommendations in the transport of dangerous goods, 8th edn. United Nations ST/SG.AC.10/REv 8:185

Weil CS, Scala A (1971) Study of intra- and inter-laboratory variability in the results of rabbit eye and skin irritation tests. Toxicol Appl Pharmacol 19:276–360

Whittle E, Barratt MD, Carter JA, Basketter DA, Chamberlain M (1996) Use of QSAR and an in vitro skin corrosivity test to investigate the corrosion/irritation potential of organic acids. Toxicol In Vitro 10:95–100

CHAPTER 20

Irritant and Allergic Contact Dermatitis Treatment 20

H. Zhai, A. Anigbogu, H. I. Maibach

Introduction

To reduce irritant contact dermatitis (ICD) and allergic contact dermatitis (ACD) in industry, application of moisturizers as well as barrier creams (BC) before or during work, wearing appropriate gloves and clothing may be indicated. Topical corticoids and other therapy approaches are critically reviewed.

Avoidance

Moisturizers

Moisturizers are frequently used to improve "dry" skin, and daily use may modify the skin surface's physical and chemical nature, so as to smooth, soften and make more pliable (Zhai 1998).

Moisturizers often contain humectants of low molecular weight and lipids. They are absorbed into the stratum corneum and there, by attracting water, increase hydration (Loden 1997). Lipids, for instance petrolatum, beeswax, lanolin and various oils in moisturizers, are incorporated into formulations on the basis of their technical and sensory properties rather than on their possible epidermal impact (Loden 1995, 1997). They may also penetrate the living epidermis, be metabolized and significantly modify endogenous epidermal lipids (Wertz 1990). A single application of a moisturizer did not cause long-lasting effects expressed as skin capacitance and conductance (Blichmann 1989; Loden 1991), whereas repeated applications of a moisturizer twice daily for 1 week produced a significant increase in the skin conductance for at least 1 week post treatment (Serup 1989).

Urea, a physiological non-allergic substance (Serup 1992a; Swanbeck 1992), can decrease reversibly the turnover of epidermal cells (Hannuksela 1996), and also may enhance the penetration of other substances into skin (Feldmann 1974; Serup 1992a; Wohlrab 1990). Other effects include binding water in the horny layer, antipruritic, and reducing irritant dermatitis (Loden 1993; Serup 1992a,b; Swanbeck 1992).

Hannuksela and Kinnunen (1992) developed a washing test method to determine the effect of moisturizers in preventing irritant dermatitis. Moisturizers decreased transepidermal water loss (TEWL), blood flow and visible dermatitis. Additionally, moisturizers significantly enhanced healing.

Halkier-Sørensen and Thestrup-Pedersen (1993) utilized a crossover study to evaluate the efficacy of a moisturizer among cleaners and kitchen assistants. Moisturizer prevented the development of skin dryness and decreased electrical capacitance (epidermal hydration).

Loden (1996) showed that repeated applications of urea-containing moisturizers influence both TEWL and the apparent susceptibility to SLS-induced irritation. Three applications of 5% urea increased TEWL, whereas treatment with 10% urea for 10 and 20 days decreased TEWL.

Gammal et al. (1996) assessed the efficacy of moisturizers with a soap-induced xerosis human model. The moisturizer-treated legs had significantly decreased dryness at all time points and conductance was also significantly increased on days 8 and 11.

Olivarius et al. (1996) evaluated the effect of moisturizing creams against water in an vivo human model, based on the color intensities when an aqueous solution of crystal violet is applied to the dorsal and volar skin of the hands of 12 subjects. The test moisturizer showed some protective effect (dorsal 57%, volar 34%) against water.

Held et al. (1999) determined the affect of long-term use of a moisturizer on normal skin. Electrical capacitance was significantly increased on the moisturizer-treated arm. After the challenge with SLS, TEWL was significantly higher on the moisturizer-treated arm. They suggested that long-term application with moisturizer on normal skin might increase skin susceptibility to irritants.

Extensive data on the physiology, pharmacology, and toxicology of moisturizers is found in Loden (1999).

Barrier Creams (BC)

BC are designed to prevent or reduce the penetration and absorption of hazardous materials, preventing skin lesions and/or other toxic effects from dermal exposure (Frosch 1993 a,b; Lachapelle 1996; Orchard 1984; Zhai 1996 a,b). Their efficacy has been investigated by in vitro and in vivo studies (Forsch 1993 a; Lachapelle 1996; Wigger-Alberti 1998; Zhai 1996 b). However, their actual benefit remains sub judice in clinical trials (Frosch 1993 a–d; Goh 1991 a,b; Goh 1994; Treffel 1994, 1996; Wigger-Alberti 1998). Inappropriate BC application may exacerbate rather than ameliorate (Forsch 1993 a–d; Goh 1991 a,b; Zhai 1996a). In practice, BC are usually recommended only for low-grade irritants (water, detergents, organic solvents, cutting oils) (Frosch 1993 d; Wigger-Alberti 1998; Zhai 1996 a). BC are also used to protect the face and neck against chemical and resinous dust and vapors (Birmingham 1969).

Minimal information on the mechanisms of BC' action exists. The frequently quoted theory is that water in oil (W/O) emulsions are effective against aqueous solutions of irritants and oil in water (O/W) emulsions are effective against lipophilic materials (Davidson 1994; Frosch 1993a; Lachapelle 1996; Mathias 1990). Some studies have demonstrated exceptions to this rule (Frosch 1993c, 1994). BC may contain active ingredients presumed to work by trapping or transforming allergens or irritants (Frosch 1994; Lachapelle 1996). Most believe they interfere with absorption and penetration of the allergen or irritants by physical blocking – forming a thin film that protects the skin (Frosch 1994; Lachapelle 1996; Marks 1995; Orchard 1984).

To avoid frequent interruptions for reapplication, BC are expected to remain effective for 3 to 4 hours. Most manufacturers claim that their products last ~4 hours. Others suggest application "as often as necessary" (Davidson 1994). Several studies document duration of action with varying results (Boman 1982; Reiner 1982; Zhai 1996 a, 1999).

Application methods may influence their effectiveness (Packham 1994). Wigger-Alberti et al. (1997) determined areas of the hands likely to be missed on self-application of BC in the workplace by a fluorescence technique. The BC application was incomplete, especially on the dorsal hands. Most manufacturers suggest rubbing thoroughly into skin; to pay special attention to cuticles and skin under nails; to let it dry for ca. 5 min; to apply a thin layer of BC to all appropriate skin surfaces 3–4 times daily.

Table 1 summarizes BC efficacy from recent experiments.

Protective Gloves and Clothing

Gloves may provide certain protective effects against corrosive agents (acids, alkalis, etc.) (Boman 1982; McClain 1992; Mellström 1994, 1996; Wigger-Alberti 1997). Protective clothing as well as other personal devices also play a critical role (Davidson 1994; Mathias 1990). It should be noted that protective clothing may trap moisture and potentially damaging substances next to the skin for prolonged periods and increase the likelihood that dermatitis will develop (Davidson 1994; Mathias 1990). The first line of defense against hand dermatitis is to wear gloves, but in many professions it is impossible to wear gloves because of the loss of dexterity. In some instances, an alternative would be to utilize BC. Note that many gloves do not resist the penetration of low molecular weight chemicals. Some allergens are soluble in rubber gloves, and may penetrate the glove and produce severe dermatitis (Estlander 1994, 1996; Mathias 1990; Mellström 1994; Wigger-Alberti 1998). Recently, allergy to rubber latex has become a growing problem (Estlander 1994, 1996; Mellström 1994; Wigger-Alberti 1998), and workers can develop contact urticaria syndrome including generalized urticaria, conjunctivitis, rhinitis, and asthma, etc. (Amin 1997; Wigger-Alberti 1998). Estlander et al. (1994) introduced the role and details of protective gloves in preventing ICD and ACD in their chapter. Mellström et al.'s (1994) documents detail this area.

Table 1. Summary of barrier cream (BC) efficacy

Models		Irritants or allergens	Barrier creams	Efficacy	Authors and reference
In vitro	In vivo (animals or humans)				
	Guinea pigs	n-Hexane, trichlorethylene, and toluene	3 water-miscible creams	Limited protective effects	Lachapelle et al. (1990)
	Guinea pigs	Cutting oil	2 barrier creams	Exacerbating the irritation	Goh (1991 a, b)
	Humans who had a history of allergic to test allergens	epoxy resin, glyceryl monothioglycolate, frullania, and tansy	One barrier cream	Minimizing the development of allergic contact dermatitis	McClain and Storrs (1992)
	Humans who had a positive patch test to Toxicodendron extract	Toxicodendron extract	Various barrier preparations	Most of them provided good protective effects	Grevelink et al. (1992)
	Guinea pigs and humans	SLS, sodium hydroxide, toluene, and lactic acid	Several barrier creams	Some of them suppressed irritation, some failed, and some even aggressive irritation	Frosch et al. (1993 b, d, 1994,)
Human skin		Dyes (eosin, methylviolet, oil red O)	16 barrier creams	Various % protection effects	Treffel et al. (1994)
	Machinists	Castrol oil	One barrier cream and one afterwork emollient	They did not appear any significant effect against cutting fluid dermatitis	Goh and Gan (1994)
	Humans who had a history of allergic to poison ivy/oak	Urushiol	Quaternium-18 bentonite (Q18B) lotion	Q-18B lotion significantly reduced reactions to the urushiol	Marks et al. (1995)
	Nickel-sensitive patients	Nickel disc	Ethylenediamine-tetra-acetate (EDTA) gels	Significantly reduced the amount of nickel in the in vitro, and significantly reduced positive reactions in vivo	Fullerton and Menné (1995)

Table 1 (continued)

Models	Irritants or allergens	Barrier creams	Efficacy	Authors and reference
Humans	Dyes (methylene blue and oil red O)	3 barrier creams	Two of them exhibited effectiveness, one enhanced cumulative amount of dye	Zhai and Maibach (1996a)
Humans	Water	2 barrier creams and a moisturizer	Various % protection effects	Olivarius et al. (1996)
Humans	10% SLS, 1% NaOH, 30% lactic acid, and undiluted toluene	4 barrier creams and white petrolatum	Very different protective effects were detectable. All products were very effective against SLS irritation	Schlüter-Wigger and Elsner (1996)
Humans	Toluene	Several barrier creams	All tested barrier creams markedly reduced the irritating effect of repetitive toluene contact	Grunewald et al. (1996)
Humans	Toluene and NaOH	Several barrier creams	None of them were able to prevent the skin erythema induced by toluene. One barrier cream as well as petrolatum and a fatty cream protected the skin significantly when against NaOH	Treffel and Gabard (1996)
Guinea pigs	Sulphur mustard	Povidone iodine (PI) ointment	PI ointment showed the powerful protective effect	Wormser et al. (1997)
Humans	Self-application of BC	An oil in water emulsion	Self-application of BC was incomplete	Wigger-Alberti et al. (1997)
	$[^{35}S]$-SLS	3 quaternium-18 bentonite (Q18B) gels	% protection effect was 88%, 81% and 65%, respectively	Zhai et al. (1999)
Humans	SLS, ammonium hydroxide (NH_4OH) and urea, Rhus	Several protectants	Most of them suppressed the SLS irritation and Rhus allergic reaction, failed to NH_4OH and urea irritation	Zhai et al. (1998)

Treatment

Corticoids

Hydrocortisone, which became available in the 1950s, was shown to be efficacious in eczematous dermatoses (Sulzberger 1957). The next major advance in topical corticoid therapy came with the introduction of triamcinolone acetonide followed shortly after by fluocinolone acetonide. The early 1970s saw the introduction of the 21-acetate derivative of fluocinolone acetonide with more biological activity than the others. Since the late 1970s many potent topically active glucocorticoids have been introduced including desoximethasone, clobetasol propionate and beta-methasone-17-dipropionate.

Mechanism of Action

Corticoids being lipophilic in nature permeate the skin by passive diffusion.

Following the penetration of the cell membrane, corticoids bind with specific cytoplasmic receptors. These receptors have been demonstrated in all target tissues including the skin (Ballard 1974; Epstein 1982).

Since inflammation is the endpoint of the immune response, the anti-inflammatory and immunosuppressive effects of corticoids may overlap (Blackwell 1980; Haynes 1985; Hirata 1980; Parrillo 1979; Thompson 1970; Vernon-Roberts 1969).

The mechanisms by which topical corticoids cause vasoconstriction remain unclear (Altura 1966; Ginsburg 1958; Juhlin 1969; Solomon 1965).

The effects of topical application of corticoids on human mast cells have been examined (Lavker 1985). Two potent corticoids, clobetasol-17-propionate and fluocinonide, produced greater than 85% decrease in histamine content over 6 weeks treatment. The first signs of cells containing sparse amounts of mast-cell granules were apparent 14 days post-steroid treatment. By 3 months, histamine levels returned to normal. This work suggested a possible treatment for one human mast cell disease, urticaria pigmentosa, and a possible additional mechanism of action of corticoids. Maibach and Surber (1992) and Korting and Maibach (1993) provide additional details.

Percutaneous Penetration

Following topical application, corticoids penetrate the stratum corneum and are absorbed into the epidermis. The efficacy and toxicity are related to corticoid penetration. Corticoids may act on the epidermis, the dermis or both.

Topical corticoids applied to diseased skin will be absorbed into the systemic circulation. When administration is chronic or when large areas of skin are involved, the absorption may be sufficient to cause systemic effects including cushingoid changes and adrenocortical suppression.

Topical corticoids are minimally absorbed from healthy skin. On the forearm, approximately 1% of the applied dose of hydrocortisone penetrates (Feldmann

1966; Malkinson 1955). Other corticoids for which data exist are not necessarily absorbed to a greater degree than hydrocortisone (Feldmann 1968) suggesting they may owe their increased efficacy to their potency rather than enhanced penetration.

Clinical Formulations and Potency of Corticoids

Corticoids form a vast range of compounds and formulations with varying effects. Table 2 groups topical corticoids according to relative potency, largely based on the vasoconstrictor assay (Stoughton 1972). The formulations in each group are only roughly equipotent. The greater the potency, is the greater the therapeutic efficacy and likelihood, therefore, of more adverse effects.

Superpotent formulations include clobetasol propionate, optimized betamethasone dipropionate, and difluorosone and must be used with caution; they have the potential for significant topical and systemic side effects far in excess of other currently utilized formulations.

Vehicles

The potency of topical corticoids can be further increased by enhancing percutaneous absorption. One way of optimizing absorption is by altering the formulation vehicle (Stoughton 1972). Ointment bases tend to give greater activity to the corticoid than do cream or lotion vehicles (Stoughton 1972).

Adverse Effects

All absorbable corticoids possess the ability to produce adrenal suppression (Carr 1968; Scoggins 1965). The degree of suppression is related to potency. Fortunately, plasma cortisol usually returns to normal within 3 days when the superpotents are discontinued – at least in short-time application studies (Levin and Maibach, in preparation).

Certain factors increase the penetration and therefore the tendency to suppression; application to large surface areas, occlusion, inflamed skin and higher concentrations. Of concern in children is growth retardation associated with excessive and prolonged use of topical corticoids (Bode 1980; Munro 1976; Vermeer 1974; Weston 1980).

Dosage and Administration

Most physicians prescribe topical corticoids with little or no thought as to the number of milligrams of material per surface area of skin. There is a dosage-response relationship, with increasing efficacy closely following increased dosage. It

Table 2. A partial list of topical corticoids available in the United States ranked according to their potencies

Drug	Potency
Lowest Potency	
Hydrocortisone	0.25–2.5%
Methylprednisolone acetate	0.25%
Dexamethasone[a]	0.04%
Dexamethasone[a]	0.1%
Methylprednisolone acetate	1.0%
Prednisolone	0.5%
Betamethasone[a]	0.2%
Low Potency	
Fluocinolone acetonide[a]	0.01%
Betamethasone valerate[a]	0.01%
Fluometholone[a]	0.025%
Aclometasone dipropionate	0.05%
Triamcinolone acetonide[a]	0.025%
Clocortolone pivalate[a]	0.1%
Flumethasone pivalate[a]	0.03%
Intermediate Potency	
Hydrocortisone valerate	0.2%
Mometasone furoate	0.1%
Hydrocortisone butyrate	0.1%
Betamethasone benzoate[a]	0.025%
Flurandrenolide[a]	0.025%
Betamethasone valerate[a]	0.1%
Desonide	0.05%
Halcinonide[a]	0.025%
Desoximetasone[a]	0.05%
Flurandrenolide[a]	0.05%
Triamcinolone acetonide[a]	0.1%
Fluocinolone acetonide[a]	0.025%
High Potency	
Betamethasone dipropionate[a]	0.05%
Amcinonide[a]	0.1%
Desoximetasone[a]	0.25%
Triamcinolone acetonide[a]	0.5%
Fluocinolone acetonide[a]	0.2%
Diflorasone diacetate[a]	0.05%
Halcinonide[a]	0.1%
Fluocinonide[a]	0.05%
Highest Potency	
Betamethasone dipropionate[a] in optimized vehicle	0.05%
Diflorasone diacetate[a] in optimized vehicle	0.05%
Clobetasol propionate[a]	0.05%

[a] Fluorinated steroids.

is therefore important to make an estimate of the quantity a patient would require in any given condition. Fortunately, most manufacturers provide a standard or regular concentration yielding the desired therapeutic result for most patients. For instance, triamcinolone acetonide is available in 0.025%, 0.1% and 0.5% formulations. Many patients with corticoid-responsive dermatoses need only the 0.025% formulations.

The standard trade concentrations suffice for most patients. In the more resistant diseases, higher concentrations should be considered. For instance, approximately 1% of a 0.25% hydrocortisone solution is absorbed from the forearm. Increasing the amount applied per unit area of skin tenfold, increases the amount absorbed 4 times (Feldmann 1967).

Regional differences in response are partially based mainly on the differences in penetration of skin in various areas. Thus, areas with increased permeability, such as the scrotum, eyelids, ears, scalp, and face respond far better to topical corticoids than such areas as the dorsa of the hands, extensor surfaces of knees and elbows, and the palms and soles (McKensie 1962).

Occlusion

Ninety-six-hour occlusion with an impermeable film, such as plastic wrap, constitutes a most effective method of enhancing penetration, yielding approximately a tenfold increase (Feldmann 1965). Specifically, with occlusion, penetration of hydrocortisone on the forearm increases from 1% of applied dose to 10%. There are, however, obvious problems associated with occlusion therapy – the plastics are sometimes uncomfortable, warm, and troublesome to use. Side effects encountered with occlusion include miliaria, bacterial and candidal infection.

Occlusion has the added advantage of keeping the drug on the skin by preventing rubbing off onto clothing. We do not have data delineating the effect of duration of occlusion on percutaneous penetration with topical corticoids.

Frequency of Application

Previously, patients applied topical corticoids 3–4 times daily. Studies on the percutaneous absorption of hydrocortisone failed to reveal a significant increase in absorption applied on a repetitive basis compared to a single dose (Lagos 1998). Clinical trials of various corticoids suggest that less-frequent applications are equally effective (Fredrickson 1980). In view of the relatively slow process of corticoid absorption, a phenomenon referred to as the "reservoir effect" (Vickers 1963), there may not be any advantage in frequent applications.

Acute tolerance (tachyphylaxis) to vasoconstriction and antimitotic effects of and suppression of epidermal DNA synthesis by topical corticoids have been demonstrated (Du Vivier 1976, 1982). This suggests that the resistance clinically observed after prolonged use might be prevented by less intensive therapy, such as daily application with short resting periods between treatment courses (Barry

1977; Miller 1980). Another study examining corticoid tachyphylaxis used fluocinolone acetonide under occlusion to the forearm and induced wheal and flare to histamine with the prick technique (Singh 1986). By the eighth day, the wheal was nonexistent, adding now a third tachyphylaxis phenomena.

Anatomic Variation

Large regional variations in percutaneous absorption of compounds are determined by factors including hair follicle density, thickness of the stratum corneum and vasculature of the region (Cronin 1962). This suggests that for areas of higher penetrability such as the face, scalp, scrotum, axilla and the groin, smaller doses are required and occlusion is not needed (Feldmann 1967).

Little quantitative information is available on how much penetration is increased in diseased skin (Aalto-Korte 1995). In initial studies, it was noted that skin with only minimally involved atopic dermatitis allowed for a several-fold increase in penetration; psoriatic plaques had no significant increase, whereas exfoliative psoriatic skin had little barrier to penetration.

Controlled Topical Efficacy Studies: Irritant and Allergic Contact Dermatitis

Irritant Dermatitis

Although most physicians employ topical corticoids in irritant dermatitis, several controlled studies in experimental irritant dermatitis's reaction to sodium lauryl sulphate show either no effect, or a negative (Van der Valk 1996) or minimal effect (Ramsing 1995).

Allergic Contact Dermatitis

Several studies document some degree of efficacy when high potency corticoids are applied after the acute phase (Funk 1994). Considering the massive amounts prescribed, the data is limited – presumably because this has long been the standard of care.

Immunosuppressives

Cyclosporin, tacrolimus, and azathioprine are used in unusual instances. See Menné and Maibach (1999) for details.

UV-Light

Most patients with ICD and ACD may be controlled by topical therapy and protective measures. But, some cases cannot be controlled either topically or by acceptable doses of systemic corticosteroids. In this situations, UV treatment should be considered. Christensen (1994) and Menné and Maibach (1999) provide the details for UV treatment regime.

Grenz-Ray

Grenz-ray may act as an adjunct topical therapy in some chronic cases. In addition, it is extremely suitable if one considers the sparing effect of grenz-radiation on hair roots, sebaceous and sweat glands, etc. Details are provided by Lindelöf (1994) and Menné and Maibach (1999).

References

Aalto-Korte K, Turpeinen M (1995) Pharmacokinetics of topical hydrocortisone at plasma level after applications once or twice daily in patients with widespread dermatitis. Br J Dermatol 133:259–263

Altura BM (1966) Role of glucocorticoids in local regulation of blood flow. Am J Physiol 211:1393–1397

Amin S, Maibach HI (1997) Immunologic contact urticaria definition. In: Amin S, Lahti A, Maibach HI (eds) Contact urticaria syndrome. CRC Press, Boca Raton, pp 11–26

Ballard PL, Baxter JD, Higgins SJ, Rousseau GC, Tomkins GM (1974) General presence of glucocorticoid receptors in mammalian tissues. Endocrin 94:998–1002

Barry BW, Woodford R (1977) Vasoconstrictor activities and bioavailabilities of seven proprietary corticosteroid creams assessed using a non-occluded multiple dosage regimen: Clinical considerations. Br J Dermatol 97:555–560

Birmingham D (1969) Prevention of occupational skin disease. Cutis 5:153–156

Blackwell GJ, Carnuccio R, DiRosa M, Flower RJ, Parente L, Persico P (1980) Macrocortin: a polypeptide causing the anti-phospholipase effect of glucocorticoids. Nature 287:147–149

Blichmann CW, Serup J, Winther A (1989) Effects of single application of a moisturizer: evaporation of emulsion water, skin surface temperature, electrical conductance, electrical capacitance, and skin surface (emulsion) lipids. Acta Derm Venereol 69:327–330

Bode HH (1980) Dwarfism following long-term topical corticosteroid therapy. J Am Med Assoc 244:813–814

Boman A, Wahlberg JE, Johansson G (1982) A method for the study of the effect of barrier creams and protective gloves on the percutaneous absorption of solvents. Dermatologica 164:157–160

Carr RD, Tarnowski WM (1968) Percutaneous absorption of corticosteroids: adrenocortical suppression with total body inunction. Acta Derm Venereol 48:417–428

Christensen OB (1994) UV-light treatment of hand eczema. In: Menné T, Maibach HI (eds) Hand eczema. CRC Press, Boca Raton, pp 293–301

Cronin E, Stoughton RB (1962) Percutaneous absorption: regional variations and the effect of hydration and epidermal stripping. Br J Dermatol 74:265–272

Davidson CL (1994) Occupational contact dermatitis of the upper extremity. Occup Med 9:59–74

Du Vivier A, Phillips H, Hehir M (1982) Applications of glucocorticosteroids: The effects of twice-daily vs once-every-other-day applications on mouse epidermal cell DNA synthesis. Arch Dermatol 118:305–308

Du Vivier A, Stoughton RB (1976) Acute tolerance to effects of topical glucocorticoids. Br J Dermatol 94, suppl 12:25–32

Epstein EH, Bonifas JM (1982) Glucocorticoid receptors of the human epidermis. J Invest Dermatol 78:144–146

Estlander T, Jolanki R, Kanerva L (1994) Protective gloves. In: Menné T, Maibach HI (eds) Hand eczema. CRC Press, Boca Raton, pp 311–321

Estlander T, Jolanki R, Kanerva L (1996) Rubber glove dermatitis: A significant occupational hazard-prevention. In: Elsner P, Lachapelle JM, Wahlberg JE, Maibach HI (eds) Prevention of contact dermatitis (Curr Probl Dermatol). Karger, Basel, pp 170–176

Feldmann RJ, Maibach HI (1965) Penetration of ^{14}C-hydrocortisone through normal human skin: The effect of stripping and occlusion. Arch Dermatol 91:661–666

Feldmann RJ, Maibach HI (1966) Percutaneous penetration of hydrocortisone in man. 2. Effect of certain bases and pretreatments. Arch Dermatol 94:649–651

Feldmann RJ, Maibach HI (1967) Regional variation in percutaneous penetration of ^{14}C cortisol in man. J Invest Dermatol 48:181–183

Feldmann RJ, Maibach HI (1968) Percutaneous penetration of steroids in man. J Invest Dermatol 52:89–94

Feldmann RJ, Maibach HI (1974) Percutaneous penetration of hydrocortisone with urea. Arch Dermatol 109:58–59

Fredrickson T, Lassus A, Bleeker J (1980) Treatment of psoriasis and atopic dermatitis with halcinonide cream applied once, two-three times daily. Br J Dermatol 102:575–577

Frosch PJ, Kurte A (1994) Efficacy of skin barrier creams. (IV) The repetitive irritation test (RIT) with a set of 4 standard irritants. Contact Dermatitis 31:161–168

Frosch PJ, Kurte A, Pilz B (1993) Biophysical techniques for the evaluation of skin protective creams. In: Frosch PJ, Kligman AM (eds) Noninvasive methods for the quantification of skin functions. Springer, Berlin, pp 214–222

Frosch PJ, Kurte A, Pilz B (1993) Efficacy of skin barrier creams. (III). The repetitive irritation test (RIT) in humans. Contact Dermatitis 29:113–118

Frosch PJ, Schulze-Dirks A, Hoffmann M, Axthelm I (1993) Efficacy of skin barrier creams. 2. Ineffectiveness of a popular "skin protector" against various irritants in the repetitive irritation test in the guinea pig. Contact Dermatitis 29:74–77

Frosch PJ, Schulze-Dirks A, Hoffmann M, Axthelm I, Kurte A (1993) Efficacy of skin barrier creams. 1. The repetitive irritation test (RIT) in the guinea pig. Contact Dermatitis 28:94–100

Fullerton A, Menné T (1995) In vitro and in vivo evaluation of the effect of barrier gels in nickel contact allergy. Contact Dermatitis 32:100–106

Funk JO, Maibach HI (1994) Horizons in pharmacologic intervention in allergic contact dermatitis. J Am Acad Dermatol 31:999–1014

Gammal CE, Pagnoni A, Kligman AM, Gammal SE (1996) A model to assess the efficacy of moisturizers – the quantification of soap-induced xerosis by image analysis of adhesive-coated discs (D-Squames®). Clin Exp Dermatol 21:338–343

Ginsburg J, Duff RS (1958) Influence of intra-arterial hydrocortisone on adrenergic responses in the hand. Br Med J 2:424–428

Goh CL (1991) Cutting oil dermatitis on guinea pig skin. 1. Cutting oil dermatitis and barrier cream. Contact Dermatitis 24:16–21

Goh CL (1991) Cutting oil dermatitis on guinea pig skin. 2. Emollient creams and cutting oil dermatitis. Contact Dermatitis 24:81–85

Goh CL, Gan SL (1994) Efficacies of a barrier cream and an afterwork emollient cream against cutting fluid dermatitis in metalworkers: a prospective study. Contact Dermatitis 31:176–180

Grevelink SA, Murrell DF, Olsen EA (1992) Effectiveness of various barrier preparations in preventing and/or ameliorating experimentally produced Toxicodendron dermatitis. J Am Acad Dermatol 27:182–188

Grunewald AM, Lorenz J, Gloor M, Gehring W, Kleesz P (1996) Lipophilic irritants: protective value of urea- and of glycerol-containing oil in water emulsions. Dermatosen 44:81–86

Halkier-Sørensen L, Thestrup-Pedersen K (1993) The efficacy of a moisturizer (Locobase) among cleaners and kitchen assistants during everyday exposure to water and detergents. Contact Dermatitis 29:266–271

Hannuksela A (1996) Moisturizers in the prevention of contact dermatitis. In: Elsner P, Lachapelle JM, Wahlberg JE, Maibach HI (eds) Prevention of contact dermatitis (Curr Probl Dermatol). Karger, Basel, pp 214–220

Hannuksela A, Kinnunen T (1992) Moisturizers prevent irritant dermatitis. Acta Derm Venereol 72:42–44

Haynes RC, Muraud F (1985) Adrenocorticotropic hormone; adrenocortical steroids and their synthetic analogs; inhibitors of adrenocortical steroid biosynthesis. In: Gilman AG, Goodman LS, Rall TW, Murad F (eds) The pharmacological basics of therapeutics. Macmillan, New York, pp 1459–1489

Held E, Sveinsdóttir S, Agner T (1999) Effect of long-term use of moisturizer on skin hydration, barrier function and susceptibility to irritants. Acta Derm Venereol 79:49–51

Hirata F, Schiffmann E, Venkatasubramanian K, Salomon D, Axelrod J (1980) A phospholipase A2 inhibitory protein in rabbit neutrophils induced by glucocorticoids. Proc Natl Acad Sci USA 77:2533–2536

Juhlin L, Michaelsson G (1969) Cutaneous vascular reactions to prostaglandins in healthy subjects and in patients with urticaria and atopic dermatitis. Acta Derm Venereol 49:251–261

Korting HC, Maibach HI (1993) Topical glucocorticoids with increased benefit/risk ratio. Karger, Basel

Lachapelle JM (1996) Efficacy of protective creams and/or gels. In: Elsner P, Lachapelle JM, Wahlberg JE, Maibach HI (eds) Prevention of contact dermatitis (Curr Probl Dermatol). Karger, Basel, pp 182–192

Lachapelle JM, Nouaigui H, Marot L (1990) Experimental study of the effects of a new protective cream against skin irritation provoked by the organic solvents n-hexane, trichlorethylene and toluene. Dermatosen 38:19–23

Lagos BR, Maibach HI (1998) Frequency of application of topical corticosteroids: an overview. Br J Dermatol 139:763–766

Lavker R, Scheckter N (1985) Cutaneous mast cell depletion results from topical corticosteroid usage. J Immunol 135:2368–2373

Lindelöf B (1994) X-ray treatment of hand eczema. In: Menné T, Maibach HI (eds) Hand eczema. CRC Press, Boca Raton, pp 303–309

Loden M (1995) Biophysical properties of dry atopic and normal skin with special reference to effects of skin care products. Acta Derm Venereol (Suppl) 192:1–48

Loden M (1996) Urea-containing moisturizers influence barrier properties of normal skin. Arch Dermatol Res 288:103–107

Loden M (1997) Barrier recovery and influence of irritant stimuli in skin treated with a moisturizing cream. Contact Dermatitis 36:256–260

Maibach HI, Surber C (1992) Topical corticosteroids. Karger, Basel

Malkinson FD, Ferguson EH (1955) Percutaneous absorption of hydrocortisone-1-C14 in two human subjects. J Invest Dermatol 25:281–283

Marks JG Jr, Fowler JF Jr, Sherertz EF, Rietschel RL (1995) Prevention of poison ivy and poison oak allergic contact dermatitis by quaternium-18 bentonite. J Am Acad Dermatol 33:212–216

Mathias CGT (1990) Prevention of occupational contact dermatitis. J Am Acad Dermatol 23:742–748

McClain DC, Storrs F (1992) Protective effect of both a barrier cream and a polyethylene laminate glove against epoxy resin, glyceryl monothioglycolate, frullania, and tansy. Am J Contact Dermatitis 13:201–205

Mckenzie AW, Stoughton RB (1962) Method for comparing percutaneous absorption of steroids. Arch Dermatol 86:603–610

Mellström GA, Johansson S, Nyhammar E (1996) Barrier effect of gloves against cytostatic drugs. In: Elsner P, Lachapelle JM, Wahlberg JE, Maibach HI (eds) Prevention of contact dermatitis (Curr Probl Dermatol). Karger, Basel, pp 163–169

Mellström GA, Wahlberg JM, Maibach HI (1994) Protective Gloves for Occupational Use. CRC Press, Boca Raton

Menné T, Maibach HI (1999) Hand eczema, 2nd edn. CRC Press, Boca Raton

Miller JA, Munro DD (1980) Topical corticosteroids: clinical pharmacology and therapeutic use. Drugs 19:119–134

Munro DD (1976) The effect of percutaneously absorbed steroids on hypothalamic-pituitary-adrenal function after intensive use in patients. Br J Dermatol 94, suppl 12:67–76

Olivarius FDF, Hansen AB, Karlsmark T, Wulf HC (1996) Water protective effect of barrier creams and moisturizing creams: a new in vivo test method. Contact Dermatitis 35:219–225

Orchard S (1984) Barrier creams. Dermatologic Clinics 2:619–629

Packham CL (1994) Evaluation of barrier creams: an in vitro technique on human skin (letter). Acta Derm Venereol 74:405

Parrillo JE, Fauci AS (1979) Mechanisms of glucocorticoid action on immune processes. Ann Rev Pharmacol Toxicol 19:179–201

Ramsing DW, Agner T (1995) Efficacy of topical corticosteroids on irritant skin reactions. Contact Dermatitis 32:293–297

Reiner R, Roßmann K, Hooidonk CV, Ceulen BI, Bock J (1982) Ointments for the protection against organophosphate poisoning. Arzneim-Forsch/Drug Res 32:630–633

Schlüter-Wigger W, Elsner P (1996) Efficacy of 4 commercially available protective creams in the repetitive irritation test (RIT). Contact Dermatitis 34:278–283

Scoggins RB, Kliman B (1965) Relative potency of percutaneously absorbed corticosteroids in the suppression of pituitary-adrenal function. J Invest Dermatol 45:347–355

Serup J (1992) A double-blind comparison of two creams containing urea as the active ingredient. Assessment of efficacy and side-effects by non-invasive techniques and a clinical scoring scheme. Acta Derm Venereol (Suppl) 177:34–43

Serup J (1992) A three-hour test for rapid comparison of effects of moisturizers and active constituents (urea). Measurement of hydration, scaling and skin surface lipidization by noninvasive techniques. Acta Derm Venereol (Suppl) 177:29–33

Serup J, Winther A, Blichmann CW (1989) Effects of repeated application of a moisturizer. Acta Derm Venereol 69:457–459

Singh G, Singh P (1986) Tachyphylaxis to topical steroid measured by histamine-induced wheal response. Int J Dermatol 25:324–326

Solomon LM, Wentzel HE, Greenberg MS (1965) Studies in the mechanism of steroid vasoconstriction. J Invest Dermatol 44:129–131

Stoughton RB (1972) Bioassay systems for topically applied glucocorticoids. Arch Dermatol 106:825–827

Sulzberger MB, Witten VH (1957) The effect of topically applied compound F in selected dermatoses. J Invest Dermatol 19:101–102

Swanbeck G (1992) Urea in the treatment of dry skin. Acta Derm Venereol (Suppl) 177:7–8

Thompson J, van Furth R (1970) The effect of glucocorticoidsteroids on the kinetics of mononuclear phagocytes. J Exp Med 131:429–442

Treffel P, Gabard B (1996) Bioengineering measurements of barrier creams efficacy against toluene and NaOH in an in vivo single irritation test. Skin Res Technol 2:83–87

Treffel P, Gabard B, Juch R (1994) Evaluation of barrier creams: An in vitro technique on human skin. Acta Derm Venereol 74:7–11

Van der Valk PGM, Maibach HI (1996) The irritant contact dermatitis syndrome. CRC Press, Boca Raton

Vermeer BJ, Heremans GFP (1974) A case of growth retardation and Cushing's syndrome due to excessive application of betamethasone-17-valerate ointment. Dermatologica 149:299–304

Vernon-Roberts B (1969) The effects of steroid hormones on macrophage activity. Int Rev Cytol 25:131–159

Vickers CFH (1963) Existence of reservoir in the stratum corneum. Arch Dermatol 88:20–23

Wertz PW, Downing DT (1990) Metabolism of topically applied fatty acid methyl esters in BALB/C mouse epidermis. J Dermatol Sci 1:33–37

Weston WL, Sams WM, Morris HG (1980) Morning plasma cortisol levels in infants treated with topical fluorinated glucocorticosteroids. Paediatrics 65:103–106

Wigger-Alberti W, Elsner P (1998) Do barrier creams and gloves prevent or provoke contact dermatitis? Am J Contact Dermatitis 9:100–106

Wigger-Alberti W, Maraffio B, Wernli M, Elsner P (1997) Self-application of a protective cream. Pitfalls of occupational skin protection. Arch Dermatol 133:861–864

Wohlrab W (1990) Effect of urea on penetration kinetics of vitamin A acid in human skin. Z Hautkr 65:803–805

Wormser U, Brodsky B, Green BS, Arad-Yellin R, Nyska A (1997) Protective effect of povidone-iodine ointment against skin lesions induced by sulphur and nitrogen mustards and by non-mustard vesicants. Arch Toxicol 71:165–170

Zhai H, Buddrus DJ, Schulz AA, Wester RC, Hartway T, Serranzana S, Maibach HI (1999) In vitro percutaneous absorption of sodium lauryl sulfate (SLS) in human skin decreased by quaternium-18 bentonite gels. In Vitro Molecular Toxicol 12:11–15

Zhai H, Maibach HI (1996) Effect of barrier creams: human skin in vivo. Contact Dermatitis 35:92–96

Zhai H, Maibach HI (1996) Percutaneous penetration (Dermatopharmacokinetics) in evaluating barrier creams. In: Elsner P, Lachapelle JM, Wahlberg JE, Maibach HI (eds) Prevention of contact dermatitis (Curr Probl Dermatol). Karger, Basel, pp 193–205

Zhai H, Maibach HI (1998) Moisturizers in preventing irritant contact dermatitis: an overview. Contact Dermatitis 38:241–244

Zhai H, Willard P, Maibach HI (1998) Evaluating skin-protective materials against contact irritants and allergens: An in vivo screening human model. Contact Dermatitis 38:155–158

CHAPTER 21

Prevention and Rehabilitation

21

J. E. WAHLBERG

Introduction

A distinction is usually made between primary prevention, i.e. inhibition of the induction and onset of a disease, and secondary prevention, i.e. inhibition of relapses. Tertiary prevention aims at inhibition of worsening ("quality of life"). The value of disease prevention is evident to individuals, the community and the medical profession. For human, social, and economic reasons, it would be of great benefit if people exposed to harmful chemicals and products, physical factors, and biological agents could be protected from developing occupational skin diseases.

When facing the current or imminent skin problems of a single patient, all of the prophylactic means listed in Table 1 should be considered. However, the responsibility for primary prevention rests mainly with manufacturers and producers of chemicals and products, governmental agencies, consumer organizations, industrial physicians and nurses, and safety engineers. Speaking of secondary and tertiary prevention, a greater responsibility is placed on physicians treating the cases (dermatologists, industrial physicians and others) and on nurses and safety engineers. In this chapter, more general aspects of prevention of occupational dermatoses will be reviewed (Table 1). The majority of these are caused by exposure to chemicals and products and will be especially addressed here, while prevention concerning physical factors, atopy, barrier creams and emollients, and protective gloves are reviewed in Chaps. 3, 15, 20, and 22/23, respectively. For biological causes, see Sadhra and Foulds (2000).

All the items listed in Table 1 should be considered, and the best results are usually achieved when several of the prophylactic means are combined judi-

Table 1. Prevention of occupational dermatoses: an outline

Subject	Source
Chemicals and products	Table 2
Physical causes	Chap. 3
Biological causes	Sadhra and Foulds 2000
Individuals	Table 3
Avoidance of contact	Table 4
Skin care program	Table 5
Miscellaneous	Table 6

Table 2. Prevention of occupational dermatoses caused by chemicals and products

Identification of allergens and irritants
Occurrence and concentration of allergens in the environment (Chap. 18)
Allergen removal or replacement
Modification or inactivation of the allergen
Predictive testing: skin irritating potential
Predictive testing: sensitising potential

ciously. To rely on just one of these recommendations – sometimes to reduce costs – is definitely less effective. However, it is up to the persons involved in preventive dermatology to demonstrate that the suggested methods and measures are efficacious and cost effective.

Prevention of Occupational Dermatoses Caused by Chemicals and Products

On some items involved in prevention of occupational dermatoses caused by chemicals and products (Table 2) additional comments are presented.

Identification of Allergens and Irritants

Allergens
In order to give a patient meaningful advice as to what chemicals and products to avoid for prevention of recurrence, the allergen responsible should be identified. Otherwise the advice will be too general and sometimes erroneous, and will make the patient's mode of life unnecessarily difficult.

In the examination of patients with contact eczema from environmental agents, tests are made with standard series and with formulated products and their ingredients (Chaps. 16, 17) to identify the allergen. The examinations should be supplemented by chemical analysis to demonstrate the degree of purity of the test compound and ensure that impurities are not the cause of an allergic reaction.

It can be concluded that, when patch-test reactions to a formulated product occur, it is also extremely important to test with each ingredient, if possible, to see where the allergenic potential exists. It is the manufacturer's responsibility to elucidate through chemical analysis whether it is the ingredient or some impurity that possesses the allergenic potential.

Irritants
There is no analogous procedure for irritants. Irritant contact dermatitis is a diagnosis of exclusion and is based on a negative patch test involving all the substances with which the patient comes into contact.

Allergen Removal or Replacement

When a new allergen has been identified (Chap. 16), the manufacturer and the governmental agencies have to decide whether the chemical should be banned or whether it can be used when specified precautions are taken. If the new chemical or drug has great advantages over those used previously, this must be balanced against the allergy risk (risk assessment). If a chemical or drug is available that lacks allergenic potential but has equal technical or therapeutic effects, this alternative should, of course, be chosen ("substitution"). Under special circumstances, potent allergens are used but precautions, such as closed processes, automation, gloves, helmets, impermeable overalls etc., are taken to avoid any skin contact.

For example, preservatives and biocides are well-known sensitisers, and the frequency of contact allergy is rather high in workers exposed to cutting fluids and to paints (Chap. 33).

Modification or Inactivation of the Allergen

Chromium by Iron Sulfate

It was demonstrated that iron sulfate added to cement reduced the chromate completely and trivalent chromium was precipitated (Fregert et al. 1979). An amount of 0.35% iron sulfate is enough to reduce 20 µg Cr + 6/g cement. In Denmark, the incidence of chromium allergy among cement workers, after addition of iron sulfate to the cement, has decreased. For details, see Chap. 31.

Inactivation of Chromium and Nickel by Ingredients in Barrier Creams

Protective creams containing various "inactivating" agents have been introduced, mainly to prevent relapses in sensitised individuals (secondary prevention). Dimethylglyoxime, diethylthiocarbamate and ethylene diamine tetraacetate (EDTA), among other substances, have been used as chelating agents for chromium absorbic acid and anionic exchangers and for nickel. For details, see Wigger-Alberti and Elsner (2000).

Inhibition of Sensitisation Reactions (Quenching)

Quenching is a process used in the perfume industry to suppress contact sensitisation from cinnamic aldehyde, citral, and phenylacetaldehyde by the addition of another agent, usually an alcohol or terpene (Opdyke 1976). More recent studies, however, have not been able to confirm the initial promising findings (Basketter and Allenby 1991).

Predictive Testing: Skin Irritating Potential

Skin irritation testing is performed to help identify chemicals, products and material that may be potential human skin irritants before their introduction into the environment. The tests may give varying results due to variation in a number of test-related factors, such as host, test dose, patch size, degree of occlusion, length of exposure, vehicle, time for reading and quality of reading. Therefore, in skin irritation tests, it is important to include a well-known positive and negative control material in order to compare the test results with those of the control materials, thereby making the results relative.

Predictive Testing: Sensitising (Allergenic) Potential

The tests are used to identify potential allergenic chemicals (hazard identification). They can be carried out in experimental animals (guinea pigs, mice) and in human volunteers. Approximately 15 guinea-pig methods have been described; the most widely used are the guinea-pig maximisation test (GPMT) and the Buehler topical closed-patch technique (Andersen and Maibach 1985). In mice, two methods have been introduced (the local node assay – LLNA, and the mouse ear swelling test – MEST). An intra- and inter-laboratorial evaluation of the LLNA has demonstrated reproducible dose-response relationships within and between the laboratories (Kimber et al. 1995; Loveless et al. 1996). The LLNA has furthermore been able to identify proven important contact allergens previously identified with the human maximisation test (Basketter et al. 1994).

For humans the most widely known methods are the human maximisation test (HMT) and the modified Draize repeated-insult patch test (Kligman 1966; Marzulli and Maibach 1973).

GPMT and HMT were developed in parallel and the results were in close conformity, which has been adduced as support for extrapolating guinea pig findings to man.

The risk of a contact allergen being missed in a correctly performed GPMT (hazard identification) must be considered minimal. The reverse is far more common, i.e. that a substance is allergenic to guinea pigs, but no clinical case of allergic contact eczema has been reported. Whether contact allergy will occur in an individual, however, does not depend solely on the substance's inherent allergenic potential, but also on exposure conditions: whether the chemical is present in high concentrations, penetrates into the skin, comes into contact with irritated or damaged skin, or whether the exposure is intermittent, continuous, or the size of the exposed area, etc.

Individuals Identified at Pre-Employment Examination or Periodic Health Screening

Examination Before Exposure ("Pre-Employment")

To identify in advance individuals who have a constitutional susceptibility to development of contact eczema is no easy task. Why some individuals are afflicted with contact eczema while others are unaffected by exactly the same exposure is still unclear; explanations advanced have been hereditary, constitutional factors and the development of tolerance (Table 3).

Table 3. Individuals identified at pre-employment examination and periodic health screening

Those with increased susceptibility or predisposition, i.e. atopics
Patients with a history of contact dermatitis
Patients with a history of other types of eczema, psoriasis, acne and others
Specific and non-specific hardening

Those with Increased Susceptibility or Predisposition, i.e. Atopics

The general view is that individuals with current, or a history of, atopic dermatitis have an inferior quality of skin with impaired barrier function. Therefore, they are more readily afflicted with irritant contact dermatitis (Chap. 15) and wet work, exposure to oils and solvents, etc. should be minimised. Regular check-ups of these individuals are recommended. The relative significance of endogenous and exogenous factors shows variation from individual to individual.

Patients with a History of Contact Dermatitis

Allergic Contact Dermatitis

It is generally believed that individuals with demonstrated contact allergy to allergens commonly occurring in the environment, such as nickel, chromium, and paraphenylene diamine, retain their sensitivity through their lives and must therefore entirely avoid the eliciting allergens to prevent relapse. The risk of recurrence is related to exposure conditions, such as dose, intermittent or continuous exposure, and barrier function at exposed skin sites.

Irritant Contact Dermatitis

For patients diagnosed with irritant (non-allergic) contact dermatitis, the prognosis is assumed to be better, but an impaired barrier function of the skin appears to exist long after it looks normal to the naked eye. This necessitates regulations governing exposure, use of protective gloves, skin care programs, etc. (Table 4). Normal barrier function is considered to be restored after several months, but the period is difficult to state on a scientifically acceptable basis. Modern, non-invasive bioengineering techniques seem to give assistance in this respect.

Table 4. Avoidance of direct contact with products and materials

Protective gloves (Chap. 22)
Aprons, sleeves, boots, glasses, masks
Barrier (protective) creams (Wigger-Alberti and Elsner 2000)
Dishwasher, washing machine, long-handled brushes
Automation, closed systems
Efficient ventilation

Patients with a History of Other Types of Eczema, Psoriasis, Acne and Others

Detailed patch testing of patients with other types of eczema (seborrhoic, discoid, stasis etc.) has demonstrated that they frequently have contact allergies to topical medicaments, preservatives or perfumes, but the relevance is usually uncertain. Whether the frequency is higher than that in the "normal" population has not been settled. It is possible that a contact dermatitis is superimposed on the original eczema, and change of topical remedies can result in clearance.

Hand psoriasis can be provoked by repeated trauma, which should be taken in consideration. Patients with severe acne should avoid contact with straight oils (Chap. 10). In cases of more severe chronic skin diseases, such as scleroderma, Raynaud's phenomenon, systemic lupus erythematosus, and light sensitivity, the patient's ordinary dermatologist should be consulted before employment.

Specific Hardening

Specific hardening is defined as a condition in which allergic contact dermatitis in sensitised persons has disappeared or failed to reappear on repeated exposure to the sensitising chemical. To prove the value of hardening today, repeated serial dilution tests would be needed to define thresholds of sensitivity to the allergen, and in vitro determination of the sensitivity would be needed (Wahlberg 1992).

Non-Specific Hardening

Non-specific hardening refers to instances in which a patient acquires a dermatitis from an irritant and, subsequently, can handle it without developing an eruption. This can take place due to continued use of mild or moderate irritants with gradual thickening and pigmentation of the skin. The hardened skin may withstand irritants, while adjacent unhardened skin remains susceptible.

Avoidance of Direct Contact with Products and Materials

Protective gloves are reviewed in Chap. 22 and barrier (protective) creams by Wigger-Alberti and Elsner (2000). Table 4 can be used as a checklist.

Skin Care Program

Soaps, detergents and other cleansing agents are known irritants. The effects of the other preventive measures suggested in Table 5 are evident and need no further comments. The table can be used as a checklist.

Table 5. Skin care program

Soaps, detergents and cleansing agents, without allergens and with low irritant potential
Hot water, shower, sauna
Soft towels
Emollient and moisturizing creams (Wigger-Alberti and Elsner 2000)

Table 6. Miscellaneous

Legislation, regulation
Labelling of products and chemicals, material safety data sheets (Chap. 19)
Information to patients, consumers, workers, supervisors, i.e. through videos, pamphlets
Training of industrial physicians and nurses, safety engineers
Training of workers in special industrial processes
Good housekeeping
Research on prevention; dissemination of results obtained

Miscellaneous

The effects of the preventive measures suggested in Table 6 are evident and need
no further comments.

Rehabilitation

Legislation concerning rehabilitation varies from country to country; only more
general principles can be reviewed. Rehabilitation is defined in Dorland's Illustrated Medical Dictionary as "the restoration of an ill or injured patient to self-
sufficiency or to gainful employment at his highest attainable skill in the shortest
possible time" (Anonymous 1988). This includes medical as well as social goals.

In the case of occupational dermatoses, there is an imperative for the cause of
the skin disease to be investigated in detail, including both workplace and leisure
time exposures, in order to obtain a correct diagnosis. The eliciting factors –
physical, biological, chemicals, products, materials etc. (Table 1) – should be considered according to the principles for prevention reviewed in this chapter. As
pointed out, the best results are achieved when the prophylactic means are combined.

A serious attempt should be made to bring the patient back to his usual place
of work. If it fails and the patient has a relapse, the exposure conditions must be
re-analysed. Has the offending allergen been removed entirely or was it met in
other products or materials? Has the patient followed the instructions on avoidance of contact (Table 4) and followed the skin care program (Table 5)? The next
attempt should be carried out after a more extended period of sick leave to guarantee that the barrier function of the skin has been restored. When contact allergens are present as dusts or vapours that cannot be controlled by ventilation or
otherwise removed, it is usually impossible to continue in the same job.

After several relapses and periods of sick leave, one has to look for alternatives. The extent of the problem varies with the worker's degree of disability, motivation, age, intelligence, and how long the individual has worked in the particular job. Proper rehabilitation involves not only medical but also social activities,
e.g. by employer, welfare officer, insurance companies involved with compensation, social institutions, labour inspectors and trade unions. Their contributions
depend largely on the legislation in a particular country. Many social and personal factors are often more decisive for change of work than is the skin disease.

Physicians can give advice based on examinations, tests, etc. and knowledge of exposure conditions, but they cannot ultimately decide on a patient's future.

References

Andersen KE, Maibach HI (1985) Contact allergy. Predictive tests in guinea pigs. Current Problems in Dermatology, vol 14. Karger, Basel

Anonymous (1988) Dorland's illustrated medical dictionary. Saunders, Philadelphia

Basketter DA, Allenby CF (1991) Studies on the quenching phenomenon in delayed contact hypersensitivity reactions. Contact Dermatitis 25:160–171

Basketter DA, Scholes EW, Kimber I (1994) The performance of the local lymph node assay with chemicals identified as contact allergens in the human maximization test. Food Chem Toxicol 32:543–547

Fregert S, Gruvberger B, Sandahl E (1979) Reduction of chromate in cement by iron sulfate. Contact Dermatitis 5:39–42

Kimber I, Hilton J, Dearman RJ et al. (1995) An international evaluation of the murine local lymph node assay and comparison of modified procedures. Toxicology 103:63–73

Loveless SE, Ladics GS, Gerberick GF et al. (1996) Further evaluation of the local lymph node assay in the final phase of an international collaborative trial. Toxicology 108:141–152

Marzulli FN, Maibach HI (1973) Antimicrobials: experimental contact sensitization in man. J Soc Cosmet Chem 24:399–421

Opdyke DLJ (1976) Inhibition of sensitisation reactions induced by certain aldehydes. Food Cosmetic Toxicol 14:197–198

Sadhra S, Foulds IS (2000) Measurement of dermal exposure. In: Kanerva L, Elsner P, Wahlberg JE, Maibach HI (eds) Handbook of occupational dermatology. Springer, Berlin Heidelberg New York, pp 81–89

Wahlberg JE (1992) Hardening. Contact Dermatitis 26:359

Wigger-Alberti W, Elsner P (2000) Barrier creams and emollients. In: Kanerva L, Elsner P, Wahlberg JE, Maibach HI (eds) Handbook of occupational dermatology. Springer, Berlin Heidelberg New York, pp 490–496

CHAPTER 22

Protective Gloves

G. A. Mellström, A. Boman

Introduction

There are both an increased occupational use of protective gloves and increased interest in their protective capacity against harmful chemicals as well as blood-borne infections, e.g. hepatitis and human immunodeficiency virus (HIV). This interest parallels new directives and regulations that have come into force in Europe concerning the use and safety requirements for protective gloves.

In order to select, purchase or use protective gloves, it is necessary to obtain information concerning current standards, quality requirements, the nature of hazards, performance data, acceptable level of exposure to hazards, and the nature of dermatologic adverse effects caused by protective gloves of rubber and plastics.

The information on the performance of protective gloves and other protective clothing is found in an increasing number of reports in the literature and from glove manufacturers. Generally, the choice of protective material can be obtained by reviewing the literature, information from manufacturers before deciding on the best suitable material.

Field of Application: Rules and Regulations

Gloves intended for protection of the user are referred to in Europe as personal protective equipment and covered by the Personal Protective Equipment Directive 89/686/EEC. However, gloves intended for use in the medical field to protect patients and user from cross-contamination are referred to as medical devices and are covered by Council Directive 93/42/EEC concerning medical devices (Mellström and Carlsson, 1994). A survey of the United States rules, regulations and standards concerning protective and medical gloves and their use has been presented by N. Henry III (1994).

Protective Gloves

The European Economic Community (EEC) Directive gives general requirements for all personal protective equipment; requirements of types of gloves have been

described (Mellström and Carlsson, 1994). Protective gloves are classified in three categories due to intended use and attestation procedures:
- Category I: Gloves of simple design – for minimal risk application
- Category II: Gloves of intermediate design (not simple nor complex design) – for intermediate risk
- Category III: Gloves of complex design – for irreversible/mortal risks

The requirements for European Community (EC)-type certification are: declaration of conformity, technical documentation file for all categories of gloves. For categories II and III, there are additional requirements: EC-type examination testing by approved laboratories, certified by approved notified bodies and manufacturing under a formal EC quality assurance system.

European Standard EN 420, for protective gloves, defines general requirements for most kinds of protective gloves. Key points are fitness of purpose, innocuousness, sound construction, storage, sizing, measure of glove hand dexterity, product information and labelling. Mellström and Boman (2000) give examples of EN and American Society for Testing and Materials (ASTM) Standards for protective gloves against chemicals.

Medical Gloves

Medical gloves for single use are gloves intended for use in the medical field to protect patients and users from cross-contamination. They are classified in categories: surgical gloves, examination and/or procedure gloves (sterile or non-sterile) and foil film gloves.

Glove Materials and Manufacturing

Today the materials used for manufacturing of protective gloves are natural rubber, synthetic rubber, textile fibres, leather and several polymeric materials (Table 1). A detailed description of the materials used for glove manufacturing as well as the different manufacturing methods and glove types was presented by Mellström and Boman (1994). The protective effect of different glove materials against hazardous chemicals is dependent on the following factors:
- *Thickness.* The breakthrough time increases as the thickness of the glove material increases but in a non-linear fashion (Schwope et al. 1988, Jencen and Hardy 1989).
- *Material composition.* The same generic material but from different manufacturers has different chemical resistance capacity due to variation in polymer formulation. The barrier effect of different generic materials is quite variable. Each combination of chemical and protective glove material has to be considered (Sansone and Tewari 1980; Mickelsen and Hall 1987). The quality and protective effect of gloves of the same material can differ due to manufacturing processes, additives and quality control (Mellström and Boman 1994; Perkins and Pool 1997).

Table 1. Survey of glove materials used for protective (*PG*) and medical (single-use) gloves (*MG*)

Material name/trade names	Intended use
Natural rubber (Latex)	PG and MG
Synthetic rubber materials	
Butyl rubber	PG
Chloroprene/Neoprene	PG and MG
Fluor rubber/Viton	PG
Nitrile rubber/Nitrilite, N-Dex	PG
Styrene-butadiene/Elastyren	MG
Styrene-ethylene-butadiene/Tactylon	MG
Plastic polymeric materials	
EMA (ethylene-methylacrylate)	PG and MG
Polyethylene, polythene (PE)	PG and MG
Polyvinyl chloride (PVC)	PG and MG
PE/EVAL/PE, laminate/4H-glove	PG
Leather	PG
Textile	PG
Cotton, nylon, jersey	PG, inner gloves
Fibre materials/Kevlar, Lycra and Spectra fibre	Used in jersey surgical inner gloves, cut resistant

Testing of the Protective Glove Barrier

To ensure that protective gloves and medical gloves for single use give an adequate level of protection the different properties have to be tested and evaluated.

Standard Test Methods

Physical Properties

In the EN and ASTM standard specifications, requirements and test methods are given. These include sampling and selection of test pieces, physical dimensions with length, strength and thickness, load for break before and after accelerating ageing. The barrier effect is also affected by storage conditions and this is particularly important for medical gloves made of natural rubber latex.

Penetration (Leakage)

This is described as the flow through closures, porous materials, seams and pinholes or other imperfections in a protective or medical glove material at a non-molecular level. Leakage can lead to uncontrolled exposure to hazardous chemicals or infectious materials, especially in the health care field. Penetration test methods for protective gloves and leakage testing for medical gloves have been described by Mellström et al. (1994). Leakage tests, as a rule, include a random sampling procedure in which a certain number of gloves are filled with a specified volume of water or air. These are pass/fail tests, and the number of gloves allowed to fail/number of gloves tested is dependent on the batch or lot size. A

sampling procedure for inspection by attributes is defined by the International Organisation for Standardisation (ISO 2859). There are several standardised leakage test methods designed for medical gloves, which have been evaluated, and all test methods show inherent limitations (Carey et al. 1989; Douglas et al. 1992). Standard quality control testing and virus penetration have been presented in an overview (Lytle et al. 1994). The standard tests for glove integrity and virus penetration testing are used and intact gloves as well as penetration through punctures in gloves are discussed. The tests used for evaluation of the barrier integrity fall into two categories:
- Those intended to assure quality during and after manufacturing
- Those that challenge the barrier with viral or chemical agents

They concluded that viral challenges to gloves indicated that latex gloves provided significant barrier protection against very small viruses. They also concluded that apparent barrier integrity cannot assure safety, although current quality control protocols do assure that medical gloves provide significant protection.

Permeation

Permeation is usually described as the process by which a chemical migrates through the protective clothing material at a molecular level, by processes including sorption, diffusion and desorption. The principle of permeation standard testing is a flow-through system in which a two-compartment permeation cell of standard dimensions is used. The test specimen acts as a barrier between the first compartment of the cell, which contains the test chemical, and the second compartment. Through this a stream of the collecting medium (gas or liquid) is passed for collection of diffused molecules of the test chemical or its component chemicals for analysis. The key parameters measured are usually:
- *Breakthrough time (BT, min).* In both the ASTM and EN standard test methods the breakthrough time is defined as the time when a specified permeation rate is reached.
- *Permeation rate (PR).* The mass of test chemical permeating the material per unit time per unit area ($\mu g/min \times cm^2$).
- *Steady-state permeation (SP).* A state that is reached when the permeation rate becomes virtually constant.

In the European Standard for protective gloves against chemicals and micro-organisms, one of the requirements is that the protective effect for a certain combination of protective glove/test chemical should be presented as protection index.

Protection index is based on breakthrough time measure at constant contact with the test chemical. (European Standard EN 374-1, 1994) (Table 2).

Biocompatibility

Over the last years there have been increasing problems with severe adverse reactions in health care workers caused by latex products, e.g. latex proteins in gloves. Also adverse reactions due to rubber chemicals, powder, lubricants, endotoxins and pyrogens are well known and more frequent than reactions to proteins. In the European standard the requirements and test methods for biological evalua-

Table 2. Index based on breakthrough times determined during constant contact with the test chemical described in European Standard EN 374-3

Protection Index	Measured breakthrough time
Class 1	>10 min
Class 2	>30 min
Class 3	>60 min
Class 4	>120 min
Class 5	>240 min
Class 6	>480 min

tion for medical glove use have been prepared and "EN 455: Medical gloves for single use. Part 3: Requirements and testing for biological evaluation" is now in force. The result of the test and applied test method shall be made available by the manufacturer of gloves, on request from the customer.

In Vivo Testing

Additional information on protective efficacy of gloves can be derived from in vivo testing in man or in experimental animals. For screening, an animal model can be used for comparative investigation of the protective effect of gloves (Boman and Mellström 1989, 1994). In work-related studies the effect of exposure to potentially hazardous chemicals used in the workplace is studied. The protective effect as well as adverse effects of gloves can be studied by patch testing of contact allergic individuals with the specific allergen together with pieces of glove (Lidén 1994; Andersson and Bruze 1999).

Protective Effect

Protection Against Micro-Organisms

A number of glove barrier studies concerning protection against micro-organisms, that used different test methods during the period 1976–1993, have been reviewed by Hamann and Nelson (1993). Their conclusions from the review were that the barrier effect of the gloves is dependent on a complex interaction of several factors:
- Type and brand of glove (latex or plastic materials)
- Condition of use (unused, stimulated use or in actual clinical situations)
- Sensitivity of the assay (water-, air-, dye-leak tests, bacterial or viral penetration)
  They also concluded that some trends could be seen from the data such as:
- The material is an important determinant of the glove barrier
- The brand of glove influences the outcome of barrier testing
- The quality of a glove is more closely related to the manufacturer than to the glove material

- Leakage rates are related to the level of use that a glove receives
- The efficacy of the glove barrier varies with the sensitivity of the testing procedure.

Protection Against Some Chemical Agents Hazardous to the Skin

Disinfectants

Disinfectants are generally used to clean surfaces and objects and to sterilise instruments. At skin disinfection and in working situations where there is a risk of acquiring blood-borne infections the use of different kinds of disinfectants is frequent. In these circumstances it is important to use gloves, both to protect the skin against infections and to prevent contact with disinfectants harmful to the skin. Some of these agents are known to cause allergic and/or irritant reactions after contact with the skin, such as ethanol, isopropyl alcohol, chlorocresol and glutaraldehyde. The effect of four disinfectants on six different brands of medical gloves has been described by Mellström et al. (1992) through measuring the permeation and Scanning Electronic Microscopy (SEM) studies of the exposed glove material surfaces. They found that gloves of latex, polyvinyl chloride (PVC) and polyethylene gave acceptable protection from contact with products containing *p*-chloro-m-cresol (Blifacid) and glutaraldehyde (Cidex) for at least 60 min, but were not giving acceptable protection from contact with isopropanol and ethanol.

Pharmaceuticals

Pharmaceutical preparations of drugs, e.g. cytostatic agents, have very heterogeneous mechanisms of action, they have potent pharmacological properties and it is well known that they can cause acute skin injuries in cases of accidental exposure (Knowles and Virden 1980). The extent of the health hazard due to chronic exposure to small amounts of cytostatic drugs for personnel handling these drugs is still not completely known and therefore it is necessary to minimise the exposure. In order to minimise the exposure when preparing, dispensing and administrating these drugs, standard procedures and appropriate techniques together with personal protective equipment, e.g. gloves, should be used. However, there are no requirements or criteria for evaluating medical glove suitability for this use (Mellström et al. 1996). Several cytostatic drugs penetrated latex gloves (Sessink et al. 1994).

Composite Materials (Bone Cement, Dental Filling Materials)

The increased use of acrylic compounds as a substitute for amalgam by dentists, dental nurses and dental technicians has caused an increasing frequency of hand eczema in these groups. This is a serious and increasing problem since there are no gloves available today that have the dexterity required and at the same time gives sufficient protection to the skin. Standard procedures, appropriate technique, packaging design together with adjusted personal protective gloves are urgently needed. In a study of the permeability of protective gloves to (di)methacrylates in resinous dental material, latex gloves were not impervious but more resistant than other glove material (Munksgaard 1991). The combined use of latex gloves with the 4H-gloves as an inner glove can be useful in some working situations. The protective efficacy of seven different non-latex gloves against a dental bonding product containing 2-HEMA was tested on eight patients with a test-verified contact allergy to 2-HEMA. Gloves made of neoprene gave the best protection and gloves of polyethylene were comparable to positive control (no glove) (Andersson et al. 1999, 2000).

Solvents

Alcohol and other aliphatic and aromatic organic solvents have a degreasing and irritating effect on the skin and can be absorbed through the skin into the blood circulation. At risk of splashes or where there is very short contact time (10–30 min), gloves made of natural rubber, PE or PVC can be useful. At occasional but intentional exposure (30–60 min) gloves made of nitrile rubber, natural or neoprene rubber can be useful and at exposure on purpose during extended periods (>60 min) gloves such as butyl rubber, Viton or a 4H-glove should be used.

Corrosive Agents

Corrosive substances, oxidising/reducing agents, acids, bases, and concentrated salt solutions can cause severe irritation to the skin, after contact with small amounts but with short repeated exposure or extended exposure. Glove materials suitable for working with these kinds of hazardous chemicals or where there is a risk for exposure to them for very short contact times (10–30 min) are natural rubber, PE and PVA. With occasional but intentional exposure (30–60 min) gloves made of neoprene, natural or nitrile rubber, can be useful. For intentional exposure during extended periods (>60 min) gloves of butyl rubber, Viton or the 4H-glove can be useful.

Detergents, Surfactants, Cleansers

Washing up-liquids, cleaning agents and soaps are usually water based and, when used in recommended concentrations, there are only mild effects on the skin; however, used in too high concentration they can cause skin injuries. Sometimes organic solvents like white spirit or isopropanol are added. Gloves made of EMA, PE or PVC can be useful, where there is a risk of splashing or very short contact time (10–30 min). With occasional but intentional exposure (30–60 min), gloves made of natural rubber, neoprene or PVC can be useful and with intentional exposure during extended periods (>60 min), gloves made of natural rubber, neoprene or PVC should be used. If an organic solvent is an ingredient then gloves made of nitrile rubber should be used as an alternative.

Oils, Cutting Fluids, Lubricant Oils

These agents often contain anti corrosive agents, bactericides and antioxidants. Used oils can contain small amounts of chromium, nickel and cobalt. With a risk from splashes or a very short contact time (10–30 min), gloves made of natural rubber or PVC gloves can be useful; with occasional but intentional exposure (30–60 min), industrial gloves made of nitrile rubber, natural rubber or neoprene can be useful and with intentional exposure during extended periods (>60 min) gloves such as nitrile rubber or the 4H-glove should be used.

Warning! When working at machinery with rotating parts, gloves can imply a risk for tear injury.

Limitations of Use Due to Side Effects

The risk of side effects from gloves are described in detail in Chap. 23.

Glove Selection

Selection Procedure for Gloves Against Chemicals

Several factors need to be taken into account when selecting a glove for a particular application. Leinster (1994) has described the selection and use of gloves against chemicals in a model based on working activity and chemical classification. The selection procedure adapted to the new EN standards for protective gloves is condensed as detailed below.

Chemical Classification: Risk of Skin Injury
A Mainly contact with chemicals less harmful and not classified as hazardous substances or requiring labelling. Minimal risk for only slight injuries.
B Mainly contact with chemicals classified as toxic, harmful or irritant. Intermediate risk for moderate, reversible injuries.
C Mainly contact with chemicals classified as highly toxic, highly corrosive, corrosive and agents causing cancer, sensitisation or those absorbed through the skin. High risk of severe or irreversible injuries.

Working Activity – Degree of Exposure
1. Risk of exposure, possible splashing.
2. Occasional, repeated and expected exposure.
3. Continuous exposure during certain times, expected or by accident.

Glove Selection – Requirements
A1:   Gloves are not essential.
A2, B1, C1:   No testing of the protective effect required (Category I).
A3, B2, B3, C2: BT and/or (PR) are required. (Category II).
C3:   Breakthrough time (BT) and/or permeation rate (PR) are required; also test results based on the glove task (Category III).

Selection Procedure for Gloves Against Micro-Organisms

A scheme for the selection and use of gloves by health care personnel in different situations based on purpose, working procedure, type of glove (medical gloves or protective gloves) and risk of exposure to infection or micro-organisms has been suggested by Burman and Fryklund (1994):
1. Protection of personnel from hepatitis (A, B, C), HIV, human T-lymphotropic virus (HTLV)
   - Surgical glove: surgery
   - Examination gloves, non sterile: dentistry, risk of contact with blood
   - Protective gloves (e.g. domestic gloves): risk of contact with blood
2. Protection of personnel and patients from various viruses and bacteria
   - Protective gloves: handling of faeces, urine, vomit etc.
3. Protection of patients from hepatitis, HIV, other viruses and bacteria
   - Surgical glove: surgery
   - Examination gloves, sterile: other invasive procedures
   - Examination gloves, non sterile: dentistry, isolation, barrier nursing
   - Protective gloves: isolation, barrier nursing, handling of faeces, urine, vomit etc.

Gloves of Synthetic Materials

Gloves of polymer materials are necessary for use in the treatment of patients and by those employees with a known allergy to latex proteins. Such gloves reduce the risk of contact dermatitis caused by rubber additives and contact urticaria caused by latex proteins. Gloves of polymer materials are also necessary for use by those employees with a known allergy to chromate in leather gloves.

Double Gloving

- Natural rubber latex gloves + inner gloves of plastic material, nylon or cotton material reduce the risk of contact dermatitis and urticaria caused by latex rubber gloves.
- Natural rubber latex gloves + synthetic fibre gloves, reduce the risk of cut and puncture injuries.
- Natural rubber latex gloves + latex or plastic gloves, reduce the risk of blood-borne infections and/or chemical permeation.

Non-Powder Gloves

Powder-free gloves should be used to reduce the risk of symptoms such as rhinitis, conjunctivitis and asthma caused by glove powder contaminated by latex proteins.

Conclusions

Factors of importance that have to be considered in the selection procedure are:
- Mechanical quality of the glove material (tensile strength, dexterity, cut, tear and puncture resistance)
- Resistance to penetration and permeation of hazardous chemicals and micro-organisms
- Risk of adverse effects when using a specific glove (allergic contact dermatitis, contact urticaria, irritation, itching etc.)
- Functionality: the gloves must not incur another risk or be a hindrance
- Comfort: the right size, pleasant to wear
- Quality uniformity and a moderate price

All of these factors show that the selection procedure can be very complicated indeed.

References

Andersson T, Bruze M (1999) In vivo testing of the protective efficacy of gloves against allergen-containing products using an open chamber system. Contact Dermatitis 41:260–263

Andersson T, Bruze M, Björkner B (1999) In vivo testing of the protection of gloves against acrylates in dentin-bonding systems on patients with known contact allergy to acrylates. Contact Dermatitis 41:254–259

Andersson T, Bruze M, Gruvberger B, Björkner B (2000) In vivo testing of the protection provided by non-latex gloves against a 2-hydroxyethyl methacrylate-containing acetone-based dentin-bonding product to acrylates. Acta Derm Venereol 80:435–437

Boman AS, Mellström GA (1989) Percutaneous absorption of three organic solvents in the guinea pig. IV. Effect of protective gloves. Contact Dermatitis 21:260–266

Boman AS, Mellström GA (1994) Percutaneous absorption studies in animals. In: Mellström GA, Wahlberg JE, Maibach HI (eds) Protective gloves for occupational use. CRC Press, Boca Raton, pp 91–107

Burman LG, Fryklund B (1994) The selection and use of gloves by health care professionals, In: Mellström GA, Wahlberg JE, Maibach HI (eds) Protective gloves for occupational use. CRC Press, Boca Raton, pp 283–292

Carey R, Herman W, Herman B, Casamento J (1989) A laboratory evaluation of standard leakage tests for surgical and examination gloves. J Clin Eng 14:133–143

Douglas AA, Neufeld PD, Wong RKW (1992) An interlaboratory comparison of standard test methods for medical gloves. In: McBriarty JP, Henry N (eds) Performance of protective clothing, 4th edn (ASTM STP 1133). American Society for Testing and Materials, Philadelphia, pp 99–113

Douglas A, Simon TR, Goddard M (1997) Barrier durability of latex and vinyl medical gloves in clinical settings. Am Ind Hyg Assoc J 58:672–676

Hamann CP, Nelson JR (1993) Permeability of latex and thermoplastic elastomer gloves to the bacteriophage Phi X 174. Am J Infect Control 21:289–296

Henry NW III (1994) Protective gloves for occupational use: US rules, regulations and standards. In: Mellström GA, Wahlberg JE, Maibach HI (eds) Protective gloves for occupational use. CRC Press, Boca Raton, pp 45–49

Jencen DA, Hardy JK (1989) Effect of glove material thickness on permeation characteristics. Am Ind Hyg Assoc J 50:623–626

Knowles RS, Virden JE (1980) Occasional review: handling of injectable antineoplastic agents. Br Med J 30:589–591

Leinster P (1994) The selection and use of gloves against chemicals. In: Mellström GA, Wahlberg JE, Maibach HI (eds) Protective gloves for occupational use. CRC Press, Boca Raton, pp 269–281

Lidén C, Wrangsjö K (1994) Protective effect of gloves illustrated by patch test testing-practical aspects. In: Mellström GA, Wahlberg JE, Maibach HI (eds) Protective gloves for occupational use. CRC Press, Boca Raton, pp 207–212

Lytle CD, Cyr WH, Carey RF, Shombert DG, Herman BA, Dillon JG, Schroeder LW, Bushar HF, Kotilainen HJR (1994) Standard quality testing and virus penetration. In: Mellström GA, Wahlberg JE, Maibach HI (eds) Protective gloves for occupational use. CRC Press, Boca Raton, pp 109–127

Mellström GA, Lindberg M, Boman A (1992) Permeation and destructive effects of disinfectants on protective gloves. Contact Dermatitis 26:163–170

Mellström GA, Boman AS (1994) Gloves: types, materials, and manufacturing. In: Mellström GA, Wahlberg JE, Maibach HI (eds) Protective gloves for occupational use. CRC Press, Boca Raton, pp 21–35

Mellström GA, Carlsson B (1994) European standards on protective gloves. In: Mellström GA, Wahlberg JE, Maibach HI (eds) Protective gloves for occupational use. CRC Press, Boca Raton, pp 39–43

Mellström GA, Carlsson B, Boman AS (1994) Testing of protective effect against liquid chemicals. In: Mellström GA, Wahlberg JE, Maibach HI (eds) Protective gloves for occupational use. CRC Press, Boca Raton, pp 53–77

Mellström GA, Wrangsjö K, Wahlberg JE, Fryklund B (1996) The value and limitation on gloves in medical health service: part II. Dermatology Nursing, 8:287–295

Mellström G, Boman A (2000). Protective gloves. In: Kanerva K, Elsner P, Wahlberg JE, Maibach HI (eds) Handbook of occupational dermatology. Springer, Berlin Heidelberg New York, pp 417–425

Mickelsen RL, Hall RC (1987) A breakthrough time comparison of nitrile and neoprene glove materials produced by different glove manufacturers. Am Ind Hyg Assoc J 48:941–947

Munksgaard EC (1992) Permeability of protective gloves to (di)methacrylates in resinous dental materials. Scand J Dent Res 100:189–192

Perkins JL, Pool B (1997) Batch lot variability in permeation through nitrile gloves. Am Ind Hyg Assoc J 58:474–479

Sansone EB, Tewari YB (1980) Differences in the extent of solvent penetration through natural rubber and nitrile gloves from various manufacturers. Am Ind Hyg Assoc J 41:527–528

Schwope AD, Costas PP, Jackson JO, Weitzman JO (1985) Guidelines for the selection of protective clothing. American Conference of Governmental Industrial Hygienists (2nd), Cincinnati

Schwope AD, Costas PP, Mond CR, Nolen RL, Conoley M, Garcia DB, Walters DB, Prokopetz AT (1988) Gloves for protection from aqueous formaldehyde: permeation resistance and human factors analysis. Appl Ind Hyg 3:167–176

Sessink PJM, van de Kerkhof MCA, Anzion RB, Bos RP (1994) Environmental contamination and assessment of exposure to antineoplastic agents by determination of cyclophosphamide in urine of exposed pharmacy technicians: is skin absorption an important exposure route? Arch Environ Health 4:165–169

CHAPTER 23

Disadvantages of Gloves 23

T. ESTLANDER, J. JOLANKI, L. KANERVA

Introduction

Protective gloves are important safeguards against factors hazardous to hands. They can be manufactured from polymers such as rubber and plastic, leather, fabric or combinations of these materials. Rubber and plastic gloves are mainly used to protect hands from chemical and biological agents, as well as products from workers' dirty hands.

Hand protection must not increase the risk of dermatitis, the risk of universal adverse effects to health, or the risk of hand accidents. Even when gloves are chosen to give the best possible protection against hazards, their use entails many problems, the most important are:
- Dirt
- Irritation and maceration of the skin
- Allergy to glove materials and donning powders
- Getting caught in moving parts of machinery.

Dirt

Chemicals may contaminate polymeric protective gloves by permeation through intact gloves. They may also be heavily soiled on the inside by chemicals or chemicals may also be accidentally spilled through the mouth of gloves, thereby causing skin damage, or the chemicals may touch the skin when soiled gloves are being pulled on or off. Noxious agents in the glove material come into direct contact with the skin and can cause allergic or irritant dermatitis. Sometimes harmful chemicals or agents are absorbed and retained in glove materials, e.g., nitroglycerin in the gloves of dynamite workers; in lubricant powders such as bacterial endotoxin in gamma sterilized gloves; or ethylene oxide (ETO), ethylene chlorhydrin, or ethylene glycol residues in glove materials. In ETO-sterilized gloves that are not sufficiently aerated before their use, ETO residues can also cause chemical burns. Allergens may also contaminate gloves in invisible amounts sufficient to provoke dermatitis in sensitized persons (Estlander et al. 2000 c).

Irritation and Maceration of the Skin

Irritation

Although irritation caused by polymeric gloves is possibly more common than allergy, there is scant data available on the subject. Corn starch, club moss (Lycopodium) powder, talc, lactose and silicone can be used as glove-donning powders. In experiments using skin replica techniques, it was suggested that mechanical rubbing of the skin by powders caused roughness of the hands (Taylor 1994; Brehler et al. 1998).

In a Japanese study, irritation was suggested as the cause of vinyl glove dermatitis, rather than allergy to the material itself. A fraction, probably an irritant, thought to be responsible for this discomfort has been found by doing animal tests on vinyl gloves sold in Japan.

Nonimmunologic contact urticaria (NICU) could explain some of the immediate itching and redness reactions attributed to gloves, as some glove powders may contain a known NICU agent, sorbic acid. Pressure urticaria or cholinergic urticaria associated with glove use may also be a cause of irritation. Tight or poorly fitting gloves can also cause skin irritation, especially in persons with considerable dermographism (Taylor 1994; Estlander and Jolanki 1988).

Occlusion caused by gloves, as well as friction from gloves rubbing against the skin, are other important causes of glove irritation. The effect of occlusion has been shown experimentally (Taylor 1994; Ramsing and Agner 1996 a, b).

Frequent hand washing using detergents and other cleaning agents, as well as hand washes containing ethyl alcohol and other disinfectants can also increase the irritant effect of gloves. The ingredients of glove materials can also cause irritation. The materials may contain residues of chemicals used in the manufacturing process. The variation in glove pH and glove chemicals may be highly responsible factors in the irritation caused by gloves. In some workplaces with strict sterility requirements, glove users may also wipe the gloves on their hands with disinfectant solutions that may permeate the glove material and cause skin irritation (Brehler et al. 1998; Estlander et al. 2000 c).

Rough leather or textile may cause friction on the skin and irritative dermatitis. Rough glove seams are especially harmful to fingers and wrists. Water and other liquids make leather slippery and cause it to deteriorate. Wet gloves are uncomfortable to wear and they may also cause skin irritation or even irritant contact dermatitis (Estlander and Jolanki 1988).

Maceration

When watertight polymeric gloves are worn for long periods without breaks, profuse sweating of the hands can cause softening or maceration and irritation of the skin. Macerated, softened skin gives poor protection against microbes and chemical injuries. In recent years, 1% of the cases reported as irritant contact dermatitis to the Finnish Register of Occupational Diseases (FROD) have been caused by maceration, mainly due to polymeric gloves (Jolanki et al. 1998 a).

Allergy to Glove Material and Donning Powder

Rubber Gloves

Rubber gloves are an important cause of occupational and non-occupational hand dermatitis. Rubber glove dermatitis may involve delayed (type-IV) allergy, leading to contact eczema, or immediate (type-I) allergy appearing as contact urticaria and protein contact dermatitis. Simultaneous type-I and type-IV allergy to rubber gloves may also occur. When occupationally related glove dermatoses are considered, allergic contact dermatitis (type-IV allergy) is probably more common than type-I allergic contact urticaria. In certain occupations, however, in which natural rubber (NRL) gloves are used daily for long periods, e.g., in hospitals, dental care, and laboratory work, contact dermatoses due to type-I allergy can be more important. Most of the reported cases of type-IV allergy to rubber gloves are due to gloves made of NRL. Reports on cases due to synthetic materials are few and usually describe allergy to neoprene gloves, but sensitization to other materials, e.g., nitrile rubber, is also possible. NRL gloves have long been the only source of type-I allergy due to rubber gloves, but also latex-free nitrile gloves and gloves made of mixtures of synthetic rubber and NRL have been reported to cause type-I sensitization and contact urticaria. NRL gloves are also the major contributor to latex aeroallergens in operating rooms ((Estlander et al. 2000c; Heese et al. 1991, 1994; Brehler 1996; Turjanmaa 1997; Jolanki et al. 1998 a, b; de Groot et al. 1998; Palosuo et al. 1998; Wigger-Alberti and Elsner 1998).

Sensitizers in Rubber Gloves

The primary ingredient in rubber gloves is rubber polymer, which is blended with various additives including vulcanizing agents, accelerators, antioxidants, pigments, fillers and oils. Rubber polymer can be a natural product (natural latex) or it can be manufactured synthetically. Neoprene and nitrile rubbers are examples of synthetic polymers used in the production of gloves. Blending NRL with neoprene or nitrile rubbers is also common in order to combine the favorable properties of both materials.

Additives, usually accelerators such as thiurams, carbamates and benzothiazoles and antioxidants are usually responsible for type-IV allergy due to gloves. Other potential type-IV sensitizers include thiourea and phenol derivatives, diphenylguanidine, mercaptobenzimidazole, quinoline derivatives, preservatives, antistatic agents, glove powder ingredients and fragrances. Organic pigments used in both rubber and plastic materials may also induce sensitization. A quaternary ammonium compound, cetylpyridinium chloride, has also been reported to be the cause of sensitization to surgical rubber gloves. Rubber polymer itself has increasingly been listed among the possible causes of delayed allergy to rubber (Heese et al. 1994; Jolanki et al. 1987; Fuchs 1995; Wilkinson and Burd 1998; Estlander et al. 2000 c).

Thiurams and carbamates have most commonly been responsible for the type-IV reactions due to rubber gloves. Mercaptobenzothiazole was the first benzothiazole accelerator used in gloves, but other derivatives can also be used. The reports on sensitization to thiourea compounds from rubber gloves are few and, for the most part, involve gloves made of neoprene rubber, which may also contain diphenylguanidine. Antioxidants are less frequent sensitizers. Allergy from gloves to *N*-isopropyl-*N*-phenyl-PPDA (paraphenylenediamine) has been cited in the literature, although PPDA derivatives are seldom used in rubber gloves except in black or dark-colored industrial gloves. Phenol derivatives are rare sensitizers in rubber gloves (Fuchs 1995; Estlander et al. 2000c).

Proteins in NRL polymers are the chief cause of type-I allergy, whereas casein and terpenes may also be possible allergens. Since the 1980s additives of rubber mixtures, both in natural and synthetic rubbers, have been increasingly reported as causes of type-I allergy to gloves. Glove powder ingredients are other potential causes of glove contact urticaria. In a study of workers at the Department of Immunology, Erasmus University, Rotterdam, none of the skin-tested participants was patch or prick-test positive to glove powder extract; nor did they test positive to a non-latex glove extract (Elastyren) used in the study. Certain polyurethane-coated surgical NRL gloves have also been reported as a possible new cause of glove contact urticaria. A life-threatening anaphylactic reaction has also been reported in an NRL allergic worker from the use of polychloroprene (neoprene) gloves, possibly caused by small amounts of NRL in the inside coating of the glove (Turjanmaa 1997; Mäkinen-Kiljunen and Turjanmaa 1995; Palosuo 1997; de Groot 1988; Hoffman-Sommargruber 1998; Estlander et al. 2000c).

Proteins with molecular weight (MW) ranging from 14 to 75 kDa are usually responsible for allergy to NRL, but allergenic proteins may also have lower or higher MW. More than 12 individual latex allergens have been identified. Enzymes, e.g., chitinases and glucanases, are possibly responsible for the latex-fruit syndrome as a result of cross-allergy between NRL and avocado, banana, kiwi and chestnut (Mäkinen-Kiljunen and Turjanmaa 1995; Alenius et al. 1996b; Palosuo et al. 1998; Hoffmann-Sommergruber et al. 1998).

Many studies conducted in the past few years also indicate that there may be considerable differences between the allergen contents of the gloves of different manufacturers, between different glove brands, and between gloves from different batches of the same manufacturer (Turjanmaa et al. 1988; Alenius et al. 1994; Palosuo et al. 1996, 1998). In many cases, powdered gloves have been shown to contain higher contents of allergens than powder-free gloves. Hamann (1993) has reviewed factors affecting antigenicity and the concentration of NRL proteins.

In addition, the manufacturing process of the gloves may cause some of the proteins to become even more allergenic. Some sensitized persons may, however, be able to use NRL gloves with low allergenicity, whereas others, especially atopic persons sensitive to NRL, seem to be more susceptible and can develop skin symptoms when wearing even these gloves. Therefore, it has been stated that NRL gloves with low allergenicity cannot always be recommended as an alternative for atopics sensitized to natural rubber (Alenius et al. 1991; Cormio et al. 1993; de Groot et al. 1998).

Rubber Gloves as Causes of Occupational Allergy

Rubber gloves have long been the main source of occupational allergy to rubber. Of all occupationally induced type-IV rubber allergy cases, 41–66% has been reported to be caused by rubber gloves. Allergy to gloves seems to be common among women, but it is also frequent among men who use them regularly. Long-standing use of rubber gloves and simultaneous exposure of hands to chemical or mechanical irritation or wet work seem to be the most important risk factors in the development of type-IV allergy to gloves. Work in medical and dental health services; laboratory work; cleaning, hair dressing, kitchen work; work in the food industry; and agricultural and industrial work are high-risk occupations (Estlander et al. 2000a,c; Fuchs 1995; Heese et al. 1994; Tarvainen 1996).

Although rubber gloves are an important cause of NRL allergy, there are also many other sources of NRL contact. Besides frequent use of NRL gloves, atopic constitution and hand dermatitis have often been connected with allergy to NRL. Allergy to NRL gloves is most frequent among hospital and dental care personnel, ranging from 2.8% to 16.9%, but it is common also in other occupations where NRL gloves are worn daily for long periods (Hamann 1993; Heese et al. 1994; Turjanmaa 1997; Palosuo 1997; Tarvainen 1996; Fuchs 1995; Mäkinen-Kiljunen and Turjanmaa 1995; de Groot 1998).

Since 1985, a worldwide increase has been reported in the cases of type-I allergy to NRL gloves. In Finland since 1990, the information from the FROD indicated a clear increase in the proportion of type-I sensitization to NRL gloves. During the period 1990–1994, 814 new cases of contact urticaria and protein contact dermatitis were reported to FROD. Natural rubber (193 cases) was the second most common cause of these dermatoses, being responsible for 23% of the cases. During 1995–1996, 118 new cases of contact urticaria or protein contact dermatitis were reported to the FROD, explaining 30% of the cases. During 1997–1999, 108 cases of type-I NRL allergy were reported to the FROD, and they were responsible for 23% of all cases of contact urticaria and protein contact dermatitis (Estlander et al. 2000a,c; Jolanki et al. 2001).

During 1997–1999, rubber chemicals were the most important cause of occupational allergic contact eczema, explaining 22% of the cases. Rubber gloves were considered to be the most common source of type-IV allergy to rubber chemicals. When all occupations were concerned, roughly 70% of the rubber-glove allergy cases were due to a delayed-type IV reaction and 30% to an immediate-type reaction (Estlander et al. 2000a,c; Jolanki et al. 2001).

Plastic Gloves

PVC, polyethylene (PE), polyvinylacetate (PVAC), polyvinylalcohol and other materials used in plastic gloves rarely cause allergic contact dermatitis. The use of plastic materials for personal protective equipment has become common since the 1950s but, in most countries, plastic gloves are possibly less used than rubber gloves. Accordingly, most of the reports on allergic contact eczema from plastic gloves are based on only one case or a few cases. Most allergy problems are connected with the use of PVC gloves. 7–10% of the examined glove allergic patients have been allergic to vinyl gloves (Estlander et al. 2000a,b,c).

A vinyl glove material may, for example, contain about 50% PVC and 50% additives. These include plasticizers, stabilizers, UV absorbers, fungicides, bactericides, flame retardants, and colorants. Although plastic materials are generally considered to be non-sensitizers, some additives may be leachable and cause contact sensitization (Jolanki et al. 1987; Estlander 1990; Estlander et al. 2000 a, b, c).

Sensitization to epoxy resin used as a plasticizer had already been reported in the 1960s. Epoxy resins can be used as plasticizers and stabilizers in PVC (gloves). A patient at the Finnish Institute of Occupational Health (FIOH) having allergic contact dermatitis from the use of certain household-type PVC gloves repeatedly reacted to bisphenol A during patch testing. Another patient, a female dentist, developed hand dermatitis after using certain disposable PVC gloves. On patch testing, she reacted to her glove material and bisphenol A. The chemical analyses of both glove materials revealed bisphenol A, which was probably the cause of their hand dermatitis (Estlander et al. 1999, 2000 b).

Plasticizers were possibly the cause of one patient's dermatitis when five patients at the FIOH were sensitized to their PVC gloves. The patient reacted to tricresyl phosphate and triphenyl phosphate, known plasticizers in PVC. In addition, colorants may be the cause of PVC-glove dermatitis. The colorant Irgalite Orange F2G (CI Pigment Orange 34) was the actual sensitizer in one of the five above-mentioned patients' gloves (Estlander et al. 2000 c).

Leather Gloves

Chrome-tanned leather gloves can induce allergy to chromium, thereby causing dermatitis. On rare occasions dyed leather gloves can also be the cause of glove dermatitis. The leather used for protective gloves is usually tanned by water-soluble chrome salts. Experiments have shown that synthetic and human sweat can release chromium from leather in amounts sufficient to induce the development of contact allergy. However, allergy to leather gloves is rare compared with that caused by rubber gloves (Estlander et al. 1995, 2000 d).

Investigations When Allergy to Gloves Is Suspected

The possibility of glove allergy should be suspected in cases in which even the careful wearing of polymer gloves seems to be of no use.

Sensitization to chromium should be considered in cases of hand dermatitis appearing in jobs in which leather gloves may often become totally wet, e.g., in many construction or forestry jobs or where there is profuse sweating of the hands in work involving high temperatures such as in welding.

Investigations should include patch testing with pieces of rubber and plastic glove materials, using the 48-h occlusion time. Tests with ultrasonic bath extracts of glove materials may also help detect the sensitizer in the materials. Further testing with a standard series, e.g., the European series (Chemotechnique Diagnostics Ab, Malmö, Sweden) is necessary to confirm an allergy to rubber. The series contains two rubber mixes; a thiuram mix; a mercapto mix, N-isopropyl-N-phenyl-4-phenylenediamine (IPPD) and mercaptobenzothiazole (MBT) which detects most cases of rubber glove allergy. The thiuram mix has been shown to be a good detector of glove allergy. It has also been suggested that it is not important to know which specific thiuram compound is the sensitizer because all thiuram-containing gloves must be avoided. Carbamates are the second most common allergens widely used in rubber gloves. It is recommended that zinc diethyldithiocarbamate, zinc dibutyldithiocarbamate and zinc dimethyldithiocarbamate are tested separately. Testing MBT separately increases the sensitivity of the test because, in addition to detecting allergy to MBT, it reveals allergies to *N*-cyclohexylbenzothiazyl sulfenamide (CBS), dibenzothiazyl disulfide (MBTS) or morpholinylmercapto benzothiazole (MOR) with the same sensitivity as mercapto mix. In the living epidermis CBS, MBTS, and MOR are converted into MBT. Cyclohexylthiophalimide (CTP) is a rather new rubber allergen, which is used as a vulcanization retarder mainly in solid rubber products such as tyres. There is no reliable data on the use of CTP in rubber gloves, but an increasing clinical experience suggests that it could also be an allergen in rubber gloves (Bruze et al. 1992; Hansson and Agrup 1993; Holness and Nethercott 1997; Geier and Gefeller 1995; Estlander et al. 1995; Estlander 2000a; Brandao 2001).

The standard series contains no thiourea compounds, but some are included in a specific rubber series, e.g., Chemotechnique Diagnostics Ab. Cross-reactivity occurs between thiourea compounds, but not all the time. Patch testing with a rubber additive series may increase the accuracy of patch testing and help to find alternative materials for patients having a specific rubber-additive allergy.

Possible sensitization to rubber polymers themselves and to glove powders should also be excluded. The fragrances used to deodorize the materials may also be the cause of glove allergy.

A series of plastics and glues containing tricresylphosphate and bisphenol A may help in cases where PVC gloves are suspected. Patch testing with all actual components of polymer gloves would give the best and the most reliable results and would also give more information on allergenic compounds found in gloves (Estlander et al. 2000a, c).

In cases where leather gloves are suspected of causing allergic dermatitis, the patch test should include, in addition to potassium dichromate in the standard series, a dilution series of potassium dichromate (and chromium chloride) to confirm sensitization to chromium. When the leather gloves are colored, sensitization to leather dye should also be kept in mind (Estlander et al. 1995, 2000c, d).

Investigations should also include tests to detect type-I allergy to polymeric glove materials and glove powders (prick tests, determinations of latex-specific IgE antibodies in serum, e.g., radioallergosorbent test (RAST), and challenges with suspected gloves). See also Turjanmaa et al. (2000).

Getting Caught in Moving or Revolving Parts of Machinery

The use of protective gloves must not increase the risk of injuries to the hands. There is considerable accident risk when the work involves wearing gloves near revolving machinery. Machines should always be tagged and locked during repair, adjustment, or mounting. The use of gloves may sometimes be necessary even though there is some risk that they might get caught in moving parts of machinery. Alternatives for gloves may be pads and cuffs that provide partial protection for the vulnerable parts of hands (Estlander and Jolanki 1988).

Prevention of the Problems of Glove Usage

All efforts to minimize the role of gloves as causes of occupational and non-occupational dermatoses, as well as accidents to hands, are necessary. A detailed job analysis should be carried out; all materials to be handled with gloves should always be checked to see whether the materials are suitable for the job in question. Also, the demands of the user should be taken into account before the gloves are selected (Estlander and Jolanki 1988; Estlander et al. 2000a, c).

New directives and regulations covering the use and safety requirements of protective gloves have come into force in Europe. Obtaining information on quality requirements and performance data, as well as an acceptable level of exposure to hazards and problems in glove usage is necessary before gloves are selected, purchased or used (Mellström and Boman 1997).

In Europe, gloves intended to protect the user are considered personal protective equipment (PPE) and covered by the personal protective Equipment Directive 89/686/EEC. Gloves that are intended for medical purposes are covered by the Council Directive 93/42/EEC concerning medical devices. The European Committee for Standardization (CEN) is responsible for establishing the necessary new standards for Europe. A survey of US rules, regulations and standards concerning protective gloves for occupational use has been completed by Henry (Henry 1994; Mellström and Boman 1997).

Glove usage should begin at the same time that handling of hazardous materials begins. One person should use each pair of gloves, and the condition of the gloves should be the user's responsibility (Estlander et al. 2000c).

Only gloves with CE markings should be used at work, at least in the countries of the European Union. Since July 1, 1995, only PPE with CE (European Community conformity) markings can be distributed inside the European Economic Area. This mark guarantees that the product fulfills the essential requirements of directive 89/686/EEC. It also implies that all PPE, except those which are used against minimal risk only, must be type examined by a notified body before the CE mark can be affixed on them. The Department of Physics at the FIOH is such a notified body. The user of the PPE is also entitled to receive information about the PPE, its classification as a PPE, and about the tests it has passed from the distributor of the PPE. This is especially important because packages of gloves no longer need to contain information on the glove material. Directive 89/656/EEC, however, obligates employers to make risk assessments and define the suitability of gloves for each job, as well as to organize a system of glove maintenance and training for glove users (Estlander et al. 1996, 2000a, c).

People who are allergic to rubber should use gloves made of plastic materials. NRL gloves are best suited for occasional use. Inner cotton or inner disposable PVC or PE gloves are recommended for use with rubber gloves. In addition, the material of NRL gloves should be of low protein content (Palosuo et al. 1996, TLT-info 1/2001, National Agency for Medicines). Lists of chemical allergens in some protective gloves can be found at http://www.gisbau.de/allergen/liste.html. Manufacturers and shops specified to distribute PPE, including gloves, can also help sensitized persons select suitable gloves.

Separate textile gloves should also be worn under unlined gloves made of polymers, especially when there are symptoms of skin irritation or dermatitis of the hands, or the hands sweat profusely. Barrier creams should not be used under NRL gloves. Skin protection creams may promote the uptake of allergens from the gloves, thus increasing allergic reactions (Baur et al. 1998).

Better protection is ensured if at least two pairs of gloves are available for every worker during every work shift. One alternative to thick gloves would be the simultaneous use of two pairs of thin gloves made of different materials (e.g., a disposable pair of PE gloves and another pair of natural rubber to be worn outermost). Special gloves made of laminated plastic materials, such as the 4H Glove or Barrier, can also be used as inner gloves (Mäkelä et al. 1999; Estlander et al. 2000 a, c).

References

Alenius H, Turjanmaa K, Palosuo T, Mäkinen-Kiljunen S, Reunala T (1991) Surgical latex glove allergy: characterization of rubber latex protein sensitivity by immunoblotting. Int Arch Allergy Immunol 96:376–380

Alenius H, Mäkinen-Kiljunen S, Turjanmaa K, Palosuo T, Reunala T (1994) Allergen and protein content of latex gloves. Ann Allergy 73:315–320

Alenius H, Kalkkinen N, Reunala T, Turjanmaa K, Palosuo T (1996a) The main IgE binding epitope of a major latex allergen, prohevein, is present in its N-terminal 43 amino acid fragment hevein. J Immunol 156:1618–1625

Alenius H, Kalkkinen N, Turjanmaa K, Mäkinen-Kiljunen S, Reunala T, Palosuo T (1996b) Significance of rubber elongation factor as a latex allergen. Int Arch Allergy Immunol 109:362–368

Baur X, Chen Z, Allmers H, Raulf-Heimsoth M (1998) Results of wearing test with two different latex gloves with and without skin protection cream. Allergy 53:441–443

Brehler R (1996) Contact urticaria caused by latex-free nitrile gloves. Contact Dermatitis 34:296

Brehler R, Sedlmayer S (1997) Contact urticaria due to rubber chemicals? Contact Dermatitis 17:125–127

Brehler R, Woss W, Müller S (1998) Glove powder affects skin roughness, one parameter of skin irritation. Contact Dermatitis 39:227–230

Brandao FM (2001) Rubber glove dermatitis: Old vs. new allergens. In: Book of Abstracts, XIII International Symposium on Contact Dermatitis. 1st Latin American Symposium on Cutaneous Allergy, 23–25 November, Uruguay

Bruze M, Trulsson L, Bendsöe N (1992) Patch testing with ultrasonic bath extracts. Am J Contact Dermat 3:133–137

Cormio L, Turjanmaa K, Talja M, Andersson LC, Ruutu M (1993) Toxicity and immediate allergenity of latex gloves. Clin Exp Allergy 23:618–623

Estlander T (1990) Occupational skin disease in Finland. Observations made during 1974–1988 at the Institute of Occupational Health, Helsinki (thesis). Acta Derm Venereol Suppl (Stockh) 155:1–85

Estlander T, Jolanki R (1988) How to protect the hands. Dermatol Clin 6:105–114

Estlander T, Jolanki R, Kanerva L (1994) Allergic contact dermatitis from rubber and plastic gloves. In: Mellström GA, Wahlberg JE, Maibach HI (eds) Protective gloves for occupational use. CRC Press, Boca Raton, pp 221–239

Estlander T, Jolanki R, Kanerva L (1995) Clothing. In: Guin JD (ed) Practical contact dermatitis. McGraw-Hill Inc, New York, pp 297–323

Estlander T, Jolanki R, Kanerva L (1996) Rubber glove dermatitis: a significant occupational hazard – prevention. In: Elsner P, Lachapelle JM, Wahlberg JE, Maibach HI (eds) Prevention of contact dermatitis. (Current problems in dermatology, vol 25). Karger, Basel, pp 170–181

Estlander T, Jolanki R, Henriks-Eckerman ML, Kanerva L (1999) Occupational allergy to bisphenol A. Contact Dermatitis 40:52–53

Estlander T, Jolanki R, Kanerva L (2000 a) Protective gloves. In: Menné T, Maibach HI (eds) Hand eczema, 2nd edn. CRC Press, Boca Raton, pp 309–322

Estlander T, Jolanki R, Henriks-Eckerman ML, Kanerva L (2000 b) Occupational contact allergy to bisphenol A. Review series Allergy 1:8–9

Estlander T, Jolanki R, Kanerva L (2000 c) Disadvantages of gloves. In: Kanerva L, Elsner P, Wahlberg JE, Maibach HI (eds) Handbook of occupational dermatology. Springer, Berlin Heidelberg New York, pp 426–436

Estlander T, Jolanki R, Kanerva L (2000 d) Occupational allergic contact dermatitis from trivalent chromium in leather tanning. Contact Dermatitis 45:114

Fuchs T (1995) Gummi und Allergie. Dustri, München-Deisenhofen, pp 1–247

Geier J, Fuchs T (1989) Kontakturtikaria durch Gummihandschuhe. Z Hautkr 65:267–272

Geier J, Gefeller O (1995) Sensitivity of patch tests with rubber mixes: results of the information network of departments of dermatology from 1990 to 1993. Am J Contact Dermat 6:143–149

de Groot H, de Jong NW, Duisjter E, van Wijk RG, Vermeulen A, van Toorenenbergen AW, Geursen L, van Joost T (1998) Prevalence of natural rubber latex allergy (type I and type IV) in laboratory workers in the Netherlands. Contact Dermatitis 38:159–163

Hamann CP (1993) Natural rubber latex protein sensitivity in review. Am J Contact Dermat 4:4–21

Hansson C, Agrup G (1993) Stability of 2-mercaptobenzothiazole (MBT). Contact Dermatitis 28:29–34

Heese A, von Hintzenstern J, Peters K-P, Koch HU, Hornstein OP (1991) Allergic and irritant reactions to rubber gloves in medical health services. J Am Acad Dermatol 25:831–839

Heese A, Peters K-P, Koch HU, Hornstein OP (1994) Allergologic evaluation and data on 173 glove-allergic patients. In: Mellström GA, Wahlberg JE, Maibach HI (eds) Protective gloves for occupational use. CRC Press, Boca Raton, pp 185–205

Henry NW III (1994) Protective gloves for occupational use. In: Mellström GA, Wahlberg JE, Maibach HI (eds) Protective gloves for occupational use. CRC Press, Boca Raton, pp 45–50

Hoffmann-Sommergruber K, Breiteneder H, Scheiner O (1998) Neue Ergebnisse zur molekularen und allergologischen Characterisierung von Hevea-brasiliensis-Latexallergenen. Allergol J 7:324–331

Holness DL, Nethercott JR (1997) Results of patch testing with a special series of rubber allergens. Contact Dermatitis 36:207–211

Jolanki R, Kanerva L, Estlander T (1987) Organic pigments in plastics can cause allergic contact eczema. Acta Dermatol Venereol Suppl (Stockh) 134:95–97

Jolanki R, Savela A, Estlander T, Kanerva L (1998 a) Causes of occupational skin diseases in Finland 1990–96 (in Finnish). Suomen Lääkärilehti (Finnish Med J) 53:409–415

Jolanki R, Estlander T, Alanko K, Savela A, Kanerva L (1998 b) Occupational contact urticaria or protein contact dermatitis from natural rubber latex by occupation. J Eur Acad Dermatol Venereol 11[Suppl 2]:207

Jolanki R, Savela A, Estlander T, Kanerva L (2001) Skin diseases according to occupational disease statistics (in Finnish). Työterveyslääkäri 1:10–16

Kanerva L, Jolanki R, Toikkanen J, Keskinen H, Savela A, Karjalainen A (1998) Occupationally induced allergies in 1995–96 (in Finnish). Työterveyslaitos, Finnish Institute of Occupational Health, Allergia ja työ-ohjelma (Allergy and work program), Helsinki, pp 9–161

Liste der Allergene in Schutzhandschuhen. http://www.gisbau.de/Allergen/Liste.html

Market surveillance study of latex gloves in Finland. National Agency for Medicines, TLT-info 1/2001, www.nam.fi/publications/medical device

Mäkelä E, Väänänen V, Alanko K, Jolanki R, Estlander T, Kanerva L (1999) Resistance of disposable gloves to permeation by 2-hydroxyethyl methacrylate and triethyleneglycol dimethacrylate. J Occup Hyg 5:121–129

Mäkinen-Kiljunen S, Turjanmaa K (1995) Latexallergene in verschiedenen Arten von Latex-Handschuhen und Sensibilisierung von Krankenhauspersonal und Patienten. Allergologie 18:366–368

Mellström GA, Boman AS (1997) Protective gloves: test results compiled in a database. In: Brune D, Gerhardsson G, Crockford GW, D'Auria D (eds) The work place, vol 1. Fundamentals of health, safety and welfare. International Occupational Safety and Health Information Centre (CIS), International Labour Office, Geneva and Scandinavian Science Publisher, Oslo, pp 716–730

Palosuo T (1997) Latex allergens. Rev Fr Allergol 37:1184–1187

Palosuo T, Turjanmaa K, Reunala T, Mäkinen-Kiljunen S, Alenius H (1996) Allergen content of latex gloves used in 1994–1996 in health care in Finland. Results of renewed market survey in 1995. Publications National Agency for Medicines 2:1–7

Palosuo T, Mäkinen-Kiljunen S, Alenius H, Reunala T, Yip E, Turjanmaa K (1998) Measurement of natural rubber latex allergen levels in medical gloves by allergen specific IgE-ELISA inhibition, RAST inhibition, and skin prick test. Allergy 53:59–67

Ramsing DW, Agner T (1996a) Effect of glove occlusion on human skin (I). Short-term experimental exposure. Contact Dermatitis 34:1–5

Ramsing DW, Agner T (1996b) Effect of glove occlusion on human skin (II). Long-term experimental exposure. Contact Dermatitis 34:258–262

Tarvainen K (1996) Occupational dermatoses from plastic composites based on polyester resins, epoxy resins and vinyl ester resins (thesis). People and Work Research Reports 11, Finnish Institute of Occupational Health, Helsinki, pp 1–66

Taylor JS (1994) Other reactions from gloves. In: Mellström GA, Wahlberg JE, Maibach HI (eds) Protective gloves for occupational use. CRC Press Inc, Boca Raton, pp 255–265

Turjanmaa K (1988) Latex glove contact urticaria (thesis). Acta Universitatis Tamperensis, Ser A, vol 254, University of Tampere, Finland, pp 1–86

Turjanmaa K (1997) Contact urticaria from latex gloves. In: Amin S, Lahti A, Maibach HI (eds) Contact urticaria syndrome. CRC Press Inc, Boca Raton, pp 173–187

Turjanmaa K, Alenius H, Mäkinen-Kiljunen S, Reunala T, Palosuo T (2000) Natural rubber latex allergy. In: Kanerva L, Elsner P, Wahlberg JE, Maibach HI (eds) Handbook of occupational dermatology. Springer, Berlin Heidelberg New York, pp 719–729

Wigger-Alberti W, Elsner P (1998) Do barrier creams and gloves prevent or provoke contact dermatitis. Am J Contact Dermat 9:100–106

Wilkinson SM, Burd R (1998) Latex: a cause of allergic contact eczema in users of natural rubber gloves. J Am Acad Dermatol 38:36–42

The Role of Skin Moisturizers in the Prevention of Irritant Contact Dermatitis: A Review   24

C. L. GOH

Introduction

Moisturizers are used by almost everybody. In wet-work occupations, the great majority of workers apply skin care products to their hands several times daily both for the prevention and treatment of dry skin and irritant contact dermatitis.

Cumulative insult dermatitis resulting from repetitive stratum corneum injury leads to chronic dermatitis, which presents as dry scaly skin. These changes are preceded subclinically by changes in skin physiological functions, e.g. decreased capacitance, increased transepidermal water loss and increased blood flow that can be measured with various devices (Barany 1999). Moisturizers have been used to repair and maintain skin hydration for many years.

Exposure to soaps, detergents, water and friction damages the cell membranes resulting in chapping and irritant contact dermatitis, and workers in wet-work occupations may therefore benefit from the use of moisturizers on their skin.

The application of moisturizers has been shown in several studies to be effective in the prevention of contact and occupational dermatitis. It is an important preventive measure where the wearing of gloves is not possible or inappropriate. Moisturizers can be seen to reinforce the natural barrier function of the skin: they increase the water content of stratum corneum directly or indirectly. Studies have shown that eczematous skin heals faster when treated for several days with a moisturizer compared to untreated, symmetrical, control skin. This article reviews studies on the efficacy of moisturizers against irritant contact dermatitis.

How Do Moisturizers Work?

The role of moisturizers is to moisten the skin. As humectants, they can help to increase stratum corneum moisture actively and as emollients they can increase stratum corneum moisture passively by occlusion. The epidermal barrier of the stratum corneum consists of free fatty acids, cholesterol and ceramides. These lipids are crucial in maintaining the hydration of the stratum corneum.

The contents of a typical moisturizer include lipids humectants, emulsifiers, preservatives, pH-adjusters and fragrances. The important role of lipids in skin moisturization can be demonstrated by studies which show that lipid removal by acetone or ether leads to dry, scaly skin; electron microscopy showed that intercellular lamellae are removed without the presence of lipids, topical application of strateum corneum lipids leads to moisturization, and ceramide creams lead to significant improvement in dry skin. Comparison of different moisturizers on sodium lauryl sulfate (SLS)-irritated skin demonstrated that the efficacy was related more to the total amount of lipids rather than to the composition of lipids (Imokawa 1986; Imokawa 1989; Imokawa 1991). Imokawa using forearm stratum corneum sheets compared the ultrastructural changes of intercellular lipids and showed that stratum corneum lipids serve as a bound-water modulator (Imokawa 1986, 1989, 1991).

Extraction of the stratum corneum sheet with acetone/ether decreased the bound-water content from 33.3% to 19.7% leading to dry and scaly skin. Further extraction with water, which released water-soluble materials, e.g. amino acids, did not change the bound-water content. Electron microscopy analysis of the acetone/ether treated stratum corneum sheet revealed selective depletion of lipids from intercellular spaces, accompanied by marked disruption of lamellar structures.

Application of the stratum corneum lipid squalane, which contains 1% alpha-monomethyl-heptadecyl glyceryl ether, to lipid-depleted stratum corneum sheet caused a significant recovery of bound-water content to the previous, almost normal level and a significant improvement in dry skin. In addition, the application of the lipids into the lipid-depleted stratum corneum sheet resulted in restoration of the lamellar structures (Imokawa 1986, 1989, 1991).

These findings strongly suggest that stratum corneum lipids serve a water-holding function through formation of lamellar structures within the stratum corneum.

Experimental Evidence on Efficacy
of Moisturizer Against Irritant Contact Dermatitis

Few studies have focused on how topically applied lipids affect the recovery phase of diseased skin in humans. Does diseased skin heal faster when a moisturizer is applied? And, does the daily use of moisturizers on normal skin influence skin barrier function?

Currently, studies used for assessing the efficacy of moisturizers include their effects on immediate acute irritation, cumulative irritation, prevention of model irritation and controlled prevention studies in the work environment.

Objective non-invasive assessment of dry skin includes measurement of skin conductance, impedance, capacitance (Corneometer) and roughness (profilometry). The damage of the stratum corneum, leading to the loss of its water retention properties, can be measured by the transepidermal water loss measurement (TEWL) (Serup 1989; de Fine-Olivarius 1996).

Several earlier studies seemed to indicate that moisturizers prevent cumulative irritant contact dermatitis (ICD). Hannuksela demonstrated that moisturizers prevent cumulative ICD and speed healing (Hannuksela 1992). Loden demonstrated that urea-containing moisture speeds healing and decreased skin susceptibility to

SLS (Loden 1996) and Loden and Andersson in 1996 reported that canola oil reduces SLS-irritation, while other lipids have no effect.

Hannuksela et al. (1992) studied the ability of eight moisturizers to prevent ICD. Twelve students washed their upper arms with liquid detergent for 1 min twice a day for 1 week. After each washing, seven different creams and one oil were applied to the left upper arm on different volunteers, while the right upper arm was left untreated. The mean TEWL increased from 7.1 to 9.3 $g/m^2/h$ ($p < 0.001$) and the mean laser doppler flowmetry value decreased from 11.8 to 10.8 units (n.s.) on the left arm but increased from 7 to 20 $g/m^2/h$ and 11 to 20 units on the right arm. No significant difference between the eight moisturizers was observed. During the second week of their study, the volunteers stopped washing their arms. The untreated right arm was treated with moisturizers 2 times a day. The mean TEWL decreased from 20.3 to 8.6 ($p < 0.001$) over 7 days. No significant difference between moisturizers was observed. Laser Doppler flowmetry values showed the same trend as TEWL. The authors concluded that the regular use of emollients can prevent irritant dermatitis from a detergent.

Loden (1996, 1997) reported that urea-containing moisture speeds healing and decreases susceptibility to SLS. In a single-blind study, a moisturizing cream was tested for its influence on barrier recovery in surfactant-damaged skin and the susceptibility of normal skin to SLS. TEWL and skin capacitance were measured. The authors found that barrier recovery and influence of irritant stimuli in skin treated with a moisturizing cream was more favorable than untreated skin. Treatment of surfactant-damaged skin with the test cream for 14 days promoted barrier recovery that was observed as decrease in TEWL. Skin capacitance also normalized more rapidly during treatment. In normal skin, the use of the test cream significantly reduced TEWL after 14 days of treatment, and irritant reactions to SLS were significantly decreased. Skin capacitance increased after only 1 application and remained elevated after 14 days. The authors concluded that the accelerated rate of recovery of surfactant-damaged skin and the lower degree of SLS-induced irritation in normal skin treated with the test cream may be of clinical relevance in attempts to reduce irritant contact dermatitis.

In another report, Barany et al. (2000) showed that emulsifiers, which are surface-active ingredients used to stabilize the emulsion, are potential irritants; they evaluated in their study, with non-invasive measurements, the influence of stearic acid, glyceryl stearate, PEG-2, -9, -40, and -100 stearate, and steareth-2, -10 and -21 on normal and irritated skin. Test emulsions were created by incorporating 5% emulsifiers in a water/mineral oil mixture (50:50). The emulsions and their vehicle were then applied to normal skin for 48 h and to SLS-damaged skin for 17 h in aluminum chambers. Twenty-four hours after removal of the chambers the test sites were evaluated for degree of irritation. In normal skin, the emulsifiers induced significant differences in TEWL but not in skin blood flow. Five of the emulsifiers increased TEWL. In SLS-damaged skin an aggravation of the irritation was expected. Three emulsifiers unexpectedly decreased TEWL. These results highlight the possibility of absorption of these emulsifiers into the lipid bilayer, which increase TEWL in normal skin and decrease TEWL in damaged skin.

Loden et al. also showed the beneficial effects of urea-containing moisturizer on the barrier properties of atopic skin. Fifteen patients with atopic dermatitis treated one of their forearms twice daily for 20 days with a moisturizing cream. Skin capacitance and TEWL were measured at the start of the study and after 10 and 20 days. On day 21 the skin was exposed to SLS, and on day 22 the irritant reaction was measured non-invasively. Skin capacitance was significantly increased by the treatment, indicating increased skin hydration. The water barrier function, as reflected by TEWL values, tended to improve, and the skin susceptibility to SLS was significantly reduced, as measured by TEWL and superficial skin blood flow ($p < 0.05$). Thus, it seems that certain moisturizers could improve skin barrier function in atopics and reduce skin susceptibility to irritants (Loden 1999).

There were other reports that further support the role of moisturizers in preventing irritant contact dermatitis. Ramsing and Agner in 1997, using the hand immersion test, showed that moisturizer tested on experimentally irritated skin of 12 volunteers prevented SLS irritation and speeded healing of irritation. The volunteers had both hands immersed in a 0.375% SLS solution for 10 min twice daily for 2 days. Before immersion one hand was treated with moisturizer; the other hand served as control. Skin barrier functions were evaluated by TEWL, LDF and Capacitance. The 12 volunteers had both hands immersed in the same way. After the final immersion one hand was treated for 5 days with the moisturizer; the other hand served as control. There was a significant preventive effect on the treated hand, compared to the control hand by all measured parameters. Skin barrier function and skin hydration on the treated hand was better than the control hand. The moisturizer prevented irritant skin reactions induced by detergent, and it also accelerated regeneration of the barrier function of irritated skin. Held and Agner (1999) also reported that moisturizer speeds healing in hand-immersion and SLS patch tests.

Protective gloves are used in the workplace to protect hands from occupational hazards, but side effects from gloves are frequently reported. These side effects include irritant skin reactions. Held et al. (1999) studied the combined use of moisturizers and occlusive gloves. The study investigated whether applying a moisturizer to compromised skin before wearing an occlusive glove could reduce skin irritation. Healthy volunteers had both hands immersed in SLS twice daily for 2 days. After each immersion, one hand had a moisturizer applied and both hands were put into occlusive gloves for 2 h. Skin barrier function was evaluated by TEWL, skin capacitance and inflammation evaluated by colorimetry. The moisturizer had a statistically significant positive effect on water barrier function and hydration. Less inflammation was observed on moisturizer-treated hands. Their findings appear to suggest that moisturizer under occlusive glove may diminish irritation from detergent.

Field Studies on the Role of Moisturizers Against Irritant Contact Dermatitis

There are few controlled prospective intervention field studies on the use of moisturizers against irritant contact dermatitis. Halkier-Sorensen and Thestrup-Pedersen in 1993 reported that moisturizer-reduced dryness in cleaners and kitchen assistants exposed to water and detergents. The efficacy of a moisturizer among cleaners and kitchen assistants during everyday exposure to water and detergents was studied. Fifty-five volunteers used the moisturizer for 2 weeks (period L), followed by a period without (period C), or vice versa. Assessment and measurement of the skin surface temperature, electrical capacitance and TEWL were performed on the fingers, hands and arms on entry to the study, after 2 weeks and 4 weeks, or at drop out. Seventy volunteers (63%) completed the study. A significant increase in dryness ($p < 0.001$) was noted during periods of no treatment (period C), and normalization of the skin texture during use of moisturizer. Electrical capacitance decreased during period C and increased to pre-study values during period L ($p < 0.001$). No significant differences were found in skin temperatures and TEWL rates. They reported that moisturizer had a positive effect in preventing skin irritation.

Goh et al (1994) showed that an after-work moisturizer appeared to reduce the incidence of irritant dermatitis, and reduced TEWL increase from cutting oil, among metal workers (Loden 1996). Point prevalence of cutting fluid dermatitis, according to severity and TEWL changes over a 30-week study period, showed a lower incidence of irritant contact dermatitis and lower TEWL increase in workers who used after-work moisturizers compared to those who did not and those using barrier creams.

In another field study, Perrenoud et al. (2001) compared the protective action of a new barrier cream to its vehicle, in hand irritation among apprentice hairdressers caused by repeated shampooing and exposure to hair-care products. Twenty-one apprentice hairdressers (20 female, 1 male) who were starting their 2nd year of studies were recruited. A double-blind, cross-over study comparing Excipial Protect (the verum, containing aluminum chlorohydrate 5% as active ingredient) against its vehicle alone (the control). The subjects were randomly assigned to 1 of 2 groups (verum followed by control and vice versa). Measurements were taken on Monday at the end of their 2-day weekly break and again on Friday (the next-to-last day of their work-week). Additionally, the back of the dominant hand was clinically evaluated for dryness, redness, and breaks in the skin. At the end of the study period, the clinical scores were generally very low: nearly everyone replied 0 (none) or 1 (mild) under either cream and there was clearly no difference between the treatments.

Only corneometric values showed a difference between the verum and the control. The averages for corneometry were significantly higher in the control period than the verum period ($p < 0.01$). Evaporimeter values increased under verum treatment, without reaching statistical significance. In the control periods, the mean corneometric values were higher than in the verum periods. This suggests that the control cream was more hydrating than the verum cream. It appeared that the base cream vehicle alone was important in the prevention of occupational irritant contact dermatitis.

In contrast to most reports, Held et al. in 1999 and 2001 reported that moisturizers, which improve stratum corneum hydration, may increase skin susceptibility to contact irritants. In her studies, a 4-week treatment of normal skin with moisturizer increased susceptibility to SLS.

What is the impact of using a moisturizer on normal skin? Most authors dealing with the testing of moisturizers agree that they hydrate the skin. But, increasing the hydration level of the stratum corneum progressively may reduce its barrier efficiency. It is speculated that the consequence is the permeation of noxious substances into the skin with greater ease. This hypothesis was investigated in 20 volunteers with normal skin (Held 1999, 2001). Held et al applied a moisturizer (with 70% lipid) 3 times a day for 27 days on 1 forearm of 20 volunteers. The other forearm, which was left untreated, acted as control. On day 28 (after stopping the moisturizer), an irritant skin reaction was elicited on each volar forearm with a patch test of SLS for 24 h. On day 30, a statistically significant higher TEWL was found on the SLS-irritated area in moisturizer-treated arms compared to their untreated symmetrical controls. An increase in TEWL is generally accepted to be a consequence of an impaired barrier function of the skin. The results suggest that long-term treatment with moisturizers on normal skin may not necessarily offer any protection against irritant trauma caused by a detergent. On the contrary, daily use of moisturizers under these conditions may increase skin susceptibility to irritants. When the stratum corneum is hydrated it may become more permeable to hydrophilic substances such as SLS. The same result was recently found in a short-term study (5 days) using the same moisturizer.

Conclusions

From the reported articles, it appears that most studies support the "protective" effects of moisturizers against skin irritants. However, in these studies, a single product is often being tested alongside a single irritant. The protective effects of moisturizers may not be "broad spectrum" and different moisturizers with different constituents may be specifically more effective against different skin irritants and in different individuals. Some reports appear to indicate that overuse of moisturizers may have harmful effects when used on normal skin. Obviously more field studies on the effects of different moisturizers against different irritants on different individuals needs to be carried out to determine the efficacy of various moisturizers.

To prevent irritant contact and occupational dermatitis an integrated preventive skin care approach is desirable, in addition to primary preventive measures, such as the use of (a) pre-work: protective creams, (b) after work: cleansers and (c) after-work moisturizers. However, dermatologists must be aware that many studies have indicated that barrier creams used as pre-work protective agents are generally not effective in preventing irritant contact dermatitis. Hence, after work moisturizers probably play a more useful role here.

Moisturizers are not without side-effects. Workers using a moisturizer must be aware that it may cause skin irritation and sensitization. Sensitizers in moisturizers include fragrances, preservatives, e.g. Kathon CG, Euxyl K 400, formaldehyde donors, emulsifiers, e.g. wool alcohol, cocoamidopropyl betaine and humectants, e.g. propylene glycol.

References

Barany E, Lindberg M, Loden M (1999) Biophysical characterization of skin damage and recovery after exposure to different surfactants. Contact Dermatitis 40:98–103

Barany E, Lindberg M, Loden M (2000) Unexpected skin barrier influence from nonionic emulsifiers. Int J Pharm 195:189–195

De Fine Olivarius F, Hansen AB, Karlsmark T, Wulf HC (1996) Water protective effect of barrier creams and moisturizing creams: a new in vivo test method. Contact Dermatitis 35:219–225

Goh CL, Gan SL (1994) Efficacies of a barrier cream and an afterwork emollient cream against cutting fluid dermatitis in metalworkers: a prospective study. Contact Dermatitis 31:176–180

Halkier-Sorensen L, Thestrup-Pedersen K (1993) The efficacy of a moisturizer (Locobase) among cleaners and kitchen assistants during everyday exposure to water and detergents. Contact Dermatitis 29:266–271

Hannuksela A, Kinnumen T (1992) Moisturizers prevent irritant dermatitis. Acta Derm Venereol 72:42–44

Held E, Sveinsdottir S, Agner T (1999) Effect of long-term use of moisturizer on skin hydration, barrier function and susceptibility to irritants. Acta Derm Venereol 79:49–51

Held E ((2001) So moisturizers may cause trouble! Int J Dermatol 40:12–13

Held E, Agner T (1999) Comparison between 2 test models in evaluating the effect of a moisturizer on irritated human skin. Contact Dermatitis 40:261–268

Held E, Jorgensen LL (1999) The combined use of moisturizers and occlusive gloves: an experimental study. Am J Contact Dermat 10:146–152

Imokawa G, Akasaki S, Hattori M, Yoshizuka N (1986) Selective recovery of deranged water-holding properties by stratum corneum lipids. J Invest Dermatol 87:758–61

Imokawa G, Akasaki S, Minematsu Y, Kawai M (1989) Importance of intercellular lipids in water-retention properties of the stratum corneum: induction and recovery study of surfactant dry skin. Arch Dermatol Res 28145–51

Imokawa G, Kuno H, Kawai M (1981) Stratum corneum lipids serve as a bound-water modulator. J Invest Dermatol 96:845–851

Loden M, Anderson AC (1996) Effect of topically applied lipids on surfactant-irritated skin. Br J Dermatol 134:215–220

Loden M (1996) Urea-containing moisturizers influence barrier properties of normal skin. Arch Dermatol Res 288:103–107

Loden M (1997) Barrier recovery and influence of irritant stimuli in skin treated with a moisturizing cream. Contact Dermatitis 36:256–260

Loden M, Andersson AC, Lindberg M (1999) Improvement in skin barrier function in patients with atopic dermatitis after treatment with a moisturizing cream (Canoderm). Br J Dermatol 140:264–267

Perrenoud D, Gallezot D, van Melle G (2001) The efficacy of a protective cream in a real-world apprentice hairdresser environment. Contact Dermatitis 45:134–8

Ramsing DW, Agner T (1997) Preventive and therapeutic effects of a moisturizer. An experimental study of human skin. Acta Derm Venereol 77:335–337

Serup J, Winther A, Blichmann C (1989) A simple method for the study of scale pattern and effects of a moisturizer – qualitative and quantitative evaluation by D-Squame tape compared with parameters of epidermal hydration. Clin Exp Dermatol 14:277–282

Prognosis of Occupational Contact Dermatitis   25

C. L. GOH

Introduction

Prognosis of occupational contact dermatitis refers to the course of dermatitis over a period of time with and without medical intervention. Understanding the prognosis of occupational contact dermatitis is important because it enables dermatologists and occupational physicians to (a) predict the course of the dermatitis in their patients; (b) implement risk management of patients who are exposed to contact irritants and allergens; (c) plan preventive measures against contact and occupational dermatitis; and (d) help the relevant authorities to prioritize implementation of preventive measures. Long-term outcome of occupational contact dermatitis has important medico-legal implications; it helps dermatologists and occupational physicians to determine the amount of medico-legal compensation. Factors that may affect the prognosis of occupational contact dermatitis include atopy, job change, the age of the patient, the nature of irritants and allergens, and the nature of the occupation.

Prognosis of Occupational Contact Dermatitis

Epidemiology studies in the 1970s and 1980s generally reported poor prognosis for occupational contact dermatitis (Skog and Tottie 1961; Agrup 1969; Burrows 1972; Fregert 1975; Christensen 1982; Coenraads 1983; Schubert et al. 1987; Pryce et al. 1989). Recent reports appear to indicate that the prognosis is better than previously thought (Chia and Goh 1991; Rosen and Freeman 1993; Nethercott and Holness 1994). The improvement in the prognosis can be attributed to improvement in diagnostic test procedures, the ability of the physicians to identify causative contact irritants and allergens, and the improvement in health education and effective preventive measures against occupational contact dermatitis.

Complete clearance of occupational contact dermatitis has been reported to range from 8% to 77% over follow-up periods ranging from 1 year to more than 10 years (Skog and Tottie 1961; Agrup 1969; Burrows 1972; Fregert 1975; Christensen 1982; Coenraads 1983; Schubert et al. 1987; Pryce et al. 1989; Chia and Goh 1991; Rosen and Freeman 1993; Nethercott and Holness 1994). Studies done between 1961 and 1989 indicated that total clearance of occupational contact dermatitis occurred in only 8–33% of patients. In contrast, studies conducted after 1990 appear to indicate that the total clearance rate is about 70%.

While Burrows, in 1972, reported that 79% of patients with occupational contact dermatitis followed-up over 10–13 years still require treatment for their dermatitis (Burrows 1972), a report from Singapore showed total clearance of dermatitis in 72% of their patients after a 1-year follow-up. In Sydney, Rosen et al. reported that improvement of occupational contact dermatitis occurred in 74% and 68% of patients with occupational irritant and allergic contact dermatitis followed up over 2–10 years, respectively (Rosen and Freeman 1993). In the United States, Nethercott et al. reported that 63% of workers had clearance of their occupational contact dermatitis when followed-up over a 4-year period, and when patients with mild eczema were included, the improvement rate was 81%. In a recent report from Switzerland, where the medical records of 88 construction workers who had occupational dichromate dermatitis between 1986 and 1989 were reviewed and the workers interviewed, 63 patients (72%) were healed in the first few years after changing jobs (Lips et al. 1996).

Most studies indicated that there is no significant sex difference in the prognosis of occupational contact dermatitis. The prognosis is also not influenced by the age of onset of contact dermatitis.

Prognosis of Occupational Irritant Versus Allergic Contact Dermatitis

Most reports indicate that irritant contact dermatitis tends to have a poorer prognosis than allergic contact dermatitis. Some occupational irritants – for example, cutting fluids – are more likely to lead to chronicity than others.

In Singapore, occupational irritant dermatitis from cutting fluids and solvents was reported to be associated with a poor prognosis. About 40% of workers with cutting-fluid dermatitis had persistent dermatitis after a 1-year follow-up, even after the workers had ceased working with the cutting fluids (Chia and Goh 1991). Similarly, Shah et al. from the UK reported that hand dermatitis from cutting fluids confers poor prognosis. A questionnaire survey conducted on 51 workers seen between 1 year and 5 years previously revealed that 82% still had hand dermatitis. There was no difference in outcome between those who continued to work with the occupational irritant and those who had changed their occupations (Shah et al. 1996).

Chia et al. observed that occupational irritant dermatitis from cement and acids/alkali tends to have a relatively better prognosis than other irritants, with all workers experiencing complete clearance of their dermatitis when they ceased contact with the irritant (Chia and Goh 1991).

Workers who continued with exposure to occupational irritants tend to have a poorer prognosis than those who cease exposure. For example, Chia et al. reported that about 60% of patients with occupational irritant dermatitis from solvents had persistent dermatitis when they continued to work with the solvents (Chia and Goh 1991). Some occupational irritants appear to cause less chronicity, e.g. irritant contact dermatitis from acids/alkali and cement appear to clear when proper preventive measures are introduced (Chia and Goh 1991). The report from Singapore showed that all workers with irritant contact dermatitis from cement had complete clearance of their dermatitis despite continuing to work with the irritant. Similarly, in Denmark, occupational irritant dermatitis from cement cleared in 80% of their workers despite the fact that they continued working at the same job (Avnstorp 1989).

Rosen and Freeman (1993), in Sydney, reported that 30% of their workers with irritant contact dermatitis had total clearance of dermatitis following a 2- to 10-year follow-up. Allergic contact dermatitis was reported to confer a slightly better prognosis, with a complete clearance rate of 38%. Similarly, Nethercott and Holness (1994), in the United States, also reported better prognosis among patients with allergic contact dermatitis (with a complete clearance rate of 70%) compared with patients with irritant contact dermatitis (with a clearance rate of 58%) after a 4-year follow-up. Chia et al. from Singapore reported that 77% of patients with occupational allergic dermatitis had complete clearance of their dermatitis after a 1-year follow-up.

Occupational allergic contact dermatitis to chromates in cement has been reported to persist even upon avoidance of cement. Burrows reported that only 8% of his patients with cement dermatitis had clearance of their dermatitis after a 10- to 13-year follow-up (Burrows 1972). In Sydney, the prognosis from occupational allergic contact dermatitis from chromate was worse than that caused by other occupational allergens; only less than 20% of such patients had clearance of their dermatitis over a 2- to 10-year follow-up period (Rosen and Freeman 1993). Another study from Perth, Australia, also reported poor prognosis from cement dermatitis, where 89% of cement workers with chromate allergy had persistent dermatitis when followed up over a period between 6 months and 9 years (Halbert et al. 1992).

In Denmark, follow-up of patients with chromate allergy after the introduction of ferrous sulphate in Danish cement to reduce hexavalent chromate concentration in cement continued to show poor prognosis. Only 30% of workers who remained on the job had total clearance of their dermatitis (Avnstorp 1989).

In contrast to the reports mentioned above, Chia et al. from Singapore reported good prognosis among construction workers with chromate dermatitis from cement if contact with cement can be avoided or reduced. In their report, all five patients with chromate allergy had clearance of dermatitis upon avoidance of contact with cement (Chia and Goh 1991). Better prognosis from chromate dermatitis was also observed in Switzerland recently, where 63 (72%) of 88 workers were healed during the first few years after changing jobs. These patients mostly changed industries and strictly avoided all contact with cement or chromium salts. The authors concluded that strict allergen avoidance, enforced by authorities, and financial support in case of job change are important factors in improving the prognosis in occupational dichromate dermatitis (Lips et al. 1996).

This improvement in prognosis could also be attributed to reduction in exposure to chromates in cement among those affected through mechanization of construction processes, health education and the reduction of the chromate content of cement as a result of changes in the manufacturing process of cement (Goh and Gan 1996).

Occupation and Prognosis of Occupational Contact Dermatitis

Construction workers with allergic contact dermatitis were reported to suffer the poorest prognosis relative to workers in other occupations (Burrows 1972; Fregert 1975; Rosen and Freeman 1993; Avnstorp 1989). The complete clearance rate of occupational dermatitis among construction workers in Sydney, Australia, was reported to be 20% when these workers were followed-up over a 2- to 9-year period, compared with a clearance rate of 40% among medical workers and 35% among hairdressers and food handlers (Rosen and Freeman 1993). When "improvement" was defined as good prognosis in all occupational groups, the improvement/clearance rate for construction workers remained low – a total of 40% compared with a corresponding rate of 80% for medical workers, hairdressers and food handlers (Rosen and Freeman 1993). Recent reports, however, indicate that workers avoiding contact with cement do have a better prognosis, with 100% clearance in Singapore (Chia and Goh 1991) and 72% clearance in Switzerland (Lips et al. 1996).

Pryce et al. (1989) reported poor prognosis among metal workers suffering from cutting-fluid dermatitis, reporting a clearance rate of about 20% during a 2-year follow-up. Similarly, Shah et al. (1996) from the UK reported that hand dermatitis from cutting fluids confers poor prognosis where 82% still have hand dermatitis after a 1- to 5-year follow-up.

Hairdressers with irritant contact dermatitis appeared to have good prognosis when they changed jobs. Matsunaga reported a 70% clearance rate for workers who ceased working as hairdressers (Matsunaga et al. 1998).

Job Change and Prognosis of Occupational Contact Dermatitis

Most patients with occupational contact dermatitis who change jobs do so for reasons other than their dermatitis (Agrup 1969; Christensen 1982; Rystedt 1985). Earlier reports indicated that job change is not associated with significant improvement in the prognosis of occupational contact dermatitis (Agrup 1969; Fregert 1975; Christensen 1982; Rystedt 1985; Hellier 1958; Keczkes et al. 1983; Williamson 1967).

Many patients preferred to continue to work despite their dermatitis. Burrows reported that only 20% of workers with occupational dermatitis stopped working because of their dermatitis (in a 10- to 13-year follow-up study). Among those who continued to work, only about 18% of workers had clearance of their dermatitis (Burrows 1972). Pryce reported the clearance rate of cutting-fluid dermatitis after a 2-year follow-up to be 12% for those who continued to be exposed to cutting fluid and 30% for those who ceased to be exposed to cutting fluid (Pryce et al. 1989). Similarly, Shah et al. (1996) from the UK reported no difference in the outcome of the poor prognosis of workers with cutting-fluid dermatitis on the hands between those who remained in the same job and those who changed their occupation.

Among hairdressers with occupational dermatitis, job change appears to confer good prognosis. Matsunaga from Japan reported clearance of occupational dermatitis in 70% of hairdressers who ceased work, compared with 20% who cleared when they continued to work as hairdressers (Matsunaga et al. 1998).

In Singapore, the prognosis of occupational allergic and irritant contact dermatitis for patients who ceased to be exposed was better than those who continued exposure to the contactants. The overall clearance rates for patients who ceased exposure and continued exposure were 73% and 69%, respectively. The clearance rates for allergic contact dermatitis were 71% (ceased exposure) and 74% (continued exposure), respectively, and for irritant contact dermatitis were 74% and 68%, respectively (Chia and Goh 1991).

In Sydney, Australia, the prognosis of occupational dermatitis was significantly poorer among patients who continued in the same job (clearance rate was 28%) than those who changed jobs (clearance rate was 43%) (Rosen and Freeman 1993). In Perth, Australia, among the 48% of construction workers with allergic contact dermatitis to chromate who changed jobs, only 31% had complete clearance of their dermatitis after a 6-month to 9-year follow-up (Halbert et al. 1992). This contrasted with the report from Switzerland, where 72% of their construction workers had clearance of their chromate dermatitis when they changed their job.

Association of Atopy and Prognosis of Occupational Contact Dermatitis

A personal history of atopy appears to significantly affect the prognosis of patients with occupational contact dermatitis. Rosen reported that the clearance rate of patients with a personal history of atopy (30%) was significantly poorer than for those without atopy (41%) (Rosen and Freeman 1993). However, Nethercott and Holness (1994) also did not observe any significant difference in prognosis between atopic and non-atopic workers with occupational dermatitis.

Conclusions

The causes of chronicity from occupational contact dermatitis are usually multifactorial. Most studies indicated that allergic contact dermatitis is less likely to lead to chronicity than irritant contact dermatitis. The risk factor for chronicity of dermatitis in patients with contact dermatitis appears to be determined by the type or causes of contact dermatitis, the presence of atopy, and job change. The prognosis of contact dermatitis appears to be better in recent years.

References

Agrup G (1969) Hand eczema and other hand dermatoses in South Sweden. Acta Derm Venereol Suppl (Stockh) 49:61
Avnstorp C (1989) Follow-up of workers from the prefabricated concrete industry after the addition of ferrous sulphate to Danish cement. Contact Dermatitis 20:365–371
Burrows D (1972) Prognosis in industrial dermatitis. Br J Dermatol 87:145–148

Chia SE, Goh CL (1991) Prognosis of occupational dermatitis in Singapore worker. Am J Contact Dermat 2:105–109

Christensen OB (1982) Prognosis in nickel allergy and hand eczema. Contact Dermatitis 8:7–15

Coenraads PJ (1983) Prevalence of hand eczema. Association with occupational exposure, especially in construction workers (M.D. thesis). University of Groningen, Groningen

Fregert S (1975) Occupational dermatitis in a 10-year material. Contact Dermatitis 1:96–107

Goh CL, Gan SL (1996) Change in cement manufacturing process, a cause for decline in chromate allergy? Contact Dermatitis 34:51–54

Halbert AR, Gebauer KA, Wall LM (1992) Prognosis of occupational chromate dermatitis. Contact Dermatitis 27:214–219

Hellier FF (1958) The prognosis in industrial dermatitis. BMJ 1:196–198

Keczkes K, Bhate SM, Wyatt EH (1983) The outcome of primary irritant hand dermatitis. Br J Dermatol 109:665–668

Lips R, Rast H, Elsner P (1996) Outcome of job change in patients with occupational chromate dermatitis. Contact Dermatitis 34:268–271

Matsunaga K, Hosokawa K, Suzuki M, Arima Y, Hayakawa R (1998) Occupational allergic contact dermatitis in beautician. Contact Dermatitis 18:94–96

Nethercott J, Holness L (1994) Disease outcome in workers with occupational skin disease. J Am Acad Dermatol 30:569–574

Pryce DW, Irvine D, English JSC et al. (1989) Soluble oil dermatitis: a follow-up study. Contact Dermatitis 21:28–35

Rosen RH, Freeman S (1993) Prognosis of occupational contact dermatitis in New South Wales, Australia. Contact Dermatitis 29:88–93

Rystedt I (1985) Hand eczema and long-term prognosis in atopic dermatitis. Acta Derm Venereol Suppl (Stockh) 117:1–59

Schubert H, Berova N, Czernielewski A et al. (1987) Epidemiology of nickel allergy. Contact Dermatitis 16:122–128

Shah M, Lewis FM, Gawkrodger DJ (1996) Prognosis of occupational hand dermatitis in metalworkers. Contact Dermatitis 34:27–30

Skog E, Tottie M (1961) Occupational eczema causing disablement. Acta Derm Venereol 41:205–212

Williamson KS (1967) A prognostic study of occupational dermatitis cases in a chemical works. Br J Ind Med 24:103–113

Part 2
Substances, Products, Occupations, Concentrations

CHAPTER 26

Computerised Product Database: Registered Chemical Contact Allergens

26

M.-A. FLYVHOLM

Introduction to the Danish Product Register Database

A product database is one way to organise product information which, compared with, for example, labelling and data sheets, has some obvious advantages when it comes to cross-sectional overviews on the distribution of contact allergens on product categories. This chapter presents a study on selected contact allergens and their occurrence in product categories covered by the Danish Product Register Database.

PROBAS is the short name for the Danish Product Register Database. It is a common register for both external environmental and work environment authorities, and it is located at the Danish Working Environment Service.

Registration in PROBAS is based on obligatory notification rules, product data submitted to the authorities for various reasons, surveys and research projects on chemical products and other relevant sources. The database includes mainly dangerous products for occupational use. Other product categories are included, but often not fully covering the products marketed. All data input is done by the Product Register staff. In general, the notification rules require complete information on all of the product's components, and the notifiers have to update changes. PROBAS is a governmental database with no public access due to confidential data, which requires special regulations for its use. The registered information on products includes ingredients, industrial area of use, product category, quantities used or marketed, physical properties, labelling etc., and administrative information. For further description and discussion on the use of product databases, see (Flyvholm et al. 1992; Flyvholm 2000; Flyvholm 1991) and chapter 18 "Sources of Information on the Occurrence of Chemical Contact Allergens" elsewhere in this book (Flyvholm 2003).

Background Data for the Investigation

This study is based on data from the general product registration in PROBAS. This includes, in general, chemical products notified by producers or importers according to obligatory notification rules or in connection with surveys and research projects. In January 2002, PROBAS had information on a total of about 75,200 chemical products registered or updated within the last 5 years. About

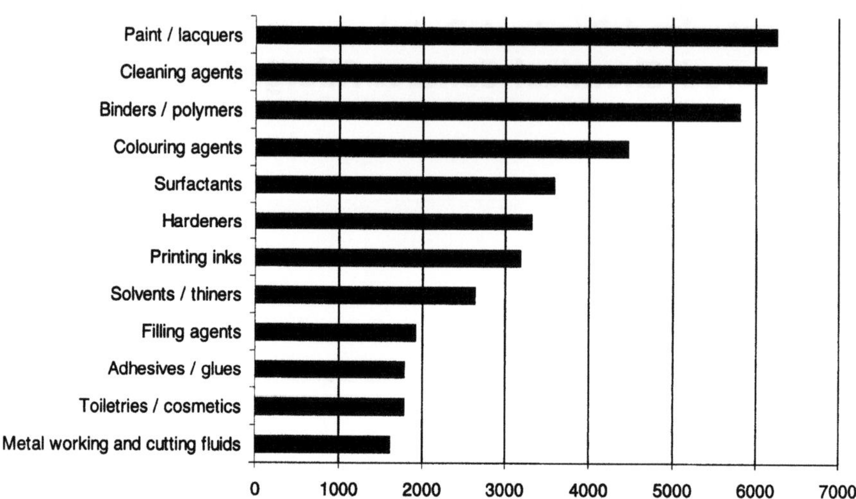

Fig. 1. The most frequently registered product categories for the general product registration in PROBAS. Based on 59,100 products active within the past 5 years and computerised with information on chemical composition and product category, January 2002

59,100 of these products were registered with information on both chemical composition and product category. Figure 1 shows the most frequently registered product categories for the general product registration in PROBAS, January 2002.

Selection of Contact Allergens for Investigation

Contact allergens relevant for chemical products were included in the study, i.e. contact allergens selected from the revised European standard series as recommended by the EECDRG 1994, the North American standard series and the list of proposed allergens for a modified international standard series (Lachapelle et al. 1997), substances classified "may cause contact sensitization by skin contact" (risk phrase R43) in lists of dangerous substances in Scandinavian countries and substances reported in textbooks on contact dermatitis. Substances registered in fewer than 30 products were excluded. All substances were identified by CAS RN (Chemical Abstract Service registry number).

Registered Chemical Contact Allergens

All products containing the selected contact allergens either as a component or in raw materials were included in the investigation. Table 1 shows the number of different products registered with the contents of each substance divided into selected product categories. In order to preserve confidentiality, data on substances registered in fewer than four products within a product category cannot be shown.

Table 1. Products registered with contact allergens divided into selected product categories. Based on 59,100 products active within the past five years and computerised with information on chemical composition and product category, January 2002. Products can be registered in more than one product category, and products can contain more than one of the allergens. Data on product categories with less than four products for each substance are not shown. (ST) substances included in the revised European standard series as recommended by the EECDRG 1994, the North America standard series or the list of proposed allergens for a modified international standard series (Lachapelle et al. 1997)

Product Categories	CAS RN	Adhesive/ Glues	Cleaning agents	Construction materials	Filling agents	Flooring agents	Hardeners	Impregnating agents	Paints/ lacquers	Polish	Printing inks	Toiletries and cosmetics	Total products for substances
Number of products registered for each product category:		1775	6126	827	1913	370	3312	497	6250	771	3176	1774	
Substances													
Aldehydes													
Formaldehyde (ST)	50-00-0	136	227	57	151	50	81	64	1157	28	311	31	3574
Glutaraldehyde	111-30-8	–	46	–	–	–	–	42	107	–	–	–	216
Amines													
Diaminodiphenylmethane	101-77-9	4	–	–	–	–	69	–	7	–	–	–	89
Diethylenetriamine	111-40-0	10	–	–	4	7	249	–	19	–	–	–	328
Ethylenediamine	107-15-3	5	5	–	7	–	56	–	59	–	–	–	192
Isophoronediamine	2855-13-2	–	–	6	8	57	398	–	47	–	–	–	502

Table 1 (continued)

Product Categories	CAS RN	Adhesive/ Glues	Cleaning agents	Construction materials	Filling agents	Flooring agents	Hardeners	Impregnating agents	Paints/ lacquers	Polish	Printing inks	Toiletries and cosmetics	Total products for substances
Tetraethylenepentamine	112-57-2	–	–	–	7	9	175	–	21	–	–	–	218
Triethanolamine	102-71-6	16	235	99	103	4	17	8	187	62	72	13	1316
Triethylenediamine	280-57-9	15	–	9	20	–	22	–	72	–	–	–	231
Triethylenetetramine	112-24-3	5	–	–	10	10	385	–	59	–	–	–	477
Epoxy Bisphenol A diglycidyl ether, monomer (ST)	1675-54-3	112	–	33	105	87	77	7	544	–	165	–	1415
Epichlorohydrin (ST)	106-89-8	188	–	43	184	140	158	9	810	–	303	–	2451
Isocyanates 2,4-diisocyanatotoluene [TDI]	584-84-9	14	–	–	35	6	46	5	194	–	128	–	475
Hexamethylene-1,6-diisocyanate [HDI]	822-06-0	22	–	–	12	6	318	–	102	–	22	–	509

Table 1 (continued)

Product Categories	CAS RN	Adhesive/Glues	Cleaning agents	Construction materials	Filling agents	Flooring agents	Hardeners	Impregnating agents	Paints/lacquers	Polish	Printing inks	Toiletries and cosmetics	Total products for substances
Isophorone diisocyanate [IPDI]	4098-71-9	14	–	–	18	7	72	–	32	–	98	–	287
4,4′-methylenebis(phenylisocyanate) [MDI]	101-68-8	127	–	15	136	12	219	–	39	–	277	–	888
Preservatives													
Benzalkonium chloride	8001-54-5	–	62	–	–	–	–	–	5	–	–	8	103
1,2-benzisothiazolin-3-one	2634-33-5	15	52	–	8	7	8	75	253	55	110	–	788
Benzoic acid	65-85-0	–	17	–	4	–	6	–	175	–	–	–	325
Benzyl alcohol	100-51-6	16	86	9	44	92	471	–	195	21	78	37	1288
2-bromo-2-nitro-1,3-propanediol [Bronopol]	52-51-7	10	97	5	–	6	–	62	177	14	–	60	514
Butylated hydroxytoluene [BHT]	128-37-0	58	69	24	110	54	107	20	1164	10	439	189	2815

Table 1 (continued)

Product Categories	CAS RN	Adhe-sive/ Glues	Cleaning agents	Con-struc-tion materials	Filling agents	Flooring agents	Harden-ers	Impreg-nating agents	Paints/ lacquers	Polish	Printing inks	Toiletries and cos-metics	Total products for sub-stances
Chloroal-lylhexami-nium chloride [Quaternium 15] (ST)	4080-31-3	–	5	–	–	–	–	–	–	5	–	16	33
CMI/MI the CMI part: 5-chloro-2-methyl-4-isothiazolin-3-one (ST)	26172-55-4	28	133	7	26	11	9	35	498	94	168	281	1907
CMI/MI the MI part: 2-methyl-4-isothiazolin-3-one (ST)	2682-20-4	26	135	7	25	11	9	35	497	89	167	279	1872
Cresol	1319-77-3	9	–	–	4	–	–	–	20	–	–	–	75
2,5 diazolidi-nylurea (ST)	78491-02-8	–	–	–	–	–	–	–	–	–	–	35	38

Table 1 (continued)

Product Categories	CAS RN	Adhesive/ Glues	Cleaning agents	Construction materials	Filling agents	Flooring agents	Hardeners	Impregnating agents	Paints/ lacquers	Polish	Printing inks	Toiletries and cosmetics	Total products for substances
1,2-dibromo-2,4-dicyanobutane (ST)	35691-65-7	–	12	–	–	–	–	–	–	–	–	36	61
Imidazolidinyl urea	39236-46-9	–	–	–	–	–	–	–	–	–	–	193	196
Mercaptobenzothiazole [MBT] (ST)	149-30-4	–	5	–	–	–	7	–	22	–	20	–	84
Parabens													
Butylparaben (ST)	94-26-8	–	–	–	–	–	–	–	–	–	–	82	101
Ethylparaben (ST)	120-47-8	–	–	–	–	–	–	–	–	–	–	59	81
Methylparaben (ST)	99-76-3	–	26	–	–	–	–	–	–	9	–	390	492
Propylparaben (ST)	94-13-3	–	24	–	–	–	–	–	–	7	–	337	430

M.-A. Flyvholm

Table 1 (continued)

Product Categories	CAS RN	Adhe-sive/ Glues	Cleaning agents	Con-struc-tion materials	Filling agents	Flooring agents	Harden-ers	Impreg-nating agents	Paints/ lacquers	Polish	Printing inks	Toiletries and cos-metics	Total products for sub-stances
Resins													
Colophony (ST)	8050-09-7	38	6	–	8	–	11	–	110	12	84	6	541
Para-tert-bu-tylphenol formaldehyde resin (ST)	25085-50-1	18	–	–	6	–	4	–	16	–	–	–	91
Phenol-form-aldehyde resin	9003-35-4	21	–	–	17	–	7	–	52	–	4	–	221
Urea-formal-dehyde resin	9011-05-6	18	–	–	–	–	–	–	110	–	–	–	179

Formaldehyde was the most frequently registered substance (3,574 products), followed by some preservatives, i.e. butylated hydroxytoluene (BHT, 2,815 products) and 5-chloro-2-methyl-4-isothiazolin-3-one and 2-methyl-4-isothiazolin-3-one (CMI/MI, 1,907 and 1,872 products) and epoxy compounds (2,451 and 1,415 products).

Substances from Standard Patch-Test Series

The European standard patch-test series from 1994 included 22 substances or mixtures (Bruynzeel et al. 1995), the North American standard series included 20 substances or mixtures, and the list of proposed allergens for a modified international standard series included 20 substances or mixtures (Lachapelle et al. 1997). A total of 10 substances or mixtures from these lists were included in the present study (15 different CAS RNs). The remaining substances from the standard patch-test series were either not relevant to chemical products (i.e. medicaments, pharmaceuticals, perfumery, rubber, metals, plants) or only sparsely registered in the product categories included in this study. Most of the contact allergens from the standard patch-test series included in this study are part of the modified international standard patch-test series as proposed by the International Contact Dermatitis Research Group. Parabens were included in a proposed list of allergens for an extended international standard patch-test series (Lachapelle et al. 1997).

Aldehydes

Formaldehyde was registered most frequently in paints/lacquers, printing inks and cleaning agents. Glutaraldehyde was registered in paints/lacquers, cleaning agents and impregnating agents.

Amines

Amines were mainly registered in hardeners and paints/lacquers. Triethanolamine was the most frequently registered amine and occurred mainly in cleaning agents, paints/lacquers, toiletries/cosmetics, filling agents and construction materials.

Epoxy

Bisphenol A diglycidyl ether monomer and epichlorohydrin were mainly registered in paints/lacquers, and product categories containing binding agents, such as printing inks, adhesives/glues and filling agents.

Isocyanates

Isocyanates were mainly registered in hardeners (HDI and MDI), printing inks (MDI, TDI and IPDI) and paints/lacquers (TDI and HDI). 4,4'-methylene-bis (phenylisocyanate) (MDI) was the most frequently registered and occurred also in filling agents and adhesives/glues.

Preservatives

Preservatives were registered in most of the product categories included in the study, although, some preservatives were mainly registered in toiletries and cosmetics. Paints/lacquers, toiletries/cosmetics, cleaning agents and printing inks were the most frequent. BHT and isothiazolinones also occurred in printing inks and benzyl alcohol in hardeners. The most frequently registered preservatives were BHT, CMI/MI and benzyl alcohol.

Resins

The resins included in the study were colophony and three formaldehyde resins. They were mainly registered in paints/lacquers and adhesives/glues. Colophony also occurred in printing inks.

Product Categories

Registration of the investigated contact allergens in selected product categories is shown in Table 1. Product categories registered with few of the investigated allergens or registered with less than four products for each substance were excluded. Among the product categories included, paints/lacquers, cleaning agents, hardeners and printing inks were the most frequently registered, followed by filling agents, adhesives/glues and toiletries/cosmetics. The registration of toiletries and cosmetics includes only a minor part of the products marketed in Denmark. Thus, the occurrence of contact allergens in toiletries and cosmetics will not show the real picture, but can give information on which contact allergens to expect both in industrial products and in toiletries/cosmetics or personal care products.

Adhesives

Among the allergens included in this study, epoxy compounds, formaldehyde and MDI were the most frequently registered in the group of adhesives/glues.

Cleaning Agents

The most frequently registered allergens in cleaning agents were triethanolamine, formaldehyde, CMI/MI and Bronopol.

Construction Materials

Triethanolamine, formaldehyde and epoxy compounds were the most frequently registered allergens in construction materials.

Filling Agents (such as Stopping, Putty)

The most frequently registered allergens in filling agents were formaldehyde, epoxy compounds, MDI, BHT and triethanolamine.

Flooring Agents

Epoxy compounds, benzyl alcohol, isophoronediamine, BHT and formaldehyde were the most frequently registered allergens in flooring agents.

Hardeners for Paints/Lacquers, Plastics

The most frequently registered allergens in hardeners were benzyl alcohol, several amines (isophoronediamine, triethylenetetramine, diethylenetriamine, tetraethylenepentamine) and isocyanates (HDI and MDI).

Impregnating Agents

The most frequently registered allergens in impregnating agents were 1,2-benzisothiazolin-3-one, formaldehyde, Bronopol and CMI/MI.

Paints/Lacquers

The most frequently registered allergens in paints/lacquers were BHT, formaldehyde and epoxy compounds, followed by CMI/MI and 1,2-benzisothiazolin-3-one.

Polish

The most frequently registered allergens in polishes were CMI/MI, triethanolamine and 1,2-benzisothiazolin-3-one.

Printing Inks

BHT, formaldehyde, epoxy compounds and isocyanates (MDI and TDI), followed by CMI/MI, were the most frequently registered allergens in printing inks.

Toiletries and Cosmetics

This product category is a combination of hair care products, skin care products and cosmetics. Among the allergens included in this study, parabens (especially methyl- and propylparaben), CMI/MI, imidazolidinyl urea, BHT and triethanolamine were the most frequently registered in toiletries/cosmetics. The selection of allergens for the present study may cause a distorted picture of the occurrence of allergens in toiletries/cosmetics, but it can show which allergens relevant in chemical products can also be found in this product category.

Discussion

It is important to remember that the distribution of allergens in product categories in a study such as the present is highly influenced by the selection of contact allergens for investigation. Thus, product categories registered as containing only a few of the studied allergens may also contain other allergens.

One way to use this information on occurrence of contact allergens in registered chemical products is either to search for allergens to patch test in patients exposed to a specific product category or to look for other sources of exposure to certain allergens.

For advising individual patients, it is always important to consult the data sheets and labelling for the specific products used at their workplaces. The labelling of chemical products is impaired by the default 1% threshold for the majority of contact allergens, which is typically too high for sensitizers of normal potency. Furthermore, the limited number of allergens classified with R43 ("may cause contact sensitization by skin contact") adds to the limitations of data sheets and labelling compared with databases with registration of complete product composition.

A study comparing the registration of contact allergens in chemical products in 1990 and 1998 showed that occurrence of isothiazolinones increased considerably during that period (Flyvholm 2000). This tendency seems to continue in the present study, although these studies cannot be compared directly due to changes in the PROBAS database and improved possibilities of excluding products that are no longer active in the marketplace.

References

Bruynzeel DP, Andersen KE, Camarasa JG, Lachapelle J-M, Menné T, White IR (1995) The European standard series. Contact Dermatitis 33:145–148

Flyvholm M-A (1991) Contact allergens in registered chemical products. Contact Dermatitis 25:49-56

Flyvholm M-A (2000) Computerized product database. Registered chemical contact allergens. In: Kanerva L, Elsner P, Wahlberg JE, Maibach HI (eds) Handbook of Occupational Dermatology. Springer, Berlin Heidelberg New York, pp 451–461

Flyvholm M-A (2003) Sources of information on the occurrence of chemical contact allergens. In: Elsner P, Wahlberg JE, Maibach HI (eds) Condensed Handbook of Occupational Dermatology. Springer, Berlin Heidelberg New York, pp 207–211
Flyvholm M-A, Andersen P, Beck ID, Brandorff NP (1992) PROBAS: The Danish Product Register Data Base – a national register of chemical substances and products. J Hazardous Mater 30:59–69
Lachapelle J-M, Ale SI, Freeman S, Frosch PJ, Goh CL, Hannuksela M, Hayakawa R, Maibach HI, Wahlberg JE (1997) Proposal for a revised international standard series of patch tests. Contact Dermatitis 36:121–123

CHAPTER 27

Fragrances   27

A.C. DE GROOT

Introduction

Perfumes are so much a part of our culture that we take them for granted, but if they were suddenly taken from us, our culture would suffer immeasurably. We do pay a price for their service, however, and part of that is dermatologic and other medical reactions. This chapter discusses contact allergic reactions to fragrance materials. For a full review of this subject see De Groot and Frosch (1997). An extended version of this chapter was published recently (De Groot 2000).

The Composition of Perfumes

Perfumery is the art of making individuals and products attractive to the olfactory sense. Of the thousands of chemical substances that have an odour, about 3000 (of which 300–400 are of natural origin) are used in the fragrance industry. A perfume is a creative composition of a few to over 300 fragrance materials. "Proper" perfumes contain approximately 12–20% of the perfume compound. They are expensive and very concentrated. The more diluted products (perfume lotion, perfume de toilette, eau de toilette, colognes) are therefore much more popular. Approximate concentrations of fragrance materials in cosmetics and other products are given in Table 1.

Widely used fragrance chemicals in perfumes, cosmetics, household products, and soap include linalool, phenylethyl alcohol, linalyl acetate, benzyl acetate, terpineol and γ-methylionone. Of the eight fragrances present in the fragrance mix (vide infra), four belong to the top 25: geraniol (>40%), eugenol (>25%) α-amyl-cinnamic aldehyde (>20%), and hydroxycitronellal (>20%) (De Groot et al 1994).

Contact with Fragrances and Fragranced Products

The use of fragrances is ubiquitous and not limited to those cosmetic products that are used primarily for their scent (such as perfumes, eaux de cologne, eaux de toilette, deodorant and aftershave). Virtually all cosmetics and toiletries contain fragrance materials; even "unscented" or "fragrance-free" products may contain a masking perfume (Scheinman 1999). A wide range of products may be scented and cause contact allergic reactions (Table 2).

Table 1. Concentrations of perfume in various products

Aerosol freshener	0.5–2%
Bathroom cleaners	≤5%
Colognes	2–5%
Compressed powder	0.5%
Dishwashing liquid	0.1–0.5%
Facial make-up	1.0%
Hair pomade	0.5%
Hair spray	0.1–0.3%
Laundry powder	0.1–0.3%
Lipstick	1.0%
Liquid detergents	0.1–1%
Masking perfume	≤0.1%
Perfume	12–20% (or higher)
Perfume lotion	5–8%
Shower and bath formulations	0.5–4%
Skin care products (emulsions)	0.3–0.5%
Soap	0.5–2%
Toilet water	5–8% (or higher)

Table 2. Fragranced products

Cosmetics not primarily used for their scent
Cosmetics used for their scent (perfume, deodorant, after-shave)
Fabrics and clothes, especially when laundered or treated with softener
Household products (cleaners, softeners, deodorizing sprays, polishes, solvents, waxes)
Industrial products (cutting fluids, electroplating fluids, paints, rubber, plastics, insecticides, air conditioning water)
Oral hygiene products (toothpaste, mouthwash, dental floss)
Paper and paper products (diapers, facial tissues, moist toilet paper, sanitary napkins)
Spices and flavours in foods and drinks (natural and synthetic)
Topical drugs
Ventilating systems

Contact with fragrances may be from direct product application to the skin or mucous membranes [toothpaste (Francalanci et al 2000), mouth fresheners, feminine hygiene sprays, perfumed eyedrops], by occasional contact with an allergen-contaminated product such as towels and pillows, contact with products used by partners, friends or co-workers (consort or connubial contact dermatitis) (Morren et al. 1992), airborne contact (Dooms-Goossens and Deleu 1991; Dooms-Goossens 1993), and systemic exposure by inhalation and ingestion (fragrances, flavours and spices in foods and drinks, cough syrup).

Any part of the body may be in contact with fragranced cosmetics.

Epidemiology of Fragrance Allergy

Adverse reactions to fragrances/fragranced cosmetics appear to be far from rare. Guin and Berry (1980) conducted a questionnaire study of 90 student nurses; 29

(32%) gave a history of cutaneous fragrance intolerance. When tested with the fragrance mix ($8\times2\%$), 15 (18%) showed a positive reaction. Of these 15, 12 (80%) had a positive history of fragrance sensitivity. In the general Danish population, 10.6% has experienced a rash from the use of scented products in a 1-year-period (Johansen et al 2000). Also in Denmark, 567 unselected individuals aged 15–69 years were tested with the fragrance mix, and 6 (1.1%) had a positive reaction (Nielsen and Menné 1992). The frequency of reactivity in men (1.1%) was identical to that in women (1.0%).

The adverse reaction seen most frequently by dermatologists in response to fragrances is allergic contact dermatitis. In most countries, the fragrance mix is positive in 6–11% of patients patch tested for suspected allergic contact dermatitis. Perfumes account for 4–18% of all reactions, and deodorants/antiperspirants account for 5–17% of all cases of allergic cosmetic dermatitis (De Groot et al. 1994).

Clinical Picture of Allergic Contact Dermatitis from Fragrances

Literature on the clinical picture of perfume dermatitis is rather scant and a good description is lacking. It can be expected, however, that the neck, skin behind the ear and axillae (Johansen et al 1998) are often implicated, given that they are exposed to products with high concentrations of fragrances (perfume, deodorant). Also, the sensitive skin of the face (Wohrl et al. 2001) and the eyelids should be particularly susceptible to developing allergic contact dermatitis to fragrances in skin care products, decorative cosmetics and cleansing preparations, and from airborne contact dermatitis (Dooms-Goossens and Deleu 1991; Dooms-Goossens 1993). Micro-traumata from shaving facilitates (photo) contact allergy to aftershave fragrances (Edman 1994).

Most reactions are erythematous, and some cases may resemble nummular eczema, seborrhoeic dermatitis, sycosis barbae, or lupus erythematosus (Meynadier et al. 1986). More acute lesions with papules, vesicles and oozing may sometimes be observed. Lesions in the skin folds may be mistaken for atopic dermatitis. Dermatitis due to perfumes or toilet water tends to be "streaky".

Hand eczema is common in fragrance-sensitive patients (Buckley et al 2000, Johansen et al. 1996). Usually, patients first have irritant dermatitis or atopic dermatitis, which is later complicated by contact allergy to products used for treatment (fragranced topical drugs) or prevention (hand creams and lotions [Johansen et al. 1998b]) of hand dermatitis, or to other perfumed products in the household, hobby, or work environment. Dyshidrotic eruptions are ascribed to ingestion of spices (Meynadier et al. 1986). Atopic dermatitis located at other body sites, perianal dermatitis, and vulvar dermatitis (Lewis et al. 1997) may also be complicated by fragrance allergy.

Detecting Allergic Contact Dermatitis from Fragrances
with the Fragrance Mix

A perfume may contain as many as 200 or more individual ingredients. This makes the diagnosis of perfume allergy by patch test procedures complicated.

Screening agents such as the fragrance mix, balsam of Peru and, to some extent, colophony have been incorporated into the standard series to overcome the problem. The fragrance mix, or perfume mix, was introduced as a screening tool for fragrance sensitivity in the late 1970s. It contains eight fragrance materials: eugenol, isoeugenol, oak moss, geraniol, hydroxycitronellal, a-amylcinnamic aldehyde, cinnamic aldehyde and cinnamic alcohol. It is estimated that this mix detects 70–80% of fragrance sensitivity cases.

The response rate in dermatological patients to the fragrance mix and its ingredients ranges worldwide from 6% to 11%, and the fragrance mix is usually the second most frequent allergen after nickel sulphate (De Groot and Frosch 1997).

Several studies have investigated the frequency of allergic reactions to the ingredients of the fragrance mix (Frosch et al. 1995a,b; Johansen and Menné 1995; Buckley et al. 2000). Although the results have varied widely, most reactions appear to be caused by oak moss, isoeugenol and cinnamic aldehyde, whereas geraniol, a-amylcinnamic aldehyde and hydroxycitronellal usually yield lower positive reaction scores.

Sensitivity to oak moss (Gonçalo et al. 1988) is frequently induced by the use of aftershave lotions, because the integrity of the epidermis is lost during shaving, facilitating sensitisation. Lichen acids (present in oak moss) that cause reactions in allergic patients include atranorin, usnic acid, evernic acid, fumarprotocetraric acid, stitic acid, physodes/physodalic acid and diffractaic acid (Fregert and Dahlquist 1983). Contact allergy to lichen acids may also be acquired from woods and plants (Stinchi et al. 1997).

The fragrance mix that is used currently ($8 \times 1\%$ with 5% sorbitan sesquioleate) is very useful, but not ideal. It may cause irritant reactions (Frosch et al. 1995a,b), irrelevant positive reactions (Frosch et al. 1995b; Johansen and Menné 1995), false-negative reactions, and leaves 20–30% of fragrance sensitivities undetected (Johansen et al. 1997). The sensitivity for detecting fragrance allergy may be enhanced by testing additional fragrances such as jasmine synthetic or absolute (Larsen 2000) and Lyral (Frosch et al 1999).

Clinical Relevance of a Positive Reaction to the Fragrance Mix

In various studies, the relevance of positive patch-test reactions to the mix has been investigated (see esp. De Groot 1999; also Frosch et al. 1995b; Marks et al. 1995; Johansen et al. 1996). However, criteria were often not provided. In cases with concomitant positive reactions to perfumes (Johansen et al 2001) or fragranced products used by the patient, interpretation of the reaction as relevant may be quite easy. Often, however, relevance may (correctly or incorrectly) only be assumed, as the role of fragrances is likely or cannot be excluded because of the ubiquitous occurrence of fragrances and multiple possible exposure moments from indirect contact, airborne exposure, inhalation or ingestion (flavours, spices).

Clinical relevance of a positive patch-test reaction may exist for at least 55–65% of positive results. Strongly positive patch test reactions (2+ or 3+) are more likely to be associated with a positive fragrance history than a weak or doubtful reaction (Frosch et al. 1995b). A positive ROAT (repeated open application test, twice daily application on the antecubital fossa for a maximum of two weeks) (Johansen et al. 1996) with fragrance ingredients makes relevance of the reaction more likely.

Less Common Fragrance Allergens

Several investigators have routinely tested one or more fragrance materials in patients suspected of contact dermatitis (Frosch et al. 1995a). Prevalence rates of greater than 1% have been observed with benzyl salicylate, carvone, citral, coumarin, farnesol, isobornyl cyclohexanol (synthetic sandalwood oil), jasmine absolute, jasmine synthetic, methyl salicylate, musk ambrette, oil of bergamot, rose oil, sandalwood oil, santalol and ylang-ylang oil. In other studies, various fragrances were tested in patients suspected to have cosmetic or fragrance allergies. In an international study (Larsen et al. 1996), most reactions were to ylang-ylang oil (17%), narcissus oil (7%), sandela (7%), sandalwood oil (7%), majantol (5%), benzyl salicylate (5%) and galbanum resin (5%). Most recently, the same investigators found the following fragrances reacting at a rate of 2% or higher in 178 fragrance allergic individuals: jasmine absolute, geranium oil bourbon, l-citronellol, spearmint oil, 1,3,4,6,7,8-hexahydro-4,6,6,7,8,8-hexamethylcyclopenta-γ-2-benzopyran, ω-6-hexadecenlactone, dimethyltetrahydrobenzaldehyde and a-amylcinnamaldehyde (Larsen et al 2001). A list of documented fragrance allergens is provided in Table 3, with their test concentrations (de Groot 2000).

Table 3. Fragrances reported as allergens (de Groot 1994; de Groot 2000)

Name of fragrance	Test concentration/vehicle
Acetylcedrene (Vertofix)	1%–5% pet
5-Acetyl-1,1,2,3,3,6-hexamethylindan (Phantolide)	3% pet
Amyl cinnamate	8% pet
a-Amylcinnamic alcohol	5% pet
a-Amylcinnamic aldehyde	3%–5% pet
Amyl salicylate	5% pet
Anethole	5% pet
Anisyl alcohol	5% pet
Anisylidene acetone	2% pet
Atranorin (in oak moss)	0.5% pet
Benzyl acetate	5% pet
Benzyl alcohol	5% pet
Benzyl benzoate	5% pet
Benzyl cinnamate	5% pet
Benzylidene acetone	0.5% pet
Benzyl salicylate	1% pet
Carvacrol (isothymol)	5% pet
Cashmeran (6,7-dihydro-1,1,2,3, 3-pentamethyl-4(5H)-indanone)	5% pet
Cedramber (cedrol methyl ether)	5% pet

Table 3 (continued)

Name of fragrance	Test concentration/vehicle
Cinnamic alcohol	3%–5% pet
Cinnamic aldehyde	1% pet
Cinnamyl benzoate	5% pet
Cinnamyl cinnamate	5% pet
Citral	2% pet
Citronellol	5% pet
Coumarin	5% pet
Cuminaldehyde	5% pet
Cyclopentadecanone[a]	5% pet
Dehydro-isoeugenol	ylang-ylang oil
Diethyl maleate	2% pet
Diffractaic acid (in oak moss)	1% pet
Dihydrocoumarin	5% pet
Dimethyl citraconate	10% pet
Dimethyltetrahydrobenzaldehyde[a]	5% pet
DMBCA (dimethylbenzyl carbinyl acetate)	3% pet
Ethyl acrylate	0.1% pet
Ethyl anisate	4% pet
Eucalyptol (1,8-cineole, cajeputol)	5% pet
Eugenol	3%–5% pet
Evernic acid (in oak moss)	0.1% pet
Farnesol	5% pet
Fixolide	3% pet
Floropal (acetaldehyde 2-phenyl-2, 4-pentane-diol acetal)	5% pet
Fumarprotocetraric acid (in oak moss)	0.1% pet
Galbanum resin	2% pet
Geranial	1%–5% pet
Geraniol	3%–5% pet
Helional (a-methyl-3,4-methylene dioxyhydrocinnamic aldehyde)	5% pet
Heliotropin	5% pet
Hexadecanolide[a]	5% pet
ω-6-hexadecenlactone[a]	5% pet
1,3,4,6,7,8-Hexahydro-4,6,6,7,8, 8-hexamethyl-cyclopenta-γ-2-benzopyran (Galaxolide)	15% pet
cis-3-Hexenyl salicylate	3% pet
a-Hexylcinnamic aldehyde	10% pet
Hexyl salicylate	12% pet
Hydroabietyl alcohol (Abitol)	10% pet
Hydroxycitronellal	3%–5% pet
Ionone	8% pet
Isobornyl cyclohexanol (synthetic sandalwood)	2% pet
Isoeugenol	3%–5% pet
Isoeugenyl acetate	2% pet
Isolongifolene ketone[a]	5% pet
Isopulegol	5% pet
Jasmine (absolute, synthetic)	5%–10% pet
Ligustral ((methyl-(2,4(3, 5)-dimethyl-3-cyclo-hexen-1-yl)-methylene anthranilate)	5% pet
Lilial (lily aldehyde, p-tert-butyl-a-methylhydro-cinnnamic aldehyde)	5% pet

Table 3 (continued)

Name of fragrance	Test concentration/vehicle
d-Limonene	2% pet
Linalool	2%–30% pet
Lyral (4–4-hydroxy-4-methylpentyl)3-cyclo-hexenel-1-carbox-aldehyde)	5% pet
Majantol (2,2-dimethyl-3-(3-methylphenyl)-propanol)	5% pet
o-Methoxycinnamic aldehyde	4% pet
Methoxycitronellal	10% pet
Methyl anisate	4% pet
Methyl heptine carbonate	0.5% pet/1% MEK
Methylionantheme	0.04% alc
γ-Methylionone	10% pet
Methyl octine carbonate	1% MEK
Methyl salicylate	2% pet
3-Methyl-5–5-(2,2,3-trimethyl-3-cyclopenten-1-yl)pent-4-en-2-ol) [a]	5% pet
Musk ambrette	5% pet
Musk moskene	5% pet
Musk xylene	5% pet
Narcissus oil	2% pet
Neral	2% pet
Nopyl acetate	10% pet
Oak moss	3%–5% pet
1-(1,2,3,4,5,6,7,8-Octahydro-2,3,8,8-tetramethyl-2-naphthalenyl)ethanone [a]	5% pet
Patchouli oil	2% pet
Phenylacetaldehyde (hyacinthin)	0.5% pet
Phenylethyl alcohol	5% pet
Physodes/physodalic acid (in oak moss)	0.1% pet
β-Pinene	15% pet
Propylidene phthalide	2% pet
Rhodinol (mixture of 1-citronellol and geraniol)	3% pet
Rose oil (Bulgarian)	2% pet
Sandalore (5-(-2,2,3-trimethyl-3-cyclopentenyl)–3-methylpentan-2-ol)	5% pet
Sandalwood oil	2% pet
Sandela (isobornyl cyclohexanol + 3-trans-isocamphyl cyclohexanol)	5% pet
Santalol	2% pet
Stitic acid (in oak moss)	0.1% pet
α-Terpineol	5% pet
1,1,6,7-Tetramethyl-6-acetyl decalene (isomers) (Iso E Super)	1%–5% pet
Thymol	1% pet
Tree moss absolute	5% pet
Tricyclodecen-4-yl 8-acetate (Cyclacet)	5% pet
Usnic acid (in oak moss)	0.1% pet
Violet leaves absolute	2% pet
Ylang-ylang oil	5% pet

Alc alcohol, *Pet* petrolatum, *MEK* methyl ethyl ketone
[a] Larsen et al (2001)

Occupational Allergic Contact Dermatitis to Fragrances

It may be expected that fragrances will cause dermatological problems for workers in the cosmetics industry (cosmetic chemists, workers handling the raw materials and the final products, salespeople), beauticians, hairdressers, and aroma therapists. Housewives, health personnel and cleaning personnel may also be endangered by frequent contact with soap, cleansers, dishwashing liquids and other fragranced products. In spite of this, surprisingly little information on occupational allergic contact dermatitis from fragrances can be found in the literature. This may be because in the majority of people at risk, a definitive relationship between dermatitis and fragrances is hard to prove. In many occupations (hairdressers, beauticians, housewives, health personnel, cleaning personnel) irritant factors may also be relevant in the aetiology of dermatitis, and sometimes other allergens are also considered of paramount importance. In addition, non-occupational exposure to fragrances occurs in virtually everybody.

Most of the pertinent information comes from studies of hairdressers. Holness and Nethercott (1990) found a very high frequency (18%) of allergic reactions to the fragrance mix in hairdressers, but the frequency in controls was as high. Reactions to cinnamic alcohol and cinnamic aldehyde occurred less frequently in hairdressers than in referents (Holness and Nethercott 1990). In Italy, Guerra et al. (1992) considered nine reactions to fragrance mix to be relevant in 184 hairdressers with allergic occupational contact dermatitis. In the Netherlands, Van der Walle and Brunsveld (1994) reported eight positive reactions in 103 hairdressers, but did not comment on the relevance of these reactions.

In Italy, Gola et al. (1992) found the fragrance mix to be the second most frequent allergen in non-occupational contact dermatitis, even though it was not one of the top 10 allergens in occupational contact dermatitis. In their occupational contact dermatitis clinic, Holness and Nethercott (1994) tested 601 patients with possible work-related dermatitis and found almost 20% positive reactions to the fragrance mix. However, in only 3% of the positive reactors was the allergy felt to be work-related. In Australia, perfume fragrances were listed as allergens in 3 of 103 women with occupational allergic contact dermatitis (Wall and Gebauer 1991); fragrances were not implicated in any of the 265 men. In Taiwan, Sun et al. (1995) found six reactions (8.8%) to the fragrance mix to be relevant in 68 patients with occupational allergic contact dermatitis: four in hairdressers, one in construction and one in medical work.

Goodfield and Saihan (1988) found a 44% prevalence of sensitivity to one or more fragrances in 35 coal miners, compared with 22% in male and 17% in female non-miner controls. The high frequency was attributed to the use of a highly perfumed body lotion provided at the pit-head bath, and to the facilitation of contact sensitisation due to the frequent occurrence of irritant dermatitis from working in the coal-mines (Goodfield and Saihan 1988).

On the basis of these data, it is concluded that fragrances may play a role in some cases of occupational contact dermatitis, but in no single profession are they a major cause of occupational allergic contact dermatitis, and rarely are they the sole aetiological factor. However, fragrances may play an important role in aggravating hand eczema of other origin (atopic hand eczema, irritant dermatitis, allergic contact dermatitis) by contact with hand cleansers, barrier creams, moisturising preparations, skin disinfectants, etc. (Uter et al 2001). In addition, flavours and spices may be involved in occupational contact dermatitis in bakers, cooks, caterers, and others working in the food industry.

Conclusions and Recommendations

Virtually everyone is exposed continuously to fragrances through contact with perfumes, cosmetics, toiletries, oral hygiene products, household products, paper products, topical drugs, industrial contact materials and through contact with flavours and spices in foods and beverages. The most frequent cutaneous adverse reaction to fragrances is allergic contact dermatitis. Considering the ubiquitous occurrence of fragrance materials, the risk of such side effects is relatively small. In absolute numbers, however, fragrance allergy is common. Approximately 1% of the unselected population is sensitised to fragrance materials. Indeed, fragrances are the most common causes of allergic contact dermatitis from cosmetics. Any part of the body may be affected. Classic locations are the face, behind the ears, the neck, and the axillae. Hand dermatitis is also frequent in fragrance-sensitive subjects. Fragrances are probably rarely the sole cause of hand eczema. These patients usually have irritant or atopic hand dermatitis first, which is later complicated by fragrance contact allergy to products used for treatment or prevention, or to other perfumed products in the household, hobby or work environment. Occupational contact dermatitis from fragrances seems to be relatively uncommon.

The currently used fragrance mix (eugenol, isoeugenol, oak moss, geraniol, hydroxycitronellal, α-amylcinnamic aldehyde, cinnamic aldehyde, cinnamic alcohol, each 1% with 5% sorbitan sesquioleate) is valuable for diagnosing fragrance sensitisation. Between 6% and 11% of patients routinely tested because of suspected allergic contact dermatitis react to the fragrance mix, and in most centres the mix is among the top 5 frequent allergens, usually ranking second after nickel sulphate. Relevance is established in 50–65% of all cases, but more strict criteria should probably be applied, and there is a need to further investigate the profile of the fragrance-sensitive patient.

References

Buckley DA, Rycroft RJG, White IR, McFadden JP (2000) Contact allergy to individual fragrance mix constituents in relation to primary site of dermatitis Contact Dermatitis 43:304–305
De Groot AC (1994) Patch testing, 2nd edn. Elsevier, Amsterdam
De Groot AC (1999) Clinical relevance of positive patch test reactions to preservatives and fragrances. Contact Dermatitis 41:224–226
De Groot AC (2000) Fragrances. In: L Kanerva, P Elsner, JE Wahlberg, HI Maibach, eds. Handbook of occupational dermatology. Springer, Berlin Heidelberg New York, pp 497–508

De Groot AC, Frosch PJ (1997) Adverse reactions to fragrances. A clinical review. Contact Dermatitis 36:57–86

De Groot AC, Weyland JW, Nater JP (1994) Unwanted effects of cosmetics and drugs used in dermatology, 3rd edn. Elsevier, Amsterdam

Dooms-Goossens A (1993) Cosmetics as causes of allergic contact dermatitis. Cutis 52:316–320

Dooms-Goossens A, Deleu H (1991) Airborne contact dermatitis: an update. Contact Dermatitis 25:211–217

Edman B (1994) The influence of shaving method on perfume allergy. Contact Dermatitis 31:291–292

Francalanci S, Sertoli A, Giorgini S, et al (2000) Multicentre study of allergic contact cheilitis from toothpastes. Contact Dermatitis 43:216–222

Fregert S, Dahlquist I (1983) Patch testing with oak moss extract. Contact Dermatitis 9:227

Frosch PJ, Johansen JD, Menné T (1999) Lyral is an important sensitizer in patients sensitive to fragrances. Br J Dermatol 141:1076–1083

Frosch PJ, Pilz B, Andersen KE, et al (1995a) Patch testing with fragrances: results of a multicenter study of the European Environmental and Contact Dermatitis Research Group with 48 frequently used constituents of perfumes. Contact Dermatitis 33:333–342

Frosch PJ, Pilz B, Burrows D, et al (1995b) Testing with the fragrance mix – is the addition of sorbitan sesquioleate to the constituents useful? Contact Dermatitis 32:266–272

Gola M, Sertoli A, Angelini G, et al (1992) GIRDCA data bank for occupational and environmental contact dermatitis. Am J Contact Dermat 3:179–188

Gonçalo S, Cabral F, Gonçalo M (1988) Contact sensitivity to oak moss. Contact Dermatitis 19:355–357

Goodfield MJD, Saihan EM (1988) Fragrance sensitivity in coal miners. Contact Dermatitis 18:81–83

Guerra L, Tosti A, Bardazzi F, et al (1992) Contact dermatitis in hairdressers: the Italian experience. Contact Dermatitis 26:101–107

Guin JD, Berry VK (1980) Perfume sensitivity in adults females. A study of contact sensitivity to a perfume mix in two groups of student nurses. J Am Acad Dermatol 3:299–302

Holness DL, Nethercott JR (1990) Epicutaneous testing results in hairdressers. Am J Contact Dermat 2:224–234

Holness DL, Nethercott JR (1994) Patch testing in an occupational health clinic. Am J Contact Dermat 5:150–155

Johansen JD, Menné T (1995) The fragrance mix and its constituents: a 14-year material. Contact Dermatitis 32:18–23

Johansen JD, Rastogi SC, Menné T (1996) Exposure to selected fragrance materials. A case study of fragrance-mix-positive eczema patients. Contact Dermatitis 34:106–110

Johansen JD, Rastogi SC, Andersen KE, Menné T (1997) Content and reactivity to product perfumes in fragrance mix positive and negative eczema patients. Contact Dermatitis 36:291–296

Johansen JD, Rastogi SC, Bruze M, et al (1998) Deodorants: a clinical provocation study in fragrance-sensitive individuals. Contact Dermatitis 39:161–165

Johansen JD, Andersen TF, Kjøller M, et al (1998b) Identification of risk products for fragrance contact allergy. A case-referent study based on patients' histories. Am J Contact Dermatitis 9:80–87

Johansen JD, Andersen TF, Thomsen LK, et al (2000) Rash related to use of scented products. A questionnaire study in the Danish population. Is the problem increasing? Contact Dermatitis 42:222–226

Johansen JD, Frosch PJ, Rastogi SC, Menné T (2001) Testing with fine fragrances in eczema patients. Results and test methods. Contact Dermatitis 44:304–307

Larsen WG (2000) How to test for fragrance allergy. Cutis 65:39–41

Larsen W, Nakayama H, Lindberg M, et al (1996) Fragrance contact dermatitis. A worldwide multicenter investigation (Part I). Am J Contact Dermat 7:77–83

Larsen W, Nakayama H, Fischer T, et al (2001) Fragrance contact dermatitis: a worldwide multicenter investigation (part II). Contact Dermatitis 44:344–346

Lewis FM, Shah M, Gawkrodger DJ (1997) Contact sensitivity in pruritus vulvae: patch test results and clinical outcome. Am J Contact Dermat 8:137–140

Marks JG, Belsito DV, DeLeo VA, et al (1995) North American Contact Dermatitis Group standard tray patch test results (1992 to 1994). Am J Contact Dermat 6:160–165

Meynadier J-M, Meynadier J, Peyron J-L, Peyron L (1986) Formes cliniques des manifestations cutanées d'allergie aux parfums. Ann Dermatol Venereol 113:31–39

Morren M-A, Rodrigues R, Dooms-Goossens A, et al (1992) Connubial contact dermatitis: a review. Eur J Dermatol 2:219–223

Nielsen NH, Menné T (1992) Allergic contact sensitization in an unselected Danish population. Acta Derm Venereol 72:456–460

Scheinman PL (1999) The foul side of fragrance-free products: what every clinician should know about managing patients with fragrance allergy. J Am Acad Dermatol 41:1020–1024

Stinchi C, Guerrini V, Ghetti E, Tosti A (1997) Contact dermatitis from lichens. Contact Dermatitis 36:309–310

Sun C-C, Guo Y-L, Lin R-S (1995) Occupational hand dermatitis in a tertiary referral dermatology clinic in Taipei. Contact Dermatitis 33:414–418

Uter W, Schnuch A, Geier J, et al (2001) Association between occupation and contact allergy to the fragrance-mix: a multifactorial analysis of national surveillance data. Occup Environ Med 58:392–398

Van der Walle HB, Brunsveld VM (1994) Dermatitis in hairdressers. (I). The experience of the past 4 years. Contact Dermatitis 30:217–221

Wall LM, Gebauer KA (1991) Occupational skin disease in Western Australia. Contact Dermatitis 24:101–109

Wohrl S, Hemmer W, Focke M, Gotz M, Jarisch R (2001) The significance of fragrance mix, balsam of Peru, colophony and propolis as screening tools in the detection of fragrance allergy. Br J Dermatol 145:268–273

CHAPTER 28

Colophony 28

A.-T. KARLBERG

Production

Colophony (rosin) is a resin obtained from different species of coniferous trees. There are three types of colophony, depending on the method of recovery: gum rosin, wood rosin and tall oil rosin. Gum rosin is obtained from various species of living pine trees. The trees are tapped for oleoresin, which is then distilled to obtain turpentine as the distillate and gum rosin as the residue. Wood rosin is produced from old pine stumps, while tall oil rosin is obtained as a by-product in the sulphate pulping of coniferous wood. The major types produced are gum rosin and tall oil rosin. In technical literature the term "colophony" corresponds to gum rosin. In dermatological literature tall oil rosin and wood rosin are also included in the term "colophony" since the resins contain the same major chemical components and allergens and are used in various technical products regardless of the source. In American literature the term "rosin" is more frequently used. China, Latin American countries and Portugal are great producers of gum rosin. The USA, Finland and the countries of the former USSR are great producers of tall oil rosin. Approximately 1.1 million tons of colophony are produced annually and the absolute majority is chemically modified to various derivatives.

Chemistry and Use

Colophony is a complex mixture of resin acids (about 90%) and neutral substances, i.e., diterpene alcohols, aldehydes and hydrocarbons (about 10%). Its composition varies with the species from which it is obtained and also depends on the recovery processes and storage conditions. The major acids are abietic acid and dehydroabietic acid (Fig. 1). Tall oil rosin contains less abietane type acids and more dehydroabietic acid than gum rosin does (Soltes and Zinkel 1989; Holmbom et al. 1974). Due to air exposure oxidized material is present in colophony. The abietan type resin acids with conjugated double bonds are more susceptible to oxidation than dehydroabietic acid and the pimarane type acids (Sadhra et al. 1998). Extensive studies have identified molecules formed at air oxidation of mainly abietic acid (Karlberg 1988, 1991; Hausen et al. 1993; Gäfvert 1994). One of the most prominent oxidation products is 15-hydroperoxyabietic acid (Fig. 1) (Karlberg et al. 1988a). The absolute majority of colophony is chem-

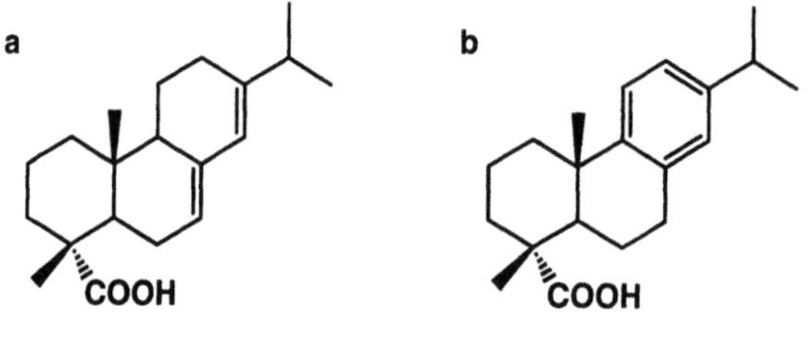

Fig. 1. Abietic acid (**a**) and dehydroabietic acid (**b**) – the main components in unmodified colophony. 15-Hydroperoxyabietic acid (**c**) – the major allergen in oxidized colophony. Maleopimaric acid (**d**) – a strong allergen present after a common derivatization of colophony

ically modified to various derivatives and different modifications are often combined (Soltes and Zinkel 1989). Maleopimaric acid (Fig. 1) is the major derivative formed in a common modification to enhance the hydrophilicity of colophony. Oxidation of colophony and the resin acids are often undesirable from a technical point of view. To prevent this, the double bonds that are susceptible to oxidation can be saturated by hydrogenation. The modifications are usually interrupted when the desired technical properties are obtained leaving unmodified colophony in the product.

Colophony has three main technical properties: it has good tackifying qualities, it can be used as an emulsifier and it has acid properties without causing corrosion. The technical properties are further modified by chemical reactions. The main areas of use for unmodified and modified colophony are listed in Table 1. The amount of unmodified colophony in different products varies from 20% or more in some adhesives, paints and soldering fluxes for electronic assemblies to small traces in products containing mainly modified colophony (Ehrin and Karlberg 1990). Since the oxidation products are the major allergens, it is desirable to be able to quantify some of them when analysing technical products suspected of causing allergic contact dermatitis. Traditionally, the major colophony components are quantified using gas chromatography (GC) (Holmbom et al. 1974), but labile compounds such as peroxides and hydroperoxides decompose due to the heat required to evaporate the compounds in the GC and will not be detected. In the high performance liquid chromatography (HPLC) method developed by Ehrin and Karlberg 1990, abietic acid and dehydroabietic acid were quantified in various technical products. However, analyses based only on the non-oxidized acids do not tell us anything about the amount of oxidized acids.

Table 1. Areas of use for unmodified and modified colophony

Colophony Type	Areas of Use
Unmodified	Soldering fluxes, paper, depilatory waxes, cosmetics, dancers' and string players' rosin, wood and gum from pine trees
Modified (modification types) Esterification with polyalcohols	Adhesive tackifiers, printing inks, bubble gum
Diels-Alder addition of maleic acid, maleic anhydride or fumaric acid	Paper size, printing inks, shoe glues
Hydrogenation	Printing inks, soldering fluxes, emulsifiers in the production of synthetic rubber, adhesive tackifiers
Polymerization/dimerization	Adhesives, printing inks, varnishes
Disproportionation/dehydrogenation	Emulsifiers in the production of synthetic rubber, paper size, adhesive tackifiers, printing inks, insulating material in electronics industry
Formaldehyde modification	Paper size, printing inks
Salt formation	Soaps, detergents, paper size, drier formulations, printing inks

A small amount of abietic acid detected might be due to a small amount of colophony present in the product or to an extensive oxidation.

Contact Allergy and Allergic Contact Dermatitis

Studies of the prevalence of contact allergy in general populations are very sparse. A Danish study (Nielsen and Menné 1992) shows that 0.7% in a population of 576 individuals were patch-test positive to colophony. In an Italian patch-test study of 539 healthy young men, only one showed a positive reaction to colophony (Seidenari et al. 1990).

Unmodified colophony is among the ten most common causes of contact allergy when tested in dermatitis patients. The prevalence of positive patch test reactions to colophony varies between 2–6% (Downs and Sansom 1999). A female dominance is seen. Patients with positive reactions to colophony usually also react to balsam of Peru and fragrance mix (Karlberg and Lidén 1985; Holness et al. 1995; Färm 1996). A slightly lower allergenic activity of tall oil rosin compared to gum rosin has been demonstrated both experimentally and clinically (Karlberg and Lidén 1985; Hausen and Loll 1993). This could be due to a difference in the composition, but since the allergenic activity is mainly due to oxidation products, the handling and storage times always affect the allergenic properties (Karlberg 1991).

The major allergen identified is the primary oxidation product, 15-hydroperoxyabietic acid (Fig. 1), while abietic acid itself is not allergenic (Karlberg et al.

1985, 1988a). Several other oxidation products have been identified as allergens (Karlberg 1988; Hausen et al. 1990; Gäfvert 1994; Khan and Saed 1994; Shao et al. 1995). The allergenic activity of colophony can be reduced by chemical modifications. Hydrogenated colophony has a very low allergenic activity (Karlberg et al. 1988b, Hausen et al. 1989). Also esterification with polyols (glycerol or pentaerythritol) reduces the allergenic activity. However, the modifications might create allergens, e.g., maleopimaric acid (Fig. 1) that do not cross-react with the allergens in unmodified colophony. Also, the unmodified colophony left after modification is still a source of sensitisation. (Karlberg et al. 1990; Gäfvert et al. 1996; Kanerva et al. 1998; Downs et al. 1999; Lyon et al. 1999; Salim and Shaw 2001).

Eighty-three patients in whom contact allergy to colophony had been diagnosed at an occupational dermatological clinic were followed up after 9–13 years. At least 30% had current hand eczema on follow-up examination. Among those in whom the dermatitis had started on the hands, there were proportionally more individuals with current hand eczema than among those in whom the onset had been on other parts of the body. At the time of the investigation 72% of the participants were still positive to colophony at patch testing and more than half had additional positive reactions to other allergens (Färm 1996).

Since colophony in modified and unmodified form is present in such a variety of products used both at work and at leisure time (Table 1), it can be difficult to trace the source of exposure and to avoid exposure. All products within the European Union (EU) containing 1% colophony or more should be labelled with an allergy warning (67/548/EEC). However, the amounts are seldom declared on the package and if modified colophony is used it can be difficult to recognise the name.

Case Reports

For references not given below see the extensive reviews on case reports in Gäfvert 1994, Färm 1997 and Downs and Sansom 1999.

Exposure from Products in Close Contact with the Skin

Several case reports deal with the clinical problems caused by colophony in products that are in close contact with the skin. Intolerance to *adhesive plasters* has been discussed since the beginning of the 1920s (Karlberg 1988). Colophony is still used, e.g., in some adhesive bandages for treatment of leg ulcers, and a high incidence of contact allergy has been observed. To minimise the allergenic effect esterified colophony is used in the bandages, but residual allergenic oxidation products can be present together with new allergens formed by modification. Colophony can also be present in *cosmetics*. There are reports of eye shadows, rouge, lip preparations and mascara causing colophony contact dermatitis. The adhesive of *bindi*, applied by Indian women on their forehead, can cause allergic contact dermatitis due to colophony derivatives. Performing artists are often extensively exposed to cosmetics in their occupation. Pharmaceutical use of oils and pitch from pines is nowadays mainly found in *folk medicine*. Colophony is present in *dental materials* such as periodontal dressings, impression materials, cavity varnishes and temporary filling materials. Cases of stomatitis and lichen planus in the mouth have been reported due to contact with colophony.

Occupational Exposure

Individuals exposed to colophony in *pine wood, sawdust and wood wool* may develop hand dermatitis but also dermatitis due to airborne exposure. The prevalence of contact allergy to colophony among the employees in a factory for production of tall oil rosin was found to be in accordance with that of dermatitis patients and thus higher than in the general population. However, the clinical symptoms were rare. A healthy worker effect cannot be excluded. Colophony in *soldering fluxes* for electronic assemblies is a well-known cause of allergic contact dermatitis. Since the allergens can be airborne, facial dermatitis is not uncommon as well as hand eczema. Paints, lacquers and glues can contain colophony, but reports of contact allergy to these products are sparse. *Cooling fluids* may contain colophony causing dermatitis among the employees in the manufacturing industry. In a study on the prevalence of hand dermatitis and contact allergy in Sweden, it was found that contact allergy to colophony was over-represented among women in *administrative work*, but the group in total showed a low prevalence of hand eczema. The content of colophony in *paper* and paper products has been investigated. So-called "environmentally friendly" paper of mechanical pulp from coniferous wood contains more colophony components than paper based on chemical pulp (Karlberg et al. 1995). The extractive material containing the colophony components is not separated from the mechanical pulp. In subjects allergic to colophony a higher response was seen to unprinted paper of mechanical pulps than to paper based on chemical pulps. When patch testing patients who suspected that their dermatitis was caused by contact with paper, only those with positive patch test reactions to colophony or maleopimaric acid (in modified colophony used for paper sizing) reacted to the paper extracts. Colophony in paper may contribute to hand dermatitis in sensitized subjects and the use of cotton gloves when in contact with paper might alleviate the dermatitis (Karlberg and Lidén 1992). Air-borne facial dermatitis caused by colophony components in the linoleum flooring and from polish on the floor among office workers has been reported. *Dancers and musicians* are exposed to colophony. The fiddler's rosin consists of unmodified colophony. Dancers use colophony on the floor, on their shoes and even on female costumes as an antislipping agent. Also colophony allergy among those who give the dancers massages is observed. Exposure to colophony has caused allergic contact dermatitis in dental personnel (Kanerva and Estlander 1999; Cockayne et al. 2001).

Patch Testing

Colophony (gum rosin from China and /or Portugal) is normally tested 20% in petrolatum (Karlberg and Lidén 1988; Sadhra et al. 1998). Investigations have shown that resin acids in petrolatum patch test preparations undergo progressive and substantial oxidation and that the dermatological activity of the preparations increases significantly with time (Sadhra et al. 1998). In the True Test gum rosin is applied in a gel in a concentration of $1.5 \ mg/cm^2$. Different colophony compounds, fractions and products have been suggested for more effective patch test diagnosis (Hausen et al. 1993, Sadhra and Foulds 1995). However, patch testing with isolated oxidation products will not detect as many cases as testing with colophony itself. Simultaneous testing with 15-hydroperoxyabietic acid methylester and colophony showed that 60–70% of the patients reacting to colophony reacted to the isolated allergen (Karlberg and Gäfvert 1996). It is not possible to isolate and patch test with all colophony allergens separately. Furthermore, primary allergens are continuously formed due to air exposure, and are further oxidized to secondary oxidation products that are also allergenic. Isolated unstable allergens are decomposed and thus the concentration can be too low in a test preparation. It is therefore recommended to patch test with a preparation of gum rosin that should be as well defined as possible with a constant and rather high level of oxidation products, since these are the main allergens.

When the history indicates that contact allergy to colophony is a possible cause of the dermatitis and the standard preparation is negative it is advisable to test with other types of colophony and with products in the patient's environment. Chemical analysis is valuable for detecting the offending agent.

Testing with identified allergens from modified colophony products and with modified colophony products will detect new cases of contact allergy (Hausen and Mohnert 1989; Gäfvert et al. 1996; Kanerva et al. 1998; Downs et al. 1999; Lyon et al. 1999; Salim and Shaw 2001). At present, no identified allergens are available for standard testing.

Other Health Effects

Colophony compounds in the fume from soldering flux rank in the top five causes of occupational asthma (Meredith and Nordman 1996). It is also reported to cause rhinitis and eye irritation (Burge 1984). Whether this is due to type I allergy or to irritation is not fully investigated. However, the occupational asthma resulting from colophony exposure usually has the features of a sensitizing reaction. There is a latent interval from first exposure to first symptom, only a proportion of similarly exposed workers are affected, and asthma is induced in affected workers with exposures which have no effect in asymptomatic exposed workers (Burge 2000).

References

21st Amendment of the Council Directive 67/548/EEC on the approximation of laws, regulations and administrative provisions relating to the classification, packaging and labelling of dangerous substances

Burge PS (1984) Occupational asthma, rhinitis and alveolitis due to colophony. Clin Immunol Allergy 4:55–82

Burge PS (2000) Colophony hypersensitivity revisited. Clin Exp Allergy 30:158–159

Cockayne SE, Murphy R, Gawkrodger DJ (2001) Occupational contact dermatitis from colophonium in a dental technician. Contact Dermatitis 44:42–43

Downs AMR, Sansom JE (1999) Colophony allergy: a review. Contact Dermatitis 41:305–310

Downs AMR, Sharp LA, Sansom JE (1999) Pentaerythritol-esterified gum rosin as a sensitizer in Granuflex hydrocolloid dressing. Contact Dermatitis 41:162–163

Ehrin E, Karlberg A-T (1990) Detection of rosin (colophony) components in technical products using an HPLC technique. Contact Dermatitis 23:359–366

Färm G (1996) Contact allergy to colophony and hand eczema. A follow-up study of patients with previously diagnosed allergy to colophony. Contact Dermatitis 34:93–100

Färm G (1997) Contact allergy to colophony. Clinical and experimental studies with emphasis on clinical relevance. Acta Derm Venereol Suppl (Stockh) 201:1–42

Gäfvert E (1994) Allergenic components in modified and unmodified rosin. Chemical characterization and studies of allergenic activity. Acta Derm Venereol Suppl (Stockh) 184:1–36

Gäfvert E, Bordalo O, Karlberg A-T (1996) Patch testing with allergens from modified rosin (colophony) discloses additional cases of contact allergy. Contact Dermatitis 35:290–298

Hausen BM, Loll M (1993) Contact allergy due to colophony (VIII). The sensitizing potency of commercial products: an investigation of French and German modified-colophony derivatives. Contact Dermatitis 29:189–191

Hausen BM, Mohnert J (1989) Contact allergy due to colophony (V). Patch test results with different types of colophony and modified-colophony products. Contact Dermatitis 20:295–301

Hausen BM, Jensen S, Mohnert J (1989) Contact allergy to colophony (IV). The sensitizing potency of commercial products. An investigation of French and American modified colophony derivatives. Contact Dermatitis 20:133–143

Hausen BM, Krohn K, Budianto E (1990) Contact allergy due to colophony (VII). Sensitizing studies with oxidation products of abietic and related acids. Contact Dermatitis 23:352–358

Hausen BM, Börries M, Budianto E et al (1993) Contact allergy due to colophony (IX). Sensitizing studies with further products isolated after oxidative degradation of resin acids and colophony. Contact Dermatitis 29:234–240

Holmbom B, Avela E, Pekkala S (1974) Capillary gas chromatography-mass spectrometry of resin acids in tall oil rosin. J Am Oil Chem Soc 51:397–400

Holness DL, Nethercott JR, Adams RM et al (1995) Concomitant positive patch test results with standard screening tray in North America 1985–1989. Contact Dermatitis 32:289–292

Kanerva L, Estlander T (1999) Occupational allergic contact dermatitis from colophony in 2 dental nurses. Contact Dermatitis 41:342–343

Kanerva L, Gäfvert E, Alanko K et al (1998) Patch testing with maleopimaric acid in an occupational dermatology clinic. Contact Dermatitis 39:329–330

Karlberg A-T (1988) Contact allergy to colophony. Chemical identifications of allergens, sensitization experiments and clinical experiences. Acta Derm Venereol Suppl (Stockh) 139:1–43

Karlberg A-T (1991) Air oxidation increases the allergenic potential of tall-oil rosin. Colophony contact allergens also identified in tall-oil rosin. Am J Contact Dermatitis 2:43–49

Karlberg A-T, Gäfvert E (1996) Isolated colophony allergens as screening substances for contact allergy. Contact Dermatitis 35:201–207

Karlberg A-T, Lidén C (1985) Clinical experience and patch testing using colophony (rosin) from different sources. Br J Dermatol 113:475–481

Karlberg A-T, Lidén C (1988) Comparison of colophony patch test preparations. Contact Dermatitis 18:158–165

Karlberg A-T, Lidén C (1992) Colophony (rosin) in newspapers may contribute to hand eczema. Br J Dermatol 126:161–165

Karlberg A-T, Bergstedt E, Boman A et al (1985) Is abietic acid the allergenic component of colophony? Contact Dermatitis 13:209–215

Karlberg A-T, Bohlinder K, Boman A et al (1988a) Identification of 15-hydroperoxyabietic acid as a contact allergen in Portuguese colophony. J Pharm Pharmacol 40:42–47

Karlberg A-T, Boman A, Nilsson JLG (1988b) Hydrogenation reduces the allergenicity of colophony (rosin). Contact Dermatitis 19:22–29

Karlberg A-T, Gäfvert E, Hagelthorn G et al (1990) Maleopimaric acid – a potent sensitizer in modified rosin. Contact Dermatitis 22:193–201

Karlberg A-T, Gäfvert E, Lidén C (1995) Environmentally friendly paper may increase the risk of hand eczema in rosin-sensitive persons. J Am Acad Dermatol 33:427–432

Khan L Saed MA (1994) 13β, 14β-Dihydroxy-13α-isopropylabietic acid, an elicitor of contact allergy. J Pharm Sci 83:909–910

Lyon CC, Tucker SC, Gäfvert E et al (1999) Contact dermatitis from rosin in footwear. Contact Dermatitis 41:102–103

Meredith SK, Nordman H (1996) Occupational asthma: measures of frequency from four countries. Thorax 51:435–440

Nielsen NH, Menné T (1992) Allergenic contact sensitization in an unselected Danish population. The Glostrup allergy study, Denmark. Acta Dermato Venereologica 72:456–460

Sadhra S, Foudls IS (1995) Allergic potential of neutrals in unmodified colophony, and a method for their separation from resin acids. Br J Dermatol 132:69–73

Sadhra S, Foulds IS, Gray CN (1998) Oxidation of resin acids in colophony (rosin) and its implications for patch testing. Contact Dermatitis 39:58–63

Salim A, Shaw S (2001) Recommendation to include ester gum resin when patch testing patients with leg ulcers. Contact Dermatitis 44:34

Seidenari S, Manzini BM, Danese P et al (1990) Pack and prick test study of 593 healthy subjects. Contact Dermatitis 23:162–167

Shao LP, Gäfvert E, Nilsson U et al (1995) 15-Hydroperoxy dehydroabietic acid – a contact allergen in colophony from pinus species. Phytochemistry 38:853–857

Soltes EJ, Zinkel DF (1989) Chemistry of rosin. In: Zinkel DF, Russel J (eds) Naval stores: production-chemistry-utilization, 1st edn, Pulp Chemicals Association, New York, pp 261–345

CHAPTER 29

Nickel

C. LIDÉN

Introduction

Nickel allergy is the most frequent contact allergy and an important cause of hand eczema (Lidén et al. 2001). Nickel allergy predominantly affects young girls and women sensitised by jewellery and other personal items. A hundred years ago, however, nickel dermatitis was an occupational disease that affected men. Occupational exposure to this metal is still a major factor in eliciting and maintaining hand eczema.

Prevalence, Use and Properties

In Nature and Production

Nickel is present in the earth's crust, in drinking water and in food. Nickel-related health problems are, however, not caused primarily by nickel in the environment but are related to industrial activity and man-made items. Ni(0) in metal nickel and its alloys, and Ni(II) are the most prevalent oxidation states. Numerous nickel salts and sulfides with different properties and uses are known. For example, nickel ions are formed when metallic nickel is in contact with sweat.

Today nickel is the fourth most-used metal after iron, chromium and lead. During the 19th century, white-nickel-containing alloys were produced in Europe as substitutes for silver and, around 1870, nickel began to be used in steels and platings. Nickel production has increased considerably since 1940, and today half the nickel produced is used in stainless steels. Nickel is used in numerous alloys and coatings, and in chemical compounds. It is also found in products for occupational and private use, many of which may come into contact with the skin.

Plating, Alloys and Corrosion

Metallurgical aspects of nickel and the corrosion of nickel-containing materials in contact with sweat have been reviewed (Flint 1998). Skin contact with homogeneous nickel is not common, but many items that are electroplated with nickel come into contact with skin. Nickel plate is often covered with a topcoat of chromium, silver, gold, tin/nickel, or different lacquers which may not be adequate to prevent contact dermatitis. Nickel used as an inter-liner under a plating of gold, silver or chromium causes dermatitis (Lidén et al. 1996).

Alloys are compounds or solid solutions of more than one element in metallic form. Common examples of nickel-containing alloys are stainless steels (iron/ nickel/chromium), copper/nickel and nickel-silver (nickel/copper/zinc). Brass (copper/zinc) and red gold (gold/silver/copper) are examples of nickel-free alloys. Resistance to corrosion on skin contact varies widely. Most stainless steels are unlikely to cause allergic contact dermatitis.

There is no relationship between the content of nickel in an alloy and its ability to cause an allergic reaction, while there is a close relationship between the rate at which ions form from nickel in contact with sweat and the potential to cause a reaction. This fact may be difficult to understand and has caused demands for "nickel-free" items instead of the generally more relevant demand for "low nickel release".

Health Effects

Toxicology

The major health effect of nickel and its compounds is contact allergy and allergic contact dermatitis. Inhalation exposure to soluble nickel and nickel oxides/ sulfides has caused nasal and pulmonary cancer in workers in nickel refineries. Inhalation of nickel compounds may induce asthma; however, nickel-induced asthma is rare.

Sensitising Capacity and Cross-Reactivity in the Guinea Pig

Nickel sulfate is moderately allergenic according to predictive studies in guinea pigs (Wahlberg 1989; Nielsen et al. 1992). To better understand the simultaneous patch-test reactivity and possible cross-reactivity often recorded in humans, cross-challenge experiments have been carried out (Wahlberg and Boman 1992; Lidén and Wahlberg 1994). It appears that the reactivity to nickel sulfate/palladium chloride is due to cross-reactivity, while cross-reactivity is not probable for nickel sulfate/cobalt chloride and nickel sulfate/potassium dichromate.

Sensitisation and Prevalence of Allergy

Sensitisation to nickel is caused by direct and prolonged skin contact with items that release nickel ions. The causes of primary sensitisation vary depending on fashion and other factors, which influence exposure. Suspenders and jeans buttons have previously been frequent sensitisers. Today, cheap jewellery is a prominent sensitiser. Piercing is over-represented in people with nickel allergy (Lars-

Table 1. Prevalence of nickel allergy in the general population and in dermatitis patients

Study population	Nickel allergy		Reference
	Men (%)	Women (%)	
General population, Finland ($n=980$)	0.8	8.0	Peltonen (1979)
Women of general population, Denmark ($n=1976$)[1]	–	14.5[1]	Menné et al. (1982)
Schoolgirls, Sweden ($n=960$)	–	9.0	Larsson-Stymne and Widström (1985)
General population, Denmark ($n=567$)	2.2	11.1	Nielsen and Menné (1992)
General population, Sweden ($n=11,000$)[1]	3.4[1]	14.9[1]	Meding et al. (2001)
Dermatitis patients, Germany ($n=36,720$)	4.8	18.3	Schnuch et al. (1997)
Occupational dermatology patients, Sweden ($n=1140$)	8	30	Lidén (1994a)

[1] Questionnaire study.

son-Stymne and Widström 1985; Nielsen and Menné 1993). Precious-metal jewellery, watches, spectacle frames, buckles, zippers, etc. are other important causes of sensitisation and elicitation of dermatitis. The nickel directive (see below) is expected to change the situation. The role of occupational exposure is discussed below.

The prevalence of nickel allergy in the general population has been shown to be 8–15% in women and 1–3% in men (Table 1). The prevalence among young females is even higher (Nielsen and Menné 1992; Meding et al. 2001).

Nickel allergy in dermatitis patients varies greatly. Publications listed in Table 1 show figures of 10–30% in female patients and 2–8% in male patients – the highest figures for occupational dermatology patients.

The role of nickel in diet, surgical implants and dental materials remains controversial and is reviewed elsewhere (Wilkinson 1989; Menné and Veien 2001).

Hand Eczema

Nickel-sensitive people run a considerably increased risk of developing hand eczema. As shown by population studies 30–43% of nickel-sensitive persons report that they have experienced hand eczema (cumulated prevalence), compared with only 15–19% among non-nickel-sensitive controls (Menné 1978; Peltonen 1979; Menné et al. 1982; Meding et al. 2001). Figures from dermatology departments on hand eczema in nickel-sensitive patients vary between 20% and 60% (Christensen and Möller 1975; Gawkrodger et al. 1986). The relationship between nickel allergy, hand eczema and atopic dermatitis has been extensively reviewed by Wilkinson and Wilkinson (1989).

Most people, in daily life and in many jobs, have repeat contact with handles, keys, coins, scissors, tools and other items that may release nickel. Wet work and other irritant factors impair the skin barrier function, facilitate the penetration of allergens into the skin, and contribute to the development of hand eczema.

Occupational Exposure

Some of the most important jobs and exposures with risk of occupational contact dermatitis due to nickel, and probably primary sensitisation, are described below, in Table 2, and in reviews by Fischer (1989), Cavelier and Foussereau (1995) and Lidén (2000).

Table 2. Prevalence of nickel allergy in selected occupational groups according to epidemiological studies and among dermatitis patients

Study population	Nickel allergy			Reference
	Men (%)	Women (%)	Total (%)	
Electroforming plant workers, UK ($n=27$)	48	–	–	Wall and Calnan (1980)
Electroplaters, Finland ($n=103$)	4	15	–	Kanerva et al. (1997)
Electronics industry workers, patients, Singapore ($n=149$, 57% male)	–	–	32.8	Tan et al. (1997)
Hairdressers, patients, Canada ($n=53$, 87% female)	–	–	17	Holness and Nethercott (1990)
Hairdressers, patients, Spain ($n=379$, 92% female)	–	–	41.4	Condé-Salazar et al. (1995a)
Junior hairdressers, the Netherlands ($n=86$)	–	27	–	van der Burg et al. (1986)
Hairdressers, Finland ($n=54$ cases of hand eczema of 355)	–	35	–	Leino et al. (1998)
Car mechanics, Sweden ($n=801$)	8	–	–	Meding et al. (1994)
Construction workers, patients, Spain ($n=408$)	10	–	–	Condé-Salazar et al. (1995b)
Hospital wet workers, Finland ($n=536$)	–	–	9.1	Lammintausta et al. (1982)
Hospital wet workers, Sweden ($n=1857$)	–	26.3	–	Nilsson and Bäck (1986)

Platers

Dermatitis due to nickel exposure was reported among platers in 1889 and, until 1930, nickel dermatitis was a frequent male occupational disease in the plating industry (Schwarz et al. 1957; Blaschko 1889). Since then, improved industrial hygiene and technical development have decreased the risk. Today much of the work may be automated, but handling of hot nickel salt solutions and heavy contamination of the work environment, skin, clothes and protective gloves are still prevalent (Aitio 1995, and personal experience).

An outbreak of occupational dermatitis in an electroforming plant in the UK was due to heavy nickel exposure (Wall and Calnan 1980) (Table 2). Improvement in industrial hygiene led to an immediate decrease in the incidence of dermatitis.

A survey was carried out in all 38 Finnish electroplating plants (Kanerva et al. 1997). Nickel allergy was found among 15% of the female workers and 4% of the male workers (Table 2). Seventy percent of those with nickel allergy reported past or present hand eczema. Sensitised workers often, but not always, were able to continue their work.

Electronics Industry

Workers in the electronics industry are exposed to skin irritants and contact allergens, among them nickel, colophony (rosin) in soldering flux, rubber chemicals, epoxy and acrylates (Koh et al. 1990). In Singapore 24% of occupational dermatology patients were from the electronics industry (Tan et al. 1997) (Table 2). Sources of contact included coolants, nickel-plated earthing straps and tools.

Metalworkers

Metalworkers are often heavily exposed to cutting fluids and cutting oils, and they are at high risk of developing irritant and allergic contact dermatitis (Rycroft 2001). The role of contamination of re-circulating fluids by metals has been discussed and may be of some importance.

Hairdressers

Hairdressers are exposed to several factors that may cause and contribute to hand eczema: wet work, nickel, fragrances, preservatives and specific occupational allergens. These factors are responsible for the high prevalence of hand eczema among hairdressers. They are exposed to nickel through handling tools and equipment.

Results from patch testing of hairdressers referred to dermatology departments have been published, some shown in Table 2. The frequency of positive reactions to nickel has varied considerably, from 17% to 42%.

Several epidemiological studies have been carried out, some of them referred to in Table 2. Some authors have doubted that the high prevalence of nickel allergy is due to occupational exposure. Current epidemiological studies will hopefully help to settle the question. In an individual case it must, however, be recognised that occupational nickel exposure might be an important factor contributing to or causing the hairdressers' hand eczema.

Car Mechanics

Car mechanics have a high prevalence of hand eczema, often related to irritants such as organic solvents and oils. In an epidemiological study of hand eczema among car mechanics, 8% were patch-test positive to nickel (Meding et al. 1994) (Table 2). Handling of tools was suggested as a contributing factor.

Construction Workers

Construction workers risk occupational contact dermatitis from exposure to irritants, chromate, cobalt, rubber and epoxy. Nickel allergy, however, is not often discussed (Coenraads et al. 1984). In construction workers it is often found together with allergy to chromate and/or cobalt.

The frequency of nickel allergy among patch-tested construction-worker dermatitis patients has been above the prevalence among many other male dermatitis patients (Table 2). Sources of nickel exposure in plumbers, carpenters, locksmiths and electricians include tools, pipes, locks and other items (Lidén 1994a; Lidén et al. 1998). Architectural aluminium such as doors and window-frames may, due to a new method for anodising aluminium, have easily-available nickel on the surface (Lidén 1994b).

Tools

Hand-held tools are used in many male and in some female occupations and metal parts may come into repeated contact with the skin often under friction and wet conditions. The Swedish tool market was surveyed, and 27% of 565 hand-held tools with metal parts that come into contact with the skin were dimethylglyoxime-test positive (Lidén et al. 1998). Tool producers should consider nickel allergy and avoid nickel-releasing materials in parts in contact with the skin, which may be parts other than the handle.

Coins

The majority of European national coins are made of copper/nickel that give high nickel release when stored in artificial sweat (Flint 1998). The Euro coinage consists of eight coins – six nickel free and two made of nickel-containing alloys (copper/nickel combined with nickel/brass). Nickel ions are readily available on the surface of used coins. Several micrograms of nickel salts may be transferred daily onto hands by intense handling of high-nickel-releasing coins (Lidén and Carter 2001).

Coins may cause or aggravate hand eczema among cashiers with nickel allergy, but handling of coins among nickel-allergic consumers is considered to be a minor problem. It is also believed that handling coins rarely induces nickel allergy. Hand eczema in nickel sensitive cashiers is a problem in clinical occupational dermatology. The magnitude of the problem is, however, not known (Lidén and Carter 2001).

Cleaning, Domestic and Hospital Wet Work

Hand eczema is common among people, especially among nickel-sensitive individuals, doing "wet work" in hospitals, cleaning and house work. Water and detergents are important skin irritants, and nickel release from frequently handled equipment, tools, handles, and keys may contribute to hand eczema. Hand eczema and nickel allergy was studied in hospital employees in Finland and Sweden (Table 2).

Miscellaneous Occupations

There are numerous reports on occupational nickel dermatitis among workers in different occupations [examples given in (Cronin 1980; Fischer 1989; Lidén 2000; Rycroft 2001)]. In individual cases, there has often been a convincing relationship between occupational nickel exposure and dermatitis, and sometimes also between the exposure and primary sensitisation. The list of examples may be extensive, but a selection is given in Table 3 to display the broad spectrum of potential hazards, which may not be shown by epidemiological studies.

Table 3. Some examples of nickel dermatitis caused by exposure in miscellaneous occupations – to display the broad variation in exposure (Lidén 2000)

Occupation	Causative nickel exposure
Bank clerk	Coins
Bartender	Measuring cups
Butchers	Metal clasps in protective gloves
Engraver	Cold-impregnated aluminium
Musicians	Parts of string instruments and wind-instruments
Offset printers	Ink-repellent solution
Pottery workers	Clay
Tailors	Needles
Teacher	Blackboard chalk
Technician	Optical instrument (black nickel)

Diagnosis

Nickel sulfate 5% in petrolatum is the standard test material in Europe, and 2.5% is used in the US.

Patch testing with serial dilution is sometimes used to gain more information on the degree of sensitivity and to discriminate between allergic reactions and irritant ones (Andersen et al. 1993; Wahlberg 2001). Open tests to study the concentration threshold have been carried out as single or repeated applications (Menné and Calvin 1993; Allenby and Basketter 1994). Intracutaneous testing is used at some centres (Möller 1989).

Patch testing with metal discs may be used as a supplement to the analysis of metal release in artificial sweat. This will give information about the ability of the materials to cause allergic contact dermatitis (Menné et al. 1987; Lidén et al. 1996).

Detection of Soluble Nickel

The Dimethylglyoxime Test

The dimethylglyoxime test (Fisher's test) is a simple screening test for nickel release. In many countries the test is commercially available.

The test is based on dimethylglyoxime (0.8–1% in alcohol) and ammonia (10%). A cotton-wool-tipped stick with 1–2 drops of each solution is rubbed for up to 30 s against the surface to be tested. A pink-red colour indicates presence of nickel ions. A modified dimethylglyoxime test with increased sensitivity by pre-treatment of the surface with artificial sweat and heat has been developed (European Committee for Standardization [CEN] 2002). The dimethylglyoxime test is a useful tool for screening purposes, but sometimes discoloration or false-negative results may occur.

Nickel Release in Artificial Sweat

Nickel release may be quantitatively determined (Flint 1998; European Committee for Standardization [CEN] 1998) by storing items in artificial sweat at 30 °C for 1 week and analysing nickel in the solution at the end of the period. Nickel release of 0.5 µg/cm^2 per week is the limit of *The Nickel Directive* (see below). The majority of nickel-sensitive persons do not react during patch testing to materials with nickel release below this limit (Lidén et al. 1996).

Prevention

The Nickel Directive

The European Union has decided on a regulation aiming at the prevention of nickel allergy, *The Nickel Directive*, which entered into full force in 2001. It restricts the use of nickel in products intended for direct and prolonged contact with the skin and for use during epithelialisation after piercing (European Parliament and Council Directive 94/27/EC [Nickel] 1994; Lidén 2001). Hopefully *The Nickel Directive* will be an effective tool for primary prevention of nickel allergy by reducing the risk of sensitisation and for secondary prevention through reduced exposure in people already sensitised, and also through increased public awareness of nickel allergy. From Denmark, where nickel release from items in contact with the skin has been limited since 1989, indications of a decrease in the sensitisation rate were reported (Duus Johansen et al. 2000). Nickel on the Swedish market in 1999 was studied, and some adaptation had been made to the requirements of *The Nickel Directive* (Lidén and Johnsson 2001).

Elimination

The dimethylglyoxime test presents a powerful tool for secondary prevention. People with contact dermatitis due to nickel allergy should limit exposure to nickel, including exposure to nickel-releasing personal items and exposure in the workplace and during leisure. Nickel-sensitive people with hand eczema and occupational hygienists, etc., may identify objects in the workplace with which skin contact should be avoided and which should possibly be exchanged for the same object made with other materials.

Protection

Soluble nickel salts, which are especially used by platers and battery workers, may heavily contaminate protective gloves and clothing. Good occupational hygiene is of great importance, as shown by the history of nickel dermatitis. Workers handling metallic items may use protective gloves of fabric, leather, rubber or plastic, but contamination as well as possible penetration by nickel ions must not be forgotten.

Barrier creams have until now been of limited value in preventing nickel contact dermatitis. Possibly useful preparations, with a specific protective effect against nickel, will be presented in the future.

Prognosis

Many mild cases of nickel dermatitis will clear when exposure to the causative object(s) is avoided and a topical treatment is applied. Hand eczema in nickel-sensitive patients is, however, considered to have a poor prognosis and may in some cases be resistant to treatment and persist for years (Fregert 1975; Christensen 1982). Nickel dermatitis in Denmark is the second most common dermatological disease, after irritant contact dermatitis, giving rise to compensation for occupational skin disease. Nickel-related hand eczema was the dermatological disease most commonly causing permanent disability from 1970 to 1976 in Denmark (Menné and Bachmann 1979a,b).

In a follow-up study of nickel-sensitive patients, the prognosis was more favourable concerning dermatitis, hand eczema and concomitant allergies in those who strictly avoided metal contact in clothing and jewellery (Kalimo et al. 1997).

References

Aitio A (1995) Nickel and nickel compounds. Arbete och Hälsa 26:1–61

Allenby CF, Basketter DA (1994) The effect of repeated open exposure to low levels of nickel on compromised hand skin of nickel-allergic subjects. Contact Dermatitis 30:135–138

Andersen KE, Lidén C, Hansen J, Vølund Å (1993) Dose-response testing with nickel sulphate using the TRUE test in nickel-sensitive individuals. Multiple nickel sulphate patch-test reactions do not cause an "angry back". Br J Dermatol 129:50–56

Blaschko A (1889) Berufsdermatosen der Arbeiter. Ein Beitrag zur Gewerbehygiene (I). Das Galvaniseur-Ekzem. Dtsch Med Wochenschr 15:925–927

Cavelier C, Foussereau J (1995) Kontaktallergie gegen Metalle und deren Salze. Teil II: Nickel, Kobalt, Quecksilber und Palladium. Dermatosen 43:152–162

Christensen OB (1982) Prognosis in nickel allergy and hand eczema. Contact Dermatitis 8:7–15

Christensen OB, Möller H (1975) Nickel allergy and hand eczema. Contact Dermatitis 1:129–135

Coenraads PJ, Nater JP, Jansen HA, Latinga H (1984) Prevalence of eczema and other dermatoses of the hands and forearms in construction workers in the Netherlands. Clin Exp Dermatol 9:149–158

Condé-Salazar L, Baz M, Guimaraens D, Cannavo A (1995a) Contact dermatitis in hairdressers: patch test results in 379 hairdressers (1980–1993). Am J Contact Dermatitis 6:19–23

Condé-Salazar L, Guimaraens D, Villegas C et al (1995b) Occupational allergic contact dermatitis in construction workers. Contact Dermatitis 33:226–230

Cronin E (1980) Metals, nickel. In: Contact dermatitis. Churchill Livingstone, Edinburgh, pp 338–367

Duus Johansen J, Menné T, Christophersen J et al (2000) Changes in the pattern of sensitization to common contact allergens in Denmark between 1985–1986 and 1997–1998, with a special view to the effect of preventive strategies. Br J Dermatol 142:490–495

European Committee for Standardization (CEN) (1998) Reference test method for release of nickel from products intended to come into direct and prolonged contact with the skin. EN 1811

European Committee for Standardization (CEN) (2002) Screening tests for nickel release from alloys and coatings in items that come into direct and prolonged contact with the skin. CR 12471

European Parliament and Council Directive 94/27/EC (Nickel) (1994) Official Journal of the European Communities 22. 7. 1994, No L 188/1–2

Fischer T (1989) Occupational nickel dermatitis. In: Maibach HI, Menné T (eds) Nickel and
the skin: immunology and toxicology. CRC Press, Boca Raton, pp 117–132

Flint GN (1998) A metallurgical approach to metal contact dermatitis. Contact Dermatitis
39:213–221

Fregert S (1975) Occupational dermatitis in a 10-year material. Contact Dermatitis 1:96–107

Gawkrodger DJ, Vestey JP, Wong W-K, Buxton PK (1986) Contact clinic survey of nickel-
sensitive subjects. Contact Dermatitis 14:165–169

Holness DL, Nethercott JR (1990) Epicutaneous testing results in hairdressers. Am J Contact
Dermatitis 1:224–234

Kalimo K, Lammintausta K, Jalava J, Niskanen T (1997) Is it possible to improve the prognosis in nickel contact dermatitis? Contact Dermatitis 37:121–124

Kanerva L, Kiilunen M, Jolanki R et al (1997) Hand dermatitis and allergic patch test reactions caused by nickel in electroplaters. Contact Dermatitis 36:137–140

Koh D, Foulds IS, Aw TC (1990) Dermatological hazards in the electronics industry. Contact
Dermatitis 22:1–7

Lammintausta K, Kalimo K, Havu VK (1982) Occurrence of contact allergy and hand eczemas in hospital wet work. Contact Dermatitis 8:84–90

Larsson-Stymne B, Widström L (1985) Ear piercing – a cause of nickel allergy in school-
girls? Contact Dermatitis 13:289–293

Leino T, Tammilehto L, Hytönen M et al (1998) Occupational skin and respiratory disease
among hairdressers. Scand J Work Environ Health 24:398–406

Lidén C (1994a) Occupational contact dermatitis due to nickel allergy. Sci Total Environ
148:283–285

Lidén C (1994b) Cold-impregnated aluminum. A new source of nickel exposure. Contact
Dermatitis 31:22–24

Lidén C (2000) Nickel. In: Kanerva L, Elsner P, Wahlberg JE, Maibach HI (eds) Handbook
of occupational dermatology. Springer, Berlin Heidelberg New York, pp 524–533

Lidén C (2001) Legislative and preventive measures related to contact dermatitis. Contact
Dermatitis 44:65–69

Lidén C, Carter S (2001) Nickel release from coins. Contact Dermatitis 44:160–165

Lidén C, Johnsson (2001) Nickel on the Swedish market before the Nickel Directive. Contact
Dermatitis 44:7–12

Lidén C, Wahlberg JE (1994) Cross-reactivity to metal compounds studied in guinea pigs
induced with chromate or cobalt. Acta Derm Venereol (Stockh) 74:341–343

Lidén C, Menné T, Burrows D (1996) Nickel-containing alloys and platings and their ability
to cause dermatitis. Br J Dermatol 134:193–198

Lidén C, Röndell E, Skare L, Nalbanti A (1998) Nickel release from tools on the Swedish
market. Contact Dermatitis 39:127–131

Lidén C, Bruze M, Menné T (2001) Metals. In: Rycroft RJG, Menné T, Frosch PJ, Lepoittevin
J-P (eds) Textbook of contact dermatitis, 3rd edn. Springer, Berlin Heidelberg New York,
pp 933–977

Meding B, Barregård L, Marcus K (1994) Hand eczema in car mechanics. Contact Dermatitis 30:129–134

Meding B, Lidén C, Berglind N (2001) Self-diagnosed dermatitis in adults. Results from a
population survey in Stockholm. Contact Dermatitis 45:341–345

Menné T (1978) The prevalence of nickel allergy among women. Dermatosen 26:123–125

Menné T, Bachmann E (1979a) Permanent disability from skin disease. A study of 564 patients registered over a six-year period. Dermatosen 27:37–42

Menné T, Bachmann E (1979b) Permanent disability from hand dermatitis in females sensitive to nickel, chromium and cobalt. Dermatosen 27:129–135

Menné T, Calvin G (1993) Concentration threshold of non-occluded nickel exposure in
nickel-sensitive individuals and controls with and without surfactant. Contact Dermatitis
29:180–184

Menné T, Veien NK (2001) Systemic contact dermatitis In: Rycroft RJG, Menné T, Frosch PJ,
Lepoittevin J-P (eds) Textbook of contact dermatitis, 3rd edn. Springer, Berlin Heidelberg New York, pp 355–366

Menné T, Borgan Ø, Green A (1982) Nickel allergy and hand dermatitis in a stratified sample of the Danish female population: an epidemiological study including a statistic appendix. Acta Derm Venereol (Stockh) 62:35–41

Menné T, Bandrup F, Thestrup-Pedersen K et al (1987) Patch test reactivity to nickel alloys. Contact Dermatitis 16:255–159

Möller H (1989) Intradermal testing in doubtful cases of contact allergy to metals. Contact Dermatitis 20:120–123

Nielsen NH, Menné T (1992) Allergic contact sensitization in an unselected Danish population. The Glostrup allergy study, Denmark. Acta Derm Venereol (Stockh) 72:456–460

Nielsen NH, Menné T (1993) Nickel sensitization and ear piercing in an unselected Danish population. The Glostrup Allergy Study, Denmark. Contact Dermatitis 29:16–21

Nielsen GD, Rohold, AE, Andersen KE (1992) Nickel contact sensitivity in the guinea pig: an efficient open application test method. Acta Derm Venereol (Stockh) 72:45–48

Nilsson E, Bäck O (1986) The importance of anamnestic information of atopy, metal dermatitis and earlier hand eczema for the development of hand dermatitis in women in wet hospital work. Acta Derm Venereol (Stockh) 66:45–50

Peltonen L (1979) Nickel sensitivity in the general population. Contact Dermatitis 5:27–32

Rycroft RJG (2001) Occupational contact dermatitis. In: Rycroft RJG, Menné T, Frosch PJ, Lepoittevin J-P (eds) Textbook of contact dermatitis, 3rd edn. Springer, Berlin Heidelberg New York, pp 555–580

Schnuch A, Geier J, Uter W et al (1997) National rates and regional differences in sensitization to allergens of the standard series. Population-adjusted frequencies of sensitization (PAFS) in 40,000 patients from a multicenter study (IVDK). Contact Dermatitis 37:200–209

Schwarz L, Tulipan L, Birmingham DJ (1957) Occupational skin diseases of the skin, 3rd edn. Lea Febiger, Philadelphia, p 274

Tan HH, Chan MTL, Goh CL (1997) Occupational skin disease in workers from the electronics industry in Singapore. Am J Contact Dermatitis 8:210–214

Wahlberg JE (1989) Nickel: animal sensitization assays. In: Maibach HI, Menné T (eds) Nickel and the skin: immunology and toxicology. CRC Press, Boca Raton, pp 65–73

Wahlberg JE (2001) Patch testing. In: Rycroft RJG, Menné T, Frosch PJ, Lepoittevin J-P (eds) Textbook of contact dermatitis, 3rd edn. Springer, Berlin Heidelberg New York, pp 435–468

Wahlberg JE, Boman AS (1992) Cross-reactivity to palladium and nickel studied in the guinea pig. Acta Derm Venereol (Stockh) 72:95–97

Wall LM, Calnan CD (1980) Occupational nickel dermatitis in the electroforming industry. Contact Dermatitis 6:414–420

van der Burg CKH, Bruynzeel DP, Vreeburg KJJ,et al (1986) Hand eczema in hair-dressers and nurses; a prospective study. Contact Dermatitis 14:275–279

Wilkinson DS, Wilkinson JD (1989) Nickel allergy and hand eczema. In: Maibach HI, Menné T (eds) Nickel and the skin: immunology and toxicology. CRC Press, Boca Raton, pp 133–163

Wilkinson JD (1989) Nickel allergy and orthopedic prostheses. In: Maibach HI, Menné T (eds) Nickel and the skin: immunology and toxicology. CRC Press, Boca Raton, pp 187–193

CHAPTER 30

Chromium

30

D. BURROWS

Chromium

Chromium is so called because of the brightness of many of its salts, hence the use of the Greek word for colour. Chromium can occur in every one of the oxidation states from –2 to +6, but the ground states 0, +2, +3, and +6 are common (Love 1983). Chromium metal itself does not act as an allergen and must do so in combination with a protein. Only the trivalent and hexavalent salts are able to act as haptens; that is, they form potentially antigenic bonds with proteins. The metal is highly resistant to corrosion in the atmosphere and many aqueous solutions and is an unlikely cause of contact allergy.

Toxicity

Trivalent chromate is not considered toxic, but hexavalent chromate has considerable toxic effects. In sufficient concentrations, it (1) causes cancer, particularly lung cancer (Bidstrup 1983), (2) causes respiratory symptoms of bronchitis (Langard 1983), (3) affects the immune system [Snyder et al. (1996) found a lower level of interleukin 6 produced by pokeweed nitrogen-stimulated mononuclear cells isolated from patients exposed to chromate in the soil], and (4) causes irritant dermatitis and chrome ulcers of the skin and mucous membranes.

Dermatitis

Irritant dermatitis is uncommon except for those in contact with high concentrations; for instance, workers whose duties include chrome plating.

Chrome Ulcers

The commonest symptom associated with the irritant effect of chromates is chrome ulcers occurring either in the skin or nasal septum. In a recent survey of 71 platers in the West Midlands of Britain, 22% were found to have permanent nasal damage, 34% had evidence of healed chrome ulcers, and 13% had evidence of new and healing ulcers. Of the 20 companies studied, 10% had at least one plater with a new ulcer (Williams 1996).

Most ulcers will heal if the patient is removed from the source. Necrosis of cartilage, but not bone, can occur; malignant change does not occur, and there is no increased incidence of chrome allergy in those with chrome ulcers.

Allergic Contact Dermatitis

Dermatitis occurs more commonly with hexavalent than trivalent chromate. Trivalent chromate binds very readily to protein and, thus, penetrates the skin poorly; little trivalent chromate gets past the stratum corneum, whereas hexavalent chromate penetrates easily and deeply into the dermis and is then transformed to trivalent chromate, whereupon it readily forms the hapten with the protein and is processed as an allergen.

Patch Testing

Potassium dichromate (0.5% in petrolatum) is the standard test material in Europe; in the United States, 0.25% is used. The concentration needed for eliciting allergy is very near that which produces irritant reactions (Burrows 1987). Patch testing with 0.5% and 0.375% potassium dichromate will produce a number of irritant reactions, whereas patch testing with lower percentages, while producing fewer irritant reactions, will miss some allergic reactions (Burrows et al. 1989). The consequence of this is that 0.25% is probably a safer percentage to use for those without much experience in patch testing.

Incidence of Chromate Allergy

The incidence of positive patch tests to chromate depends on which population is studied. In normal, healthy volunteers without apparent contact with chromate, Peltonen and Fraki (1983) found only 0.5% were positive, whereas healthy volunteers in contact with chromate had an incidence of 1.8%. Decaestecker et al. (1990) found a similar incidence (1.7%) in chromate-pigment workers, and Goh et al. (1986) found 2.9% in prefabrication-construction factory workers with normal skin. Nethercott (1982), in a review of the world literature, found an incidence of 7.9% positive chromate sensitivity in routine testing in a patch-test clinic. Peltonen and Fraki (1983) found that, in their routine patch testing, 6.8% of 1159 men and 2.8% of 1823 women reacted to dichromate. Of these, 16.1% of the men and 18.1% of the women had a present or past history of atopic dermatitis but, of 390 patients with atopic dermatitis as a primary diagnosis, only 1.3% showed a positive reaction to dichromate. These high figures of apparent allergy to dichromate must be accepted with a certain amount of reserve, bearing in mind the potentially irritant nature of 0.5% potassium dichromate, which could give irritant reactions in those with active skin disease. Indeed, Fischer and Rystedt (1985) found that only 40% of their positive chromium patch tests were relevant. The incidence of positive patch tests in routine testing in a skin clinic probably runs nearer to 1–2% and, if the figures are higher, then some special reason should be sought.

Exposure to Chromium

Exposure to chromium is possible in contact with the following compounds (Burrows and Adams 1990):
- Metals
- Analytic standards/reagents
- Anticorrosion agents
- Batteries
- Catalysts (for hydrogeneration, oxidation, polymerization)
- Ceramics
- Cement (See Chap. 71)
- Drilling muds
- Chromium lignosulphonates (from sodium dichromate using lignosulphate waste)
- Electroplating and anodizing agents
- Engraving
- Explosives
- Fire retardant
- Galvanised sheeting
- Hardeners and resins in the aircraft industry
- Leather
- Magnetic tapes
- Metallic chromium
- Milk preservatives
- Paints and varnishes
- Paper
- "Chrome cake" (containing sodium sulphate and small amounts of sodium dichromate)
- Photography
- Roofing
- Stainless steel
- Sutures
- Tanning leather
- Textile mordants and dyes
- Television screens
- Welding
- Wood preservatives
- Detection of Chromate

Chromate is often a hidden allergen, and in any situation where a patient has a positive patch test to chromate and has contact dermatitis, one should always suspect that they are in contact with chromate, and spot testing for chromate can be helpful.

Spot Test for Detection of Hexavalent Chromium (Chromate)

Reagents
Reagent I: 1,5-diphenylcarbazide (1% weight/volume in ethanol)
Concentrated sulfuric acid

Investigative Procedures
- *Chromate on the surface of a solid object:* a few drops of each reagent are applied on a cotton swab. The cotton swab is thereafter rubbed against the surface of the object for 1 min. If chromate is present, a red-violet colour appears.
- *Chromate in solutions:* to a sample of approximately 10 ml a few drops of each reagent are added. If chromate is present, a red-violet colour appears.
- *Chromate in powders insoluble in water (cement):* G cement is mixed with 10 ml water for some minutes. The mixture is then filtered and the filtrate is handled in the same way as described for chromate in solutions.

Reagent I must be prepared immediately before the investigation. Spot testing is not so accurate or easily carried out as the dimethylglyoxime test for nickel.

Prognosis

It is well documented that prognosis in chromium dermatitis is probably worse than in any other form of dermatitis. Burrows (1972) found that a very small percentage were clear after 10–15 years. Halbert et al. (1992) confirmed this, and Hogan et al. (1990), in a review of the prognosis of occupational contact dermatitis of the hands, again confirmed the poor prognosis in chromate dermatitis.

Change of Occupation

There is very little clear data on the beneficial effect of a change of occupation, but common sense and clinical experience would suggest that it would be beneficial. Halbert et al. (1992), in a review of 122 patients with chromate allergy followed up for 6–9 years found 62 (52%) were in the same occupation and, of these, 55 (89%) had ongoing dermatitis, 7 (11%) had completely cleared despite continuing chromate exposure, 58 (48%) had completely changed their type of work since initial presentation and, despite this, changing dermatitis persisted in 40 (69%). A significant factor in improvement appeared to be the length of time the person had continued in employment with their dermatitis prior to changing work.

Prevention, Protection, Treatment

Prevention

Reduction of exposure is clearly the best method of prevention. Mechanisation in the construction industry and allergen replacement – for instance, changes to trivalent chromate for plating – produce a significant improvement (Burrows and Cooke 1980). A survey in the chrome plant industry showed that there is considerable room for improvement, and Dornan (1981) showed that efforts in improving hygiene were quite worthwhile. Changing trivalent chromate into hexavalent chromate in cement is taking place in four countries (Norway, Sweden, Finland, and Denmark), and there has been a reduction in chromate dermatitis in the cement industry in these countries.

Barrier Creams

It is doubtful that ordinary barrier creams have any protective effect. Specific barrier creams that change hexavalent chrome into trivalent chrome have been suggested, including ascorbic acid (Valsecchi and Cainelli 1994), ascorbic acid with ethylenediamine tetraacetic acid (Romaguera et al. 1985), dithionate (Wall 1982), tartaric acid plus glycine (Romaguera et al. 1985), and sodium metabisulphite (Burrows and Calnan 1965). Romaguera has also found a preparation containing silicone, glyceryl lactate, glycine, and tartaric acid to be effective in a clinical trial. Niklasson et al. (1996) reported a polymer resin with a chelating agent that was effective in depressing nickel patch tests. This is also effective in chelating chromate (B. Niklasson, personal communication).

Treatment

One of the most important steps in improving prognosis is to remove the patient from the source of the chromate as soon as possible (Halbert et al. 1992). A discussion must take place with the patient, because improvement of their dermatitis cannot be guaranteed, and many patients will continue to experience discomfort even though they have no obvious further contact with chromate. There has never really been any satisfactory explanation for this; it may be that chromate remains a long time in the skin or that it only requires minute quantities of chromate, such as are found in soil, paper, etc., to keep the dermatitis going. Nevertheless, it is ideal for the patient to be moved to another area of the company where they do not have contact with chromate-containing compounds. Otherwise, the treatment is the same as that for any eczematous condition: emollients and use of local steroids, when necessary.

References

Bidstrup PL (1983) Effects of chrome compounds on the respiratory system. In: Burrows D (ed) Chromium: metabolism and toxicity. CRC Press, Boca Raton, pp 31–51

Burrows D (1972) Prognosis in industrial dermatitis. Br J Dermatol 87:145–148

Burrows D (1987) Comparison of 0.25 and 0.5% potassium dichromate in patch testing. Bull Dermatol Allerg Profess 2:117–120

Burrows D, Calnan CD (1965) Cement dermatitis. Trans St Johns Hosp Dermatol Soc 51:27–39

Burrows D, Cooke MD (1980) Trivalent chrome plating. Contact Dermatitis 6:222

Burrows D, Andersen KE, Camaras JG, et al (1989) Trial of 0.5% versus 0.375% potassium dichromate. Contact Dermatitis 21:351

Decaestecker AM, Marez T, Jdaini J, et al (1990) Hypersensitivity to dichromate among asymptomatic workers in a chromate pigment factory. Contact Dermatitis 23:52–53

Dornan JD (1981) Occupational dermatoses amongst chrome platers in the Sheffield area 1977–80. Contact Dermatitis 7:354–355

Fischer T, Rystedt I (1985) False positive follicular and irritant patch test reactions to metal salts. Contact Dermatitis 12:93–98

Goh CL, Wong PH, Kwok SF, et al (1986) Chromate allergy: total chromium and hexavalent chromium in the air. Derm Beruf Umwelt 34:132–134

Halbert AR, Gebaver KA, Wall LM (1992) Prognosis of occupational chromate dermatitis. Contact Dermatitis 27:214–219

Hogan DJ, Dannaker W, Lal S, et al (1990) An international survey of the prognosis of occupational contact dermatitis of the hands. Derm Beruf Umwelt 38:143–147

Langard S (1983) The carcinogenicity of chrome compounds in man and animals. In: Burrows D (ed) Chromium: metabolism and toxicity. CRC, Boca Raton, pp 13–31

Love G (1983) Chromium – biological and analytical considerations. In: Burrows D (ed) Chromium: metabolism and toxicity. CRC, Boca Raton, pp 1–12

Nethercott JR (1982) Results of routine patch testing of 200 patients in Toronto, Canada. Contact Dermatitis 8:389–395

Niklasson B, Bjorkner B, et al (1996) In vivo evaluation of an active barrier cream in nickel contact allergy. Jadassohn Centenary Congress, London

Peltonen L, Fraki J (1983) Prevalence of dichromate sensitivity. Contact Dermatitis 9:190–194

Romaguera C, Grimalt F, Vilaplana J, Carreras E (1985) Formulation of a barrier cream against chromate. Contact Dermatitis 13:49–52

Snyder CA, Udasin I, Waterman SJ, Taioli E, Gochfield M (1996) Reduced IL-6 levels among individuals in Hudson County, New Jersey, an area contaminated with chromium. Arch Environ Health 51:26–28

Valsecchi R, Cainella T (1984) Chromium dermatitis and ascorbic acid. Contact Dermatitis 10:252–253

Wall LM (1982) Chromate dermatitis and sodium dithionate. Contact Dermatitis 8:291–293

Williams N (1996) A survey of respiratory and dermatological diseases in the chrome plating industry in West Midlands, UK. Occup Med 46:432–434

CHAPTER 31

Cement

31

C. Avnstorp

Introduction

Irritant and allergic cement eczema has been found to be one of the most serious occupational health problems in building trades and industries. This has been illustrated more recently by the high frequency of cement dermatitis in underground workers during construction of the English Channel tunnel between England and France (Irvine et al. 1994), among workers from the construction industry in Taiwan (Sun et al. 1995; Guo et al 1999), construction workers in Spain (Condé-Salazar et al. 1995), in Germany (Geier and Schnuch 1995) and in Singapore (Wong et al. 1998). In the United States, the Occupational Health Foundation has recently focused on the problem (Occupational Health Foundation 1996).

Allergic cement eczema is caused by water-soluble chromate in the cement. Chromium allergy very often develops into chronic eczematous disadvantage.

In Singapore allergic contact dermatitis was more common than irritant contact dermatitis in the construction industry. Of the patients with allergic contact dermatitis in this industry, 104/110 or 94.5% were allergic to chromate in cement (Goon and Goh 2000).

By adding ferrous sulfate to the cement, it is possible to prevent the development of allergic cement eczema. This was illustrated in an epidemiological intervention study from Denmark (Avnstorp 1992) and in reports from Finland and Sweden (Roto et al. 1996).

Further information about those being affected by cement eczema is detailed in Chap. 114 (Cement Workers) and Chap. 120 (Construction Workers) in Kanverva et al. (2000).

The Evolution of Cement

Cement is a material which binds together solid bodies (aggregate) by hardening from a plastic state. The Latin word "cementum" means crushed stone. Portland cement consists of hydraulic calcium silicates, usually containing one or more of the forms of calcium sulfate as an interground addition. It is produced when a raw mixture of limestone and clay is heated to high temperatures (Mehta 1986). The chemical reactions taking place in the cement kiln system can be approximately represented as shown in Fig. 1.

Clay (SiO_2, Al_2O_3, Fe_2O_3), Limestone ($CaCO_3$), Cr(III), $\longrightarrow$
$3CaO \cdot SiO_2$, $3CaO \cdot Al_2O_3$, $4CaO \cdot Al_2O_3 \cdot Fe_2O_3$, Cr(VI)

Fig. 1. Basic chemical reactions taking place in the cement kiln system

Concrete is a mixture of Portland cement, sand, stones and water. Mortar consists of a mixture of Portland cement, sand, and water and often also hydrated lime. The exact composition depends on the purpose for which the product is to be used.

Chromate in Cement

The Origin of Chromate

The potential source of water-soluble hexavalent chromate [Cr(VI)] in cement is the trivalent [Cr(III)] compound (Cr_2O_3) in the raw materials from which it is produced. Cr(III) compounds are oxidised to Cr(VI) compounds (CrO_4^{2-}) when heated in the kilns to temperatures of approximately 1400 °C. The Cr(VI) content of cement varies from country to country according to variations in the amount of chromium in the raw materials (Fregert and Gruvberger 1972).

Reduction and Solubility

Ferrous sulfate reduces Cr(VI) in cement to Cr(III) (Fig. 2).

$$CrO_4^{2-} + 3\,Fe^{2+} + 4\,OH^- + 4\,H_2O \longrightarrow Cr(OH)_3 + 3\,Fe(OH)_3$$

Fig. 2. The chemical reaction in the reduction of water-soluble chromate by the addition of ferrous sulfate

In 1981, Aalborg Portland A/S (Ltd), the only manufacturer of cement in Denmark, patented a method whereby the amount of chromate in the cement could be reduced using this method, thus reducing the content of water-soluble chromate in cement to not more than 2 ppm at a cost of about 1% of the total value of the cement. Legislation stating that the content of water-soluble chromate in dry cement must not exceed 2 mg/kg (2 ppm) was passed in Denmark in 1983 (Danish Working Environment Service 1983). Since then, Finland, Sweden, Norway and Iceland have all established the same regulation. In Germany bagged cement has been regulated.

Recently the European Communities have decided that cement-products containing more than 2 ppm water soluble chromate should be labelled with a health warning because of the risk of developing chromium allergy. This directive came into effect on 30 July 2002 (Commission Directive 2001/60/EC).

The chromate in both bagged cement and bulk cement will remain in a reduced state, as Cr(III) compounds, for 8 weeks. The type of storage conditions used is essential, because if the bagged cement is stored in open sacks or exposed to moisture the Cr(VI) will not be reduced when the cement is subsequently mixed with water (Bruze et al. 1990b).

Clinical Patterns of Cement Eczema

Cement eczema may be of an irritant nature, allergic or both.

Irritant Cement Eczema

Depending on exposure, concentration and time, and individual factors, different clinical manifestations of irritant cement eczema are seen (Avnstorp 1995).

Acute Reactions

Cement eczema may initially develop as a result of daily irritation of the skin by contact with cement. The skin of those who have daily contact with wet cement becomes irritated by the hygroscopic and alkaline constitution of the cement. Erythema and dry skin on the dorsal aspects of the hands and fingers are the most frequent findings. Itching of the hand and fingers is the most important symptom (Avnstorp 1983). Acute reactions may develop within weeks. Cement burns are mostly seen in those, who are not familiar with the handling of cement products (Vickers and Edwards 1976; Spoo and Elsner 2001).

Chronic Reactions

Repeated and continual contact with wet cement products in combination with other physical traumas due to the work processes may lead to the development of chronic irritant cement eczema. This may take months or years. The efflorescences may vary with time. These are erythema, lichenification and hyperkeratoses on the dorsal and volar aspects of the hands, fingers and fingertips, and also on the wrists. The eczema may be nummular in morphology (Fig. 3) or in-

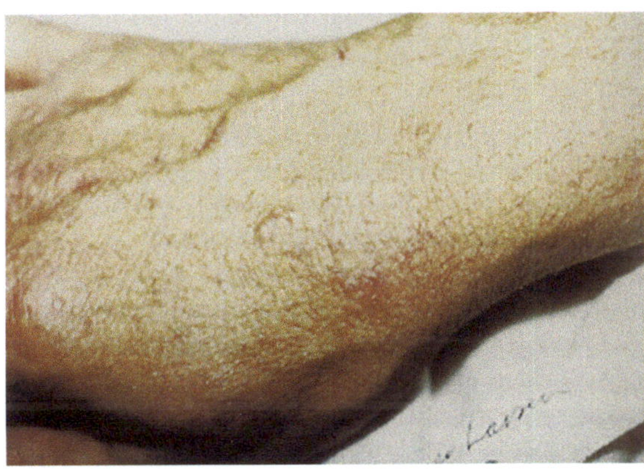

Fig. 3. Nummular cement eczema

clude the whole skin on the affected area. Vesicles are seldom found (Calnan 1960; Høvding 1970; Avnstorp 1983).

Noneczematous Skin Changes
Minor skin complaints are accepted as normal among workers who have daily contact with wet cement products (Avnstorp 1983). Mechanical traumas from the handling of bricks, tools and machines cause occupational stigmata in the form of hyperkeratoses, with fissures on the palmar aspects of the hands and fingers. This phenomenon is particularly seen among individuals working outdoors in cold weather (Avnstorp 1992).

Allergic Cement Eczema

In general, allergic cement eczema cannot be differentiated from irritant cement eczema clinically. This differentiation should be made after patch testing. If the test reveals a positive reaction to chromate, the eczema must be classified as allergic cement eczema (Avnstorp 1992). The severity of irritant cement eczema with respect to extension has been found to be mild to moderate, whereas allergic cement eczema has tended to be more severe (Avnstorp 1991).

Allergic cement eczema is primarily located on the hands, fingers and wrists (Burrows and Calnan 1965; Høvding 1970; Avnstorp 1983). Furthermore, allergic cement eczema has been found to have a greater extent of involvement than irritant cement eczema (Avnstorp 1991). Allergic cement eczema may also spread to the forearms, the feet and sometimes the face and parts of the trunk (Fig. 4).

Concomitant Sensitisations

Concomitant sensitivities to cobalt and rubber chemicals have been found significantly more often among chromium-hypersensitive workers than among those not hypersensitive to chromium (Fregert and Rorsman 1966; Høvding 1970; Fregert 1975; Avnstorp 1983). Among 172 chromium-allergic workers from the Spanish building industry, 82 (47.6%) were sensitised to rubber chemicals (Condé-Salazar et al. 1995). A similar correlation has been described among workers from a factory in Singapore manufacturing pre-cast concrete building components (Goh and Gan 1987).

Cobalt occurs in cement as water-insoluble oxides, but forms complexes with amino acids in eczematous skin, thereby possibly forming haptens (Fregert and Gruvberger 1978). In cement eczema, cobalt sensitivity is therefore probably secondary to the chromium hypersensitivity.

Nickel is a contaminant of cement in the form of insoluble NiO, which, in contrast to the cobalt oxides, is not allergenic (Wahlberg et al. 1977).

Epoxy sensitivity has been observed with relatively high frequency. Bricklayers and workers engaged in pre-cast concrete building component factories are exposed to products containing epoxy resins (van Putten et al. 1984; Avnstorp 1992; Condé-Salazar et al. 1994).

Fig. 4. Allergic cement eczema on the leg of a construction worker

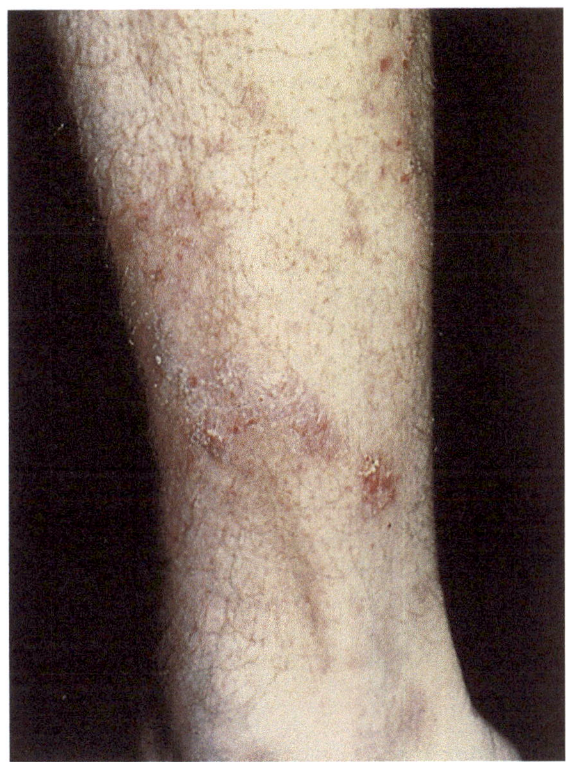

Hereditary Factors

Combined influences of endogenous and exogenous factors may lead to the development or to aggravation of hand eczema (Nilsson 1985).

In a prevalence study among concrete workers from the building industry, up to 13% of the workers reported previous episodes of eczema other than hand eczema; among those, approximately 50% developed hand eczema (Avnstorp 1983).

Psoriasis may be triggered by repeated mechanical traumas from handling bricks, tools and machines, and from daily contact with wet cement products.

Prophylaxis

The risk of developing allergic cement eczema can be brought to a very low level by the addition of ferrous sulfate to the cement (Avnstorp 1992). The concentration of water-soluble chromate in the cement should not exceed 2 ppm. In Scandinavian countries, this intervention has shown to be a significantly effective method in the prevention of allergic cement eczema (Avnstorp 1992; Roto et al. 1996; Zachariae et al. 1996).Experimental studies in humans, investigating the threshold for allergic reactivity, support this concentration level (Basketter et al. 2001). Reduced numbers of statements and approved claims of cement eczema have been found following the addition of ferrous sulfate to cement in Denmark and Finland (Avnstorp 1992; Roto et al. 1996). This economic benefit should be included in the calculation together with smaller costs for medical support, fewer lost working days and less personal suffering for the workers who develop allergic cement eczema.

Individual Prophylaxis

The dynamics of the development of occupational hand eczema are not fully understood, but irritation and contact sensitivity, together with individual constitutional factors, influence its development. Theoretically, at least one of the triggering factors could be eliminated if the workers used individual preventive measures. Use of gloves, protective hand creams and hand washing were not found to influence the propensity for developing irritant cement eczema (Avnstorp 1991). The absence of influence from individual preventive measures could be explained by the possibility that the work processes are so hazardous that they overwhelm the protective effect. It could also be that the preventive initiatives were not conducted systematically or carefully enough.

References

Avnstorp C (1983) Cement eczema in Danish workers engaged in the building trades and industries (PhD thesis). University of Copenhagen, Denmark (In Danish with English summary)

Avnstorp C (1991) Risk factors for cement eczema. Contact Dermatitis 25:81–88

Avnstorp C (1992) Cement eczema. An epidemiological intervention study. Acta Derm Venereol Suppl (Stockh) 179:14–17

Avnstorp C (1995) Irritant cement eczema. In: van der Valk PGM, Maibach HI (eds) The irritant contact dermatitis syndrome. CRC Press, Inc. Boca Raton, pp 111–119

Basketter D, Horev L, Slodovnik D, Merimes S, Trattner A, Ingber A (2001) Investigation of the threshold for allergic reactivity to chromium. Contact Dermatitis 44:70–74

Bruze M, Gruvberger B, Hradil E (1990) Chromate sensitization and elicitation from cement with iron sulfate. Acta Derm Venereol Suppl (Stockh) 70:160–162

Burrows D, Calnan CD (1965) Cement dermatitis. 2. Clinical aspects. Trans St John's Hosp Derm Soc 51:27–39

Calnan CD (1960) Cement dermatitis. J Occup Med 2:15–22

Commission Directive 2001/60/EC of 7 August 2001

Condé-Salazar L, Gonzalez MA, Guimaraens D (1994) Sensitization to epoxy resin systems in special flooring makers. Contact Dermatitis 31:157–160

Condé-Salazar L, Guimaraens D, Villegas C, Romero A, Gonzalez MA (1995) Occupational allergic contact dermatitis in construction workers. Contact Dermatitis 33:226–230

Danish Working Environment Service (1983) Order on water-soluble chromate in cement. Order no. 661 (in Danish)

Fregert S (1975) Occupational dermatitis in a 10-year material. Contact Dermatitis 1:96–107

Fregert S, Gruvberger B (1972) Chemical properties of cement. Dermatosen 20:238–248

Fregert S, Gruvberger B (1978) Solubility of cobalt in cement. Contact Dermatitis 4:14–18

Fregert S, Rorsman H (1966) Allergy to chromium, nickel and cobalt. Acta Derm Venereol 46:114–118

Geier J, Schnuch A (1995) A comparison of contact allergies among construction workers and nonconstruction workers attending contact dermatitis clinics in Germany: Results of the information network of departments of dermatology from November 1989 to July 1993. AJCD 6:86–94

Goh CL, Gan SL (1987) Rubber allergy among construction workers in a prefabrication construction factory. Clin Exp Dermatol 12:332–334

Goon AT-J, Goh C-L (2000) Epidemiology of occupational skin disease in Singapore 1989–1998. Contact Dermatitis 43:133–136

Guo YL, Wang B-J, Yeh K-C, Wang J-C, Kao H-H, Wang M-T, Shih H-C, Chen C-J (1999) Dermatoses in cement workers in southern Taiwan. Contact Dermatitis 40:1–7

Høvding G (1970) Cement eczema and chromium allergy, an epidemiologic investigation (thesis). University of Bergen, Norway

Irvine C, Pugh CE, Hansen EJ, Rycroft RJG (1994) Cement dermatitis in underground workers during construction of the channel tunnel. Occup Med 44:17–23

Kanerva L, Elsner P, Wahlberg J, Maibach HI (eds) (2000) Handbook of occupational dermatology. Springer, Berlin Heidelberg New York

Mehta PK (1986) Concrete: structure, properties and materials. Prentice-Hall, Inc., Englewood Cliffs

Nilsson E (1985) Contact sensitivity and urticaria in "wet" work. Contact Dermatitis 13:321–328

Occupational Health Foundation (1996) How to save your skin: preventing skin problems in the construction industry. Symposium findings and recommendations. Washington DC

Roto P, Sainio H, Reunala T, Laippala P (1996) Addition of ferrous sulfate to cement and risk of chromium dermatitis among construction workers. Contact Dermatitis 43:43–50

Spoo J, Elsner P (2001) Cement burns: a review, 1960–2000. Contact Dermatitis 45:68–71

Sun CC, Guo YL, Lin RS (1995) Occupational hand dermatitis in a tertiary referral dermatology clinic in Taipei. Contact Dermatitis 33:414–418

van Putten PB, Coenraads PJ, Nater JP (1984) Hand dermatoses and contact allergic reactions in construction workers exposed to epoxy resins. Contact Dermatitis 10:146–150

Vickers HR, Edwards DH (1976) Cement burns. Contact Dermatitis 2:73–78

Wahlberg JE, Lindsted G, Einarsson Ö (1977) Chromium, cobalt and nickel in Swedish cement, mould and cutting oils. Dermatosen 25:220–228

Wong S-S, Chan MTS, Gan S-L, Ng S-K, Goh C-L (1998) Occupational chromate allergy in Singapore: a study of 87 patients and a review from 1983 to 1995. AJCD 9:1–5

Zachariae COC, Agner T, Menné T (1996) Chromium allergy in consecutive patients in a country where ferrous sulfate has been added to cement since 1981. Contact Dermatitis 35:83–85

CHAPTER 32

Epoxy Resins   32

R. Jolanki, L. Kanerva, T. Estlander

Chemistry and Properties

Epoxy resins are normally used in what is called an epoxy-resin system. This system consists of the epoxy resin and a hardener, and reactive diluent or other additives, such as fillers, modifiers, pigments and reinforcements.

Epoxy Resins

Epoxy resins contain at least two cyclic three-membered ring structures containing oxygen, called epoxy groups, oxirane or epoxide groups, in their molecules. The term "epoxy resin" may refer to the resins in both the uncured thermoplastic and cured thermoset state. The uncured resins can be cross linked through the use of a variety of curing agents or hardeners to form cured plastics with insoluble three-dimensional structures.

The reaction products of epichlorohydrin [CAS 106–89–8] and bisphenol A [CAS 80–05–7] resulted in the first commercial epoxy resins, which are generally mixtures of monomeric diglycidyl ether of bisphenol A (DGEBA), with a molecular weight (MW) of 340 Da, and oligomers with a higher MW (Fig. 1). Apart from the DGEBA and higher oligomers, side reactions result in the formation of low levels of impurities.

DGEBA epoxy resins with a low average MW of 350–400 Da are liquids with a relatively high viscosity, and they contain up to and more than 90% monomeric DGEBA. Resins with a high average MW of over than 900 Da are solids (Muskopf and McCollister 1987), but may contain more than 15% DGEBA (Henriks-Eckerman and Laijoki 1986b).

DGEBA epoxy resins account for about 75% of the epoxy resins used worldwide. Non-DGEBA epoxy resins possess special properties that have made them competitive with DGEBA resins for certain applications. A list of chemical names and CAS numbers of available epoxy resins is given in Table 1. The resin or mixture of resins chosen for a particular application depends on the desired balance of properties. For example, brominated epoxy resins are semisolids and resistant to ignition, and epoxy resins based on diglycidyl ether of bisphenol F (DGEBF) are less viscous and exhibit better chemical resistance than DGEBA epoxy resins (Pontén and Bruze 2001). Triglycidyl isocyanurate (TGIC) is one of the non-DGE-

bisphenol A

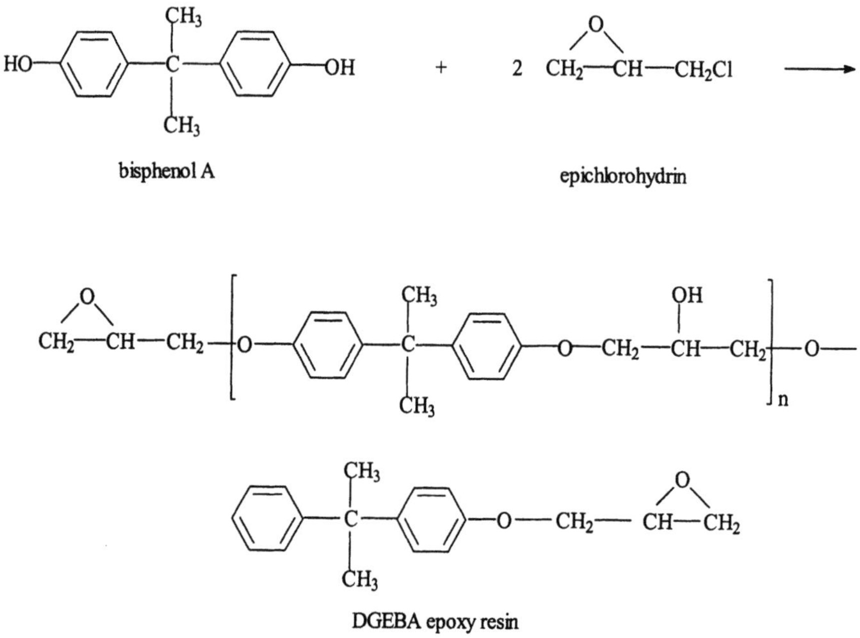

+

epichlorohydrin

DGEBA epoxy resin

Fig. 1. Diglycidyl ether of bisphenol A (DGEBA) epoxy resin

BA epoxy resins (Table 1), but is mainly used as a hardener in thermosetting one-component powder polyester paints (Muskopf and McCollister 1987).

Reactive Diluents

Reactive diluents are used principally to reduce the viscosity of the resin, e.g. in paints and adhesives. The reactive diluents are generally glycidyl ethers and sometimes glycidyl esters; structurally, they are aliphatic or aromatic, and they also contain epoxy groups in their molecules (Table 2). It has been estimated that more than half of the epoxy-resin products contain varying (0.1–20%) amounts of reactive diluents (Henriks-Eckerman and Laijoki 1986b; Jolanki et al. 1987).

Hardeners

A wide variety of curing agents is currently available (Tables 3–6).

When epoxy resins are used in two-component products, the hardeners are added to the resins immediately before the application, and the subsequent cross linking occurs at either an ambient or an elevated temperature. Aliphatic and cycloaliphatic polyamines react readily with epoxy resins at ambient temperatures; aromatic polyamines require an elevated curing temperature (Muskopf and McCollister 1987).

Table 1. Epoxy resins [CAS number] (Muskopf and McCollister 1987; Guin and Work 1995)

Diglycidyl ether of bisphenol A based epoxy resins
  Diglycidyl ether of bisphenol A (DGEBA) [1675-54-3]
Brominated bisphenol A based epoxy resins
  Diglycidyl ether of tetrabromo bisphenol A [68928-70-1, 26265-08-7, 40039-93-8]
Phenol and cresol epoxy novolacs
  Cresol epoxy novolacs [37382-79-9]
  Diglycidyl ether of bisphenol F [54208-63-8]
  2,2',2'',2'''-[1,2-ethanediylidenetetrabis(4, 1-phenyleneoxymethylene)]tetrabisoxiran
  [7328-97-4]
  Phenol epoxy novolacs [9003-36-5]
  Resorcinol diglycidyl ether [101-90-6]
  Trisphenol novolac epoxy resin [66072-38-6]
Glycidyl ethers of phenol-aldehyde adducts
  1,1,2,2-tetrakis[4-[(2,3-epoxypropyl)phenyl]ethane [27043-37-4]
  Tris[4-(2,3-epoxypropoxy)phenyl]methane [66072-39-7]
Glycidyl ethers of phenol-hydrocarbon novolacs
  2,5-bis[(2,3-epoxypropoxy)phenyl]octahydro-4,7-methano-5H-indene [13446-85-0]
Glycidyl ethers of aliphatic diols
  Ethylene glycol diglycidyl ether[2224-15-9]
  Diglycidyl and triglycidyl ether of glycerol
  Diglycidyl ether of polypropyleneglycol [16096-30-3]
  Diglycidyl ether of hydrogenated bisphenol A [30583-72-3]
  Sorbitol polyglycidyl ether [68412-01-1]
Aromatic glycidyl amines
  4-glycidyloxy-N,N-diglycidylaniline
  N,N'-tetraglycidyl-4,4'-methylenedianiline (TGMDA) [28768-32-3]
  Triglycidyl-p-aminophenol (TGPAP) [5026-74-7]
Heterocyclic glycidyl imides
  1,3-*bis* (2,3-epoxypropyl)-5,5-dimethylhydantoin; dimethyl hydantoin epoxy resin
  [15336-81-9]
  3-(2-glycidyloxypropyl)-1-glycidyl-5,5-dimetylhydantoin [32568-89-1]
  Triglycidyl isocyanurate (TGIC) [2451-62-9]
Glycidyl esters
  Diglycidyl ester of hexahydrophthalic acid [5493-45-8]
  Diglycidyl ester of phthalic acid [7195-45-1]
  Glycidyl ester of dimerized linoleic acid and epiclorohydrin
Fluorinated epoxy resins
Epoxidized cycloaliphatic olefins
  3',4'-epoxycyclohexylmethyl-3,4-epoxycyclohexanecarboxy-
  Late (cycloaliphatic epoxy resin) [2386-87-0]
  4-epoxyethyl-1,2-epoxycyclohexane (vinyl cyclohexene diepoxide) [25550-49-6]

Polyamines (Table 3) are often troublesome to work with because of their reactivity and volatility, and also because of their irritating and sensitising properties to the skin and respiratory tract. To overcome these problems, polyamides and amine-epoxy adducts have been developed. Polyamides are prepared by combining aliphatic polyamines, e.g. diethylenetriamine (DETA) or triethylenetetramine (TETA), with fatty acids. Amine-epoxy adducts are formed in a reaction between epoxy resin and an excess of polyamine, mostly DETA, TETA or isophoronediamine (IPDA) (Bauer 1985). The content of free amine is about 5% in the amine-

Table 2. Reactive diluents [CAS number] (Muskopf and McCollister 1987; Angelini et al. 1996; Jolanki 1996) there is a 1988 in the reference list but not 1996 and 88 doesn't feature anywhere

Aliphatic glycidyl ethers
  Allyl glycidyl ether (AGE) [106-92-3]
  1,4-butanediol diglycidyl ether (BDDGE) [2425-79-8]
  n-butyl glycidyl ether (*n*-BGE) [2426-08-6]
  t-butyl glycidyl ether (*t*-BGE) [7665-72-7]
  Diethyleneglycol diglycidyl ether (DEGDGE)
  Diglycidyl ether of pentaerythritol
  2-ethyl hexyl glycidyl ether
  Glycidyl ether of aliphatic alcohols (Epoxide 8) [68609-97-2]
  Glycidyl ether of polypropyleneglycol [9072-62-2]
  1,6-hexanediol diglycidyl ether (HDDGE) [16096-31-4]
  Neopentyl glycol diglycidyl ether (NPGDGE) [17557-23-2]
Cycloaliphatic glycidyl ethers
  Cyclohexanedimethanol diglycidyl ether
Aromatic glycidyl ethers
  tert-Butylphenyl glycidyl ether [3101-60-8]
  Cresyl glycidyl ether (CGE) [26447-14-3]
  p-Fluorphenyl glycidyl ether
  Alpha-naphthyl glycidyl ether
  Phenyl glycidyl ether (PGE) [122-60-1]
Glycidyl esters
  Castor oil glycidyl ether [74398-71-3]
  Glycidyl ester of neodecanoic acids (Cardura E 10) [26761-45-5]
  Glycidyl methacrylate [106-91-2]
  Glycidyl neodecanoate [26761-45-5]

epoxy adduct hardeners used in metal paints, but for those used in floor and concrete coatings the corresponding figure is about 20% (Bäck and Saarinen 1986). Free DGEBA is not found in amine-epoxy adducts (Henriks-Eckerman and Laijoki 1986 b).

When DGEBA epoxy resins are cured by polyamine-bearing hardeners at room temperature, the amounts of unreacted DGEBA and polyamine diminish rapidly within 1–2 days, but thereafter the decrease is slow. Nevertheless, after 1 week's cure, 0.02–12% of free DGEBA and 0.01–1% of free DETA were found when epoxy resin products were experimentally cured by DETA (Henriks-Eckerman and Laijoki 1986 a). The use of an elevated curing temperature is more effective in reducing the DGEBA concentration than simply waiting until the next day (Hansson 1994).

One-component products contain curing agents which are inactive at storage temperatures, but which initiate a curing process when heated. Typical latent curing agents include organic acid anhydrides, e.g. phthalic anhydride (PA) and PA derivatives (Table 4), which are used mainly in the electrical industry. Other examples of one-component epoxy products are powder paints, one-pack glues and prepreg-laminates. With the anhydrides, the cross-linking reaction is achieved using tertiary amines (Table 6) as catalysts and an elevated curing temperature (50–200 °C). The typical latent curing agents in powder epoxy paints are com-

Table 3. Polyamine hardeners [CAS number] (Muskopf and McCollister 1987; Guin and Work 1995; Kanerva et al. 1996)

Aliphatic polyamines
  N'-(3-aminopropyl)-N,N-dimethyl-1,3-propanediamine
  Diethylenetriamine (DETA) [111-40-0]
  Diethylamino propylamine (DEAPA) [104-78-9]
  3-dimethylaminopropylamine (DMAPA) [109-55-7]
  Dipropylene triamine (DPTA) [56-18-8]
  Ethylene diamine (EDA) [107-15-3]
  p-Menthane-1,8-diamine [80-52-4]
  Poly(oxypropylene diamine) [9046-10-0]
  Poly(oxypropylene-triamine) [39423-51-3]
  Tetraethylene pentamine (TEPA) [112-57-2]
  Triethylenetetramine (TETA) [112-24-3]
  2,2,4-Trimethylhexamethylene 1,6-diamine [3236-53-1]
  2,4,4-Trimethylhexamethylene 1,6-diamine [3236-53-2]
Cycloaliphatic polyamines
  1,2-Cyclohexanediamin [694-83-7]
  3-Cyclohexylaminopropylamine [3312-60-5]
  1,4-Diaminocyclohexane [3114-70-3]
  Isophoronediamine (IPDA) [2855-13-2]
  2,2'-Dimethyl-4,4'-methylenebis(cyclohexylamine) [6864-37-5]
Aromatic polyamines
  4,4'-Diaminodiphenylmethane (DDM) [101-77-9]
  4,4'-Diaminodiphenyl sulfone (DDS) [80-08-0]
  Diethyltoluenediamine [75389-89-8]
  m-Phenylenediamine (MPDA) [108-45-2]
  o-Tolyl biguanide [93-69-6]
  m-Xylene diamine [1477-55-0]
Polyamide diamines
  Polymeric amido-amine alkoxylated trietylene tetramine
  Adducts of aliphatic amines with mono- and diepoxides and
  Ketones (i.e. amine-epoxy adducts)
  Diethylenetriamine-ethylene oxide adduct
  Ethylene diamine adduct to solid epoxy
  Triethylenetetramine-propylene oxide adduct

posed of hardeners, such as dicyandiamide (Table 5) or pyromellitic anhydride. TGIC is used to cure powder polyester paints. The polymerisation of the powder paints occurs in a curing oven at about 200 °C. Blocked isocyanates are latent curing agents used in water-borne coatings (Muskopf and McCollister 1987). Polysulfides and hexavalent chromate (Table 5) are constituents found especially in the curing agents of epoxy sealants used in the aircraft industry (Handley and Burrows 1994; Bruze et al. 1996).

Use

Epoxy resins are used mostly in two-component paints and other protective coatings, and two-component adhesives. Epoxy resins are also used to insulate or encapsulate and they are used in the assembly of a wide variety of electrical and

Table 4. Organic acid anhydride hardeners [CAS number] (Guin and Work 1995; Jolanki et al. 1997 b)

Chlorendic anhydride [115–27–5]
cis-Cyclohexane-1,2-dicarboxylic anhydride [13149–00–3]
Dodecenylsuccinic anhydride (DDS) [25377–73–5]
Hexahydrophthalic anhydride (HHPA) [85–42–7]
Maleic anhydride (MA) [108–31–6]
Methyl endo-methylene-tetrahydrophthalic anhydride
Methylhexahydrophthalic anhydride (MHHPA) [19438–60–9]
Methyl nadic anhydride [25134–21–8]
Methyltetrahydrophthalic anhydride (MTHPA) [26590–20–5]
Phthalic anhydride (PA) [85–44–9]
Polyazelaic polyanhydride
Polysebacic polyanhydride [26776–29–4]
Pyromellitic dianhydride (PMDA) [89–32–7]
Succinic anhydride [108–30–5]
Tetrahydrophthalic anhydride (THPA) [85–43–8]
Trimellitic anhydride (TMA) [552–30–7]

Table 5. Miscellaneous curing agents [CAS number] (Muskopf and McCollister 1987; Guin and Work 1995; Bruze et al. 1996; Kanerva et al. 1996)

N-Aminoethylpiperazine [140–31–8]
Cyanoethyl modified aliphatic amine
2,4-Diamino-6-(2′-alkylimidazol-1-yl)ethyl-s-triazine
Dicyandiamide [461–58–5]
Di- and polyisocyanates
Diethylene glycol diaminopropyl ether
Hexavalent chromate
Melamineformaldehyde resins [9003–08–1]
Phenolformaldehyde resins [9003–35–4]
Polycarboxylic acid polyesters
Polysulfides
Ureaformaldehyde resins [9011–05–6]

electronic devices, in the manufacture of glass fibres as sizing agents (Heino et al. 1996) and in the manufacture of composite products or other plastic items. They can also be used as injection resins to repair cracks in concrete, and in flooring materials (Condé-Salazar et al. 1994) and stone work (Angelini et al. 1996). Powder paints, microscopy immersion oils (Kanerva et al. 2001) and even nail polishes (Jolanki et al. 1996 a) may contain epoxy-resin compounds. For special applications, epoxy resins are used as lamination resins and in prepreg laminates (Kanerva et al. 2000 b, 2002 a).

Both solvent-less and solvent-borne epoxy coatings have been employed mainly as anticorrosion protection for metals (marine and maintenance coatings), as waterproof protection for concrete, and as chemical-resistant protection for floors and walls (Bauer 1985; Muskopf and McCollister 1987). Two-component coatings can be cured at ambient temperatures with polyamines, polyamides and

Table 6. Catalyst-curing agents [CAS number] (Guin and Work 1995; Kanerva et al. 1996)

Aliphatic thioester
Boron trichloride-amine complex
Boron trifluoride-benzylamine complex [696–99–1]
Boron trifluoride:monomethylamine
1-Cyanoethyl-2-(alkyl or phenyl)imidazoles
1-Cyanoethyl-2-(alkyl or phenyl)imidazole-trimellitates
1-Cyanoethyl-2-phenyl-4,5-di(cyanoethoxymethyl)imidazole
Dimethylaminomethylphenol [25338–55–0]
2,4,6-Tris-(dimethylaminomethyl)phenol (tris-DMP)
[CAS 90–72–2]
Tris(dimethylaminomethyl)phenol-tri(2-ethylhexoate)
N,N-Dimethylbenzylamine [CAS-103–83–3]
Imidazolinealkyl imidazoles
Ketimine [P-83–0735]
2-(Methyl or phenyl)imidazole-isocyanuric acid adduct
4,4'-Methylene-*bis*(2-ethyl-5-methylimidazole)
Morpholine salt of *p*-toluenesulfonic acid
2-Phenylimidazole [670–96–2]
Thioether
Trifunctional mercaptan terminated polymer

amine-epoxy adducts. Tertiary amines, e.g. tris-DMP, are frequently used to accelerate the curing rates (Kanerva et al. 1991). Most epoxy surface coatings are based on DGEBA epoxy resins, but coatings based on DGEBF epoxy resins have also been used increasingly (Pontén and Bruze 2001). Epoxy resins with a low average MW are used in two-component solvent-less coatings. Waterborne epoxy coatings are prepared by the dispersion of epoxy resins modified with water-soluble functional groups or by the emulsification of DGEBA epoxy resins with surfactants (Bauer 1985; Muskopf and McCollister 1987).

Epoxy adhesives range from those used as two-package, ambient-cure, general adhesives in domestic applications to high-performance one-component sheet adhesives for aircraft assembly (Gardiner et al. 1992). Araldite is a well-known, old trademark of Ciba Geigy for consumer epoxy adhesives. Liquid DGEBA epoxy resins are used in most of the one- and two-component epoxy adhesives. The curing agent generally consists of polyamides or aliphatic polyamines, e.g. DETA and TETA.

Epoxy resins are used in the manufacture of composite products (Tarvainen and Kanerva 2000). Epoxy composites are used, e.g. for sporting goods, automotive, boat-building and aircraft industries, and for military and aerospace applications (Jolanki et al. 2000; Tarvainen and Kanerva 2000).

Casting resins are liquid and solvent-less mixtures of low-MW epoxy resin, a curing agent, and additives. The mixture is poured into moulds and cured to solid structures. The casting resins are used mainly as electrical insulating material in the manufacture of transformers, switching gear, circuit breakers, conductors and insulators. Anhydride-cured cycloaliphatic epoxy resins are commonly used to improve arc-track resistance and durability particularly to changes in weather, e.g. in outdoor electrical insulators (Muskopf and McCollister 1987; Jolanki et al. 2000).

Epoxy moulding compounds are solid mixtures of epoxy resin (epoxy novolac), a curing agent and catalyst, mould-release compounds, fillers and other additives. The moulding compounds become liquid at relatively low temperatures (150–200 °C) (Adams 1983; Muskopf and McCollister 1987). Epoxy moulding compounds are used, for example, in the manufacture of models and engine covers and in the encapsulation of electrical components (Fregert 1981 b).

Epoxy resins were introduced in 1956 in the preparation of samples for electron microscopy and they are still widely used (Glauert 1991).

Epoxy Dermatitis

Delayed Allergic Epoxy Dermatitis

The first reports of sensitisation to epoxy compounds were published in the 1950s, shortly after large-scale production of epoxy resins began (Jolanki et al. 2000).

In Finland, the most common causes of occupational allergic contact dermatitis in 1997–1999 were rubber chemicals (22.2%), plastic chemicals (20.8%) and metals (16.0%) (Jolanki et al. 2001 b). Plastic chemicals have been common causes of occupational allergic contact dermatitis in Finland since the 1960s and 1970s. At first, most of the cases were due to phenol-formaldehyde resins. By the beginning of the 1970s, epoxy-resin compounds began to cause increasing numbers of occupational dermatoses. In the 1990s, the epoxy-resin compounds were clearly more frequent causes than other plastic chemicals. They have induced about 10% of the cases of occupational allergic contact dermatitis (Jolanki et al. 2000; Jolanki et al. 2001 b).

The component causing sensitivity, while most often the DGEBA epoxy resin, is probably determined more by the opportunity for exposure. The 22-year statistics on patients diagnosed at the Finnish Institute of Occupational Health showed that most of the 182 patients who had occupational allergic contact dermatitis from epoxy-resin compounds were sensitised to DGEBA epoxy resins (Jolanki et al. 2001 a). DGEBA resin allergy was found in 80% of the cases. Contact allergy from non-DGEBA epoxy resins was found in about 9% of the patients, contact allergy from polyamine hardeners in 23% and from reactive diluents in 16%. Of the 182 patients, 95 (52%) had an isolated contact allergy to DGEBA epoxy resins, 16 (9%) to non-DGEBA epoxy resins, 6 to polyamine hardeners and 6 to reactive diluents. Six patients had allergic contact dermatitis from TGIC and one from PA hardeners. Simultaneous contact allergy to two or more epoxy-resin compound categories was found in 29% of the patients (Jolanki et al. 2001 a).

Roughly 1% of the exposed workers, annually, developed an occupational dermatosis due to epoxy-resin compounds (Jolanki 1991). Holness and Nethercott (1993) found 18% of patients with a history of potential exposure to the epoxy-resin system to exhibit a positive response to DGEBA epoxy resin. Even higher risks of contact allergy from exposure to epoxy resin compounds are found for individual groups of workers constantly exposed to epoxy resin compounds, e.g.

56% in aircraft manufacturing workers (Burrows et al. 1984), 45% in marble workers (Angelini et al. 1996), and 27% in ski-factory workers (Jolanki et al. 1996 b).

In some instances, the latent period before onset of contact allergy to epoxy-resin compounds may be quite short, ranging from less than 1 month to several years (Jolanki 1991). Even a single accidental exposure may induce primary sensitisation to epoxy resin (Kanerva et al. 2000 a). Most of the patients contracting epoxy-compound dermatosis are men.

Epoxy compounds can induce direct or airborne contact dermatitis, but the skin symptoms are located mainly on the patients' hands or arms. The fingers and interdigital spaces, forearms and wrists, and the eyelids are the most typical locations of the skin disorders due to epoxy compounds (Jolanki et al. 1990). Reactive diluents and hardeners have been considered the most probable causes of airborne epoxy-resin compound dermatitis because the substances are more volatile than DGEBA epoxy resins (Dahlquist and Fregert 1979). In another study, facial dermatitis was found in 60% of the patients, but it was not especially common among patients allergic to reactive diluents or hardeners (Jolanki et al. 1990).

Diglycidyl Ether of Bisphenol A (DGEBA) Epoxy Resins

Thorgeirsson and Fregert (1977) confirmed that the main sensitiser during the handling of components of the epoxy system was DGEBA, with an MW of 340 Da. In the guinea-pig maximisation test, the oligomer with an MW of 624 Da was also a sensitiser, but it had a minor sensitising capacity, whereas oligomers with an MW of more than 900 Da did not induce sensitivity (Thorgeirsson et al. 1978).

The DGEBA epoxy resin was included in the European standard patch-test series in 1966 (Jolanki 1991). In general, in the patch-test series performed, the frequency of positive responses to epoxy resin ranged from 0.4% (Enders et al. 1989) to about 3%. The percentage positives from occupational dermatology clinics in Toronto and Helsinki were as high as 3.7%, corresponding to the selectivity of the patients in the clinics (Jolanki 1991; Holness and Nethercott 1992).

Paints, varnishes and other surface coatings as well as exposure in the electronics industry are common causes of DGEBA epoxy-resin sensitisation. Epoxy sensitisation is also often due to exposure to two-component glues and bonding agents. Several reports describe workers sensitised to epoxy resins used as binders in carbon- or glass-fibre-reinforced plastic products (Jolanki et al. 2000). Epoxy resin used as a sizing agent in glass fibres has also induced contact allergy during the production (Heino et al. 1996) or the use of composite products (Tarvainen and Kanerva 2000), as well as epoxy resin used in electron microscopy (Dannaker 1988).

Furthermore, numerous case reports present epoxy sensitisation due to hidden sources of epoxy resin, such as a one-pack epoxy glue, oil painting, lamination of glass products, adhesive plaster, bowls polish, a billiard cue, and microscopy immersion oils (Jolanki et al. 2000; Kanerva et al. 2001). Solid, completely polymerised resins rarely cause dermatitis, but traces of unhardened monomeric DGEBA epoxy resin have been identified on sign-boards, bottle caps, film cassettes, metal packages and brass doorknobs (Fregert 1981 a). Tooling, e.g. sawing and drilling, of epoxy resin in the cured state, especially, promotes the release of epoxy allergens (Hansson 1994). Allergic contact dermatitis has also been induced by unhardened epoxy resin in several finished products. In addition, a few cases of allergic contact dermatitis due to DGEBA epoxy resins with a high average MW have been reported, even though the amount of DGEBA has been as low as 0.2% in the causative products. Epoxy resins used as stabilisers and plasticisers for polyvinyl chloride have also been shown to be sensitisers (Jolanki et al. 2000).

Non-Diglycidyl Ether of Bisphenol A

Most of those who have contact allergy to epoxy resins have been sensitised to DGEBA epoxy resins. Since the 1980s, allergic contact dermatitis has also been reported from non-DGEBA epoxy resins, such as *N-N'*-tetraglycidyl-4,4'-methylene dianiline and *ortho*-diglycidyl phthalate, 4-glycidyloxy-*N,N'*-diglycidylaniline, vinyl cyclohexene dioxide and a triglycidyl derivative of *para*-aminophenol. In addition, cycloaliphatic epoxy resins based on diglycidyl ester of hexahydrophthalic acid, heterocyclic dimethyl hydantoin epoxy resins, phenol novolac epoxy resins, and brominated epoxy resins have been found to be causes of allergic contact dermatitis. Many of the patients sensitised to non-DGEBA epoxy resins do not have contact allergy to DGEBA epoxy resin (Bruze et al. 1996; Jolanki et al. 2000; Kanerva et al. 2000b, 2002a).

TGIC is a known skin irritant (Nishioka et al. 1988), but has also been shown to be an allergen. Workers may become sensitised to TGIC from short-term exposure to the chemical during its production, in the manufacture and use of TGIC-containing powder polyester paints, and from silk-screen printing coatings in the manufacture of circuit boards (Jolanki et al. 1994; Wigger-Alberti et al. 1997).

Reactive Diluents

Reactive diluents have been shown to be common contact allergens among exposed patients (Jolanki 1991; Tosti et al. 1992; Angelini et al. 1996). Contact allergy to reactive diluents without contact allergy to epoxy resins is also possible. These materials are more volatile than DGEBA epoxy resin, and may cause an airborne dermatitis pattern (Dahlquist and Fregert 1979; Angelini et al. 1996). Most patients sensitised to reactive diluents are allergic to phenyl glycidyl ether (PGE), cresyl glycidyl ether, hexanediol diglycidyl ether, butanediol diglycidyl ether or butyl glycidyl ether, and cross-sensitisation between reactive diluents is common (Tosti et al. 1992; Condé-Salazar et al. 1994; Angelini et al. 1996; Jolanki et al. 2000). Rare reactive diluent contact allergens are allyl glycidyl ether, cyclohexanedimethanol glycidyl ether, neopentyl glycol diglycidyl ether, Cardura E10, Epoxide 8, diethyleneglycol diglycidyl ether and alpha-naphthyl glycidyl ether and *p*-fluorphenyl glycidyl ether (Jolanki et al. 2000). Allyl glycidyl ether has also caused allergic contact dermatitis in the plastics industry from the use of epoxy silane in a single-component sealant (Dooms-Goossens et al. 1995).

Hardeners

Most of the patients with contact allergy to epoxy hardeners react to 4,4'-diaminodiphenyl methane (DDM), DETA and TETA (Jolanki 1991; Tosti et al. 1992). In addition, cases of contact allergy to IPDA (Kanerva et al. 1998; Tarvainen et al.

1998), trimethyl hexamethylene diamine, tetraethylenepentamine (TEPA), xylylene diamine (Kanerva et al. 1998), or other cyclohexylamines (Gordon and McLelland 1998) have been reported. Polyamides and amine-epoxy adducts induced sensitisation probably only due to the polyamine remnants. Cross-reactivity between polyamine hardeners is possible.

Isolated contact allergy to epoxy hardeners is unusual, but possible. Tris-DMP has been reported to be probably a more common allergen than expected (Kanerva et al. 1996; Brooke and Beck 1998). Allergic patch-test reactions to DDM or ethylene diamine (EDA) are not necessarily an indication of sensitivity from exposure to epoxy-resin hardeners. The relevance of DDM allergy is sometimes difficult to detect. For example, a positive patch-test reaction to DDM may represent allergy to *para*-amino compounds, e.g. *para*-phenylene diamine (Gailhofer and Ludvan 1989), or exposure to diphenyl methane diisocyanate (Jolanki et al. 1990). EDA allergy may be due to exposure, for example, to rubber, synthetic coolants or topical creams (Rietschel and Fowler 1995). Another aliphatic polyamine hardener, DMAPA, is an impurity responsible for cocamidopropylbetaine allergy from cosmetics (Angelini et al. 1995).

A few reports of contact allergy to non-amine hardeners have been published in the case of dicyandiamide (Senff et al. 1988), dodecenyl succinic anhydride (Göransson 1977), methylhexahydrophthalic anhydride (Kanerva et al. 1997), hexavalent chromate, an accelerator additive (Handley and Burrows 1994; Bruze et al. 1996) and polysulfides (Bruze et al. 1996).

Bisphenol A and Epichlorohydrin

Occupational contact dermatitis due to epichlorohydrin and bisphenol A is uncommon (Jolanki 1991). In epoxy-resin plants, despite closed manufacturing systems, workers may have a rather high risk of becoming sensitised to epichlorohydrin, but they do not generally become sensitised to bisphenol A (van Joost et al. 1990).

The group of van Joost (van Joost et al. 1990; Jolanki et al. 2000) found very few cases of bisphenol A allergy in workers at epoxy-resin plants, although several patients had been sensitised to epichlorohydrin. Cases of allergy to bisphenol A have been reported from, e.g. bis-GMA-based dental composite resins, semi-synthetic waxes, plastic footwear, and plastic gloves (Estlander et al. 1999; Estlander et al. 2000; Jolanki et al. 2000). The contact allergy to bisphenol A may also be a cross reaction with compounds responsible for phenol-formaldehyde resin allergy, such as dihydroxydiphenyl methanes (bisphenol F) (Bruze and Zimerson 1985; Jolanki 1991).

Contact Urticaria

Only a few cases of immediate-type contact urticaria caused by epoxy-resin compounds have been reported. In particular, organic acid anhydride hardeners and epoxy resins (Jolanki et al. 1997a,b; Jolanki et al. 2000; Kanerva et al. 2002b) should be regarded as potential causes of the contact-urticaria syndrome. In Finland in the period between 1997 and 1999, 10 cases of contact urticaria from organic acid anhydrides and one from DGEBA were reported to the Finnish Register of Occupational Diseases (Jolanki et al. 2001 b).

Irritant Epoxy Dermatitis

Irritative, low-MW degradation products may be produced in the tooling of epoxy products and in heating processes (Engström and Henriks-Eckerman 1988). Polyamine hardeners and epichlorohydrin, in particular, irritate the skin and conjunctivae. In addition to causing irritant contact dermatitis, epichlorohydrin, as a highly reactive compound, and aliphatic polyamines, as highly alkaline compounds (pH 13–14), can cause corrosive burns on the skin. Organic acid anhydrides, when cold, are not very harmful to dry skin, but hot compounds may cause severe chemical burns. On sweating skin, anhydrides are hydrated to the corresponding acids and can cause caustic dermatitis and burns (Adams 1983; Jolanki et al. 2000).

Other Skin Disorders Caused by Epoxy Compounds

Purpuric allergic contact dermatitis, scleroderma-like disorders, atypical psoriasis and erythema multiforme have been described as being caused by exposure to epoxy compounds (Holness and Nethercott 1989); Bachurzewska and Borucka (1986) reported Raynaud's-disease-type ailments. Rycroft (1980) reported on a patient whose epoxy-resin sensitisation was followed by atypical psoriasis, while Lichter et al. (1992) described a patient whose sensitisation to epoxy resin and hardener was followed by lichenoid contact dermatitis. Photosensitivity has been reported in relation to the heating of DGEBA epoxy resin and the use of epoxy powder paints (Göransson et al. 1984). Photosensitivity is considered probably to be due to bisphenol A contained in the resin (Maguire 1988).

Skin Testing and Chemical Investigations

No single chemical can be used alone to screen for sensitisation to several different contact allergens of epoxy compounds. About one third of the patients who have developed contact allergy to epoxy-resin compounds have been found to be sensitive to more than one of the three main epoxy-resin compound groups, i.e., resins, hardeners and reactive diluents (Jolanki et al. 2001 a). In addition, individual contact allergies to hardeners, reactive diluents and non-DGEBA epoxy resins without simultaneous contact allergy to the standard epoxy resin are rather common among workers exposed to epoxy-resin compounds (Jolanki et al. 2000; Jolanki et al. 2001 a). Thus, it might be recommended that patients suspected of contracting contact dermatitis from epoxy-resin compounds also be tested with the individual allergenic compounds, hardeners, reactive diluents and non-DGE-BA epoxy resins, according to the contents of the epoxy-resin compounds used by the patients. The patients should also be tested with their own specific materials, to which they have been exposed, especially if there is no response to the standard epoxy resin (Holness and Nethercott 1993; Chap. 17, this book).

A patch-test concentration of 0.25 for DGEBF epoxy resins (Pontén and Bruze 2001) and 0.5% for other non-DGEBA epoxy resins is probably preferable to 1% when low viscosity resins are being tested, because 1% non-DGEBA may irritate (Jolanki et al. 2000; Pontén and Bruze 2001). Patch testing with the resinous part alone does not exclude contact allergy to reactive diluents if the patient is also sensitive to the resin. The test concentration of 0.25% in petrolatum has been found to be suitable for testing reactive diluents.

On patch testing, cross allergy has been found between compounds that are chemically closely related, especially between reactive diluents. PGE and 1,4-butanediol diglycidyl ether (BDDGE) are probably enough to also screen contact allergy to reactive diluents (Jolanki 1991). Reactive diluents do not produce cross allergy with DGEBA epoxy resins, and contact allergy to reactive diluents is not revealed by testing with the standard epoxy resin. Patients who are allergic to cycloaliphatic epoxy resins often react to reactive diluents, and vice versa.

Patch testing with DETA, TETA, DDM, IPDA and tris-DMP should be performed when allergy to polyamine hardeners is suspected. All but tris-DMP are available from the test substance suppliers. The recommended test concentration for tris-DMP is 0.5–1% in petrolatum (Kanerva et al. 1996; Brooke and Beck 1998). Because of the vast variety of hardeners used, it is highly recommended also to test patients with the hardeners that they have been exposed to; a test concentration of about 1% is the most suitable for polyamine-type hardeners; test concentrations of up to 10% should be used for the amine-epoxy adducts.

In general, petrolatum seems to be a good vehicle for epoxy-resin compounds. For solid materials containing uncured epoxy resins, it is preferable to use acetone instead of water for ultrasonic cleaning bath extractions or to soften the material in the patch test chamber (Jolanki et al. 2000; Chap. 17, this book).

In problematic cases, skin-prick testing with epoxy compounds, consultations with industrial hygienists, visits to the patients' work sites and analyses of the materials handled by the patients are important. Thin-layer chromatography and other chromatographic methods (gas chromatography and high-performance liquid chromatography) can be used to demonstrate the presence or absence of particular allergens (Gruvberger et al. 2000; Jolanki et al. 2000).

Prevention of Epoxy Dermatitis

Most patients who have acquired occupational allergic contact dermatitis from epoxy resin compounds have to quit their work. Quitting may also be beneficial for the prevention of possible respiratory allergy or contact urticaria following by the skin sensitisation (Kanerva et al. 2000 a,b). Allergic epoxy dermatitis nevertheless has a good prognosis. Skin problems generally clear up shortly after exposure has ended (Rosen and Freeman 1993).

Those working with epoxy compounds should be aware of the risk of sensitisation. Gloves made of laminated, multilayered plastic (4H-glove), developed especially for the handling of epoxy compounds, give the best protection against them (McClain and Storrs 1992). The use of any type of gloves, however, seems to reduce the exposure to epoxy resin compounds and helps to protect against the risk of sensitisation, although the use of protective gloves may, in some individual cases, even promote contact allergens to come into contact with the skin (Jolanki et al. 1990). Unhealthy skin, including even small wounds and abrasions, should be protected from epoxy-compound exposure because of increased skin penetration. The use of less-sensitising products may reduce the possibility of developing allergy to epoxy, as high-MW epoxies do not sensitise readily. The use of one-bag epoxies, which mix in the package (Van Putten et al. 1984), may reduce the possibility of skin contact. The airways should also be protected from exposure to the epoxy compounds, because the compounds can be considered potential causes of asthma. An automatic process, as such, does not guarantee protection against skin contact and exposure of the respiratory tract to the compounds because, for example, of exposure during maintenance, repair or sampling (Jolanki 1991).

References

Adams RM (1983) Occupational skin disease. Grune Stratton Inc, New York, pp 238–266

Angelini G, Foti C, Rigano L, Vena GA (1995) 3-Dimethylaminopropylamine: a key substance in contact allergy to cocamidopropylbetaine? Contact Dermatitis 32:96–99

Angelini G, Rigano L, Foti C, Grandolfo M, Veña GA, Bonamonte D, Soleo L, Scorpinitti AA (1996) Occupational sensitization to epoxy resin and reactive diluents in marble workers. Contact Dermatitis 35:11–16

Bachurzewska B, Borucka I (1986) Gefässläsionen bei Eisenbahnarbeiterinnen, die mit Epoxidharzen in Berührung kommen. Dermatosen 34:77–79

Bäck B, Saarinen L (1986) Free amines in epoxy hardeners and in workplace air (in Finnish with English summary). Työterveyslaitoksen tutkimuksia 1:31–36 (Summary p 69)

Bauer RS (1985) Epoxy resins. In: Tess RW, Poehlein GW (eds) Applied polymer science, 2nd edn. American Chemical Society, Washington, pp 931–961

Brooke R, Beck MH (1998) Contact allergy to 2,4,6-tris(dimethylaminomethyl)phenol. Contact Dermatitis 38:284–285

Bruze M, Zimerson E (1985) Contact allergy to dihydroxydiphenyl methanes (bisphenol F). Dermatosen 33:216–220

Bruze M, Edenholm M, Engström K, Svensson G (1996) Occupational dermatoses in a Swedish aircraft plant. Contact dermatitis 34:336–340

Burrows D, Fregert S, Campbell H, Trulsson L (1984) Contact dermatitis from the epoxy resins tetraglycidyl-4,4′-methylene dianiline and o-diglycidyl phthalate in composite material. Contact Dermatitis 11:80–82

Condé-Salazar L, Conzalez de Domingo MA, Guimaraens D (1994) Sensitization to epoxy resin system in special flooring workers. Contact Dermatitis 31:157–160

Dahlquist I, Fregert S (1979) Allergic contact dermatitis from volatile epoxy hardeners and reactive diluents. Contact Dermatitis 5:406–407

Dannaker CJ (1988) Allergic sensitization to a non-bisphenol A epoxy of the cycloaliphatic class. J Occup Med 30:641–643

Dooms-Goossens A, Bruze M, Buysse L, Fregert S, Gruvberger B, Stals H (1995) Contact allergy to allyl glycidyl ether present as an impurity in 3-glycidyloxypropoxyltrimethoxysilane, a fixing additive in silicone and polyurethane resins. Contact Dermatitis 33:17–19

Enders F, Przybilla B, Ring J, Burg G, Braun-Falco O (1989) Patch test results in 1987 compared to trends from the period 1977–1983. Contact Dermatitis 20:230–232

Engström B, Henriks-Eckerman M-L (1988) Welding and paint (in Finnish). Työterveyslaitos (Työolot 68.), Helsinki

Estlander T, Jolanki R, Henriks-Eckerman M-L, Kanerva L (1999) Occupational contact allergy to bisphenol A. Contact Dermatitis 40:52–53

Estlander T, Jolanki R, Henriks-Eckerman M-L, Kanerva L (2000) Occupational contact allergy to bisphenol A. Allergy Review 2:8–9,22

Fregert S (1981a) Epoxy dermatitis from the non-working environment. Br J Dermatol 105[Suppl 21]:63–64

Fregert S (1981b) Manual of contact dermatitis, 2nd edn. Munksgaard, Copenhagen

Gailhofer G, Ludvan M (1989) Zur Wertigkeit positiver Epikutantestreaktionen auf 4,4'-Diamino-diphenylmethan. Dermatosen 37:17–22

Gardiner TH, Waechter JM Jr, Wiedow MH, Solomon WA (1992) Glycidyloxy compounds used in epoxy resin systems: a toxicology review. Regul Toxicol Pharmacol 15:S1

Glauert AM (1991) Epoxy resins: an update on their selection and use. Eur Microsc Analysis September:13–18

Göransson K (1977) Allergic contact dermatitis to an epoxy hardener: dodecenyl-succinic anhydride. Contact Dermatitis 3:277–278

Göransson K, Andersson R, Andersson G, Marklund S, Anderson K, Östbye P, Zingmark P-A (1984) An outbreak of occupational photodermatosis of the face in a factory in northern Sweden. In: Berglund B, Lindvall T, Sundell J (eds) Indoor air, vol 3. Swedish Council for Building Research, Stockholm, pp 367–375

Gordon PM, McLelland J (1998) Contact sensitivity to Ancamine 2280 (p-aminocyclohexylamine) following a change in work practice. Contact Dermatitis 38:54

Gruvberger B, Bruze M, Fregert S (2000) Physicochemical methods for detection of occupational contact allergens. In: Kanerva L, Elsner P, Wahlberg JE, Maibach HI (eds) Handbook of occupational dermatology. Springer, Berlin Heidelberg New York, pp 384–391

Guin JD, Work WJ (1995) Plastics: Epoxy resins. In: Guin JD (ed) Practical contact dermatitis. A handbook for the practitioner. McGraw-Hill, USA, pp 433–446

Handley J, Burrows D (1994) Dermatitis from hexavalent chromate in the accelerator of an epoxy sealant (PR1422) used in the aircraft industry. Contact Dermatitis 30:193–196

Hansson C (1994) Determination of monomers in epoxy resin hardened at elevated temperature. Contact Dermatitis 31:333–334

Heino T, Haapa K, Manelius F (1996) Contact sensitization to organosilane solution in glass filament production. Contact Dermatitis 34:294

Henriks-Eckerman M-L, Laijoki T (1986a) Aliphatic polyamines and epoxy oligomers in cold cured epoxy products (in Finnish with English summary). Työterveyslaitoksen tutkimuksia 4:37–40 (Summary, p 69)

Henriks-Eckerman M-L, Laijoki T (1986b) Glycidyl ethers in epoxy resin products (in Finnish with English summary). Työterveyslaitoksen tutkimuksia 4:41–46 (Summary, p 70)

Holness DL, Nethercott JR (1989) Occupational contact dermatitis due to epoxy resin in a fiberglass binder. J Occup Med 31:87–89

Holness DL, Nethercott JR (1992) Results of testing with epoxy resin in an occupational health clinic population. Am J Contact Dermat 3:169–174

Holness DL, Nethercott JR (1993) The performance of specialized collections of bisphenol A epoxy system components in the evaluation of workers in an occupational health clinic population. Contact Dermatitis 28:216–219

Jolanki R (1991) Occupational skin diseases from epoxy compounds. Epoxy resin compounds, epoxy acrylates and 2,3-epoxypropyl trimethyl ammonium chloride (doctoral dissertation). Acta Derm Venerol Suppl 159:1–80

Jolanki R, Estlander T, Kanerva L (1987) Contact allergy to an epoxy reactive diluent: 1,4-butanediol diglycidyl ether. Contact Dermatitis 16:87–92

Jolanki R, Kanerva L, Estlander T, Tarvainen K, Keskinen H, Henriks-Eckerman M-L (1990) Occupational dermatoses from epoxy resin compounds. Contact Dermatitis 23:172–83

Jolanki R, Kanerva L, Estlander T, Tarvainen K (1994) Concomitact sensitization to triglycidyl isocyanurate, diaminodiphenylmethane and 2-hydroxyethyl methacrylate from silkscreen printing coatings in the manufacture of circuit boards. Contact Dermatitis 30:12–15

Jolanki R, Kanerva L, Estlander T (1996a) Allergic patch test reactions to diglycidyl ether of bisphenol A in hardened nail base and top coat. Contact Dermatitis 35:246–247

Jolanki R, Tarvainen K, Tatar T, Estlander T, Henriks-Eckerman M-L, Mustakallio KK, Kanerva L (1996b) Occupational dermatoses from exposure to epoxy resin compounds in a ski factory. Contact Dermatitis 34:390–396

Jolanki R, Kanerva L, Estlander T (1997a) Contact urticaria from epoxy resins. In: Amin S, Lahti A, Maibach HI (eds) Contact urticaria syndrome. CRC Press LLC, Boca Raton, FL, pp 143–147

Jolanki R, Kanerva L, Estlander T, Tarvainen K (1997b) Skin allergy caused by organic acid anhydrides. In: Amin S, Lahti A, Maibach HI (eds) Contact urticaria syndrome. CRC Press LLC, Boca Raton, FL, pp 217–224

Jolanki R, Kanerva L, Estlander T (2000) Epoxy resins. In: Kanerva L, Elsner P, Wahlberg JE, Maibach HI (eds) Handbook of occupational dermatology. Springer, Berlin Heidelberg New York pp 570–590

Jolanki R, Estlander T, Kanerva L (2001a) 182 patients with occupational allergic epoxy contact dermatitis over 22 years. Contact Dermatitis 44, 121–123

Jolanki R, Savela A, Estlander T. Kanerva L (2001b) Ihotaudit ammattitautitilastojen mukaan. (Occuptional dermatoses according to the statistic on occupational diseases, in Finnish). Työterveyslääkärilehti 19:10–16

Kanerva L, Jolanki R, Estlander T (1991) Allergic contact dermatitis from epoxy resin hardeners. Am J Contact Dermatitis 2:88–97

Kanerva L, Estlander T, Jolanki R (1996) Occupational allergic contact dermatitis caused by 2,4,6-tris-(dimethylamino-methyl)phenol, and a review of sensitizing epoxy resin hardeners. Int J Dermatol 35:852–856

Kanerva L, Hyry H, Jolanki R, Hytönen M, Estlander T (1997) Delayed and immediate allergy caused by methylhexahydrophthalic anhydride. Contact Dermatitis 36:34–38

Kanerva L, Jolanki R, Estlander T (1998) Occupational epoxy dermatitis with patch test reactions to multiple hardeners including tetraethylenepentamine. Contact Dermatitis 38:299–301

Kanerva L, Estlander T, Keskinen H, Jolanki R (2000a) Occupational allergic airborne contact dermatitis and delayed bronchial asthma from epoxy resin revealed by bronchial provocation test. Eur J Dermatol 10:475–477

Kanerva L, Jolanki R, Estlander T, Henriks-Eckerman M-L, Tuomi M-L, Tarvainen K (2000b) Airborne occupational allergic contact dermatitis from triglycidyl-p-aminophenol and tetraglycidyl-4,4′-methylene dianiline in preimpregnated epoxy resin product in the aircraft industry. Dermatology 201:29–33

Kanerva L, Jolanki R, Estlander T (2001) Active sensitization caused by epoxy in Leica® immersion oil. Contact Dermatitis 44:194–196

Kanerva L, Jolanki R, Estlander T, Henriks-Eckerman M-L, Tuomi M-L, Tarvainen K (2002a) Airborne occupational allergic contact dermatitis from triglycidyl-p-aminophenol and tetraglycidyl-4,4′-methylene dianiline in preimpregnated epoxy resin product in the aircraft industry. Allergy Review Series No 1, 19–21, 24

Kanerva L, Pelttari M, Jolanki R, Alanko K, Estlander T, Suhonen R (2002b). Occupational contact urticaria from diglycidyl ether of bisphenol A epoxy resin. Allergy 57:1205–1207

Lichter M, Drury D, Remlinger K (1992) Lichenoid dermatitis caused by epoxy resin. Contact Dermatitis 26:275

Maguire HC (1988) Experimental photoallergic contact dermatitis to bisphenol A. Acta Derm Venerol 68:408–412

McClain DC, Storrs FJ (1992) Protective effect of both a barrier cream and a polyethylene lamintate glove against epoxy resin, glyceryl monothioglycolate, frullania, and tancy. Am J Contact Dermat 3:201–205

Muskopf JW, McCollister SB (1987) Epoxy resins. In: Gerhartz W, Yamamoto YS, Kaudy L, Rounsaville JF, Schulx G (eds) Ullmann's encyclopedia of industrial chemistry, vol A9. 5th compl rev edn. VCH Verlagsgesellschaft, Weinheim, pp 547–563

Nishioka K, Ogasawara M, Asagami C (1988) Occupational contact allergy to triglycidyl isocyanurate (TGIC, Tepic®). Contact Dermatitis 19:379–380

Pontén A, Bruze M (2001) Contact allergy to epoxy resin based on diglycidylether of bisphenol F. Contact Dermatitis 44:98–99

Rietschel RL, Fowler JF, Jr (1995) Fisher's Contact Dermatitis, 4th edn. Williams Wilkins, Philadelphia

Rosen RH, Freeman S (1993) Prognosis of occupational contact dermatitis in New South Wales, Australia. Contact Dermatitis 29:88–93

Rycroft RJG (1980) Atypical psoriasis following epoxy resin sensitization. J Soc Occup Med 30:132–134

Senff H, Kuhlwein A, Hausen BM (1988) Allergisches Kontaktekzem auf Dicyandiamid. Dermatosen 36:99–101

Tarvainen K, Jolanki R, Henriks-Eckerman M-L, Estlander T (1998) Occupational allergic contact dermatitis from isophoronediamine (IPDA) in operative-clothing manufacture. Contact Dermatitis 39:46–47

Tarvainen K, Kanerva L (2000) Plastic composites. In: Kanerva L, Elsner P, Wahlberg JE, Maibach HI (eds) Handbook of occupational dermatology. Springer, Berlin Heidelberg New York, pp 611–621

Thorgeirsson A, Fregert S (1977) Allergenicity of epoxy resins in the guinea pig. Acta Derm Venerol 57:253–256

Thorgeirsson A, Fregert S, Ramnäs O (1978) Sensitization capacity of epoxy resin oligomers in the guinea pig. Acta Derm Venerol 58:17–21

Tosti A, Guerra L, Bardazzi F (1992) Occupational contact dermatitis from exposure to epoxy resins and acrylates. Clin Dermatol 10:133–140

Van Joost T, Roesyanto ID, Satyawan I (1990) Occupational sensitization to epichlorohydrin (ECH) and bisphenol-A during the manufacture of epoxy resin. Contact Dermatitis 22:125–126

Van Putten PB, Coenraads PJ, Nater JP (1984) Hand dermatoses and contact allergic reactions in construction workers exposed to epoxy resins. Contact Dermatitis 10:146–150

Wigger-Alberti W, Hofmann M, Elsner P (1997) Contact dermatitis caused by triglycidyl isocyanurate. Am J Contact Dermat 8:106–107

CHAPTER 33

Paints, Lacquers and Varnishes 33

T. Estlander, R. Jolanki, L. Kanerva

Introduction

The manufacture and chemistry of paints have undergone profound changes since the 1940s. Nowadays paints, lacquers and varnishes are complex mixtures of several components. The detailed composition of a paint, lacquer or varnish is planned to meet the special requirements of its use as well as the expectations concerning health and safety requirements (Fischer and Adams 1990; Rose and Vance 1997).

Composition

The paints can be liquids or powders that are applied to surfaces to make a dry coating for protective or decorative purposes. The basic constituents of modern paints include pigments, film formers, solvents and additives. Varnishes and lacquers have the same composition as paints, but lack pigments (Mathias 1984; Rose and Vance 1997).

Pigments

Pigments are fine powders that give the paints their colour. They also cover and hide surfaces. Limited solubility in water and in solvents, as well as good colour fastness are characteristics of pigments. They must also be dispersed in a paint formulation containing a resin binder to bind the pigment to the painted surface (Mathias 1984; Rose and Vance 1997).

Examples of inorganic pigments found in paints and coatings are shown in Table 1. Nowadays, paint manufacturers usually supply only some oil-based or emulsion-type basement paints, from which thousands of shades of colour can be produced by adding a combination of pigment pastes according to a special shading chart (Fischer and Adams 1990).

Solvents

Solvent-based paints (SBPs) dominated the market for construction paints until the 1970s. SBPs contain about 50% organic solvents. Since the 1980s aliphatic hydrocarbon solvents have replaced turpentine in construction paints. The first

Table 1. Examples of inorganic pigments found in paints and coatings (Mathias 1984; Fischer and Adams 1990)

Color	Pigment
White	Titanium dioxide, zinc oxide, white lead, lithopone, antimony trioxide
Black	Carbon black, mineral black, black iron oxide
Red	Synthetic iron oxide, red lead oxide, cadmium red
Yellow	Chrome yellow, strontium yellow, zinc yellow, nickel titanate yellow, zinc chromate, earthen iron oxide (ochre)
Orange	Chrome orange, molybdate orange, lead molybdate, cadmium mercurate orange
Green	Chrome green, chromium oxide
Blue	Iron blue (Prussian Blue), Ultramarine Blue
Violet	Mineral violet (manganese)

Table 2. Differences between solvent-based (alkyd paint) and water-based paints (acrylic dispersion paint) (Van Faassen and Borm 1991)

Component	Acrylic dispersion	Alkyd paint
Binder	Yes (polyacrylate)	Yes (alkyd resin)
Pigment	Yes	Yes
Filler	Yes	Yes
Organic solvent	Yes (0–15%)	Yes (about 50%)
Ammonia	Yes	No
Amine	Yes	No
Preservative	Yes	No
Surfactant	Yes	No
Corrosion inhibitor	Yes	No
Thickener	Yes	Yes
Drier	Yes	Yes
Anti-skinning agent	Yes	Yes
Ultraviolet-absorber	Yes	No

water-based latex-type paint was introduced in 1957 as an exterior paint. Because of the health hazards to the nervous system connected with SBPs, they have gradually been replaced by water-based paints (WBP) whenever possible. During the past 10 years, WBPs have constituted more than 90% of the construction paints in Scandinavia (Mathias 1984; Hansen et al. 1987; van Faassen and Borm 1991; Wieslander et al. 1994; Rietschell and Fowler 1995; Rose and Vance 1997; Estlander et al. 2000).

Water-based paints are dispersions based on synthetic polymers. Dispersions of polyacrylates are the most common. Water-based paints can also contain water-soluble alkyd resin and a mixture of polyacrylate and polyurethane. Although water is the main solvent in these types of paints, about 10% organic solvents are added (Hansen et al. 1987; van Faassen and Borm 1991; Wieslander et al. 1997). The differences between SBP and WBP can be seen in Table 2.

Table 3. Examples of film formers/binders and other plastic chemicals found in paints

Naturally drying oils
Alkyds
Epoxy-resin compounds
Formaldehyde resins
Vinyl resins
Acrylic resins
Urethane resins
Other synthetic resins
Polyester resins
Cyclohexanone resin
Other compounds (polyfunctional azidine hardeners, dipropylene glycol diacrylate, para-tertiary-butylcatechol)

Nowadays, coatings that are free from organic or other solvents are also increasingly used. Powder paints are composed of pigments, binders and additives which are melted together, cool set and ground into a powder which is applied by electrostatic spray (Mathias 1988; Rose and Vance 1997).

Film Formers

Resins or binders are the film-forming agents in paints. The resin hardens and keeps the pigments bound and permanently dispersed on the painted surface. Examples of resins used in paints and coatings are given in Table 3 (Mathias 1984; Rose and Vance 1997).

Naturally Drying Oils

Naturally drying oils, including dammar, Japanese lacquer and shellac, are suitable for lacquers and varnishes. Copal is a fossil resin that can be used in varnishes. Other natural oils include, e.g. flaxseed or linseed oil and pine oil or tall oil, which are used in oil-based paints. Since the 1980s, synthetic alkyd resins have widely replaced naturally drying oils (Mathias 1984; Fischer and Adams 1990).

Alkyds

Alkyds are condensation products of polyalcohols, e.g. glycerol, trimethylol propane pentaerythritol and polycarboxylic acids such as phthalic acid or its anhydride. Alkyd resins are formed by modifications with oils containing unsaturated fatty acids. These include, e.g. linseed and tall or pine oil. Linseed oil and similar drying oils can be combined with colophony (rosin). Epoxidized alkyd resins are alkyds modified with epoxidized oils (Mathias 1984; Fischer and Adams 1990).

Epoxy-Resin Compounds

Paints, varnishes and lacquers based on epoxy resins are used in various industrial applications. Two-component epoxy paints need a hardener added before their use. One-component epoxy paints that are heat-cured contain a hardener that can be activated only by heating. Polyfunctional aliphatic amines, aromatic amines, solid polyamides and anhydrides can be used as curing agents. Epoxy-ester-resin paints are formed by the reaction of epoxy resin with unsaturated fatty acids in drying oils (Mathias 1984, 1988). See the chapter on epoxy resins in this book (Chap. 17).

Formaldehyde Resins

Urea, melamine, phenol or substituted phenols can be modified with formaldehyde to produce corresponding resins. An excess of free formaldehyde must be removed in order to prevent interference with the film-forming properties of the paint. These resins can also be used to cross-link alkyd resins (Mathias 1984; Bruze 1985; Fischer and Adams 1990).

Vinyl Resins

Vinyl resins consist of polymers, copolymers or derivative products of vinyl acetate and vinyl chloride. Polyvinyl acetate resins are used in latex paints. Resins derived from polyvinyl chloride (PVC) can be dissolved or dispersed in organic solvents (Mathias 1984).

Acrylic Resins

Acrylic resins are used in latex paints. The latex binders are copolymers of two to five monomers, e.g. butyl acrylate, acrylic acid and styrene. Lattices are made by emulsion polymerization of the monomers dispersed in water as droplets. Polymerization is initiated by, for example, benzoyl peroxide. The lattices may contain small amounts of ammonia (0.3% w/w), formaldehyde (0.06% w/w) or other biocides (e.g. a mixture of isothiazolinones), surfactants and polymerization inhibitors (e.g. *p*-methoxy phenol or hydroquinone) (Mathias 1984; Hansen et al. 1987; Fischer and Adams 1990).

Industrial acrylate paints and coatings may contain polyfunctional acrylics, e.g. trimethylolpropane triacrylate and pentaerythritol acrylate and photoinitiators, e.g. benzophenones. Polyfunctional acrylates can also be combined with aziridine cross-linking agents (Mathias 1984). Before use a polyfunctional aziridine (PFA) hardener or cross-linker is added to the aqueous acrylic- or water-based urethane polymers. PFA is used to cross-link a variety of products (Kanerva et al. 1995; Estlander et al. 2000).

Urethane Resins

Urethane resins are formed by the reaction of isocyanate groups with hydroxyl groups of polyalcohols. In the reaction, diisocyanates, e.g. toluene diisocyanate, are used. The resins can be modified with natural drying oils, resulting in coatings which dry in air and are polymerizable like alkyd resins. Two-component systems harden when a diisocyanate curing agent, e.g. an amine, is added to prepolymerized polyurethane (PU) resin before application (Mathias 1984; Fischer and Adams 1990).

Other Synthetic Resins

Polystyrene resins are made from polymerized styrene. Synthetic rubber, known as styrene-butadiene rubber or chlorinated rubber latex, can be used in paints for floor coverings or tank linings (Fischer and Adams 1990).

Cyclohexanone resin (C-R) can be added to increase the hardness and water resistance of any paint but is most often used in floor paints. A paint can contain 5% C-R. There are several C-Rs from various manufacturers (Bruze et al. 1988).

Additives

Several additives can be used in paints in small percentages, e.g. to ensure the stability, quality and desired application properties of a paint. A list of additives is given in Table 4. The most important of these, in terms of their effects on the skin, are biocides and hardeners (Mathias 1984; Fischer and Adams 1990; van Faassen and Borm 1991; Rose and Vance 1997).

Hardeners are used to cure a paint system and include amines, peroxides and polyamides.

The other additives include extenders, driers, emulsifiers or surfactants, antifoaming agents, thixotropic agents or thickeners, plasticizers, coalescing agents, stabilizers, antioxidants or antiskinnning agents and photoinitiators (Mathias 1984; Fischer and Adams 1990).

Biocides are used to prevent the growth of bacteria and fungi mainly in water-based latex paints. Oil-based paints do not usually contain antimicrobials, but some exterior paints can contain an antimildew agent. A great number of biocides are available for use in paints (Table 5) (Fischer and Adams 1990; Hansen et al. 1987; Geier et al. 1996). Antifouling agents are used in marine paints. These include, for example, copper, organic tin, tetramethylthiuram disulfide and zinc carbamates (Fischer and Adams 1990).

Corrosion inhibitors in paints protect metallic surfaces from oxidation. Coating primers are used, e.g. in marine applications. Examples are coal-tar derivatives, epoxy resins and coal-tar modified epoxies. Primers that inhibit corrosion by anodic or cathodic polarization contain inorganic metallic pigments such as chro-

Table 4. Examples of additives in paints

Hardeners
Extenders
Driers
Emulsifiers
Antifoaming agents
Thixotropic agents
Plasticisers
Stabilizers
Biocides
Corrosion inhibitors
Photoinitiators

Table 5. Examples of biocides used in paints and glues (Fischer and Adams 1990; Geier et al. 1996)

Biocide	Paint	Glue
Bronopol	Yes	Yes
Chlorocresol	Yes	No
Chloroacetamide	Yes	No
1,2-Benzisothiazolinon-3-one	Yes	Yes
2-Chlor-*N*-hydroxymethyl acetamide	Yes	Yes
Zineb	Yes	No
2-*n*-Octyl-4-isothiazolin-3-one	Yes	No
5-Chloro-2-methyl-4-isothiazolin-3-one	Yes	Yes
Biopan P 1487	Yes	Yes
Biopan CS 1246	Yes	Yes
Biopan CS 1135	Yes	Yes
1,2-Dibromo-2,4-dicyanobutane	Yes	Yes
o-Phenylphenol	Yes	Yes
Benzylhemiformal	Yes	Yes
Propylene glycol hemiformal	Yes	Yes
Hexahydro-1,3,5-triethyl-s-triazine	Yes	–
2-(4-Thiazolyl)benzimidazole	Yes	–
Tributyltin oxide	Yes	No
N-(Trichloromethylthio)phthalimide (Folpet)	Yes	–
N-(Trichloromethylthio)-4-cyclohexane-1,2-dicarboximide (Captan)	Yes	–
Formaldehyde in raw materials	Yes	Yes

mates or leads or both. Composite pigments containing calcium oxide, zinc, silica, and oxides of phosphorus and boron can also be used. Nowadays, powder paints such as polyester and epoxy powder paints can also be used for corrosion inhibition (Mathias 1984, 1988; Rose and Vance 1997).

Paint and Varnish Removers

Paint and varnish removers can be in the form of liquids or pastes used to remove old coatings before refinishing a surface. They can contain volatile solvents, caustic agents and special chemicals (Kanerva et al. 1998; Fischer and Adams 1990; Vincent et al. 1994).

Prevalence of Dermatitis Caused by Paints, Lacquers and Varnishes

Piirilä (1947) was the first to investigate paint-factory workers, painters, polishers and varnishers in the mid-1940s. Within a period of 1 year, 10.7% of the paint workers and 3.7% of the painters had had contact dermatitis. In the 1950s, Schwartz et al. (1957) estimated that dermatitis among painters constituted about 3% of all compensated cases of occupational dermatoses, and was most frequent among painters in the building trade.

Between 1976 and 1977, Högberg and Wahlberg (1980) conducted a survey of Swedish house painters. A prevalence of 3.9% contact dermatitis was suggested. Irritant dermatitis was more common than allergic dermatitis.

Despite major changes in the contents of paints, lacquers and varnishes, as well as changes in the methods of application and the use of hand protection, the professionals using these products still belong to occupations with increased risk of occupational diseases. According to a Finnish study based on skin and other occupational diseases reported to the Finnish Register of Occupational Diseases between 1986 and 1991, painters and lacquerers had the greatest variety of occupational diseases.

The painters and lacquerers were eleventh in order among 25 occupations with an elevated risk of contracting an occupational skin disease [standardized rate ratio (SRR) greater than 1]. The risk of contracting allergic dermatitis was 3.5 times as common as in all occupations (SRR 3.52) and the risk of contracting irritant dermatitis was fourfold compared with that in all occupations.

However, in certain groups of painters exposed mainly to less irritating and sensitizing products, hand eczema is not more common than in the average population (Fischer et al. 1995; Estlander T et al. 2000).

Causes of Irritant Dermatitis

Skin irritation and irritant dermatitis are usually caused by repeated or prolonged contact with agents noxious to the skin. Both chemical and physical factors are involved. Important causes include soaps, detergents, acids, organic solvents, remnants of monomers and biocides as well as putties, plasters and cement (Mathias 1984; Fischer and Adams 1990; Estlander et al. 2000).

Biocides

Tri-N-butyl tin oxide (TBTO) can be used as a biocide (antifouling agent) in marine paints and other paints. It is known to be a strong skin irritant and has been shown to be corrosive to the skin in a 0.1% aqueous solution. The use of organic tin compounds is, however, decreasing because of the toxicity of the compound to marine life (Fischer and Adams 1990).

Most other biocides also have skin-irritating properties (Fischer and Adams 1990; Fischer et al. 1995; Geier et al. 1996).

Dusts and Mechanical Irritation of the Skin

Dust that irritates the skin and airways is created by the removal of old wallpapers, manual filling and sanding of walls and the hanging of fiberglass fabrics, especially during renovation of old buildings. Epoxy or polyester powder paints can also irritate the skin. *Mechanical irritation* of the skin associated with the last-mentioned operations may also promote the development of skin irritation (Mathias 1984; Jolanki 1991; Wieslander et al 1994; Fischer and Adams 1990; Fischer et al 1995).

Organic Solvents

Organic solvents induce dermatitis mostly by skin irritation, except in some cases caused by exposure to turpentine, glycols and citrus solvent. Glycols or glycol ethers are rare sensitizers, but a few cases of allergy to hexylene glycol have been reported. Solvents used as thinners or to remove grease and dirt from products to be spray painted, or to clean hands and tools are more important causes of irritant contact dermatitis than the solvents contained in paints (Pirilä 1947; Cronin 1980; Fischer and Adams 1990; Karlberg et al. 1992).

Nowadays, the most commonly used solvents are mineral or white spirits. Other solvents include a wide variety of alcohols, esters and ketones. Often, a mixture of different solvents is used to ensure the desired outcome, e.g. in thinners (Mathias 1984; Rose and Vance 1997; Leira 1997).

Other Solvents and Irritants

Water-based paints contain, in addition to solvents, other skin irritants including *monomers* from binders, *preservatives* and *surface-active agents* (*polyphosphates*), and *triethylamine* and *ammonia*. Monomers include, for example, butyl acrylate and various other acrylates. The solvents used in these products are also called coalescing solvents or cosolvents. They include hydrocarbon mixtures, alcohols, esters, glycols and glycol ethers/esters, e.g. ethylene glycol ethyl ether. Occupationally related contact dermatitis is not, however, common among painters using mainly these types of paints (Mathias 1984; Hansen et al. 1987; Fischer and Adams 1990; Fischer et al. 1995; Wieslander et al. 1997; Rose and Vance 1997).

Paint and Varnish Removers

Paint and varnish removers are especially noxious to the skin because they may contain, in addition to irritating solvents, many caustic chemicals, such as sodium phosphate, sodium silicate and caustic soda, as well as special chemicals such as dibutylthiourea. Solvents include, e.g. methylene chloride, methyl alcohol, ethyl alcohol and toluene (Kanerva et al. 1988; Fischer and Adams 1990).

Causes of Allergic Contact Dermatitis

Allergic contact dermatitis is the most important occupational skin disease among painters. Since the 1970s, synthetic resins have been the most important causes of sensitization caused by paints. Other causes include biocides and other additives such as hardeners or accelerators and inhibitors of polymerization. There are also several other potential causes, including plasticizers, dryers and chromates. Formaldehyde and rubber chemicals, as well as turpentine and other natural products, can also be included in the list of potential allergens (Mathias 1984; Jolanki 1991; Holmes et al. 1993; Kanerva 1995; Fischer and Adams 1990; Fischer et al. 1995).

At the Finnish Institute of Occupational Health (FIOH) between 1974 and 1997, a total of 85 cases of allergic contact dermatitis were diagnosed in different kinds of painters, lacquerers, parquet installers and paint-factory workers. Synthetic resins caused 68 of the cases, 54 of them in paints, lacquers or raw materials of paints, 5 in floor coverings, 5 in car painters' filling cements, 4 in parquet lacquers and one in a glue. The other agents included chromium, formaldehyde, cobalt, colophony, a mixture of isothiazolinones, and rubber chemicals. No cases of type 1 sensitization to natural rubber latex were found.

Film Formers/Synthetic Resins

Epoxy-Resin Compounds

Most cases of allergic contact dermatitis are caused by epoxy compounds contained in solvent-based and water-based paints, but powder paints have also been responsible for contact sensitization due to epoxy compounds. Of the above-mentioned 68 cases of allergic contact dermatitis caused by synthetic resins detected in painters, lacquerers, parquet layers and paint factory workers, 56 cases were caused by epoxy compounds. Bisphenol A diglycidyl ether epoxy resins were most often the responsible compounds. Epoxy isocyanurate (triglycidyl isocyanurate, TGIC) compounds caused five of the cases. TGIC can also cause asthma. Epoxy-reactive diluents and hardeners are also important sensitizers. Phthalic anhydride and its derivatives used in heat-cured paints may cause urticaria, even airborne contact urticaria, rhinitis and asthma, though type IV allergy is rare (Jolanki 1991; Tarvainen et al. 1993; Tarvainen et al. 1995; Kanerva et al. 1997; Piirilä et al. 1998). See the chapter on epoxy resins in this book (Chap. 17).

Formaldehyde Resins

Formaldehyde resins are also potential sensitizers. Sensitization most commonly develops from exposure to phenolformaldehyde resin (PFR). At least some previous cases of allergy to PFR have been reported from varnish coatings. In these cases the resin itself was considered to be the sensitizer. Bruze's investigations (1985) later confirmed that formaldehyde is not one of the main sensitizers in PFR. At the FIOH, one parquet lacquerer developed work-related allergic contact dermatitis, and in patch testing he reacted to formaldehyde and PFR as well as to melamine formaldehyde resin. In addition, a painter was sensitized to *p*-tertiary butylphenol formaldehyde resin from a contact glue that he used in his work (Pirilä 1947; Cronin 1980; Estlander et al. 2000).

Acrylic Resins

Acrylic polymers and copolymers in water-based latex paints can contain free monomers. The content of monomers in lattices is usually less than 0.3%, and they may consist of various acrylate and methacrylate compounds. All are skin irritants and sensitizers. In a Swedish factory manufacturing binders for use in, e.g. water-based latex paints, three out of 16 occupationally sensitized production workers were allergic to various methacrylates. In a study of Swedish construction painters (Fischer et al. 1995) *n*-butyl acrylate was considered to be the most common residual monomer in water-based latex paints, but none of the workers in the study reacted to the chemical. Butyl acrylate has also been determined in the air of workplaces where water-based latex paints have been used. Asthma, rhinitis and other mucosal symptoms have also been reported to be associated with exposure to acrylates (Hansen et al. 1987; Fischer et al. 1995; Gruvberger et al. 1998; Piirilä et al. 1998).

PFA Hardeners and Polyfunctional Acrylates

Allergic contact dermatitis from PFA hardeners (cross-linkers) and residual polyfunctional acrylates has been reported from various exposures to solvent-free products. Four patients have been reported to develop hand and face dermatitis from exposure to residual TMPTA in a PFA hardener used in a polyurethane floor topcoating. Another patient contracted an extensive dermatitis when exposed to a paint primer (undercoating) used to protect wood siding. In addition to allergic contact dermatitis, PFA hardeners can also cause asthma, allergic rhinitis and contact urticaria. In the FIOH, 11 patients have been detected who have been sensitized to a PFA hardener, and seven of them have had allergic contact dermatitis. Six of the patients were parquet lacquerers who used two-component solvent-free lacquers. No one reacted to acrylates (Kanerva et al. 1995; Estlander et al. 2000).

Dipropylene Glycol Diacrylate

Dipropylene glycol diacrylate (DPGDA) is a new acrylate sensitizer in UV-curable wood coatings. A male worker was sensitized to DPGDA by canning a paint containing the chemical. During the canning process, droplets of the paint splashed onto his clothes and also contaminated his skin (Estlander et al. 1998).

Urethane Resins

Urethane resins may contain free diisocyanates, which are usually respiratory irritants and sensitizers that cause rhinitis and asthma (Estlander et al. 1992). 2,4-Toluene diisocyanate (TDI) and hexamethylene diisocyanate (HDI) are important respiratory sensitizers, whereas 4,4'-diphenylmethane diisocyanate (MDI) is the most important skin sensitizing diisocyanate (Estlander et al. 1992). See also the chapter on polyurethane resins in Kanerva et al. (2000).

Other Synthetic Resins

No cases of sensitization have been reported from alkyd resins. Cyclohexanone resin (C-R) has caused allergic contact dermatitis in painters and floor installers. The sensitizer(s) responsible for contact allergy to C-R have not been identified, but they are probably to be found among the monomers and dimers formed when cyclohexanone is condensed in the production of C-R (Bruze et al. 1988).

Para-Tertiary-Butylcatechol

Para-tertiary-butylcatechol (PTBC) is a potential sensitizer in the paint industry. It can be considered a strong skin sensitizer capable of inducing active sensitization. It is also a skin irritant and a depigmenting agent. It is used as a stabilizing agent in monomeric styrene, butadiene and vinyl toluene. It prevents the polymerization of polyester resin, butadiene and PVC. Sensitization and allergic dermatitis have been reported from various exposures (Estlander et al. 1998).

Unsaturated Polyester Resins

Unsaturated polyester (UP) resins are made by condensation of a di- or polyhydric alcohol with a di- or polybasic acid or anhydride. Propylene, diethylene or ethylene glycol are the most common alcohols and phthalic, maleic or fumaric acid the most common acids used in the manufacture of UP resins. The curing reaction occurs when an unsaturated cross-linking monomer, such as styrene or methyl methacrylate, and an oxidizing catalyst, most often benzoyl peroxide, are mixed together. In addition, many potentially sensitizing auxiliary compounds, including pigments, fillers, inhibitors, accelerators, UV-protecting agents, stabilizers and flame retardants, are used to manufacture UP resin for different purposes. UP resins have been extensively used for coatings, finishes, cements and glues, as well as in the reinforced-plastics industry. Allergic dermatitis has been reported, e.g. from paints and cements, and the causative agents have been the auxiliary ingredients and cross-linking agents of UP resins. Six cases of allergic dermatitis from car-repair painting due to UP-resin cements have been reported. Allergic reactions were found to UP-resin chemicals in the cements. Diethylene glycol maleate (DGM) was purified and identified as an allergen from the UP resin in a cement (Tarvainen et al. 1993; Kanerva et al. 1999).

Turpentine and Other Natural Products

Turpentine is an extract of pine trees; alpha-pinene and beta-pinene are the main ingredients, but some products contain also delta-carene and camphene. Turpentine peroxides, especially delta-carene, have been considered to be the main sensitizers in turpentine. The content of turpentine oxides is high, e.g. in the turpentine from Finland, Sweden, Russia, India and Indonesia, whereas oil of turpentine from Portugal, Spain and southern France contains less delta-carene, and the gum turpentine from the USA contains practically no delta-carene (Pirilä et al. 1969; Cronin 1980; Mathias 1984; Ippen 1998).

Turpentine is still used in some countries, e.g. in Portugal; its main sensitizers are dipentene and alpha-pinene (Moura et al. 1994). In the 1990s, *dipentene*, which is a racemic mixture of D-limonene and L-(–)limonene has been offered for sale as solvent for the paint industry (Karlberg et al. 1992; Karlberg et al. 1997; Ippen 1998). Allergic contact dermatitis due to dipentene in various products has been reported. Artists and craftsmen may also use turpentine or related terpenes (Estlander et. al 2000).

Naturally drying oils are regarded as products with low sensitizing capacity. Some new natural paints may contain *linseed oil*. According to the information obtained from the material data sheets of two Finnish manufacturers, such paints can be composed of linseed oil varnish, coloured pigments and turpentine or white spirits. Sensitivities to *shellac, dammar* and *tung oil* may also occur (Pirilä 1947; Schwartz et al. 1957).

Colophony (rosin, pine rosin, wood rosin) is obtained from various species of pine tree. It has a complex chemical composition, of which about 90% is resin acids and the rest is corresponding esters, aldehydes and alcohols. Colophony is not used alone as a drying resin but is used to modify other resins, such as alkyds. Colophony is an important contact sensitizer. See the chapter on colophony in this book.

In the beginning of the 1990s, *citrus solvent* (D-limonene) and the racemic form of dipentene, in concentrations of 20–100%, found new applications because they are able to replace chlorinated hydrocarbons, chlorofluorocarbons and other organic solvents as less toxic substances. Products containing up to 95% D-limonene can be used in factories for degreasing metal surfaces before painting. D-limonene is the main ingredient of the oil from several citrus fruits. The distillate, peel oil, usually contains more than 95% D-limonene (Karlberg and Dooms-Goossens 1997; Ippen 1998). The oxidation products of D-limonene, e.g. limonene oxide, l-carvone and limonene hydroperoxides, found after prolonged air exposure of D-limonene, are potent sensitizers (Karlberg et al. 1992; Karlberg et al. 1994), whereas the sensitizing potential of D-limonene itself has been shown to be low (Karlberg et al. 1991). In the study of Karlberg et al. (1992), five main oxidation products – carvone, the *cis* and *trans* isomers of limonene oxide-(1,2) and of carveol, were identified. Of these, (R)-(+)carvone and a mixture of *cis* and *trans* isomers of limonene oxide-(1,2) were found to be potent sensitizers. In a two-center study where dermatitis patients in Stockholm and in Leuven (Belgium) were tested with D-limonene hydroperoxides, positive reactions were obtained in 2.4% and 1.1%, respectively.

Additives

Biocides

Biocides are the second most common cause of allergic contact dermatitis after synthetic resins. The problem of sensitization to biocides has become more common because of the increased use of water-based latex paints. Table 5 gives a list of the biocides used in paints. Similar biocides are also used in the glues needed by wallpaper hangers.

Isothiazolinones

Isothiazolinones are commonly used preservatives in water-based paints. In a Swedish study, construction painters, were found to react on patch testing to

chloromethyl isothiazolinone, benzisothiazolinone (BIT) and 2-*n*-octylisothiazoli-
none. Chloromethyl isothiazolinone is used as a preservative in binders used in
latex paints. Sensitization caused by the chemical has been reported from a Swedish factory manufacturing such binders. In the FIOH, one worker had allergic
contact dermatitis from chloromethyl isothiazolinone used as a slimicide in a varnish (unpublished) (Fischer et al. 1995; Geier et al. 1996; Gruvberger et al. 1998).

Chloromethyl isothiazolinone is a potent allergen, which has caused sensitization in concentrations as low as 7 ppm in stay-on cosmetics. The active ingredients are a mixture of two isothiazolinones: methylchloroisothiazolinone and
methylisothiazolinone. The isothiazolinone derivatives have more than 30 trade
names, including Kathon CG and Kathon 886 MW (de Groot and Weyland 1988;
Cronin et al. 1988; Hunziker 1992; Gruvberger et al. 1998).

In Sweden, benzisothiazolinone is a leading preservative incorporated into
most Swedish water-based paints and putties. Many cases of sensitization from
various exposures to 1,2-benzisothiazolin-3-one (1,2-BIT, Proxel) have been reported (Estlander et al. 2000).

N-octyl-isothiazolinone (Skane M-8) has been used mainly as a mildewcide in
latex paints and sometimes also in oil-base paints. Skane M-8 is supplied as 50%
concentrate in propylene glycol, which contains about 45% active ingredients and
5% impurities, for use as a paint mildewcide. *n*-Octyl-isothiazoline is also marketed as Kathon 4200 and Kathon LM, and is supplied as 25% and 5% concen-
trates for use as a mildewcide for fabrics. The same active ingredient is also marketed as Kathon 893 and recommended as an industrial multipurpose biocide
and mildewcide (Estlander et al. 2000).

Allergic contact dermatitis caused by *n*-octyl-isothiazolinone has been reported in paint-factory workers. It is chemically related to 1,2-benzisothiazolin-3-
one. One of the seven Swedish construction painters who were patch-test positive
to 1,2-benzisothiazolin-3-one also reacted to *n*-octyl-isothiazolinone (Fischer et
al. 1995).

Formaldehyde and Formaldehyde Releasers
Formaldehyde was previously used as a biocide. Nowadays, small amounts of
formaldehyde can be present in many water-based products, either as a contaminant from the raw material or from the formaldehyde-liberating compounds contained in the paints. Bronopol and Preventol ON are formaldehyde releasers used
to preserve, for example, binders intended for use in water-based latex paints
(Gruvberger et al. 1998). Benzylhemiformal, propylene glycol hemiformal, Biopan
P 1487, Biopan CS 1246, Biopan CS 1135 and methylen-bis-5-methyl-oxazolinone
are other examples of such biocides used in paints (Geier et al. 1996). In the
FIOH, three painters and one parquet installer had been sensitized to formaldehyde (unpublished research).

Chloracetamides
Chloracetamide and *N*-methylol-chloracetamide have caused occasional cases of
sensitization from various sources. Chloracetamide was also the main contact allergen in Swedish house painters. It has also caused allergic dermatitis in a paint
factory to a forklift driver who also reacted to Mergal K6N containing *N*-meth-

ylol-chloracetamide. Cross-reactions between the two chloracetamides are also possible. Airborne allergic contact dermatitis has also been reported in a chloracetamide-sensitive patient from exposure to a home-decorating paint containing the chemical as a preservative (Estlander et al 2000).

Euxyl K400

Euxyl K400 is a rather new preservative, which has in many cases replaced chloromethyl isothiazolinone as a less sensitizing alternative. It consists of two active ingredients, 2-phenoxyethanol (PE) and 1,2-dibromo-2,4-dicyanobutan (BCB) of which the last one is the main sensitizer in the product. As a product with the trade name Tektamer 38, it has also caused allergic dermatitis. Tektamer 38 can also be used in latex paints (Bruze et al. 1988; Fuchs et al. 1991; Aalto-Korte et al. 1996; Estlander et al. 2000).

Chlorocresol

Chlorocresol, or *p*-chloro-*m*-cresol, e.g. Preventol CMK, is a rare sensitizer which can be found in adhesives, glues, inks, paints and varnishes, in addition to packaging materials, textile finishes, leather and tanning agents, industrial oils and emulsions, cosmetics and medications (Dooms-Goossens et al. 1981).

Chlorothalonil

Tetrachloroisophthalonitrile (chlorothalonil) is a fungicide which is a skin irritant and a sensitizer and has caused contact dermatitis to workers in producing it. Allergic dermatitis has been reported from exposure to the chemical used as a wood preservative and as a pesticide in paints. Recently, a patient who contracted immunologic contact urticaria from a latex paint due to chlorothalonil has been reported (Jolanki et al. 2000.)

N-(Trichloromethylthio)phthalimide (Folpet, Fungitrol, Cosan P, Phaltal) is a pesticide sensitizer. Solitary cases of sensitization in painters have also been reported (Fischer et al. 1995).

Butylated Hydroxytoluene

Butylated hydroxytoluene (BHT), 2,6-di-(tert-butyl)-*p*-cresol is a commonly used antioxidant. The Danish Product Register (PROBAS) had registered BHT in 400 products by March 1990. The main categories were one- and two-component paints and lacquers, hardeners for two-component paints, glues, fillers, and binders for paints. Allergic contact dermatitis due to BHT has been reported only in solitary cases (Flyvholm and Menne 1990).

Other Additives

Hardeners such as amines and anhydrides include many sensitizers. See the sectionson epoxy, acrylate and urethane resins. Triethylamine may irritate and sensitize. Benzoyl peroxide, *p*-methoxy phenol and hydroquinone are used as *accelerators* and *inhibitors* of polymerization (see the chapters on epoxy resin compounds and acrylics in this book). Of the other additives, *dioctyl sodium sulfosuccinate*, a surfactant, is a potential, rare sensitizer, as are *dibutyl phthalate* and *triphenyl phosphate*, used as plasticizers (Estlander et al. 2000).

Metals and Metal Salts

Chromate corrosion inhibitors such as zinc chromate in primer paints have caused allergic contact dermatitis in painters. Cobalt in paint dryers is a potential sensitizer. In the FIOH between 1974 and 1990, three painters and a tinter in a paint factory were primarily sensitized to chromates and two to cobalt (unpublished).

Nickel has caused sensitization, e.g. from contact with nickel-plated tool handles. Allergic contact dermatitis has also been reported from exposure to a powder paint containing nickel. A female nickel-allergic decorative painter, investigated at the FIOH, noted worsening of her sensitization from exposure to nickel in the paint she used (unpublished research).

Phenyl mercuric derivatives have previously caused some skin damage to painters. Mercury has also caused sensitization from exposure to an interior latex paint (Agocs et al. 1990).

Pigments

Because the pigments in paints and coatings occur as insoluble particles, they very seldom sensitize, with the exception of chromates (see Chap. 30, this book). Organic pigments, especially azo derivatives, should be considered as potential skin sensitizers (Mathias 1984).

Paint and Varnish Removers

Dibutyl thiourea (DBTU) is a chemical used in paint and glue removers. Two workers were sensitized to the chemical when using a paint remover, namely Stripper 100. DBTU is also a rubber allergen and has caused allergic contact dermatitis from exposure to various rubber articles (Kanerva et al. 1988; Estlander et al. 2000).

Miscellaneous

Protective gloves, especially rubber gloves made of natural rubber latex or synthetic rubber (e.g. neoprene rubber), as well as rubber parts of respiratory masks used with certain industrial solvent-based paints should also be remembered as potential causes of sensitization in painters. Preservatives in barrier creams, hand ointments and hand cleansers are other potential causes of dermatitis (Mathias 1984; Estlander et al. 2000).

Investigations

The investigations should include exploration of exposure to chemicals, clinical examination of dermatitis, and patch testing. In addition to the test substances contained in the European standard series (e.g. Hermal, Kurt Herrmann, Rhinebeck, Germany; TRUE test, Pharmacia Research Center AS, Denmark; Chemo-technique Diagnostics AB, Malmö, Sweden), a series of epoxy chemicals (see also Chap. 32, this book), plastics and glues also containing MDI, TDI and HDI (Estlander et al. 1992), a series of antimicrobials and an extensive rubber-chemical series also containing thiourea compounds (Kanerva et al. 1994a) should be investigated. Patch testing should be supplemented with test substances made of actual paints the patient has been exposed to and with the ingredients of the paint when possible. Patch tests should also include the materials of all polymer gloves used at work and rubber parts of masks or tools, hand creams and cleansers used at work. Material data sheets are useful in clearing the exposure, but often the information given is too scarce (Kanerva et al. 1997). Contact with manufacturers or distributors is sometimes necessary. Chemical analysis of a suspected product may also be necessary to determine the actual sensitizer (Tarvainen et al. 1993; Kanerva et al. 1997).

Prevention

Personal protective equipment (PPE) is important in the prevention of hazards caused by handling paints, lacquers and varnishes. PPE includes safety helmets, eye and face protectors, hearing protectors, respiratory protective equipment, protective gloves, safety footwear and other protective clothing, as well as fall-arresting systems. Overalls or separate long-sleeved shirts or coats and long pants made of cotton fabrics or blends of cotton and synthetic fibres should be used, as well as caps or safety helmets to protect the head. Hand protection with appropriate gloves is essential. Long-sleeved protective gloves made of PVC or rubber materials (natural or synthetic) or combinations of leather and cotton, or disposable cotton gloves, depending on the type of paints handled, should be used (Mellström and Boman 1997). Protective footwear may also be necessary, as well as eye protection using spectacles, goggles, visors, or hoods (Korhonen 1997).

When highly sensitizing epoxy paints or UV-radiation-curable acrylate coatings are used, special protective gloves and disposable overalls should be used. Control of the UV-radiation curing process is also necessary, as well as regular industrial hygiene assessments to prevent chemicals in aerosols or vapours from coming into contact with the airways and the skin. Special preventive measures must also be taken when paints containing low-molecular-weight epoxy compounds are handled. A single exposure, e.g. a paint splash onto the skin or absorbed in a worker's clothes next to the skin, may lead to primary sensitization and allergic eczema (Holmes et al. 1993; Kanerva et al. 1994b).

Careful working techniques, especially in the prevention of paint splashes coming into contact with skin, are essential. Organic solvents should be used only temporarily. Skin moisturizers should be used daily to prevent drying of the skin. White petrolatum is a rather effective barrier and greatly facilitates skin cleansing (Mathias 1984).

In addition, depending on the type of chemicals and type of exposure, the respiratory tract should be protected against inhalation of airborne contaminants. Also, hearing protectors should not be forgotten (Korhonen 1997).

References

Aalto-Korte K, Jolanki R, Estlander T, Alanko K, Kanerva L (1996) Occupational allergic contact dermatitis caused by Euxyl K 400. Contact Dermatitis 35:193–194

Agocs MM, Etzel R, Gibson-Parrish R, Paschal C, Campagna PR, Cohen S, Kilbourne EM, Hesse JL (1990) Mercury exposure from interior latex paint. N Engl J Med 323:1096–1101

Bruze M (1985) Contact sensitizers in resins based on phenol and formaldehyde (thesis). University of Lund, Lund, pp 1–200

Bruze M, Gruvberger B, Agrup G (1988) Sensitization studies in the guinea pig with active ingredients of Euxyl K®400. Contact Dermatitis 18:37–39

Cronin E (1980) Contact dermatitis. Churchill Livingstone, Edinburgh, pp 614–621

Cronin E, Hannuksela M, Lachapelle J-M, Maibach HI, Malten K, Meneghini CL (1988) Frequency of sensitization to the preservative Kathon®CG. Contact Dermatitis 18:274–279

De Groot AC, Weyland JW (1988) Kathon CG: a review. J Am Acad Dermatol 18:350–358

Dooms-Goossens A, Degreef H, Vanhee J, Klerkhofs I, Chrispeels MT (1981) Chlorocresol and chloracetamide: allergens in medications, glues, and cosmetics. Contact Dermatitis 1:51–52

Estlander T, Keskinen H, Jolanki R, Kanerva L (1992) Occupational dermatitis from exposure to polyurethane chemicals. Contact Dermatitis 27:161–165

Estlander T, Kostiainen M, Jolanki R, Kanerva L (1998) Active sensitization and occupational allergic contact dermatitis caused by para-tertiary-butylcatechol. Contact Dermatitis 38:96–100

Estlander T, Jolanki R, Kanerva L (2000) Paints, laquers and varnishes. In: Kanerva L, Elsner P, Wahlberg JE, Maibach HI (eds) Handbook of occupational dermatology. Springer, Berlin Heidelberg New York, pp 662–678

Fischer T, Adams RM (1990) Paints, varnishes, and laquers. In: Adams RM (ed). Occupational skin disease, 2nd edn. Saunders, Philadelphia, pp 426–438

Fischer T, Bohlin S, Edling C, Rystedt I, Wieslander G (1995) Skin disease and contact sensitivity in house painters using water-based paints, glues and putties. Contact Dermatitis 32:39–45

Flyvholm M-A, Menne T (1990) Sensitizing risk of butylated hydroxytoluene based on exposure and effect data. Contact Dermatitis 23:341–345

Fuchs T, Enders F, Przybilla B, Ippen H, Aberer W, Bauer R, Böhm I, Schulze-Dirks A, Frosch PJ, Peters K-P, Steffan M-A, Wassilew SW, Hensel O, Gehring W, Lischka G, Agathos M, Breit R, Bahmer F, Stary A, Brasch J (1991) Contact allergy to Euxyl K 400, results of a multi-center study of the German Contact Allergy Group (DKG). Derm Beruf Umwelt 39:151–153

Geier J, Kleinhans D, Peters K-P (1996) Kontaktallergien durch industriell verwendete Biozide. Egebnisse des Informationsverbunds Dermatologicher Kliniken (IVDK) und der Deutschen Kontaktallergiegruppe. Derm Beruf Umwelt 44:154–159

Gruvberger B, Bruze M, Almgren G (1998) Occupational dermatoses in a plant producing binders for paints and glues. Contact Dermatitis 38:71–77

Hansen MK, Larsen M, Cohr K-H (1987) Waterborne paints, a review of their chemistry and toxicology and the results of determinations made during their use. Scand J Work Environ Health 13:473–485

Högberg M, Wahlberg JE (1980) Health screening for occupational dermatoses in house painters. Contact Dermatitis 6:100–106

Holmes N, Pearce P, Simpson G (1993) Prevention of epoxy resin dermatitis: failure of manufacturers to use available research information. Am J Ind Med 24:605–617

Hunziker N (1992) The 'isothiazolinone story'. Dermatology 184:85–86

Ippen H (1998) Limonen – Dipenten, Citrus-Öle und Citrus-Terpene. Teil I: Allgemeines, Vorkommen, Verwendung, Penetration, Kinetik, Metabolismus. Derm Beruf Umwelt 46:18–25

Jolanki R (1991) Occupational skin diseases from epoxy compounds, epoxy resin compounds, epoxy acrylates and 2,3-epoxypropyl trimethyl ammonium chloride (thesis). Acta Derm Venereol Suppl (Stockh) 159:1–80

Jolanki R, Alanko K, Estlander T, Laukkanen A, Kanerva L (2000) Occupational contact urticaria from latex paint due to fungicide tetrachloroisophthalonitrile (TCPN). Contact Dermatitis 42 (Suppl 2):54

Kanerva L, EstlanderT, Jolanki R (1994a) Occupational allergic contact dermatitis caused by thiourea compounds. Contact Dermatitis 31:242–248

Kanerva L, Tarvainen K, Pinola A, Granlund H, Estlander T, Jolanki R, Förström L (1994b) A single accidental exposure may result in chemical burn, primary sensitization and allergic contact dermatitis. Contact Dermatitis 31:229–235

Kanerva L, Estlander T, Jolanki R, Tarvainen K (1995) Occupational allergic contact dermatitis and contact urticaria caused by polyfunctional aziridine hardener. Contact Dermatitis 33:304–309

Kanerva L, Hyry H, Jolanki R, Hytönen M, Estlander T (1997) Delayed and immediate allergy caused by methylhexahydropthalic anhydride. Contact Dermatitis 36:34-38

Kanerva L, Estlander T, Alanko K, Jolanki R (1998) Occupational airborne allergic contact dermatitis from dibutylthiourea. Contact Dermatitis 38:347–348

Kanerva L, Estlander T, Alanko K, Pfäffli P, Jolanki R (1999) Occupational dermatitis from unsaturated polyester resin in a car repair putty. Int J Dermatol 38:447–452

Karlberg A-T (1988) Contact allergy to colophony, chemical identification of allergens, sensitization experiments and clinical experiences (Thesis). National Institute of Occupational Health, Stockholm, pp 1–43

Karlberg A-T, Dooms-Goossens A (1997) Contact allergy to oxidized D-limonene among dermatitis patients. Contact Dermatitis 36:201–206

Karlberg A-T, Boman A, Melin B (1991) Animal experiments on the allergenity of D-limonene – the citrus solvent. Ann Occup Hyg 35:419–425

Karlberg A-T, Magnusson K, Nilsson U (1992) Air oxidation of D-limonene (the citrus solvent) creates potent allergens. Contact Dermatitis 26:332–340

Karlberg A-T, Shao LP, Nilsson U (1994) Hydroperoxides in oxidized D-limonene identified as potent contact allergens. Arch Dermatol Res 286:97–103

Korhonen E (1997) Personal protective equipment. In: Brune D, Gerhardsson G, Crockford GW, D'Auria D (eds) Fundamentals of health, safety and welfare (The workplace, vol 1). International Occupational Safety and Health Information Centre (CIS) International Labour Office, Geneva and Scandinavian Science Publishers, Oslo, pp 685–715

Leira HL (1997) Organic solvents. In: Brune D, Gerhardsson G, Crockford GW, Norbäck D (eds) Major industries and occupations (The workplace, vol 1). International Occupational Safety and Health Information Centre (CIS) International Labour Office, Geneva and Scandinavian Science Publishers, Oslo, pp 650–660

Mathias CGT (1984) Dermatitis from paints and coatings. Dermatol Clin 2:585–602

Mathias CGT (1988) Allergic contact dermatitis from triglycidyl isocyanurate in polyester paint pigments. Contact Dermatitis 19:67–68

Mellström G, Boman A (1997) Protective gloves: test results compiled in a database. In: Brune D, Gerhardsson G, Crockford GW, D'Auria D (eds) Fundamentals of health, safety and welfare. (The workplace, vol 1) International Occupational Safety and Health Information Centre (CIS) International Labour Office, Geneva and Scandinavian Science Publishers, Oslo, pp 716–730

Moura C, Dias M, Vale T (1994) Contact dermatitis in painters, polishers and varnishers. Contact Dermatitis 31:51–53

P, Kanerva L, Keskinen H, Hytönen M, Tuppurainen M, Estlander T, Nordman H (1998) Occupational respiratory hypersensitivity caused by acrylates in dental personnel. Clin Exp Allergy 28:1404–1411

Pirilä V (1947) On occupational disease of the skin among paint factory workers, painters, polishers, and varnishers in Finland (thesis). Acta Derm Venereol 27[Suppl 26]:1–163

Pirilä V, Kilpiö O, Olkkonen A, Pirilä L, Siltanen E (1969) On the chemical nature of the eczematogens in oil of turpentine V. Pattern of sensitivity to different terpenes. Dermatologica 139:183–194

Rietschel RL, Fowler JF Jr (1995) Fisher's contact dermatitis, 4th edn. Williams & Wilkins, Baltimore, pp 563–565

Rose FG, Vance CJ (1997) The paint industry. In: Brune D, Gerhardsson G, Crockford GW, Norbäck D (eds) Major industries and occupations. (The workplace, vol 2) International Occupational Safety and Health Information Centre (CIS) International Labour Office, Geneva and Scandinavian Science Publishers, Oslo, pp 350–360

Schwartz L, Tulipan L, Birmingham DJ (1957) Dermatoses caused by paints, varnishes and lacquers. In: Occupational diseases of the skin, 3rd edn. Lea Febiger, Philadelphia, pp 527–534

Tarvainen K, Jolanki R, Estlander T (1993) Occupational contact allergy to unsaturated polyester resin cements. Contact Dermatitis 28:220–224

Tarvainen K, Jolanki R, Estlander T, Tupasela O, Keskinen H, Pfäffli P, Kanerva L (1995) Immunologic contact urticaria due to airborne metylhexahydrophthalic anhydride and metyltetrahydrophtalic anhydride. Contact Dermatitis 32:204–209

Van Faassen A, Borm PJA (1991) Composition and health hazards of water-based construction paints: results from a survey in the Netherlands. Environ Health Perspect 92:147–154

Vincent R, Poirot P, Subra I, Rieger P, Cicolella A (1994) Occupational exposure to organic solvents during paint stripping and painting operations in the aeronautical industry. Int Arch Occup Environ Health 65:377–380

Wieslander G, Norbäck D (1997) Water-based paints in the construction industry. In: Brune D, Gerhardsson G, Crockford GW, Norbäck D (eds) Major industries and occupations. (The workplace, vol 2) International Occupational Safety and Health Information Centre (CIS) International Labour Office, Geneva and Scandinavian Science Publishers, Oslo, pp 690–696

Wieslander G, Norbäck D, Edling C (1994) Occupational exposure to water-based paints and symptoms from the skin and eyes. Occup Environ Med 51:181–186

CHAPTER 34

Phenol-Formaldehyde Resins

34

E. ZIMERSON, M. BRUZE

Introduction

Phenol-formaldehyde resin was developed as the first wholly synthetic polymer at the beginning of the 20th century and was called Bakelite. From the first resins others varieties have been developed and phenol-formaldehyde resins now designates a group of resins with varying properties made from different phenols and aldehydes.

Chemistry

The most used phenol-formaldehyde resins are based on phenol or p-*tert*-butylphenol and formaldehyde. However, other phenols can be used, such as resorcinol, cresols, guayachol (2-methoxy phenol), p-phenylphenol, xylenols, amylphenol, octylphenol, nonylphenol and bisphenol A. Aldehydes other than formaldehyde are occasionally used, such as furfural. In modified phenol-formaldehyde resins other components such as colophony, terpenes, fatty acids, amines or epoxy resins are added.

Formaldehyde reacts with phenols giving methylol (hydroxymethyl)-substituted phenols and also creates chemical bonds between monomers forming dimers, trimers, tetramers and so on. Phenol-formaldehyde resins can be produced in two ways, either as resol or novolac resins. Resol resins are produced by the reaction of phenols with a molecular excess of formaldehyde under alkaline conditions and the resins are cured by applying pressure and/or heat. Novolac resins are produced when formaldehyde reacts with a molecular excess of phenol under acidic conditions. Curing of novolac resins requires the addition of a formaldehyde releaser such as paraformaldehyde or hexamethylenetetramine. Curing transforms resins based on phenol into a rigid network polymer while cured resins based on p-*tert*-butylphenol have thermoplastic properties.

Use

The resins are mainly used as binders in different products and large quantities are used, for example, in the building, construction, car, leather, shoe, moulding and electric industries.

Resins based on phenol are used in many glues and adhesives for decorative boards, laminated boards for floors, plywood, water resistant boards, glass and mineral fibres for insulating, brake and clutch linings, abrasive cloth and paper, grinding wheels and moulds for casting metal and plastic.

p-*tert*-Butylphenol-formaldehyde resin is used in adhesives where flexibility of the joint or when extra water resistance is needed. The resin is frequently used in glues for shoes and other leather products, such as watch straps.

Modified resins or resins based on p-*tert*-butylphenol or other alkyl-substituted phenols are used for surface coatings as protective and isolating varnishes for packing due to their water-repellent properties and can be used as binders in inks, typewriter correction papers, and different laminates.

Contact Dermatitis and Allergy

Irritant contact dermatitis (Fregert 1980) and chemical burns (Fisher 1973) have been attributed to phenol-formaldehyde resins. The low or high pH of the resin, excess phenol and/or aldehyde can contribute to irritant contact dermatitis. Depigmentation can be caused by certain resins and is likely due to remaining phenols such as p-*tert*-butylphenol (Malten et al. 1971; Stevenson 1981). Contact urticaria has been ascribed to phenol-formaldehyde resins (Kalimo et al. 1980).

Among workers in laminate productions a high frequency of allergies to resins based on phenol has been reported (Bruze and Almgren 1988). Reports on occupational sensitisation have also included a secretary handling typewriter correction paper (Jordan and Bourlas 1975), a newspaper dealer (Castelain et al. 1980), painters (Hjort and Fregert 1967), a worker in a rubber factory (van der Willingen 1987), bricklayers (Sonneck 1964), workers producing abrasive paper (Bompart and Smagghe 1959), a worker manufacturing gasoline filters (Gaul 1967), and workers sawing masonite or using grinding wheels (Fregert and Tegner 1972).

p-*tert*-Butylphenol-formaldehyde resin is used both in industry and in personal products. In 1958, contact allergy was described among cobblers (Malten 1958). Since then more patients working with shoe manufacturing or shoe repairing have been reported (Mancuso et al. 1996) as well as patients with shoe dermatitis (Freeman 1997). Contact allergies have also been reported among workers in a car factory (Engel and Calnan 1966), painters (Högberg and Wahlberg 1980), and glue users (Moran and Martin-Pascual 1978; Cronin 1980). Other causes of sensitisation and/or allergic contact dermatitis can be leather watch straps (Foussereau et al. 1968; Mobacken and Hersle 1976), plastic finger nail adhesives (Rycroft et al. 1980), athletic tapes (Shono et al. 1991), an hearing aid (Matrolonardo et al. 1993), a lip liner (Angelini et al. 1993), a knee guard (Vincenzi et al. 1992), a derotation brace and a rain coat (Hayakawa et al. 1994), a waist support, and leather glues (Tarvainen 1995), marking pens (Hagdrup et al. 1994) and a prosthetic device (Romaguera et al. 1985). The frequency of positive patch test reactions has varied between 0.3% and 2.6% among dermatological patients (Tarvainen 1995; Handley et al. 1993). In Portugal, frequencies between 1.4% (1984) and

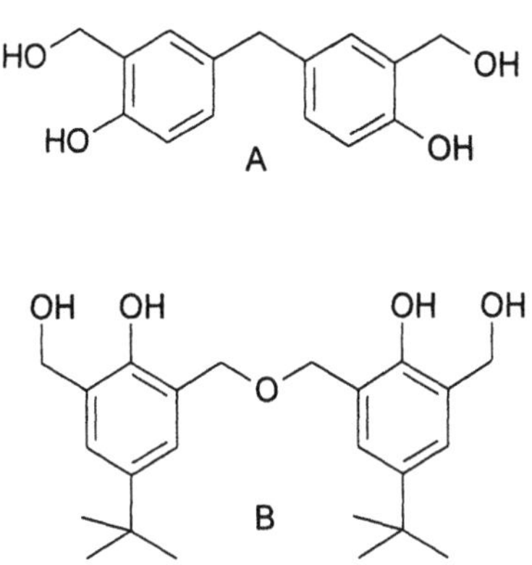

Fig. 1 A, B. Chemical structures of main allergens **A** 4,4'-dihydroxy-3,3'-dihydroxymethyl-diphenylmethane from phenol-formaldehyde resin and **B** 4-*tert*-butyl-2-(5-*tert*-butyl-2-hydroxy-3-hydroxymethyl-benzyloxymethyl)-6-hydroxymethyl-phenol from p-*tert*-butylphenol-formaldehyde resin

3.8% (1992) are reported, with an increasing tendency mainly in woman (Marques et al. 1994).

Free formaldehyde in phenol-formaldehyde resins it is not a major sensitiser (Hjort and Fregert 1967; Bruze et al. 1985). Free phenols also seem to be of little or no significance concerning allergic reactions to the resins (Fregert and Hjort 1969; Bruze et al. 1985). Monomers and dimers in the resins have been shown to be allergens and main allergens have been found among the dimers (Bruze 1985; Bruze et al. 1986; Agatha and Schubert 1979; Schubert and Agatha 1979; Zimerson and Bruze 2000a; Zimerson and Bruze 2000b). Two of these main allergens are shown in Fig. 1.

Connections to Other Sensitisers

In 1967, a possible relation between contact allergy to phenol-formaldehyde resin and coal tar was noted (Hjort and Fregert 1967). Some simple phenols have been shown to be probable cross-reacting substances in patients hypersensitive to phenol-formaldehyde resin, for example, o-cresol (Bruze and Zimerson 1997). o-Cresol is also a known component in coal and wood tar (Snell and Ettre 1973; Richardson 1993) and it has been identified as an allergen in phenol-formaldehyde resin (Bruze and Zimerson 2002). This could explain the connection to coal tar. It also indicates a possible connection to other sources of o-cresol, for example, tobacco smoke (Jeanty et al. 1984).

In patients hypersensitive to phenol-formaldehyde resin (resol) simultaneous patch test reactions to formaldehyde, colophony, hydroabietyl alcohol, balsam of Peru, perfume mixture and p-*tert*-butylphenol-formaldehyde resin have been reported. In patients hypersensitive to p-*tert*-butylphenol-formaldehyde resin (resol) simultaneous patch test reactions to hydroabietyl alcohol, balsam of Peru and phenol-formaldehyde resin have been reported (Bruze 1986).

Simultaneous patch test reactions to p-*tert*-butylphenol-formaldehyde resin and p-*tert*-butylcatechol have been reported (Estlander et al. 1998) and p-*tert*-butylcatechol has been shown to be a component in at least some resins based on p-*tert*-butylphenol (Zimerson and Bruze 1999). p-*tert*-Butylcatechol is used as an antioxidant (Gellin et al. 1970) and as a stabilizer in different plastic monomers (Macfarlane et al. 1990).

Treatment and Prevention

In many cases of occupationally related allergic dermatitis caused by phenol-formaldehyde resin, the person cannot continue the job. However, the prognosis is usually good when they can change their job to one with less exposure to the allergen. Work including handling of cured products can be tolerated if the sensitivity is not too high.

For patients hypersensitive to p-*tert*-butylphenol-formaldehyde resin for whom no clinically relevant contact to this resin can be found, patch testing with p-*tert*-butyl catechol is indicated.

Patch testing with p-*tert*-butylphenol-formaldehyde resin is not sufficient to detect hypersensitivity to phenol-formaldehyde resins based on other phenols. Patch testing should include phenol-formaldehyde resin and the patients' own resins/materials. Extracts of cured/finished products can be useful for patch testing. Resins based on phenol and p-*tert*-butylphenol can be tested as a mix (Bruze 1988; Bruze 1985).

Phenol-formaldehyde resins included in standard or supplementary test series should be of the resol type as they contain higher levels of allergens than novolac resins.

References

Agatha G, Schubert H (1979) Untersuchungen zur Allergen-Identifizierung bei der p-tertiären Butylphenol-Formaldehydharz-Allergie. Dermatol. Monatschr. 165:337–345

Angelini E, Marinaro C, Carrozzo AM, Bianchi L, Delogu A, Gianello G, Nini G (1993) Allergic contact dermatitis of the lip margins from para-tertiary-butylphenol in a lip liner. Contact Dermatitis 28:146–148

Bompart PV, Smagge G (1959) Quelques remarques d'ardre pratique à propos d'une application industrielle des résines formo-phénolique. Arch Mal Prof 20:64–67

Bruze M (1985) Contact sensitizers in resins based on phenol and formaldehyde. Acta Dermatol Venereol Suppl (Stockh) 119:1–83

Bruze M (1986) Simultaneous reactions to phenol-formaldehyde resins colophony/hydroabietyl alcohol and balsam of Peru/perfume mixture. Contact Dermatitis 14:119–120

Bruze M (1988) Patch testing with a mixture of 2 phenol-formaldehyde resins. Contact Dermatitis 19:116–119

Bruze M, Almgren G (1988) Occupational dermatoses in workers exposed to resins based on phenol and formaldehyde. Contact Dermatitis 19:272–277

Bruze M, Zimerson E (1997) Cross-reaction patterns in patients with contact allergy to simple methylol phenols. Contact Dermatitis 37: 82–86

Bruze M, Zimerson E (2002) Contact allergy to o-cresol – a sensitizer in phenol-formaldehyde resin. Am J Contact Dermat 13:198–200

Bruze M, Fregert S, Zimerson E (1985) Contact allergy to phenol-formaldehyde resins. Contact Dermatitis 12:81–86

Bruze M, Persson L, Trulsson L, Zimerson E (1986) Demonstration of contact sensitizers in resins and products based on phenol and formaldehyde. Contact Dermatitis 14:146–154

Castelain PY, Pirious A, Raulot-Lapointe H, Rabaglia JL (1980) Sensitization to abieto-for-mo-phenolic resin in printing ink. Contact Dermatitis 6:145

Cronin E (1980) Contact Dermatitis. Churchill Livingstone, Edinburgh, pp 617–619

Engel HO, Calnan CD (1966) Resin dermatitis in a car factory. Br J Ind Med 23:62–66

Estlander T, Kostiainen M, Jolanki R, Kanerva L (1998) Active sensitization and occupational allergic contact dermatitis caused by para-tertiary-butylcatechol. Contact Dermatitis 38:96–100

Fisher AA (1973) Contact Dermatitis, 2nd edn. Lea and Febiger, Philadelphia, pp 16–18

Freeman S (1997) Shoe Dermatitis. Contact Dermatitis 36:247–251

Fregert S (1980) Irritant dermatitis from phenol-formaldehyde resin powder. Contact Dermatitis 6:493

Fregert S, Hjort N (1969) Results of standard patch tests with substances abandoned. Contact Dermatitis Newslett 5:85–86

Fregert S, Tegner E (1972) Allergic contact dermatitis due to phenolic resin in ready products. Contact Dermatitis Newslett 12:328

Foussereau MJ, Petitjean J, Barré JG (1968) Eczema aux bracelets-montres par allergie a des résines formol-p.t.butylphénol des colles pour cuir (résines du type c.k.r. 1634) Bull Soc Fr Dermatol Syphiligr 75:630–633

Gaul LE (1967) Absence of formaldehyde sensitivity in phenol formaldehyde dermatitis. J Invert Dermatol 48:485–486

Gellin GA, Possick PA, Perone VB (1970) Depigmentation from 4-tertiary butyl catechol: an experimental study. J Invest Dermatol 55:190–197

Hagdrup H, Egsgaard H, Carlsen L, Andersen KE (1994) Contact allergy to 2-hydroxy-5-*tert*-butyl benzylalcohol and 2,6-bis(hydroxymethyl)-4-*tert*-butylphenol, components of a phenolic resin used in marking pens. Contact Dermatitis 31:154–6

Handley J, Todd D, Bingham A, Corbett R, Burrows D (1993) Allergic contact dermatitis from para-tertiary-butylphenol-formaldehyde resin (PTBP-F-R) in Northern Ireland. Contact Dermatitis 29:144–146

Hayakawa R, Ogino Y, Suzuki M, Kaniwa M (1994) Allergic contact dermatitis from para-tertiary-butylphenol-formaldehyde resin (PTBP-F-R). Contact Dermatitis 30:187–188

Hjort N, Fregert S (1967) Sensitivity to formaldehyde and formaldehyde resins. Contact Dermatitis Newsletter 2:18–19

Högberg M, Wahlberg J E (1980) Health screening for occupational dermatoses in house painters. Contact Dermatitis 6:100–106.

Jeanty G, Massé J, Bercot P, Coq F (1984) Quantitative analysis of cigarette smoke condensate monophenols by reverse-phase high-performance liquid chromatography. Beitr Tabakforschung Int 12:245–250

Jordan WP, Bourlas M (1975) Contact dermatitis from typewriter correction paper. Cutis 15:594–595.

Kalimo K, Saarni H, Kytta J (1980) Immediate and delayed type reactions to formaldehyde resin in glass wool. Contact Dermatitis 6:496.

Macfarlane AW, Yu RC, King CM (1990) Contact sensitivity to para-tertiary-butylcatechol in an artificial limb. Contact Dermatitis 22:56–57

Malten KE (1958) Occupational eczema due to para-tertiary butylphenol in a shoe adhesive. Dermatologica 117:103–109

Malten KE, Seutter E, Hara I, et al (1971) Occupational vitiligo due to p-*tert*-butylphenol and homologues. Trans St John's Hosp Dermatol Soc 57:115–134

Mancuso G, Reggiani M, Berdondini RM (1996) Occupational dermatitis in shoemakers. Contact Dermatitis 34:17–22

Marques C, Goncalo M, Goncalo S (1994) Sensitivity to para-tertiary-butylphenol-formaldehyde resin in Portugal. Contact Dermatitis 30:300–301

Matrolonardo M, Loconsole F, Conte A, Rantuccio F (1993) Allergic contact dermatitis due to para-tertiary-butylphenol-formaldehyde resin in a hearing aid. Contact Dermatitis 28:179

Mobacken H, Hersle K (1976) Allergic contact dermatitis caused by paratertiary butylphenol-formaldehyde resin in watch straps. Contact Dermatitis 2:59

Moran M, Martin-Pascual A (1978) Contact dermatitis to para-tertiary-butylphenol formaldehyde. Contact Dermatitis 4:372–373

Richardson M L (ed) (1993) The dictionary of substances and their effects. Cambridge Royal Society of Chemistry, Cambridge pp 675–678

Romaguera C, Grimalt F, Vilaplana J (1985) Paratertiary butylphenol formaldehyde resin in prosthesis. Contact Dermatitis 12:174

Rycroft R J G, Wilkinson J D, Holmes R, Hay R J (1980) Contact sensitization to p-tertiary-butylphenol (PTBP) resin in plastic nail adhesive. Clin Exp Dermatol 5:411–445

Schubert H, Agatha G (1979) Zur Allergennatur der para-tert. Butylphenol-formaldhydharze. Dermatosen 27:49–52

Shono M, Ezoe K, Kaniwa M-A, Ikarashi Y, Kojima S, Nakamura A (1991) Allergic contact dermatitis from para-tertiary-butylphenol-formaldehyde resin (PTBP-FR) in athletic tape and leather adhesive. Contact Dermatitis 24:281–288

Snell F D and Ettre L S (1973) Encyclopedia of industrial chemical analysis, vol 17. Interscience Publishers, USA, pp 9–10

Sonneck H J (1964) Hautschäden durch Kunstharzäurekitte. Berufsdermatosen 12:42–48

Stevenson C J (1981) Occupational vitiligo: clinical and epidemiological aspects. Br J Dermatol 105 [suppl 21]:51–56

Tarvainen K (1995) Analysis of patients with allergic patch test reaction to a plastics and glue series. Contact Dermatitis 32:346–351

Vincenzi C, Guerra L, Peluso AM, Zucchelli V (1992) Allergic contact dermatitis due to phenol-formaldehyde resin in a knee-guard. Contact Dermatitis 27:54

van der Willingen AH, Stolz E, van Joost T (1987) Sensitization to phenol formaldehyde in rubber glue. Contact Dermatitis16:291–292

Zimerson E, Bruze M (1999) Demonstration of the contact sensitizer p-*tert*-butylcatechol in p-*tert*-butylphenol-formaldehyde resin. Am J Contact Dermat 10:2–6

Zimerson E, Bruze M (2000a) Contact allergy to 5,5′-di-*tert*-butyl-2,2′-dihydroxy-(hydroxymethyl)-dibenzyl ethers, sensitizers in p-*tert*-butylphenol-formaldehyde resin. Contact Dermatitis 43:20–26

Zimerson E, Bruze M (2000b) Sensitizing capacity of 5,5′-di-*tert*-butyl-2,2′-dihydroxy-(hydroxymethyl)-dibenzyl ethers in the guinea pig. Contact Dermatitis 43:72–78

CHAPTER 35

Occupational Contact Dermatitis to Plants 35

J. D. GUIN

Contact dermatitis to plants is extremely common among the general population in the United States, and occupational contact dermatitis to plants may well be more common than reported. Examples of situations where risk is high would include poison-ivy dermatitis in American agriculture, irritant dermatitis in food processing, and protein contact dermatitis to latex protein in healthcare. Some of the more prevalent forms of plant dermatitis will be addressed in more detail followed by reactions found in certain occupations that are more at risk for plant dermatitis.

Toxicodendron dermatitis is exemplified by poison-ivy dermatitis where the antigen, urushiol, comprises mostly pentadec(en)yl catechols. This is found in small canals in the roots, phloem, leaflets, etc. below the surface, requiring injury to be released. Usually the sap contaminates the hands from which it is transferred to sites that absorb better, causing characteristic streaks and fingerprints of erythema and vesiculation (Fig. 1). The time of onset is delayed but it may occur as early as a few hours on the face and up to several days where the skin is thicker. This pattern can also occur with other strong antigens such as other toxic Anacardiaceae, phytophotodermatitis, *Primula obconica*, *Phacelia*, English ivy, etc. While *Toxicodendron* dermatitis is largely found in North America and Japan,

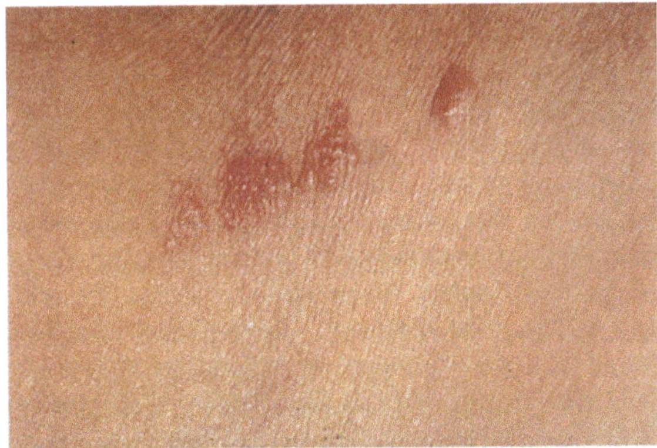

Fig. 1. Typical acute eczematous streak of poison-ivy dermatitis caused by hand transfer of the antigen. Note the separation caused by the pattern of the fingers that transferred the antigen

other toxic Anacardiaceae occur in Central and South America, the Caribbean, South Africa, Asia and Australia. Plant recognition is the best preventive method, as most cases are caused by failure to identify the plant. Barriers such as protective clothing or Ivy Block can be used prophylactically, and disposable vinyl (not latex) gloves provide a simple, effective and inexpensive barrier. Once exposed, soap and water or solvents (or in an emergency, water) can be used to reduce the contamination, provided this is done within a few minutes or up to 30 minutes for moderately sensitive persons. Hyposensitization is no longer feasible, as effective agents are not available, although natural hardening occurs in some workers.

Treatment of the eruption is largely through oral, or parenteral corticosteroids, e.g., prednisone tapered from 30–60 mg daily over 14–21 days. For those unable to take systemic corticosteroids, occlusive therapy with category 2–5 topical steroids for at least two 24-h periods.

Compositae dermatitis is called weed dermatitis in Texas, bush dermatitis in Australia and, because of the allergenic component, sesquiterpene lactone dermatitis by many authors. This condition, usually chronic, occurs in several distinct patterns that may overlap including pseudo-photodermatitis, atopic eczema-like, localized, exfoliative erythroderma and hand eczema. Plants from some other plant families, e.g., *Frullania*, *Magnolia*, and *Laurus* contain SQTLs and may cause sensitization or may cross-react with other SQTL containing plants. Patch testing is best done to specific plants, as a 1% ether or acetone extract in petrolatum, but screening tests using Benezra's sesquiterpene lactone mix (in the European series) or a group of specific plants are often used as a screen. Treatment is often successful provided the patient avoids known sources of exposure, which requires some instruction. PUVA therapy is often helpful.

Alstroemeria and tulip typically cause an eruption in the grip area of the fingers of florists and especially the thumb, index and middle fingers. Fissures are commonly present within a hyperkeratotic eczema starting at the free edge of the nail and progressing to the finger-tips and proximally to the periungual area. Persons who work with tulip bulbs regularly have a very high prevalence of sensitivity. Exposure to cut flowers seems to be associated with sensitization less often, but it does occur. Tulip sensitivity is caused by allergy to alpha-methylene gamma-butyrolactione or tulipalin A, which is derived from the glycoside tuliposide A. Both tuliposide A and its hydroxy derivative, tuliposide B have fungistatic and bacterostatic properties. Contact sensitivity to tulip often occurs after long periods of exposure of handling the bulbs, but it can also occur from contact with other parts as well. The allergen in Alstroemeria is especially concentrated in the petals. The allergenic chemical is found in several of the Lilyflorae, including not only *Alstroemeria* (Peruvian or Inca lily), but also tulip, *Erythronium dens canis* (dog's tooth violet), *E. americanum* (trout lily, adder's tongue), *Bomarea*, *Gagea* and at least one species of onion (*Allium triquetrum*). Minor amounts can be found in a few other genera. Tuliposides A and B have antifungal properties but only the former produces the allergen, alpha-methylene gamma-butyrolactone by hydrolysis. In tulip, the allergen is found in greatest concentration in the bulb with decreasing concentrations in the stem, leaf, and petal. In one series, 9/10 varieties of tulip were equally potent with Red Emperor variety, slightly less allergenic. The high concentration, on the scale that the bulb contains, can cause airborne contact dermatitis. Patch testing is done to a commercial antigen, alpha-methylene-gamma-butyrolactone (0.01% petrolatum). Treatment for retail florists involves the use of nitrile gloves, but incidental contact with antigen contaminating the work area can occur.

Primula dermatitis can be occupational, but usually one sees an older housewife with a dermatitis of the fingertips and streaks and patchy eczema on the hands, face (especially the eyelids) and arms. *Primula obconica* is such a common contact allergen in Europe that ca. 1.0–1.8% of persons routinely patch tested react to the causative allergen, primin, 0.01% in petrolatum, as part of the European screening series The eruption may not be suspected until the positive patch test appears, and a nondescript pattern may suggest an endogenous cause. Rarely does one see a reaction to the plant when the patch test to primin is negative.

The allergy apparently develops when the person growing the houseplant pinches off dying blooms to encourage the plant to bloom again. The allergen is present in shorter "hairs" on the plant surface (and more concentrated in smaller leaves), so contact is extremely easy. Primin is such a strong antigen and is in such variable concentration in the plant that it is wise to patch test to the commercial antigen. Delayed readings up to 7 days are important.

Treatment is principally avoidance. A primin-free strain of *Primula obconica* is now available as seed.

Phytophotodermatitis is usually phototoxic, although photosensitivity can be found concomitantly with Compositae dermatitis. Poison-ivy like streaks or vesicles and bullae in light-exposed sites can be caused by photocontact dermatitis, and when produced by psoralens, the acute eruption is typically followed by pigmentation. There are multiple mechanisms of phytophotodermatitis, but most such reactions are caused by plants containing furanocoumarins or psoralens, including certain members of the Umbelliferae and Rutaceae (citrus) combined with sun exposure. There are also photosensitizing plants that do not contain psoralens, e.g., St. John's wort (*Hypericum perforatum*).

Irritant Reactions

An "irritant" is a nonallergic response, which can have any one or more of many causes. Irritant reactions tend to occur rapidly, often within a few minutes, and they are more likely to burn rather than itch. They can also occur on first exposure and they tend to be dose-related. Allergic reactions should not occur on first exposure and prominent reactions can sometimes result from very small amounts of antigen, especially in highly sensitive subjects. The mechanism for nonallergic reactions can be greatly variable ranging from mechanical injury from cactus to urticaria from stinging nettles and painful inflammation from bull nettles to strong vesiculation from Euphorbiaceae such as manchineel.

Physical injury can be seen from splinters, glochids of certain cacti, awns of certain grasses, burrs of many shrubs, the bark of some trees, woody spines and almost any plant component sharp and firm enough to penetrate the skin. Thorns of plants from roses and blackberry to locust and Hawthorn trees to *Euphorbia* spp. may cause mechanical and sometimes chemical injury. Some grains, e.g., barley, have prominent awns that can be irritating. Many of the Cactaceae also produce mechanical injury. The list of such plants is long, but normally one can easily make the diagnosis.

Sabra dermatitis from *Opuntia Ficus-indica* can sometimes resemble scabies. The bunny's ears cactus *Opuntia microdasys*, a commonly grown ornamental, also has collections of tiny spines called glochides which are a source of immediate irritation, and sometimes progress to granuloma formation.

Calcium oxalate is a common source of plant irritation found in a number of irritant plants including dumbcane (*Dieffenbachia*), daffodils, *Hyacinth*, *Arisaema*, lily, pineapple and other species. The chemical is contained in intracellular crystals called raphides, and is ejected from the cell on contact with water. When leaves of dumbcame are chewed, a burning sensation develops almost immediately followed by salivation and perhaps a dermatitis. Mustards including radish, horseradish, etc., contain sinigrins which become irritating when they are enzymatically converted into isocyanates. Buttercup (*Ranunculus* spp.) contains proto-anemonin as does columbine (*Aquilegia*), marsh marigold (*Caltha*), *Clematis*, *Delphinium*, and *Anemone*.

Many but not all members of the Euphorbiaceae are irritant and some (e.g., snow on the mountain) are grown for use as decorative plants. Some spurges (*Euphorbiaceae*) contain phorbol esters in the latex, which are not only strong vesicants, but contain co-carcinogens as well. Many are tropical plants such as the infamous manchineel tree, but equally irritant latex may be found in some related houseplants such as the candelabra cactus (*Euphorbia lactea*). Croton oil is obtained from *Croton Tiglium* a member of the Euphorbiaceae.

Photosensitivity

Plants known to cause phytophotodermatitis include Persian limes (*Citrus aurantium*), fig trees (*Ficus carica*), gas plant (*Dictamnus albus*), giant hogweed (*Heracleum Mantegazzianum*), common rue (*Ruta graveolens*), *Ruta montana*, *Ruta chalepensis*, *Ruta corsica*, bishop's weed (*Ammi majus*), wild parsnip (*Pastinica sativa*), angelica (*Angelica archangelica*), and the scurf pea (*Psoralea corylifolia*).

Light absorbing chemicals in lichens or oak moss (from a lichen) are said to cause photoallergic dermatitis, although this is not experimentally reproducible, at least not with atranorin and lichen mix.

Occupations

Occupational plant dermatitis obviously tends to occur more often in certain vocations, the prevalence depending upon the opportunity for exposure, the population at risk, and the sensitizing capacity of the plant. Reactions to plants and plant products might occur in any occupation with exposure to sensitizing plants or plant products, but one should be aware of several clinical pictures within specific occupational groups.

Agricultural workers may experience reactions to poison ivy, oak and sumac that go unreported. Exposure can occur in clearing fence-rows and sometimes in handling domestic animals. These plants are not usually found with the crops where herbicides are used for weed control but are more often seen on fence-rows. Compositae dermatitis is seen in farmers in the United States, especially, but may be seen in other countries. Some reactions to the Compositae are irritant and some are allergic. Very likely some are both. An epidemic of bullous irritant dermatitis (and one with erythema multiforme) was seen in 14 farm workers pulling weeds (chiefly *Anthemis cotula*) in a field of sugar beets. Allergy to *P. hysterophorus*, while seen in the United States, has been, since the 1950s, far more common in India. This eruption typically involves older males engaged in outdoor work, and about 4% will become sensitive in 3–12 months. The eruption goes through stages with progressive severity and a more and more widespread distribution. Sunflower (*Helianthus annuus*) causes allergic contact dermatitis of the hands and other exposed sites in agricultural workers engaged in growing the plant for commercial purposes. This sensitivity may produce a cross reaction to arnica. Chicory dermatitis has been seen from April until September, when the plant is harvested.

Pyrethrum, derived from *Chrysanthemum cinerariifolium* and used as a pesticide, can induce contact dermatitis in farmers, and chervil, *Anthriscus Cerefolium*, has been reported several times to induce contact allergy.

Tobacco, *Nicotiana tabacum*, may induce either contact urticaria, or contact dermatitis. This plant can also cause airborne contact dermatitis. Coffee workers have experienced contact dermatitis to the leaf of the coffee plant and to the unroasted coffee bean. Urticaria also occurs in those handling coffee beans, which sometimes may be due to castor beans included in the harvested material.

Contact dermatitis has been reported in grape workers, to a kiwi (*Actinidia chinensis*) orchard operator, and a farmer reacted to salicyl alcohol in aspen. Okra (*Hibiscus esculentus*) may cause either irritant or allergic contact dermatitis. Harvesters can develop a pruritic eruption shortly after starting to pick the plant, and continued exposure leads to fissures and flattening of the finger ridges. *Frullania* sensitivity was reported in fruit pickers in Portugal, and lichens caused contact dermatitis in rural agricultural workers. A mushroom gatherer developed hand eczema that later spread to involve the extremities, face and trunk. Opium poppy, *Papaver somniferum*, reportedly caused allergic contact dermatitis to codeine in producers.

Photosensitivity may occur from figs, certain plants of the Umbilleriferae and Rutaceae, but the best-known example in agricultural workers is perhaps the reaction to celery (*Apium graveolens*) affected with pink rot caused by the fungus organism, *Sclerotinia sclerotiorum*. However, several epidemics of phytophotodermatitis have been reported from celery that was not infected.

Automobile mechanics have little exposure to plants but may become allergic to latex gloves used to try to protect the hands.

Bakers, chefs and food service workers are subject to several types of eruptions. Protein contact dermatitis, an eczenatous response to immediate type allergens, appears more rapidly than contact allergy. It can be as early as 30 minutes, and there is usually a positive scratch, prick, rub or RAST test and often, but not always, a negative patch test. Sometimes a scratch chamber is used to confirm the diagnosis, and sometimes a rub test will reproduce it. Testing for protein contact dermatitis is done by both prick testing for urticaria and either patch testing, or scratch chamber methodology. Some grain-sensitive patients experience aggravation of atopic eczema, some experience contact urticaria, some contact eczematous reactions, some protein contact dermatitis and some more than one of these. Bakers with dermatitis from grain sensitivity seem to demonstrate reactivity towards antigens with molecular weights higher than 50 kD. Grains include wheat, bran, oats, rye, barley, rice and corn. Bakers with immediate sensitivities have an increased chance of having respiratory allergy to whole wheat.

Contact dermatitis can occur from endive (*Cichorium endivum*), chicory, parsley (*Cichorium Intybus*), chervil (*Anthriscus Cerefolium*), and lettuce (*Lactuca sativa*).

Reactions may be seen to *Cynara scolymus* in workers cleaning artichokes, market gardeners, food handlers, and vegetable sellers, and to parsley and parsnip in kitchen workers. In Japan, persons who wrap leaves of the beefsteak plant, *Perilla frutescens* (shiso), are prone to develop allergic contact dermatitis apparently from l-perillaldehyde. Mustard caused contact dermatitis in a salad maker. Patch testing can be done with synthetic oil of mustard (0.1% allylisothiocyanate).

Immunologic and nonimmunologic contact urticaria can occur with exposure to many different plants. Contact dermatitis to spices often accompanies sensitivity to fragrances. Dooms-Goossens found reactions to nutmeg and mace (from *Myristica fragrans* Myristaceae), cardamom (from *Elettaria cardamomum* Zingiberaceae), tumeric (from *Curcuma longa* Zingiberaceae), coriander (from *Coriandrum sativum* Umbelliferae), curry (from a mixture of several spices including pepper, cloves, cinnamon, cardamom, coriander, nutmeg, mace and tumeric), cinnamon (from *Cinnamomum zeylanicum* Lauraceae), and bay leaves (*Laurus nobilis* Lauraceae). Vanilla and paprika may also cause sensitivity. Colophony, balsam of Peru, fragrance mix and wood tars are used as a screen for such reactions.

Food service workers and cooks may have reactions to many plants including lettuce, potato, and protein contact, citrus, tomato and carrot, cauliflower, kiwi, onion, chicory, and parsnip.

Of all forms of contact dermatitis in *chefs*, sensitivity to garlic is perhaps best known and recognizable, and while it is usually thought of as causing delayed hypersensitivity reactions, immediate sensitivity is also reported. Actually in some countries seemingly non-specific hand dermatitis in housewives (if one considers this occupational) may be caused by garlic exposure. However, most such reactions are seen as occupational dermatitis, especially in caterers and other food service occupations. Caterers and chefs also are at risk for sensitization to flavors for which balsam of Peru is one marker.

Mushroom dermatitis, can be seen in those exposed occupationally, as the allergy seems to be limited to the uncooked material. In Japan and certain other countries, a characteristic eruption follows consumption of an edible mushroom *Lentinus edodes*, if it is uncooked. This begins with an erythematous, papular rash in lines suggestive of finger marks, some 1–2 days after the mushrooms are consumed. Externally it fits a hand transfer pattern, but it is best known as an eruption following ingestion. Histologically one sees spongiosis with dermal edema and a perivascular lymphocytic infiltrate. This does not occur from cooked mushrooms. This may have multiple underlying mechanisms, as both patch tests for delayed hypersensitivity and prick tests for immediate hypersensitivity are positive. Sometimes a generalized toxic erythema is seen. Symptomatology is not limited to cutaneous problems as respiratory symptoms occur sometimes in persons who work in commercial production.

Bartenders can be exposed to citrus peels (lemon, lime, and orange) and mint *Menthus citrata (aquatica)* and other decorations such as stirring instruments. Contact urticaria to beer was reported in a waitress who was most sensitive to malt on RAST test. Psoralens in lime may produce photosensitivity.

Basketmakers may develop an irritant reaction from Osler (*Salix viminalis*), the plant used.

Beekeepers may be exposed to allergens found in propolis, poplar extract and balsam of Peru. Persons sensitive to propolis are frequently sensitive to balsam of Peru, and there is an overlap of reactivity with poplar buds. Routine testing shows positive responses to balsams of Peru and Tolu.

Botanists working in both the field and herbaria are at risk to develop or elicit plant-induced contact dermatitis, but there are relatively few reports. Perhaps this is because this occupation is uniquely equipped to know the cause of the eruption and to avoid contact through recognition. One might look for Urticaceae (*Urtica, Laportea*), *Phacelia*, exotic Anacardiaceae, Umbelliferae (where phototoxicity is likely), and almost any other plant known to cause irritant or allergic contact dermatitis.

Construction workers who work on roads and bridges often encounter irritant plants as well, such as nettles, thorns, etc. They may also encounter almost any potentially allergenic plant that grows in the geographic area where they are working, such as, for instance, toxicodendrons or Compositae.

Cosmetics workers, cosmetologists, etc have been exposed to plant materials in cosmetics for a long time. However, they have a potential in today's world to become allergic to thousands of plants, as today botanicals are so commonly incorporated into cosmetics. This has not appeared in quantity in the literature although many patients react to plant materials in cosmetics, so those exposed in industry are likely to follow.

Dock-workers are reported to break out in response to castor bean as a contaminant in coffee beans, barley in cattle fodder, and a warehouseman developed urticaria from *Cinchona* from burlap bags of the dried bark. I have seen persons in shipping who were allergic to cashew-nut shell oil (Anacardiaceae) that they had handled.

Food processing workers handling nuts may break out on contact with macadamia nuts, or develop cashew dermatitis due to contaminants from the shell. Both immediate (especially from green coffee beans) and delayed allergy may occur in coffee workers. This is sometimes, but not always, from castor beans. Plantation workers may develop lupus erythema-like periungual telangiectasia.

Of the Cruciferae, mustards are known irritants, and contact urticaria and/or protein contact dermatitis may occur to mustard (*Brassica nigra*) and cauliflower

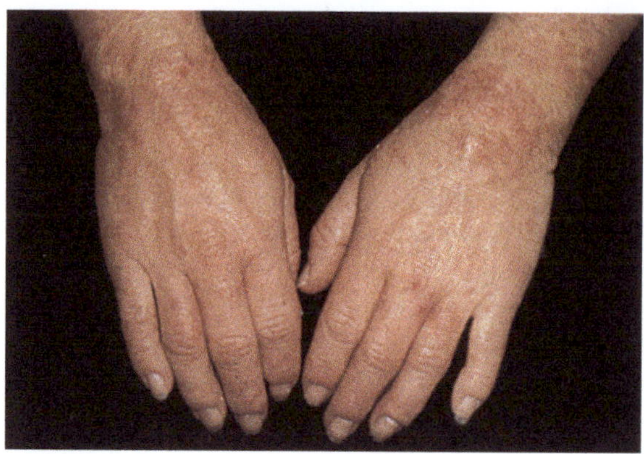

Fig. 2. Contact dermatitis to *Frulliania* from exposure to hardwood cut for firewood

(*Brassica oleracea*) in chefs, salad makers and others preparing and handling food. Celery dermatitis can occur in a food-processing worker. Radish (*Raphanus sativus*) contains allyl and benzyl isothiocyanates that may cause allergic contact dermatitis in a waitress mixing salads.

Many spices, e.g., rosemary, (*Rosmarinus officinalis*), may induce allergic contact dermatitis (see discussion of bakers above). Workers in corn processing plants commonly develop an irritant prurigo-like eruption of the hands, forearms and unprotected areas.

Forestry fire fighters in the United States are at risk to develop Toxicodendron dermatitis. Frullania is a problem in *woodcutters* in Portugal, Italy, Spain, Czechoslovakia, and the Pacific Northwest (Fig. 2). Woodcutters working in the forests of the Pacific northwest are prone to develop sensitivity to sesquiterpene lactones because of exposure to *Frullania nisquallensis*, (a liverwort) living on decaying timber.

Lichen sensitivity to "reindeer moss" (*Cladonia stellaris*) is sometimes called woodcutter's disease in Europe and "cedar poisoning" or "pine poisoning" in the United States. The risk for sensitization to this plant is considered low, but there are probably more cases among "lichen pickers". Sensitizing components include atranorin, fumarprotocetraric acid, evernic acid, (–) and (+) usnic acid, and stictic acid. Lichens and oakmoss are also potentially photosensitizing.

Grain workers and elevator operators commonly itch after exposure to dust from barley and oat dust, but this is of a relatively short duration.

Grocery workers, several years ago, experienced an epidemic of phytophotodermatitis to psoralens in cut stalks of celery combined with UV exposure from tanning salons or sun. Grocers may also become sensitive to produce, or grain in animal feed.

Healthcare workers tend to become allergic to latex protein, especially if they are atopic. This represents an allergy to *Hevea brasiliensis* in most cases and sometimes to cornstarch, the principal ingredient of glove powder. Up to 9% of dental assistants have immediate contact allergy to latex. Cross reactions are said to occur from banana, avocado, peach, kiwi, and pineapple but a more extensive list might also include chestnut, hazel nut, peanut, celery, melon, potato, papaya, figs, passion fruit, tomato, grapes, cherries, apricot, nectarines, and plums.

Lawn-care workers are at risk to develop *Toxicodendron* dermatitis in North America. They are also at risk for Compositae dermatitis, including reactions to ragweed, dandelion and other weeds.

Massage therapists or their customers may become sensitive to natural materials used in massage therapy. *A metalworker* with occupational hand eczema broke out in response to the chamomile tea used to treat his rash. *Musicians* may break out in response to cane reed, colophony, or therapeutic agents. Woods are covered elsewhere.

Nursery workers and florists are at risk to develop both irritant and allergic reactions to plants. The most prevalent cause varies with the country in question but Alstroemeria and tulip, Compositae and daffodil are considered common sources. Other sources include Compositsae, e.g., Chrysanthemum, elecampane, Gebera and *Tanacetum parthenium* or fevergew, Lilaceae (tulip and hyacinth), Amaryllidaceae (narcissus) and Carophyllaceae (carnation), to name a few.

Those allergic to toxicodendrons may react to *Philodendron* spp., seed of *Ginkgo biloba*, cashew (*Anacardium occidentale*), mango (*Mangiferica indica*), *Grevillea robusta* and *Grevillea Robyn Gordon* (Proteaceae). Other taxons reported include Araliaceae, e.g., *Hedera helix, Hedera canariensis, Schefflera*, and *Fatsia. Chrysanthemum, Dahlia*, Elecampane (*Inula helenium*), *Liatris spicata, Trachelium*, chamomile, sunflower, magnolia and laurel, and *Tetrapanax* (Campanulaceae) *Gaillardia*, as with sunflower, can cross react with *Arnica*. Other species at risk include *Anthemis nobilis* and *Sisymbrium officinale* (Brassicaceae), *Dianthus caryophyllus*, Caryophyllaceae), African violet, *Cotoneaster* sp. (Rosaceae), *Coleus* sp. Labiatae (flame nettle), *Trachelium caeruleum* (Campanulaceae), *Wedelia trilobata*, Wild artichoke (*Cynara cardunculus*), firebush (*Ixodia achillaeoides*), *Paeonia* (Paeoniaceae), and *Verbena* (Verbenaceae).

A *hobby gardener* developed delayed urticaria from elm, *Ulmus* sp., with inhibition by aluminum sulphate. Other plants causing contact urticaria in this group include *Lily longifolium* and tulip, *Limonium tartaricum* (from dried flowers), and *Chrysanthemum*.

Irritant reactions may take many forms. Calcium oxalate in some plants, e.g., *Dieffenbachia* and hyacinth, and daffodils, causes irritation in those harvesting them. Spurges contain phorbol and diterpene esters that are quite irritating. *Apalochlamys spectabilis, Wisteria sinensis* and some *Grevillea* species were irritant causing "plant hair dermatitis," and called attention to penetrating and irritating pod spines of *Brachychiton* spp. (kurrajongs and relatives) and *Lagunaria patersonii* (Norfolk Island hibiscus or pyramid tree), often planted as ornamental street trees. Phytophotodermatitis may occur to plants listed in that section, and pseudophytophotodermatitis may occur from pesticides.

Laboratory workers have experienced phytophotodermatitis from psoralens in *Cachrys libanotis* (Umbelliferae) and urticaria from *Cannabis sativa*.

Office workers may break out in response to plants kept at the office such as Araceae (Diffenbachia, Philodendron, etc.), Araliaceae (*Hedera helix* and *H. canariensis, Schefflera arboricola, Brassasia actinophyla, Polyscias fruticosa*), Gesneriaceae (*Saintpaulia*), and Cactaceae (*Opuntia microdasys*).

Pharmaceutical workers are reported to have reacted to *Arnica longifolia*, and *A. montana*, Atropine (*Duboisia* spp.), Psyllium (*Plantago* sp.), *Vinca* alkaloids, and Codeine.

Textile workers may experience irritant dermatitis more often from wool than plant fibers but may break out working with linseed oil and flax.

Tobacco workers handling cigars may develop hand eczema. The cause for the rare cases of allergic contact dermatitis has not been identified, but it is not nicotine.

Servicemen may react to a wide variety of plants that are found in their sphere of operation. Some of the best-known examples are urticaria from certain grasses, irritant reactions to manchineel, and dermatitis from toxic Anacardiaceae.

Tree surgeons may experience allergy to propolis, to toxicodendrons in North America, and to other toxic Anacardiaceae and cross reacting Proteaceae in other geographic regions. In Hawaii *Philodendron* may even be a problem.

Woodworkers in Japan who tend to become sensitive to lacquer from *Toxicodendron vernicifluum*, develop hardening with time. Heat treatment of the lacquer seems to render the substance less allergenic.

Suggested Reading

Guin JD (2000) Occupational contact dermatitis to plants. In: Handbook of occupational dermatology. Kanerva L, Elsner P, Wahlberg J, Maibach HI (eds) Springer, Berlin Heidelberg New York, pp 730–766

Guin JD, Beaman JH (1986) Plant dermatitis. Clin Dermatol 4:1–226

Hansen BM (2000) Woods. In: Handbook of occupational dermatology. Kanerva L, Elsner P, Wahlberg J, Maibach HI (eds) Springer-Verlag, Berlin Heidelberg New York, pp 771–780

Mitchell J, Rook A (1979) Botanical dermatology: plants and plant products injurious to the skin. Greengrass Pub, Vancouver, Canada

Kingsbury JM (1964) Poisonous plants of the United States and Canada. Prentice-Hall, Inc., Englewood Cliffs, New Jersey

Lampe KF, McCann MA (1985) AMA handbook of poisonous and injurious plants. American Medical Association, Chicago

Benezra C, Ducombs G, Sell Y, Foussereau C (1985) Plant contact dermatitis. Decker, Toronto, pp 200–203

Hjorth N, Wilkinson DS (1968) Contact dermatitis. 4. Tulip fingers, hyacinth itch and lily rash. Brit J Dermatol 80:696–698

Hogan DJ, Dosman JA, Li KY, Graham B, et al. (1986) Questionnaire survey of pruritus and rash in grain elevator workers. Contact Dermatitis 14:170–175

CHAPTER 36

Polyurethane Resins

36

T. Estlander, L. Kanerva, R. Jolanki

Introduction

The occupational hazards of polyurethane (PU) chemicals affect mainly the airways and eyes, and can cause rhinitis, asthma, hypersensitive pneumonitis or alveolitis, conjunctivitis, and chronic obstructive lung disease. Isocyanates are also toxic and poisonous chemicals (Cronin 1980; Adams 1983; Israeli et al 1981).

Exposure to isocyanates and auxiliary chemicals may also result in both allergic and irritant contact dermatitis, as well as urticaria (Malten 1964; Rothe 1976; Israeli et al. 1981; Fisher 1986; Kanerva et al. 1989, 1991; Estlander et al. 1992, 2000).

Composition

PUs are formed as a result of a condensation or an adduction reaction between isocyanates and polyols. Many auxiliary substances are also used in the manufacture of PU products. The hardening process can be modified by heat or with a catalyst [diamino diphenylmethane or methylenedianiline (MDA), triethylenediamine, triethylamine, cobalt naphthenate or nickel salts]. Figure 1 lists the isocyanates used in the production of PU plastics (Estlander et al. 2000).

The most commonly used difunctional isocyanates are TDI, MDI and 1,6-hexamethylene diisocyanate or 1,6-diisocyanatohexane (HDI). TDI often contains mixtures of the isomers 2,4-TDI and 2,6-TDI. MDI is industrially used as a mixture of 4,4'-MDI with 2,4'-MDI and 2,2'-MD which is also called polymethylene polyphenyl isocyanate (PAPI or PMPPI). Phenyl isocyanate is usually a trace constituent in commercial MDI products. Examples of other diisocyanates include isophorone diisocyanate (IPDI), trimethylhexamethylene diisocyanate (TMDI), naphthalene diisocyanate (NDI), triphenylmethane triisocyanate (TPMTI), and DMDI (Malten 1984a,b, 1987a,b; Björkner 1992; Elvers et al. 1991; Estlander et al. 1992, 2000).

Isocyanates are increasingly used in the manufacture of various PU products, such as elastic and rigid foams, paints, lacquers, varnishes, other surface coatings, adhesives, binding and impregnation agents, joint sealants, insulation materials, textile finishes, synthetic rubbers, and elastomeric fibers. Elastic foams are used for mattresses, car seats, cushions, dashboards and packages (Adams 1983; White et al. 1983; Wilkinson et al. 1991; Björkner 1992; Estlander et al. 1992, 2000).

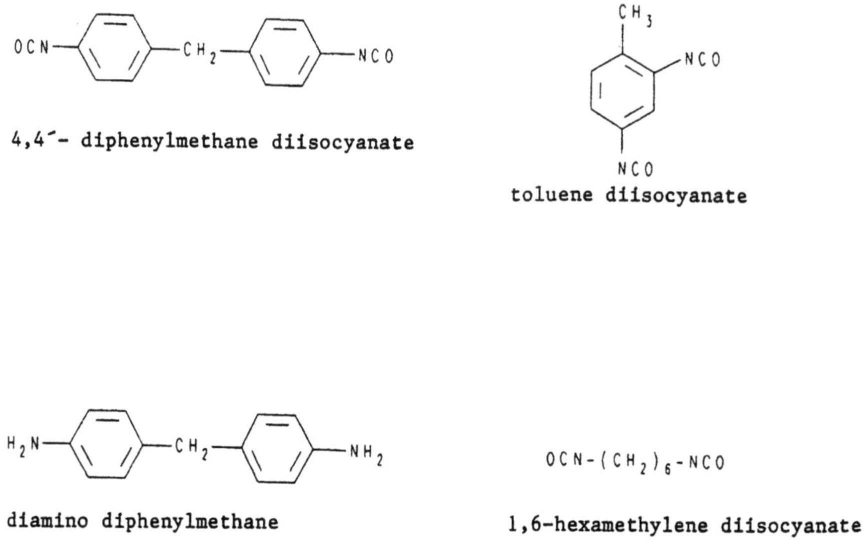

$OCN-C_6H_4-CH_2-C_6H_4-NCO$

4,4´- diphenylmethane diisocyanate

toluene diisocyanate

$H_2N-C_6H_4-CH_2-C_6H_4-NH_2$

diamino diphenylmethane

$OCN-(CH_2)_6-NCO$

1,6-hexamethylene diisocyanate

Fig. 1. Chemical structure of isocyanates used in the production of polyurethane plastics

Skin Problems Caused by PU Chemicals

Allergic Contact Dermatitis

The reports on allergic contact eczema are few. Polyols are not considered to be sensitizers. Allergy caused by PU chemicals has been reported mainly from occupational exposure to the various diisocyanates, although cases caused by accelerators have also been reported. Contact allergy is most often reported to be caused by various MDI and DMDI, as summarized by Malten 1987 a,b. Cases due to TDI, IPDI, NDI, and HDI have also been reported, as well as cases due to MDA used as an accelerator, and from exposure to MDI (Malten 1984 a,b; Cronin 1980; White et al. 1983; Tanaka et al. 1987; Kanerva et al. 1989; Huang et al. 1991; Estlander et al. 1992, 2000).

Workers exposed to PU chemicals and prepolymers in laboratories and in the manufacture of PUs, e.g., car spray painters, adhesive workers – such as those exposed to two-part glues used by floor layers as well as lacquer workers and insulation installers – and those accidentally exposed to pyrolysis products are at risk of developing dermatitis (Rothe 1976; Kanerva et al. 1989; Estlander et al. 1992; Björkner 1992). Some rare sources of sensitization to PU chemicals have also been reported (Rothe 1995; Estlander et al 2000).

Allergic Contact Dermatitis and Urticaria

Allergic Contact Dermatitis

In the period from 1974 to 1997, nine cases of allergic contact dermatitis and one case of urticaria due to PU chemicals were diagnosed at the Finnish Institute of

Occupational Health (FIOH) (Kanerva et al. 1989, 1991; Estlander et al. 1992, 2000).

The first three patients with allergic contact dermatitis were exposed for 2–8 months to PU chemicals containing different diisocyanates before they developed dermatitis. On patch testing, they reacted to IPDI, TMDI, TDI, HDI and MDA. Two of the patients also had diisocyanate-induced asthma confirmed by bronchial challenge, in one case with MDI and in the other with HDI (Kanerva et al. 1989).

The next three patients had been exposed to MDI or a mixture of MDI and PAPI during periods ranging from 2 weeks to 19 years before they acquired dermatitis. On patch testing, all but one reacted to MDI. All three individuals, however, reacted to MDA, and one also reacted to TDI (Estlander et al. 1992).

One of the last three patients (unpublished) was an industrial worker who developed dermatitis after 1 week of mixing a PU hardener containing MDI and traces of TDI and a polyol. The second was a car electrician who acquired dermatitis on his face after 4 years of having occasionally handled two adhesives/insulating materials containing MDI and TDI. The last one was a worker finishing circuit boards with a lacquer containing TDI, MDI and MDA. On patch testing, the industrial worker reacted to the PU hardener containing 100% MDI, and to MDA, as well as to TDI. The car electrician was patch-test positive only to TDI, and the circuit-board worker to MDI and MDA but not to TDI (Estlander et al. 2000).

A structural similarity or cross allergy between MDI and MDA has been considered as an explanation for simultaneous reactions to MDI and MDA. MDA may also have formed as a result of hydrolysis of MDI. The positive TDI reactions in patients exposed to MDI can be explained by cross-reactions between MDI and TDI or be due to concomitant sensitization to the chemicals. Commercial MDI and PAPI may contain TDI (Fregert 1967; Rother 1976; Buist and Gudgeon 1970).

Insufficient hand protection is also an important factor in the development of sensitization to diisocyanates. Some of our patients did not use protective gloves at all, or glove contamination and penetration had even increased allergen contact with their skin (Estlander et al. 1992, 2000; Dooms-Goossens et al 1995; Forsberg and Olsson 1985).

Urticaria

Other skin symptoms, except contact dermatitis, have seldom been reported to be caused by isocyanates. Urticaria has been described by Schürmann (1955) and Israeli et al. (1981). Our patient was a welder who had been welding mild steel profiles for 10 years and, occasionally, Forster Therm steel-PU profiles. The inside of the steel profile was made of PU, which was synthesized from MDI and other substances.

After welding the profiles for 2 weeks, he developed a generalized urticaria associated with edema of the lids and face, and fever up to 40 °C. The symptoms disappeared 2 days after he stopped welding the profiles. All skin tests to show type-I or -IV allergy to isocyanates were negative. Welding the profile for 30 min in the provocation chamber, however, provoked a symmetrical urticarial reaction on the hands and knees, and on the following night his temperature rose to 38.5 °C.

The lung-function tests were normal. Provocation tests with pure MDI and MDA were negative. Possibly the reaction was caused by product(s) formed and inhaled while welding PU, although contact urticaria from airborne chemicals was not excluded (Kanerva et al. 1991).

Irritant Contact Dermatitis

Isocyanates are described as mild to strong skin irritants and listed in industrial safety data sheets as skin-irritating substances. Liquid monomer coming into contact with the skin has been reported to cause edema and redness (Fisher 1986). Irritant contact dermatitis seems to be more common than allergic contact dermatitis, and small epidemics have occurred in certain plants using isocyanates.

Itchy rash-like eruptions on exposed skin areas in the factory workers who coat car badges with the resin have been reported from exposure to DMDI (White et al. 1983). The same was reported in workers at a glass-bottle factory, where DMDI was used to coat the bottles (Israeli et al. 1981), as well as in the workers of a PU-molding plant (Emmett 1976). Irritant dermatitis appearing in a laboratory technician within a few hours of contact with TDI and in a repair-man have also been described (Rothe 1976).

After heavy exposure to TDI, pulmonary symptoms followed by thrombocytopenia and purpura have been reported (Jennings and Rower 1963). Irritant dermatitis, in addition to allergic dermatitis from HDI, occurred in the workers of two clothing mills handling cloths previously coated with an anti-pill finish containing HDI (Wilkinson et al. 1991).

Skin irritation can also be caused by amine accelerators, e.g., MDA, triethylenediamine and triethylamine. Concentrated liquids may even be corrosive. The irritant effect of diisocyanates in the hardeners, glues and paints may also be attributed to the solvents used in these products. Completely hardened PU products usually do not cause skin problems. During machining and cutting, PU dust containing isocyanate is produced. When heated to above 250 °C, PU polymers decompose into isocyanates and nitrogen oxides, and may then cause dermatitis (Björkner 1992; Estlander et al. 2000).

Examination of Dermatoses Caused by PU Chemicals and Their Prevention

Examinations should include clinical examination and patch testing. Patch tests should include at least MDI, TDI, HDI and MDA, in addition to actual chemicals to which the workers have been exposed (Estlander et al. 1992). Besides the chemicals, patch tests with the suspected products and the chemical analyses of the products are often necessary.

An impurity, not the monomers or additives themselves, may also be the actual cause of allergic dermatitis (Dooms-Goossens et al. 1995). In the case of urticaria, prick tests with MDI, TDI and HDI human serum albumin conjugates and the determinations of the same diisocyanate IgE-specific antibodies should be included in the examinations (Keskinen et al. 1988). However, a challenge test in an exposure chamber (Kanerva et al. 1991) is probably the most reliable method of confirming the diagnosis of diisocyanate-induced urticaria.

In the prevention of dermatoses induced by PU chemicals, it is important to inform all exposed workers about all the health hazards of PU chemicals and to give detailed instructions on how the chemicals or products should be handled. This means using appropriate personal protective equipment, such as EC conformity-marked chemical protective gloves, masks, eye and face protectors and other protective clothing. Good ventilation, local exhausts and general cleanliness are also essential.

References

Adams RM (1983) Plastics. In: Occupational skin disease. Grune and Stratton, New York, pp 238–266

Björkner B (1992) Plastic materials. In: Rycroft RJG, Menné T, Frosch PJ, Benezra C (eds) Textbook of contact dermatitis, Springer, Berlin Heidelberg New York, pp 557–559

Buist JM, Gudgeon H (eds) (1970) Advances in polymer technology. Elsevier, London, pp 311–385

Cronin E (1980) Contact dermatitis. Churchill Livingstone, Edinburgh, pp 637–642

Dooms-Goossens A, Bruze M, Buysse L, Fregert S, Gruvberger B, Stals H (1995) Contact allergy to allyl glycidyl ether present as an impurity in 3-glycidyloxypropyltrimethoxysilane, a fixing additive in silicone and polyurethane resins. Contact Dermatitis 33:17–19

Elvers B, Hawkins S, Schulz G (eds) (1991) Ullmans's encyclopedia of industrial chemistry, 5th edn, vol A19. VCH Verlagsgesellschaft GmbH, Weinheim, Basel, pp 371–385

Emmett EA (1976) Allergic contact dermatitis in polyurethane plastic moulders. J Occup Med 18:802–804

Estlander T, Jolanki R, Kanerva L (2000) Disadvantages of gloves. In: Kanerva L, Elsner P, Wahlberg JE, Maibach HI (eds) Handbook of occupational dermatology. Springer, Berlin Heidelberg New York, pp 597–601.

Estlander T, Keskinen H, Jolanki R, Kanerva L (1992) Occupational dermatitis from exposure to polyurethane chemicals. Contact Dermatitis 27:161–165

Fisher AA (1986) Contact dermatitis, 3rd edn. Lea and Febiger, Philadelphia, pp 562–565

Fregert S (1967) Allergic contact reaction to diphenyl-4,4'-diisocyanate. Contact Dermatitis Newslett 2:17

Forsberg K, Olsson KG (1985) Selection of chemical protective gloves (in Swedish). Förening Teknisk Företagshälsovard, FTF Stockholm

Huang J, Wang XP, Chen BM, Ueda A, Aoyma K, Matsushita T (1991) Allergologic evaluation for workers exposed to toluene diisocyanate. Ind Health 29:85–92

Israeli R, Smirnov V, Sculsky M (1981) Vergiftungerscheinungen bei Dicyclo-methan-4-4'-Diisocyanat-Exposition. Int Arch Occup Environ Health 48:179–184

Jennings GH, Rower ND (1963) Thrompocytopenic purpura in toluene di-isocyanate workers. Lancet 1:406–408

Kanerva L, Lähteenmäki M-T, Estlander T, Jolanki R, Keskinen H (1989) Allergic contact dermatitis from isocyanates. In: Frosch PJ, Dooms-Goossens A, Lachapelle J-M, Rycroft RJG, Scheper RJ (eds) Current topics in contact dermatitis. Springer, Berlin Heidelberg New York, pp 368–373

Kanerva L, Estlander T, Jolanki R, Lähteenmäki M-T, Keskinen H (1991) Occupational urticaria from welding polyurethane. J Am Acad Dermatol 24:825–826

Keskinen H, Tupasela O, Tiikkainen U, Nordman H (1988) Experience of specific IgE in asthma due to isocyanates. Clin Allergy 18:597–604

Malten KE (1964) Occupational dermatoses in the processing of plastics. Trans St John's Hosp Dermatol Soc 59:78–113

Malten KE (1984a) Dermatological problems with synthetic resins and plastics in glues, part I. Derm Beruf Umwelt 32:81–86

Malten KE (1984b) Dermatological problems with synthetic resins and plastics in glues, part II. Derm Beruf Umwelt 32:118–125

Malten KE (1987a) Printing plate manufacturing processes. In: Maibach HI (ed) Occupational and industrial dermatology, 2nd edn. Year Book Medical Publishers Inc, Chicago, pp 351–366

Malten KE (1987b) Old and new, mainly occupational dermatological problems in the production and processing of plastics. In: Maibach HI (ed) Occupational and industrial dermatology, 2nd edn. Year Book Medical Publishers, Chicago, pp 290

Rothe A (1976) Zur Frage arbeitsbedingter Hautschädigungen durch Polyurethanchemikalien. Derm Beruf Umwelt 24:7–24

Rothe A (1995) Gefahren bei der Injektion von Rissen in Betonbauwerken. Bau 2:72–75

Schürmann D (1955) Gesundheitsschäden durch neuartige Lacke und Schaumstoffe. Die DD (Desmodur/Desmophen) Lacke und Schaumstoffe als Ursache beruflicher Gesundheitsschädigungen. Dtsch Med Wochenschr 45:1661–1663

Tanaka K-I, Takeoka A, Nishimura F, Hanada S (1987) Contact sensitivity induced in mice by methylene bisphenyl diisocyanate. Contact Dermatitis 17:199–204

White IR, Stewart JR, Rycroft AJ (1983) Allergic contact dermatitis from an organic di-isocyanate. Contact Dermatitis 9:300–303

Wilkinson SM, Cartwright PH, Armitage J, English JSC (1991) Allergic contact dermatitis from 1,6-diisocyanatohexane in an anti-pill finish. Contact Dermatitis 25:94–96

CHAPTER 37

Organic Solvents

37

A. Boman, J. E. Wahlberg

Introduction

Industrial solvents are volatile organic liquids commonly used to dissolve other organic materials such as oils, fats, resins, rubber, lacquers, waxes, perfumes and plastic. They have a wide variety of uses, including:
- Painting
- Paint manufacturing
- Floor-laying
- Production of glass-fiber inforced polyester
- Surface coating
- Graphic industries, rotogravure printing
- Dyeing of paper, plastics, fabrics
- Metal degreasing
- Dry cleaning
- Cleansing
- Spotting agents
- Carriers and intermediates in organic synthesis
- Medium for extraction processes
- Analytical chemistry

Technical-grade organic solvents are reasonably inexpensive; considerable volumes are used yearly and numerous workers are exposed daily. Although mainly treated as a group due to their general properties solvents are chemically diverse (Fig. 1) and can be classified in different categories according to their physico-chemical characteristics. Threshold limit values (TLVs) are inter alia proposed by the American Conference of Governmental Industrial Hygienists (ACGIH) and various national government agencies (The Swedish Work Environment Authority 2000) and have had great influence in many industrialised countries when reviewing health hazards from solvents and implementing preventive measures. Information on water and lipid solubility and volatility is also of great value when discussing potential risks from solvent exposure. Steadily increasing knowledge of the various adverse effects seen in man has resulted in a gradual decrease in TLVs over the years. The relative importance of the percutaneous route of absorption of solvents has increased as result of these regulatory activities concerning inhalation of solvents. Awareness of environmental and human effects has also

Organic solvents

Aliphatic

$CH_3(CH_2)_4CH_3$
n-Hexane

Halogenated aliphatics

CH_2Cl_2
Methylenechloride

$CHCl_3$
Chloroform

CCl_4
Carbon tetrachloride

$CHCl=CCl_2$
Trichloro ethylene

$CCl_2=CCl_2$
Tetrachloro ethylene

CCl_3CH_3
Methyl chloroform

Miscellaneous solvents

CS_2
Carbon disulphide

$HCON(CH_3)_2$
Dimethyl formamide

Aromatic

Benzene 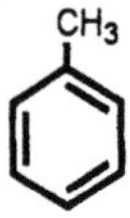   Toluene

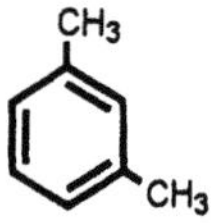

Xylene 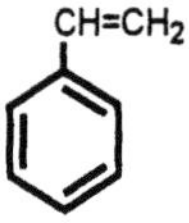   Styrene

Ketones

CH_3COCH_3
Acetone

$CH_3COCH_2CH_3$
Methylethyl ketone

$CH_3COCH_2CH_2CH_2CH_3$
Methyl-n-butyl ketone

Glycol ethers

$CH_3CH_2OCH_2CH_2OH$
Ethoxyethanol

Alcohols

CH_3CH_2OH
Ethanol

$CH_3CHOHCH_3$
iso-Propanol

$CH_3CH_2CH_2CH_2OH$
n-Butanol

Ethers

$CH_3CH_2OCH_2CH_3$
Diethyl ether

Esters

$CH_3COOCH_2CH_3$
Ethyl acetat

Petroleum distillates

Gasoline

White Spirit

Fig. 1. Structural formulas for selected solvents

led to a change from chlorinated solvents to biologically degradable solvents with altered risk spectra.

Adverse Effects Resulting from Skin Exposure

The various signs, disorders, diseases and other effects seen at skin exposure to solvents are summarized in Table 1.

The systemic effects of solvents are in some cases on specific target organs and the adverse effects may be caused by the solvent itself or reactive more toxic metabolites.

In addition to irritancy the various adverse effects (Table 1) can often be linked to a particular solvent. However, the main side effect in the skin – different degrees of defatting – is uniform and in general toxicology related to concentration, dose and duration of exposure. It has been demonstrated (Klauder and Brill 1947) that the low-boiling-range ($<250\,°C$) petroleum solvents have the greatest defatting action and dermatitis potential. Irritant action such as defatting action decreases as the boiling range increases. A worker is rarely exposed just to one solvent; more often he/she is exposed to mixtures of several solvents with a varying degree of purity. Mineral spirits, kerosene, gasoline and thinners are examples of widely used mixtures. From a clinical point of view it is hard to demonstrate the relative importance of one ingredient in a mixture of solvents.

With the exception of generalised dermatitis and Steven-Johnson syndrome from trichloroethylene (see below) the dermatoses caused by solvent exposure are considered to be comparatively benign and rarely a cause for job change or pension. In a Danish publication of notified occupational eczematous diseases 1984–1991 (Halkier-Sørensen 1996) exposure to solvents was the cause in 991 cases (3.6%) and was placed fifth in the ranking list.

Table 1. Adverse effects of solvents at skin exposure

Subjective irritation Irritancy
Contact urticaria
Flushing, generalised dermatitis and Steven-Johnson syndrome – from trichloroethylene
Whitening
Irritant contact dermatitis
Chemical burns
Allergic contact dermatitis
Scleroderma
Dermatoses from higher boiling petroleum distillates
Percutaneous absorption – systemic toxicity
Enhancing absorption of other toxic chemicals

Subjective Irritation

The affected workers report a stinging, tingling and/or burning sensation from a skin area exposed to a solvent or to a mixture of solvents. The site looks normal to the naked eye. This phenomenon is not restricted to solvents only; it has been reported, for example, from skin exposure to lactic acid ("the stinging test").

Irritancy

Solvents that quickly evaporate from the skin if not occluded are not as likely to damage the skin as solvents that do not evaporate, i.e. they will act for a longer period of time. Erythema, oedema and drying are the most common side effects seen from single or repeated exposures to solvents. These signs are sometimes transient or may develop into irritant contact dermatitis (see below). The course is related to the type of solvent, concentration, dose, and exposure time.

Erythema

In attempts to study and differentiate the erythema – inducing capacity of solvents in man the objective laser Doppler technique was used to measure skin blood flow (Wahlberg 1984a). This technique is three or four times more sensitive than the naked eye (Wahlberg 1989) (Table 2).

Oedema

Oedema caused by repeated skin exposure to solvents can be quantified with a rather unsophisticated device: the caliper (Wahlberg 1984b). Results from measurements of skin fold thickness in experimental animals treated once daily with

Table 2. Increase in skin blood flow from exposure to solvents (neat) as an expression of irritancy - objectively recorded by laser Doppler flowmetry (Wahlberg 1984a)

Solvent	0.1 ml pipetted onto the skin	Whitening after rubbing with cotton (exposure in excess of 1.5 ml/3.1 cm^2)	Duration in min required to get an increase
Dimethylsulfoxide	Increase	No	1
Trichloroethane	No increase	Yes	1
n-Hexane	No increase	Yes	5
Carbon tetrachloride	No increase	Yes	5
Toluene	No increase	Yes	5
1,1,1-Trichloroethane	No increase	Yes	5
1,1,2-Trichloroethane	No increase	Yes	5
Dodecane	No increase	Yes	15
Methyl ethyl ketone	No increase	Yes	No increase
Propylene glycol	No increase	No	No increase
Ethanol	No increase	Yes	No increase
Water	No increase	No	No increase

Table 3. Ranking of oedema-inducing capacity of solvents (neat) at skin exposure in experimental animals. Method: skin fold thickness measurements (Wahlberg 1984)

Solvent	Guinea pig	Rabbit
Trichloroethylene	1	1
Toluene	2	1
1,1,2-Trichloroethane	3	1
Carbon tetrachloride	4	2
1,1,1-Trichloroethane	4	2
Dimethylsulfoxide	5	Not tested
n-Hexane	6	4
Methyl ethyl ketone	7	3
Ethanol	7	5

neat solvents are summarized in Table 3. However, daily open treatments with solvents (neat) for 10–18 days on human volar forearms did not cause any increase in skin fold thickness (Wahlberg 1993).

Histopathology
The histopathological picture after epicutaneous administration of solvents to guinea pigs also demonstrated great variation in potency (Kronevi et al 1977, 1979, 1981).

Contact Urticaria

Several solvents e.g. alcohols, have been shown to cause immunologic as well as non-immunologic contact urticaria (Fisher 1978, Rilliet et al 1980, Varigos and Nurse 1986, Goodfield and Saihan 1988, Ophaswongse and Maibach 1994).

From a clinical point of view is it important to know that oral provocation with alcohol can elicit anaphylaxis (Ophaswongse and Maibach 1994).

Testing. To diagnose immunologic contact urticaria open tests with gas-chromatographically-pure ethanol ("as is") is recommended (Ophaswongse and Maibach 1994). With other solvents where data is lacking it is recommended to use graded concentrations as well as a great number of controls to verify the specificity.

Generalized Dermatitis, Steven-Johnson Syndrome and Flushing from Trichloroethylene

Exposure to trichloroethylene has been associated with cases of generalised dermatitis (Bauer and Rabens 1974) and of Steven-Johnson syndrome (Phoon et al 1984). Several of the patients had signs of liver dysfunction (toxic hepatitis) and one fatal case was reported (Nakayama et al 1988). From the case reports, however, it is somewhat hard to judge what route of absorption – inhalation or percutaneous absorption – had dominated.

Flushing. There are some case studies where exposure to trichloroethylene and to dimethyl formamide followed by ingestion of alcohol resulted in outbred flushing of the skin ("degreasers flush") and nausea (Stewart et al 1974).

Whitening

When some solvents are applied to human skin followed by gentle rubbing with e.g. cotton the site will turn white ("whitening"). In a comparative study this phenomenon was observed for 9 solvents (Goldsmith et al 1988) (Table 2). No decrease in skin blood flow – evaluated by laser Doppler flowmetry – was found indicating that the whitening was not due to vasoconstriction but rather to lipid extraction.

Irritant Contact Dermatitis

There is a general agreement that solvents are important skin irritants and that repeated exposure may develop into irritant contact dermatitis. As previously mentioned there is a great variation in the degree of irritancy produced (Tables 2, 3); in addition concentration, aromatic content, duration of exposure, occlusion, temperature, humidity and individual factors such as atopic diathesis, history of contact dermatitis, barrier function are supposed to interact and contribute to irritant contact dermatitis. Examples of predisposition and individual susceptibility are exemplified in Table 4. Individuals with past or current atopic dermatitis are more susceptible to irritants; among those individuals wet work are considered to be of great importance for relapses and deteriorations. Pre-employment examination and vocational guidance are recommended for these categories (Table 5).

Table 4. Individual susceptibility at skin exposure to organic solvents

History of atopic dermatitis	Predisposition/increased susceptibility
History of asthma/rhinitis	Not settled
History of contact dermatitis	Dry or senile skin;
	Considerable variation – even in non-atopics
Recommendation	Pre-employment examination, vocational guidance

Table 5. Adverse effects at skin exposure to solvents – preventive measures (Wahlberg and Boman 1996)

Reduce exposure
Appropriate selection – great variation in potency (irritancy, percutaneous absorption, systemic toxicity)
Gloves- some protection. Sleeves
Barrier creams- questionable protection. Still matter for debate
Individual susceptibility
Skin care program, cleansing, moisturisers etc.
Legislation, labelling, information, education

A common affected site is the hands and especially the back of the hands and the finger webs but any skin site contaminated by solvents can develop an irritant contact dermatitis. When the face is affected vapours are suspected as well as contamination by hands.

Scleroderma

There are some case reports on scleroderma related to exposure to various solvents (Yamakage and Ishikawa 1982, Walder 1983, Bottomley et al 1993, Czirják et al 1994).

Dermatoses from Higher Boiling Petroleum Distillates

Petroleum distillates obtained at temperatures above 315 °C are mainly oils (lubricating, spindle, transformer, machine and cutting oils) and have less defatting but more keratogenic action. They can cause comedones, acne, photosensitivity, melanosis, keratoses and epitheliomas.

Chemical Burns

Extensive and prolonged skin exposure to solvents – especially under occlusion – may cause severe skin damage including blisters, bullae, oozing or necrosis. Solvent-soaked clothing in direct and prolonged contact with skin is an often-mentioned cause of these burns.

Solvents that have been implicated are according to the literature: tetrachloroethane, trichloroethylene, methylene chloride, carbon disulphide, Stoddard solvent, gasoline, kerosene, benzene, toluene but probably many more have this potential if the exposure conditions are unfavourable for the worker (concentration, duration, occlusion).

Perchloroethylene used in dry cleaning may to some extent remain in clothing and cause skin irritation especially on legs, wrists and neck. It has been suspected that this residue may cause or contribute to chemical burns.

Allergic Contact Dermatitis

Solvents as Contact Allergens

There are rather few case reports on allergic contact dermatitis to solvents, considering their extensive use and the size of the exposed population. This may partly be due to the inherent problems encountered when patch testing with solvents (see below) but also to ignorance or lack of suspicion by the examining physician and partly to the solvents relative chemical inertness. Examples are turpentine (Hellerström et al 1955, 1957, Rudzki et al 1991), D-limonene (Karlberg et al 1991, Karlberg and Dooms-Goossens 1997), and alcohols (Ophaswongse and Maibach 1994).

Patch Testing with Solvents – Feasibility

The irritant properties and volatility of some solvents make patch testing highly problematic and since they are potent skin irritants even after short exposure times (Table 2) it is thus probably impossible to demonstrate allergenicity by the conventional patch test technique.

Information regarding test concentrations and vehicles are rarely available – for the examining dermatologist the testing is a question of trial and error. If a "positive" reaction is obtained it is crucial to carry out serial dilution tests and to test a sufficient number of controls (>25).

Percutaneous Absorption – Systemic Toxicity

As a consequence of observed risks for systemic toxicity, carcinogenicity, etc. from inhalation of solvents a gradual decrease in TLVs has taken place and, therefore, the percutaneous route of uptake has become more prominent. Skin absorption from exposure to solvent vapours is negligible for most common solvents. However, those that contain a lipophilic and a hydrophilic part (glycol ethers and DMF) are readily absorbed and skin exposure to solvent vapours may contribute to the total uptake. Glycol ethers have low volatility and high boiling points compared with other organic solvents.

2-Chloroethanol, 2-butoxyethanol, carbon tetrachloride, 1,1,2-trichloroethane, dimethylformamide and dimethylsulfoxide gave rise to mortality in guinea pigs exposed percutaneously (Wahlberg and Boman 1979). Fatalities in man has also been reported.

An important aspect is thus that percutaneous absorption contributes to the total body burden and there are strong motives to reduce skin exposure as well as airway exposure of solvents.

In the national occupational hygiene standards, several of the industrial solvents have notations for skin absorption. In the recent Swedish standard (The Swedish Work Environment Authority 2000) the solvents given this notation are marked with "H" ("hud", Swedish for "skin") indicating that they are readily absorbed through the skin.

A defective skin barrier is considered to facilitate percutaneous penetration. However, in an experimental study in guinea pigs (Boman and Wahlberg 1989), it was demonstrated this was not uniformly so but that the lipophilic and hydrophilic properties of a particular solvent also influenced the absorption over injured skin.

Penetration Enhancing Action

Several solvents have an absorption promoting effect: glycol ethers, aprotic solvents such as DMF, DMSO, and DMAA. Alcohols and propylene glycol are used in many topical medicaments and are supposed to have several functions, including facilitating penetration of other ingredients.

Prevention

The preventive measures are summarized in Table 5.

Reduced Exposure

Reduced exposure is of great importance due to the considerable systemic toxicity of some solvents. As a result of increasing awareness of their adverse effects, also skin exposure will also hopefully be reduced due, inter alia, to automation, enclosed manufacturing systems and avoidance of direct contact.

Appropriate Selection

Quantitative data on skin irritant properties (Table 2), percutaneous absorption and systemic toxicity must be balanced against the technical requirements on a solvent. It is self-evident that those with the most favourable toxicity profile should be chosen.

Protective Gloves

Gloves, if selected according to recommendations, may provide a protection which allows for direct contact with solvents for several hours. The basis for these recommendations is data gathered in technical testing or in vitro studies (Mellström et al 1994, Mellström and Boman 1998; see also Chap. 22, this book, by Mellström and Boman). The varying efficacy of gloves and barrier creams and the importance of using proper skin protection when working with a solvent with low vapour pressure and high skin absorption conditions was clearly demonstrated for dimethyl formamide (DMF). A glycerol-based barrier cream was clearly demonstrated to be less protective than gloves (Lauwerys et al 1980).

Barrier Creams

Barrier creams are generally considered to be less protective than gloves to reduce penetration of solvents. In a human study using bioengineering techniques to assess skin reactions it was found that the barrier creams studied did not affect the irritant properties of toluene (Frosch and Kurte 1994). General aspects of barrier creams were recently reviewed (Lachapelle 1996, Berndt et al. 2000; see also Wigger-Alberti and Elsner 2000).

Skin Care Program

The use of moisturisers is crucial in all professions in which workers are exposed to irritants, including solvents. According to some recent findings, moisturisers seem to be more efficacious than barrier creams in preventing the irritation and appearance irritant contact dermatitis. Personal hygiene, proper agents for cleansing, soft towels, etc. are general recommendations applicable to every work place in which exposure to irritants occurs. Solvents should not be used for skin cleansing! However, if this is the only way to remove dirt, paint, oil, adhesives the use of moisturisers afterwards is necessary.

Legislation, Labelling, Information, Education

Legislation, labelling, information and education are applicable to all kind of exposures to chemicals and products at the workplace. Threshold limit values (TLVs) and notations on skin absorption are basic knowledge supplemented with information on the irritant properties of solvents on skin exposure (Tables 2, 3).

References

Bauer M, Rabens S (1974) Cutaneous Manifestations of Trichloroethylene toxicity. Arch Dermatol 110:886–890

Berndt U, Wigger-Alberti W, Gabard B, Elsner P (2000) Efficacy of a barrier cream and its vehicle as protective measures against occupational irritant contact dermatitis. Contact Dermatitis 42:77–80

Boman A, Wahlberg JE (1989) Percutaneous absorption of 3 organic solvents in the guinea pig. I. Effect of physical and chemical injuries to the skin. Contact Dermatitis 21:36–45

Bottomley WW, Sheehan-Dare RA, Hughes P, Cunliffe WJ (1993) A sclerodermatous syndrome with unusual features following prolonged occupational exposure to organic solvents. Br J Dermatol 128:203–206

Czirják L, Pócs E, Szegedi G (1994) Localized scleroderma after exposure to organic solvents. Dermatology 189:399–401

Fisher A (1978) Immediate and delayed allergic contact reactions to polyethylene glycol. Contact Dermatitis 4:135–138

Frosch PJ, Kurte A (1994) Efficacy of skin barrier creams. The repetitive irritations test (RIT) with a set of 4 standard irritants. Contact Dermatitis 31:161–168

Goldsmith LB, Friberg SE, Wahlberg JE (1988) The effect of solvent extraction on the lipids of the stratum corneum in relation to observed immediate whitening of the skin. Contact Dermatitis 19:348–350

Goodfield MJD, Saihan EM (1988). Contact urticaria to naphtha present in a solvent. Contact Dermatitis 18:187

Halkier-Sørensen L (1996) Occupational skin diseases. Contact Dermatitis 35, suppl. 1:11

Hellerström S, Thyresson N, Blohm S-G, et al (1955) On the nature of the eczematogenic component of oxidized D3-carene. J Invest Dermatol 24:217

Hellerström S, Thyresson N, Widmark G (1957) Chemical aspects on turpentine eczema. Dermatologica 115:277

Karlberg A-T, Boman A, Melin B (1991) Animal experiments on the allergenicity of d-limonene – the citrus solvent. Ann Occup Hyg 35:419–426

Karlberg A-T, Dooms-Goossens A (1997) Contact allergy to oxidized d-limonene among dermatitis patients. Contact Dermatitis 36:201–206

Klauder JV, Brill F A (1947) Correlation of boiling ranges of some petroleum solvents with irritant action on skin. Arch Dermatol 56:197–215

Kronevi T, Wahlberg JE, Holmberg B (1977) Morphological lesions in guinea pigs during skin exposure to 1,1,2-trichloroethane. Acta Pharmacol Toxicol 41:298–305

Kronevi T, Wahlberg JE, Holmberg B (1979) Histopathology of skin, liver, and kidney after epicutaneous administration of five industrial solvents to guinea pigs. Environ Res 19:56–69

Kronevi T, Wahlberg JE, Holmberg B (1981) Skin pathology following epicutaneous exposure to seven organic solvents. Int J Tissue Reac 3:21–30

Lachapelle J-M (1996) Efficacy of protective creams and/or gels. Curr Probl Derm (25):182–192

Lauwerys RR, Kivits A, Lhoir M, Rigolet P, Houbeau D, Buchet J-P, Roels H (1980) Biological surveillance of workers exposed to dimethylformamide and the influence of skin protection on its percutaneous absorption. Int Arch Occup Environ Health 45:189–203

Mellström G, Wahlberg JE, Maibach HI (1994) Protective gloves for occupational use. CRC, Boca Raton

Nakayama H, Kobayashi M, Takahashi M, Ageishi Y, Takano T (1988) Generalized eruption with severe liver dysfunction associated with occupational exposure to trichloroethylene. Contact Dermatitis 19:48–51

Ophaswongse S, Maibach HI (1994) Alcohol dermatitis:allergic contact dermatitis and contact urticaria syndrome. Contact Dermatitis 30:1–6

Phoon WH, Chan MO, Rajan VS, Tan KJ, Thirumoorthy T, Goh CL (1984) Stevens-Johnson syndrome associated with occupational exposure to trichloroethylene. Contact Dermatitis 10:270–276

Rilliet A, Hunziker N, Brun R (1980) Alcohol Contact Urticaria Syndrome (Immediate-type Hypersensitivity). Dermatologica 161:361–364

Rudzki E, Czernielewski A, Grzywa Z, Hegyi E, Jirasek J, Kalensky J, Michailov P, Nebenfuhrer L, Rothe A, Schubert H, Stransky L, Szarmach H, Temesvá ri E, Ziegler V, (1991) Contact allergy to oil of turpentine:a 10-year retrospective view. Contact Dermatitis 24:317–318

Stewart RD, Hake CL, Peterson JE (1974) "Degreasers' Flush" Dermal response to trichloroethylene and ethanol. Arch Environ Health 29:1–5

The Swedish Work Environment Authority (2000). Occupational exposure limit values. Statute book of the Swedish National Board of Occupational safety and Health. Ordinance 2000:3

Varigos GA, Nurse DS (1986) Contact urticaria from methyl ethyl ketone. Contact Dermatitis 15:259–260

Wahlberg JE, Boman A (1979) Comparative percutaneous toxicity of ten industrial solvents in the guinea pig. Scand J Work Environ Health 5:345–351

Wahlberg JE (1984a) Erythema-inducing effects of solvents following epicutaneous administration to man- Studied by laser Doppler flowmetry. Scand J Work Environ Health 10:159–162

Wahlberg JE (1984b) Edema-inducing effects of solvents following topical administration. Derm Beruf Umwelt 32:91–94

Wahlberg JE (1989) Assessment of erythema: a comparison between the naked eye and laser Doppler flowmetry. In: Frosch PJ, Dooms-Goossens A, Lachapelle J-M, Rycroft RJG, Scheper RJ (eds) Current topics in Contact Dermatitis. Springer, Berlin Heidelberg New York, pp 549–553

Wahlberg JE (1993) Measurement of skin-fold thickness in the guinea pig. Contact Dermatitis 28:141–145

Wahlberg JE, Boman A (1996) Prevention of contact dermatitis from solvents. Curr Probl Derm (25):57–66

Walder BK (1983) Do solvents cause scleroderma? Int J Derm 22:157–158

Wigger-Alberti W, Elsner P (2000) Barrier creams and emollients. In: Kanerva L, Elsner P, Wahlberg JE, Maibach HI (eds) Handbook of occupational dermatology. Springer, Berlin Heidelberg New York, pp 490–496
Yamakage A, Ishikawa H (1982) Generalized morphea-like scleroderma occurring in people exposed to organic solvents. Dermatologica 165:186–193

CHAPTER 38

Adhesives and Glues

38

J. Spoo, M. Gebhardt, P. Elsner

Introduction

Exposure to adhesives and glues is common in occupation, leisure time and household activities. Several types of glues and adhesives are in use, depending on the materials to be joined. Today almost any type of materials can be fixed to each other.

In the majority of glues, the action is simply due to removal of solvents, cooling or crystallization. In these cases, it is not the action of the macromolecular molecules but rather the preservatives, detergents and other additives added to the adhesive preparation that may cause dermatological problems, although this is rare. There is, however, a constantly growing second group of glues in which the adhesive is a polymerisation product formed by a complex chemical reaction between the macromolecules. This second group may cause many more irritant and allergic reactions on the skin (Malten 1984).

In this instance, two component systems are common that react only after being mixed. Other ways to start the reaction include heating, UV irradiation, oxygen and air exposure, pressure-induced rupture of catalyst reservoirs, etc. This chapter mainly focuses on this second group of adhesive chemicals and their occupational use.

Formaldehyde Resins

Phenol-formaldehyde resins resemble a group of chemicals that contain the formaldehyde structure, but are not necessarily associated with formaldehyde allergy. Among them, para-tertiary butylphenol formaldehyde resin (PTBP-FR) is a well-known allergen with particular use as neoprene-based leather glue. An Italian survey revealed PTBP-FR-containing neoprene adhesives to be the major allergens in a shoe factory (Manusco et al. 1996). Apart from PTBP-FR, mercaptobenzothiazole (MBT), two-component-polyurethane- and epoxy resin-based glues were also found in the same study as relevant glue allergens with special applications each in shoe manufacture. PTBP-FR-based glues have also been reported for their use in car manufacturing (Schubert and Agatha 1979). Non-occupational relevance is given in foot dermatitis elicited by shoes, in wrist dermatitis by watchstraps and in other leather articles (Freeman 1997). Nine of 839 Finnish patients patch tested with a glue series reacted to PTBP-FR, which turned out to be the most common relevant glue allergen (Tarvainen 1995).

PTBP is used in the production of PTBP-FR. Formerly, PTBP was added in excess, which might have caused concomitant reactions, whereas nowadays this is no longer relevant. Toxic exposure to PTBP-FR may cause chemical burns and even toxic leukoderma. Vitiligo-like leukoderma on the hands of PTBP-FR-exposed shoe-manufacturing workers has been found in the Italian study cited above. For patch-test purposes, PTBP-FR is available 1% in petrolatum from all well-known suppliers, either in a special plastic and glue or in the shoe series.

Urea-formaldehyde resin and melamine-formaldehyde resin are used as glues in the wood industries to make furniture press plates. Despite a low constant release of formaldehyde from these plates into the indoor air, the health effects for individuals living or working in the room is way overestimated in our opinion. Melamine-FR has also been reported as a relevant contact allergen for workers in the fibre industries (Finch et al. 1999; Isaksson et al. 1999). Both resins are currently available from Chemotechnique, Sweden, urea-FR as a 10% petrolatum and melamine-FR as a 70% preparation in the textile colour and finishes series.

If nail varnishes are considered to be adhesives, then toluene-sulfonamide-formaldehyde resin (TS-FR) should be included in this chapter. A very common ingredient of nail lacquers and hardeners, it may be an occupational allergen for cosmetologists, beauticians and, in a wider sense, those who use these products and who are in public service, such as bank clerks, office employees and salespersons. Among patients with cosmetic-related contact dermatitis, TS-FR was found to be relevant in 12.6% of the cases, second only to skin care products (De Groot et al. 1988). Typically, TS-FR allergy involves the eyelids, lateral aspects of the neck and, more seldom, the truly exposed periungual area. Because traces of the allergen are easily transferred to the eyelids, it has been included in the topical eye preparation series of several allergen providers. Almost all brands of nail polishes contain TS-FR (Hausen et al. 1995; Sainio et al. 1997). TS-FR has recently been included in most cosmetic patch-test trays. In addition to TS-FR, acrylates are gaining more and more importance in nail varnishes and lacquers. Chemotechnique provides a separate acrylic nail test series for this purpose.

Epoxy Resins

When used for industrial adhesive purposes, epoxy resins occur mostly in the construction industry, the assembly of cars, ships and aeroplanes, the manufacturing of sports equipment, as well as in the optical and electronic industries. The chemistry of epoxy resins and acrylates is similar. Both are (often) two-component systems. They are not sensitising when fully cured but frequently contain an amount of remaining monomer, which is enough to boost a pre-existing sensitisation. Both penetrate regular gloves, which makes skin protection a real problem, especially for sensitised people. Epoxy resins are usually based on bisphenol A and epichlorhydrin, a highly reactive epoxy group, which is responsible for the allergenicity of the compound.

Many different chemicals may be added to improve or adapt the material to the required condition. Hardeners of the amine or acid anhydride type are cross-linking agents for the resin. They are usually dissolved in organic solvents. Some of those additional chemicals, such as glycidyl ether, benzol and toluene, are skin irritants, which may enhance skin damage and thereby boost the induction or elicitation of an allergic reaction.

A patch testing series with plastic and glue allergens revealed 5.1% sensitisation to novolac epoxy resin and 3.2% allergic reactions to diglycidil ether of bisphenol A in 360 patients exposed to plastics for occupational reasons (Kanerva et al. 1999). Workers in the electronics, optical, paint and glue industries are most likely to acquire occupational allergy to epoxy resins (Richter 1974; Tosti et al 1993). A Dutch survey among employees of several companies that specialise in epoxy resin-related work in the construction industry revealed hand eczema in 23 of 135 persons. Of these, 61% of the eczema population and 12% of the healthy skin group had positive patch-test reactions. Almost all positive patch-test reactions were due to epoxy resin. This shows the tremendous relevance of epoxy resin as an occupational allergen (van Putten et al 1984). Epoxy resin coated fibreglass fibres have been reported as a cause of dermatitis in this particular field of industry (Holness and Nethercott 1989).

We recommend limiting patch tests with epoxy chemicals to the standardised test series because of the danger of active sensitisation. Once proven, epoxy resins should not be re-tested. When testing epoxy-exposed individuals, never forget to include chemical additives such as the broad range of hardeners.

Acrylates

Apart from their use in plastics, colours, lacquers, coatings, dental materials, orthopaedic appliances etc., acrylates are now increasingly used in adhesives (Kanerva and Manko 1999; Table 1) because of their excellent properties, such as strong adhesion – even to metals, ceramics, glass and other building materials – fast curing and easy handling. Stickers, tapes and office material may also be based on acrylic adhesives. The most common allergenic ingredient of such tapes is 2-ethylhexyl acrylate. Occupational problems can arise from workplaces where stickers and labels are put on the final products or, theoretically, in medicine. However, compared with epoxy and colophony rosin, which have been preferred

Table 1. Adhesives based on acrylates, methacrylates and epoxy diacrylates according to Kanerva and Manko (1999)

Anaerobic sealants
Cyanoacrylates
Ultraviolet-cured sealants
Methyl methacrylate
Metal and glass glues
Epoxy diacrylates (vinyl resins)
Acrylic dental bonding agents

in the past, acrylate-based tape adhesives are less sensitising and reports are based on single cases. There are one- and two-component acrylic adhesive systems. Other macromolecular substances can be included into acrylates, such as epoxy resins, to form epoxy acrylates.

Hazardous health effects on the skin are allergic sensitisations and irritation to several acrylates. Glue-induced adherence of contaminated skin (finger, eyelids) may be very difficult to separate. If possible, wait for spontaneous resolution; gentle teasing with repeated moistening of the skin is best in this otherwise harmless condition. Asthma and rhinitis have also been reported when handling acrylics (Savonius et al. 1993; Kopferschmidt-Kubler et al. 1996).

As known from other fields of (meth)acrylate use (dental prostheses, daily plastic wear), allergy can only be initiated and elicited by uncured monomers. In contrast to plastic wear, monomers are always available when using glues, so the rate of sensitisation could be rather high and similar to that of momomeric acrylate use in other occupational fields. A 0.22% rate of occupational contact allergy to (meth)acrylates among a population of 13,833 patients suspected of contact dermatitis between 1978 and 1999 was reported by Geukens and Goosens (2001). Among dental personnel, a high-risk group for occupational dermatitis to (meth)acrylates, the prevalence of contact allergy was reported to be 3% (Ohlson et al 2001) and has been increasing (Kanerva et al. 2000).

In occupational medicine, acrylates are important sensitisers to keep in mind. Sometimes it may be hard to find suitable personal protective equipment for sensitised people because most acrylates do penetrate gloves easily.

Cyanoacrylates are among the most common ingredients of acrylate glues (Loctite is a well-known brand example). Eyelid eczema, nummular eczema on the hands and periungual dermatitis are typical features of allergic contact dermatitis caused by cyanoacrylate glue used to fix artificial nails. Aluminium test chambers should be avoided when testing cyanoacrylates, because they may contain catalysts for the polymerisation process. The vehicle acetone further enhances the tendency to polymerise spontaneously (Bruze et al. 1995). Due to their excellent adhesive properties with various materials, cyanoacrylate glues may occur in many different occupations.

For patch-test purposes, a test screening with several acrylates should therefore be carried out when suspecting acrylate allergy. Chemotechnique has the most diverse patch-test tray on methacrylates; however, other companies also provide a suitable screening composition. Accelerators, inhibitors and catalysts, which may be added to the acrylates, can also sensitise. We recommend reading the chapters that deal with that problem.

Colophony

Colophony rosin, a naturally occurring rosin from trees, is another natural base of glues and adhesives. Abietic acid, also available as a test allergen, and its oxidative derivatives are the causative allergens (Guin et al. 1995). It ranks high on hit lists of contact allergens because of widespread exposure from occupational use in wood, paper, paint, electronics and cosmetics industries to household contacts and to natural exposure (Sadhra et al. 1994). Some tackifiers for heel and toe stiffeners in shoes are based on colophony and may therefore be relevant allergens in shoe manufacturers (Freeman 1997).

Medical use of rosin derivatives on tapes, bandages, surgical and dental dressings, wart paints (Lachapelle and Leroy 1990) and hydrocolloid dressings has been reported (Sasseville et al. 1997). Most patients with a sensitisation to colophony report intolerance of brown coloured tapes. Occupational sensitisation to colophony seems to be a rare condition, but has been reported for dental personnel (Kanerva and Estlander 1999; Cockayne et al. 2001).

For patch testing, a routine analysis of rosin preparations is recommended since oxidation by air and light has been proved to increase the allergenicity of raw colophony rosin due to an increase in concentration of oxidised resins (Sadhra et al. 1998).

Others

A very special kind of biological adhesives are the so-called fibrin tissue glues. They are two-component systems consisting of fibrinogen and factor XIII in one syringe and thrombin in the second syringe. By adding thrombin to the fibrinogen/factor-XIII mixture, there is a coagulation reaction. Tissue adhesives are used to re-combine skin and organ cuts (liver, spleen, etc.), to seal wounds in surgically opened body cavities or vascular prostheses and to stop bleeding. We are not aware of any report of either occupational contact dermatitis or immediate-type contact reactions to this product because skin contact to the medical person is usually prevented by gloves worn for hygienic reasons.

Patch Testing with Adhesives and Glues

The most important part of allergological diagnosis is to think about possible exposure to glues and adhesives. Optimally, one should only consider patch tests with possible allergenic glue ingredients when the chemical composition of the glue or adhesive is known. This can be determined by asking the manufacturer or, to a lesser extent, by looking at the material data safety sheets. In daily practice, however, this very often fails. Therefore, a glue-screening series makes good practical sense. For detailed information on available glue contact allergens, plastic allergens, accelerators, inhibitors and UV adsorbers, we refer to this chapter in the extended version of this book.

Under special circumstances we also recommend testing the glue itself. When the complete composition is known and the single allergenic ingredients are available, testing the native glue is avoidable. We warn against testing unknown epoxy resin based glues because of possible active sensitisation. Active sensitisation is also well known for acrylics and has been reported even after one single exposure. However, by leaving the glue exposed to air and letting it dry on the patch-test chamber, the risk of strong patch-test reactions is minimised.

The easiest way to patch test a patient's own products is using tapes and medical self-adhesive dressings. Simply cut a small piece and stick it to the skin for 24–48 h. For further information, refer to the other chapters in this book that deal with acrylates and epoxy resins.

References

Bruze M, Björkner B, I.epoittevin JP (1995) Occupational allergic contact dermatitis from ethyl cyanoacrylate. Contact Dermatitis 32:156–159

Cockayne SE, Murphy R, Gawkrodger DJ (2001) Occupational contact dermatitis from colophonium in a dental technician

De Groot AC, Bruynzeel DP, Bos JD, et al (1988) The allergens in cosmetics. Arch Dermatol 124:1525–1529

Freeman S (1997) Shoe dermatitis. Contact Dermatitis 36:247–251

Finch TM, Prais L, Foulds IS (1999) Allergic contact dermatitis from medium-density fibreboard containing melamine-formaldehyde resin

Geukens S, Goosens A (2001) Occupational contact allergy to (meth)acrylates. Contact Dermatitis 44:153–159

Guin JD (1995) Colophony (rosin) In: Guin JD (ed) Practical contact dermatitis. McGraw-Hill, New York, pp 115–124

Hausen BM, Milbrodt M, König WA (1995) The allergens of nail polish. Contact Dermatitis 33:157–164

Holness DL, Nethercott JR (1989) Occupational contact dermatitis due to epoxy resin in a fiberglass binder. J Occup Med 31:87–89

Isaksson M, Zimerson E, Bruze M (1999) Occupational dermatoses in composite production. J Occup Med 41:261–266

Kanerva L, Jolanki R, Alanko K, Estlander T (1999) Patch-test reactions to plastic and glue allergens. Acta Derm Venereol 79:296–300

Kanerva L, Alanko K, Estlander T, et al (2000) Statistics on occupational contact dermatitis from (meth)acrylates in dental personnel. Contact Dermatitis 42:175–176

Kanerva L, Estlander T (1999) Occupational allergic contact dermatitis from colophony in 2 dental nurses

Kopferschmidt-Kubler MC, Stenger R, Blaumeiser M, et al (1996) Rev Mal Respir 13:305–307

Lachapelle JM, Leroy B (1990) Allergic contact dermatitis to colophony included in the formulation of flexible collodion BP, the vehicle of a salicylic and lactic acid wart paint. Dermatol Clin 8:143–146

Malten KE (1984) Dermatological problems with synthetic resins and plastics in glues, part I. Dermatosen 32:81–86

Manusco G, Reggiani M, Berdondini RM (1996) Occupational dermatitis in shoemakers. Contact Dermatitis 34:17–22

Ohlson CG, Svensson L, Mossberg B, Hok M (2001) Prevalence of contact dermatitis among dental personnel in a Swedish rural county. Swed Dent J 25:13–20

Richter G (1974) Zur Epidemiologie des Epoxidharzekzems. Derm Monatsschr 160:785–789

Sadhra S, Foulds IS, Gray CN, Koh D, Gardiner K (1994) Colophony: uses, health effects, airborne measurement and analysis. Ann Occup Hyg 38:385–396

Sadhra S, Foulds IS, Gray CN (1998) Oxidation of resin acids in colophony (rosin) and its implications for patch testing. Contact Dermatitis 39:58–63

Sainio E-L, Engström K, Henriks-Eckerman M-L, Kanerva L (1997) Allergenic ingredients in nail polishes. Contact Dermatitis 37:155–162

Sasseville D, Tennstedt D, Lachspelle JM (1997) Allergic contact dermatitis from hydrocolloid dressings. Am J Contact Dermat 8:236–238

Savonius B, Keskinen H, Tuppurainen M, Kanerva L (1993) Occupational respiratory disease caused by acrylics. Clin Exp Allergy 23:416–424
Schubert H, Agatha G (1979) Zur Allergennatur der para-tert. Butylphenolformaldehydharze. Dermatosen 27:49–52
Tarvainen K (1995) Analysis of patients with allergic patch test reactions to a plastics and glue series. Contact Dermatitis 32:346–351
Tosti A, Guerra L, Vincenzi C, Peluso AM (1993) Occupational skin hazards from synthetic plastics. Toxicol Ind Health 9:493–502
van Putten PB, Coenraads PJ, Nater J (1984) Hand dermatoses and contact allergic reactions in construction workers exposed to epoxy resins. Contact Dermatitis 10:146–150

CHAPTER 39

Rubber Chemicals 39

D. V. BELSITO

Introduction

Rubber-based products permeate our lives, forming part of the many materials used for personal, domestic and industrial purposes. Rubber may be natural, synthetic or a mixture of the two. Since the vast majority of rubberized materials are unlabeled, it is difficult to determine whether a product contains natural or synthetic rubber. The overlap between "rubber" and "plastic" further complicates the matter, since plastics contain many of the same catalysts, stabilizers, antioxidants and pigments/dyes present in rubber products. Fregert (1981) listed a number of naphthylamines, substituted para-phenylenediamines, alkylphenols, and hydroquinone derivatives that are utilized in manufacturing both rubber and plastic. Although completely cured plastics rarely sensitize, fully cured rubber products produce allergic reactions because the allergens in rubber can leach out or "bloom" over time.

Natural rubber is based on the polymer 1,4-polyisoprene, a substance extracted from several plant sources, especially *Hevea brasiliensis*. A variety of synthetic rubbers exists, each based on different polymers (Table 1). Although as a percentage of all rubber goods, those made of natural rubber are declining, the absolute use of natural rubber continues to increase due to the expanding use of rubber worldwide. About 60% of all natural and synthetic rubber production is utilized in the tire industry. The remaining 40% is processed into thousands of different products. The widespread use of rubber has been facilitated by the development of new rubber polymers with varying properties of industrial value (Table 1).

Rubber Related Chemicals

Natural Rubber

Natural rubber is based on *isoprene* monomers derived from various plants. The principal source is latex obtained from *Hevea brasiliensis*, which belongs to the Euphorbiaceae family. Other commercial sources of natural rubber include *Parthenium argentatum* (guayule rubber) and plants of the Sapotaceae family (gutta-percha). These plants produce a viscous substance that contains about 30%

Table 1. Commonly encountered synthetic rubbers[a]

Common Name	Polymer	Usage
Polyurethane (i.e., Spandex)	Isocyanates + polyesters	Elasticized clothing, shoes, sealants/caulkings, adhesives, industrial products resistant to abrasion
Neoprene	Chloroprene	Clothing/gloves, latex foams, industrial products
Nitrile	Acrylonitrile + butadiene	Shoes/gloves, waterproof clothing, adhesives, artificial leathers, industrial products designed to resist solvents and oils
Styrene-Butadiene	Styrene + butadiene	Widely used in industrial rubber products, especially tires
Butyl	Isobutylene + isoprene or butadiene	Gas impermeable products (inner tubes, hoses, electrical insulation, etc.)
Polysulfide (i.e., Thiokol)	Polysulfide + organic dichlorides	Sealants, adhesives, protective clothing and other oil-resistant materials
Ethylene-propylene-diene terpolymer	Ethylene-propylene-diene monomer (EPDM)	Automobile hoses, gaskets, belts and industrial rubber resistant to weathering
Silicon elastomer	Dimethyl siloxane	Gaskets, seals, hoses and insulating tapes designed to resist high temperature

[a] Abstracted from Rubber World Magazine's Blue Book (2001).

isoprenes; the remainder consists of water, proteins, resins, and sugars (Rogers 1974). The 1,4-polyisoprenes chemically occur in two different isomeric forms: the *cis* form is found in latex and guayule rubber; gutta percha and balata, which are less frequently used, contain the *trans* form (Adams 1983).

Delayed-type hypersensitivity reactions to natural latex were once considered rare. Sidi and Hincky (1954) suggested that latex may be a delayed-type allergen based on their study of patients with allergic reactions to latex gloves, but without evident allergy to the accelerators or anti-oxidants likely to be present in the gloves. Subsequently, Wilson (1960) had similar experiences in 2 of 42 patients, all of whom tested positive to gloves. Substantiated reports of isoprene allergy include those of Wyss et al. (1993) and Wilkinson and Beck (1996). In this latter study of 822 patients, 10 (1.2%) exhibited positive patch test reactions to latex. Despite the increasingly more frequent reports of allergic contact dermatitis (ACD) to natural latex, the exact chemical nature of the allergen(s) remains unknown. In contrast, proteins present in latex obtained from the *Hevea brasiliensis* tree are the cause of the IgE-mediated hypersensitivity/allergic contact urticaria (ACU) to natural latex rubber (Turjanmaa et al. 2000). Since *Hevea brasiliensis* accounts for >99% of natural rubber used worldwide, ACU to latex is a significant problem.

It is unknown whether the polyisoprene containing sap from *Parthenium* and *Sapotacea* spp. contains the chemical responsible for inducing ACU and/or ACD to latex. However, it has been reported that the sap from *Parthenium argentatum*, a member of the *Compositae* family, contains a cinnamic acid ester of sesquiterpene, which is a potent sensitizer for delayed-type hypersensitivity in the guinea pig (Rodriguez et al. 1981). Perhaps for this reason, guayule rubber has not become a significant source of rubber worldwide. Although the sap of *Sapotaceae* spp is apparently free of sensitizers, it is highly irritating (Mitchell and Rook 1979).

Artificial Rubber

Isoprene can now be synthesized from petroleum derivatives. Thus, multiple types of synthetic rubbers with specific properties can be manufactured (Table 1). Despite the proliferation of these synthetic rubbers, allergic reactions to the synthetic monomers/polymers are quite rare. To date, there have only been case reports of possible ACD to isocyanates present in shoes (Shackelford and Belsito 2002), to synthetic plastic/rubber wound dressings (Helland et al. 1983; Kilpikari and Halme 1983), and to polysulfides in sealants (Wilkinson and Beck 1993).

Vulcanization and Rubber Additives

The monomers of both artificial and natural rubber must be polymerized into a three-dimensional network to obtain the finished product. Different processes are used, although they are all quite similar. Polymerization (vulcanization) involves the reaction between rubber isomers and sulfur to produce a polymer with enhanced elasticity and reduced plasticity. The reaction between the monomers and sulfur is enhanced by the addition of accelerators and activators. Other chemicals that can be added to both natural and synthetic rubber include: retardants, antioxidants, curing agents, reinforcers, fillers, ultraviolet inhibitors, softeners/extenders, stabilizers, blowing agents and colorants. Readers are referred to Rubber World Magazine's "Blue Book" (2001), which extensively surveys the various additives to both natural and synthetic rubbers. Those additives of principal interest to occupational dermatologists include certain *accelerators* (viz., thiazoles, thiurams, thiocarbamates and thioureas) and *anti-oxidants* (viz., derivatives of *p*-phenylenediamine). In addition, natural rubber latex is of increasing importance. In contrast, allergic reactions to the other components of rubber, except for reactions to the phenol formaldehyde resins (used as tackifiers/reinforcing agents) and epoxy resins (used as stabilizers) are rare (Condé-Salazar et al. 1993) (Table 2).

Accelerators

Vulcanization of rubber consists of heating the molecules of polyisoprene so that they polymerize into a product that maintains its elasticity over a range of temperatures. Chemical accelerators are added to speed vulcanization at lower temperatures. The original accelerators were metallic oxides. In the 1920s, 2-mercaptobenzothiazole (2-MBT) was introduced and revolutionized the process. Subse-

Table 2. Vulcanization materials and other rubber additives[a]

Auxiliary and surface materials
Adhesives and bonding/sealing agents
Blowing agents and blow promoters
Dusting, dipping and washing materials
Finishes
Lubricants
Odorants and anti-staining agents
Polymerization materials
Reclaiming materials
Solvents
Extenders, fillers and reinforcers
Carbon blacks
Other black materials
Non-black materials
Fiber reinforced materials
Processing materials
Homogenizing agents
Peptizers
Plasticizers and softeners
Processing aids and dispersing agents
Tackifiers
Protective materials
Anti-oxidants, anti-ozonants and inhibitors
Chemical and heat stabilizers
Vulcanization materials
Accelerators
Activators
Retarders
Vulcanizers

[a] Data abstracted from Rubber World Magazine's Blue Book (2001).

quently, numerous other accelerators have been identified including thiurams, thiazoles, dithiocarbamates, guanadines, thioureas and amine aldehydes (Table 3). While some synthetic rubbers (e.g., butyl and nitrile) can be polymerized with organic peroxides without the addition of sulfur, others (e.g., styrene-butadiene) require much greater amounts of sulfur-donors (viz., 2-MBT and thiuram) than natural rubber (Feinman 1987).

The principal *thiurams* used industrially are: tetramethylthiuram monosulfide (TMTM), tetramethylthiuram disulfide (TMTD), tetraethylthiuram disulfide (TETD), and dipentamethylenethiuram disulfide (PTD). Thiurams are among the more frequently used rubber accelerators, especially in the manufacturing of gloves. Numerous other consumer products also contain thiurams (Table 4).

Thiazoles are derivatives of benzothiazole compounded with sulfenamides. The benzothiazoles include 2-mercaptobenzothiazole (MBT), dibenzothiazyl disulfide (MBTS) and the zinc salt of 2-mercaptobenzothiazole (ZMBT). The sulfenamides are principally *N*-tert-butyl-2-benzothiazyl sulfenamide (TBBS), *N*-cyclohexyl-2-benzothiazyl sulfenamide (CBS) and morpholinylmercaptobenzothiazole (MOR). Because of their greater capacity to sensitize, thiazoles are less frequently used in

Table 3. Accelerators in natural and synthetic rubbers likely to cause allergic contact dermatitis[a]

Chemical Class	Allergen(s) Present in Standard Patch Test Series
Thiazoles	2-Mercaptobenzothiazole
	Mercapto mix
	N-Cyclohexyl-2-benzothiazyl sulfenamide
	2,2′-Dibenzothiazyl disulfide
	Morpholinylmercaptobenzothiazole
Thiurams	Thiuram mix
	Tetramethylthiuram disulfide
	Tetramethylthiuram monosulfide
	Tetraethylthiuram disulfide
	Dipentamethylenethiuram disulfide
Dithiocarbamates	Carba mix
	Zinc diethyldithiocarbamate
	Zinc dibutyldithiocarbamate
Guanadines	Carba mix
	1,3-Diphenylguanadine
Thioureas	No
Amine aldehydes	No

[a] For a more complete listing of the many available accelerators, see Rubber World Magazine's Blue Book (2001).

Table 4. Thiurams: potential exposures

Adhesives
Animal repellents
Crepe soles (neoprene)
Disinfectants
Food wrappings
Fungicides
Germicides
Insecticides
Medications (anti-alcohol, scabicide, fungicides, sunscreens, surgical wraps)
Pesticides
Polyolefin plastics (anti-oxidant)
Preservatives (woods, paints, lubricating oils, greases, etc.)
Putty
Rubber products, especially gloves
Veterinary soaps and shampoos

gloves than are thiurams. However, MBT remains the commonest accelerator for industrial rubber (Feinman 1987). Thiazoles are also widely used in other industries (Table 5). Sensitization to thiazoles among consumers is less frequent than it is to thiurams. Most consumers sensitized to thiazoles are exposed to the chemical in shoes (Shackelford and Belsito 2002).

The *dithiocarbamates* include zinc dibutyldithiocarbamate (ZDBC), zinc diethyldithiocarbamate (ZDEC) and zinc dimethyldithiocarbamate (ZDMC). In

Table 5. Thiazoles: potential exposures

Adhesives (neoprene-based)
Anti-freeze
Caustic cleansers (automotive cooling systems)
Cutting oils/Greases
Detergents (granulated and tablets)
Fungicides
Germicides
Paints
Photographic film emulsion
Refrigerants
Rubber products, especially tires or other industrial rubber items and boots/shoes
Veterinarian medicaments
Waterproof cements/glues

Table 6. Carbamates: potential exposures

Anti-oxidants
Fungicides
Pesticides
Rubber products

Table 7. Thioureas: potential exposures

Adhesives
Anti-corrosives
Anti-oxidants
Cleaning products
Detergents (acidic)
Diazo paper
Fungicides
Impermeable rubbers
Neoprene and foam rubbers
Paint/glue remover
Photocopy paper
Textile elastic

the rubber industry, the carbamates are principally used in gloves, condoms and elastic bands. In a recent study of single use medical gloves, ZDEC and ZDBC, along with ZMBT, were among the most frequent accelerators found by chemical analysis (Knudsen et al. 2000). Due to their chemical similarity with thiurams, the potential for cross-reactivity between these groups exists (Condé-Salazar 1990a; Knudsen and Menné 1996). The greatest use of carbamates is not in rubber but in pesticides and fungicides (Table 6).

Thioureas include dibutylthiourea (DBTU), diethylthiourea (DETU), diphenylthiourea (DPTU) and ethylenethiourea (ETU). These chemicals are frequently used, especially in the manufacture of neoprene and foam rubbers. In addition to being accelerators, thioureas have other uses as anti-corrosives and anti-oxidants (Table 7). Important sources of sensitization to thioureas have been the foam and impermeable rubbers used in sporting equipment (sport shoes, diving masks, swimming goggles, wet suits, etc.).

Anti-Oxidants

Although the various rubber accelerators account for the vast majority of allergic reactions to rubber among consumers, anti-oxidants are by no means rare causes of sensitivity, especially occupationally acquired (Feinman 1987). Also referred to as anti-degradants or anti-ozonants, anti-oxidants retard the deterioration of rubber by ozone. The most common anti-oxidants are derivatives of amines (alkylamines and quinolines), phenols (hydroquinones), and phosphites (Table 8). The most important from the aspect of sensitization are the following phenylenediamine derivatives: N'-isopropyl-N'-phenyl-p-phenylenediamine (IPPD), N-phenyl-N'-cyclohexyl-p-phenylenediamine (CPPD), N,N'-diphenyl-p-phenylenediamine (DPPD), and N-(1,3-dimethylbutyl)-N'-phenyl-p-phenylenediamine (DMPPD). Of these, CPPD and DPPD are more strongly sensitizing than IPPD (Hervé-Bazin et al. 1977). These phenylenediamine derivatives are found principally in industrial rubbers (Table 9) and in almost any rubber of black color. Their capacity to sensitize is very high and they easily bloom from the surface of rubber with heat or friction. Another highly sensitizing anti-oxidant, monobenzyl ether of hydroqui-

Table 8. Anti-oxidants in natural and synthetic rubber causing ACD

Chemical Class	Allergen(s) Present in Standard Patch Test Series
Amines	
Phenylenediamines	Black rubber mix:
	N-phenyl-N'-cyclohexyl-p-phenylenediamine
	N-isopropyl-N'-phenyl-p-phenylenediamine
	N,N'-diphenyl-p-phenylenediamine
Quinolines	No
Phenols	
Hydroquinones	No
BHT	No
Phosphites	No

Table 9. Amine anti-oxidants: potential exposures

Acrylates
Black rubbers
Cutting oils/fluids
Gasoline (inhibitor/antiozonant)
Industrial and automotive rubbers
Orthopedic bandages
Rubber cements

none, also causes contact leukoderma (Oliver et al. 1939) and is now rarely used in the manufacture of rubber (Feinman 1987). Other anti-oxidants such as the hydroquinones (Norris and Storrs 1990), styrenated phenol (Kaniwa et al. 1994a), dialkylamines (Kaniwa et al. 1994b), piperidines (Kaniwa et al. 1994b), dihydroquinolines (Hansson 1994), butylhydroxyanisole (Rich et al. 1991) and 4,4'-thiobis(6-tert-butyl-m-cresol) (Rich et al. 1991) have a much reduced capacity to sensitize. Although the naphthylamines also appear to have low rates of sensitization, they are rarely used in consumer goods because they may contain trace amounts of the carcinogen β-naphthylamine (Feinman 1987).

Incidence

The incidence of ACD to rubber in the general population is difficult to evaluate. Due to genetic variations, differing exposure patterns, and other demographic factors, the incidence of allergic reactions to the various chemicals within rubber will vary among countries. Of 274 non-dermatologic patients undergoing arthroplasty in Sweden, 1.1% had allergic reactions to thiuram mix and carba mix (both accelerators), and 0.4% had reactions to black rubber mix (anti-oxidant) and mercapto mix (accelerator) upon routine patch testing (Magnusson and Möller 1979). Since these patients were randomly selected as opposed to those referred for patch testing, the incidence rates of allergic reactions to rubber additives in this study are more representative of those in the Swedish population.

Because of automation and other preventive measures, cases of sensitization to rubber among workers manufacturing it are rare and account for no more than 20% of all rubber allergy (Fregert 1975; Toeppen-Sprigg, 1999). Individuals most likely to be sensitized are those exposed to rubber in other industries. The release or "blooming" of allergens from rubber is particularly likely with direct skin contact since sweat and humidity are liberating factors.

Most available data on incidence rates are generated from patients referred for evaluation of suspected contact dermatitis; thus, these rates, as they pertain to the general population, are overstated. In studies of the North American Contact Dermatitis Group (Rudner et al. 1975; Storrs et al. 1989; Nethercott et al. 1991; Marks et al. 1995; Marks et al. 1998; Marks et al. 2000), a significant percentage of North American patients referred for patch testing had allergic reactions to one or more rubber additives tested. Of note, the percentage of patients reacting to the thiazoles has been relatively constant over time. In contrast, the percentage reacting to p-phenylenediamine derivatives and thiurams seems to be increasing. An increase in the rate of ACD to rubber chemicals, especially thiurams, has been reported worldwide (Nurse 1979; Themido and Brandão 1984; Lammintausta and Kalimo 1985; Estlander et al. 1986; Gibbon et al. 2001). Condé-Salazar et al. (1993) noted that reactions to thiuram mix accounted for the majority of rubber allergies (83%), followed by carba mix (22.3%), black rubber mix (17.8%), mercapto mix (16.0%) and naphthyl mix (2.4%). It has been suggested that reactivity rates for black rubber mix are indicative of the rate of sensitization from industrial exposure, while those for thiuram are indicative of the rate of sensitization from non-industrial exposures, especially gloves (Cronin 1980).

In studies performed outside the rubber/tire industry, the principal source of exposure to rubber-related chemicals is gloves: in a Finnish study, gloves accounted for 58.3% of rubber-related eczema (Estlander et al. 1986). Similar results were seen in Germany where, out of 3,851 patients, allergic reactions to rubber additives were seen in 145 individuals; in 80/145 (55%), the source of exposure was occupational (von Hintzenstern et al. 1991). Of the occupational cases, 84% of workers acquired the dermatitis from use of rubber gloves. Those workers most likely to develop glove dermatitis were those engaged in health/laboratory services or homemaking activities (von Hintzenstern et al. 1991). However, non-occupational exposure to items such as condoms, shoes, boots, elasticized garments, belts and watchbands are also important sources for the development of ACD to rubber (Wilson 1960; Condé-Salazar 1990a; Condé-Salazar 1990b).

Construction workers represent another occupational group with a high incidence of rubber-related dermatoses (Ko et al. 2001). In their study of 408 construction workers, Condé-Salazar et al. (1995) found that 104 (25.4%) of the workers were sensitized to one or more of the rubber mixes on their standard screening series: Ninety-seven workers (23.7%) were allergic to thiuram mix, which ranked second to chromate as a cause of ACD in these workers. In all workers, the source of sensitization was either gloves and/or boots used for personal protection (Condé-Salazar et al. 1995).

Workers in the basic rubber industries are another obvious high-risk group for rubber-related dermatoses. The annual risk of allergic plus irritant dermatitis among these workers has historically ranged from 0.31% in Britain (Calnan 1978) to 0.56% in Finland (Kilpikari 1982). The apparently lower risk of developing ACD among workers in basic rubber industries relates in part to the reporting of risk as an annual rate rather than as the total percentage of workers with occupationally related dermatitis. In addition, increasing automation within the rubber industry minimizes direct chemical contact and reduces sensitization rates. An important difference between ACD in rubber workers and that among other workers is the high percentage of ACD due to amine anti-oxidants (e.g., *p*-phenylenediamine derivatives) in the former (Alfonzo 1979; Kilpikari 1982). 2-mercaptobenzothiazole and carbamates also have relatively high sensitization rates in this industry (Nethercott 1982; Vestey et al. 1986).

Skin Disease in Rubber Workers

Dermatitis among rubber plantation workers who harvest latex has been little studied. Occupational ACD occurs more frequently in the manufacturing of finished rubber goods, since the major delayed-type allergens are found among the chemicals subsequently added to natural and synthetic rubbers (Toeppen-Sprigg 1999). Although ACD is rare due to automation, workers who weigh the ingredients added to pre-cut chunks of natural or synthetic rubber in large mixers (Banbury mixers) and skilled laborers involved in the fabrication of tires are most likely to develop allergic sensitization. Other workers, such as those operating the Banbury mixers, the calenders (two or more steel drums used to produce sheets of rubber or to ply rubber to other materials), the extruders (devices which produce lengths of rubber with specific cross-sectional characteristics), and the molding machines, are also at some risk, as are those workers involved in packing and shipping the final product. Derivatives of *p*-phenylenediamine (PPD) are the main sensitizers among these workers (Alfonzo 1979; Cronin 1980; Kilpikari 1982; Ancona et al. 1982). Other causes of ACD in the rubber industry (Brandão, 1990; Kanerva et al. 1996) have included the plasticizers (dialkyl phthalates), the peptizers (tricresyl phosphate), the blowing agents (e.g., N,N'-pentamethylenetetramine and other amines) and the retarders (e.g., N-[cyclohexylthio] phthalimide).

Irritant dermatitides are common among rubber workers (Kilpikari 1982; Varigos and Dunt 1981; White 1988). The most common irritants are the alkalis, solvents, activators (e.g., stearic acid and other fatty acids), soaps, and dusting/dipping/washing materials (e.g., calcium carbonate, calcium stearate, etc.) encountered in the workplace. Mechanical friction is another important source of irritation. In an Australian tire factory, Varigos and Dunt (1981) noted that 3.7% of the 1,000 workers had dermatitis, of which 34% was irritant dermatitis.

Curious reactions can occasionally be seen among rubber workers. Plotnick and Birmingham (1993) reported an epidemic of pronounced facial flushing, typically appearing after lunch, among 10 of 20 Banbury mixers. Patch testing to an expanded rubber tray was completely negative. The cause was tetramethylthiuram disulfide used as the accelerator together with alcohol consumed at lunch. It was surmised that when sweat-tainted with alcohol contacted the airborne accelerator, a localized disulfiram-like reaction occurred.

The presence of *carcinogenic compounds* within the rubber industry has been a controversial issue in the field of occupational medicine (Condé-Salazar 1987; Condé-Salazar 1990a). Both 1,3-butadiene and styrene, which are used extensively in synthetic rubber, are known carcinogens (reviewed in Fishbein 1992). Significant levels of butadiene [0.06–39 ppm (NIOSH 1984; IARC 1986; de Meester 1988)] and styrene [2.4 ppm (WHO 1983)] can be found in factories where these synthetic rubbers are produced; however, due to automation and safety precautions, workers are not routinely exposed to significant levels (IARC 1979; Fajen et al. 1990). Other carcinogens in the rubber industry may be present in minimal concentrations as either contaminants of the raw materials or as newly formed compounds due to uncontrolled reactions during manufacturing; e.g., *n*-nitrosamines can be found in parts per billion (ppb) in some accelerators. Disulfiram, a thiuram, is controversial since, in experimental studies, it has been identified as a potentiator of carcinogenesis: rats exposed simultaneously to ethylene dibromide and to disulfiram in the diet had a 10-fold increase in hepatocellular carcinoma as compared to animals exposed only to ethylene dibromide (Plotnick 1978).

Occupational Skin Disease Outside the Rubber Industry

Allergic Contact Dermatitis (ACD)

In some workers outside the rubber industry, the sources of sensitization are the same raw ingredients to which workers in the rubber industry are exposed. For example, the carbamate-based pesticides among agricultural workers. However, for most workers, the sources of sensitization are the protective barriers (such as gloves, boots and masks) used to avoid other sensitizers and irritants. As a result, sensitization to components of rubber can not only be the direct cause of acute dermatitis, but can also aggravate an existing allergic or non-allergic eczema. When it coexists with another dermatitis, ACD to rubber can be difficult to diagnose and may be suspected only after patch testing (Duarte et al. 1998). The components of a typical patch-testing tray for detecting rubber allergies is detailed in Table 10. Other allergens such as the anti-oxidants monobenzyl ether of hydroquinone (1% in petrolatum) and piperazine (1% in petrolatum) can also be purchased commercially (Trolab, Hermal Kurt Herrmann, Reinbeck/Hamburg, Germany). PPD, present on most standard screening trays, is not an adequate screen

Table 10. Rubber additive series[a]

Allergen	Conc/veh[b]
Tetramethylthiuram disulfide (TMTD)	1.0% pet
Tetramethylthiuram monosulfide (TMTM)	1.0% pet
Tetraethylthiuram disulfide (TETD)	1.0% pet
Dipentamethylenethiuram disulfide (PTD)	1.0% pet
N-Cyclohexyl-N-phenyl-4-phenylenediamine (CPPD)	1.0% pet
N,N'-Diphenyl-4-phenylenediamine (DPPD)	1.0% pet
N-Isopropyl-N-phenyl-4-phenylenediamine (IPPD)	0.1% pet
2-Mercaptobenzothiazole (MBT)	2.0% pet
N-Cyclohexyl-2-benzothiazylsulfenamide (CBS)	1.0% pet
Dibenzothiazyl disulfide (MBTS)	1.0% pet
4-morpholinylmercaptobenzothiazole (MOR)	1.0% pet
Diphenylguanidine (DPG)	1.0% pet
Zinc diethyldithiocarbamate (ZDEC)	1.0% pet
Zinc dibutyldithiocarbamate (ZDBC)	1.0% pet
N,N'-Di-β-naphthyl-4-phenylenediamine	1.0% pet
N-Phenyl-2-naphthylamine (PBN)	1.0% pet
Hexamethylenetetramine	2.0% pet
Diaminodiphenylmethane	0.5% pet
Diphenylthiourea (DPTU)	1.0% pet
Zinc dimethyldithiocarbamate (ZDMC)	1.0% pet
2,2',4-Trimethyl-1,2-dihydroquinoline	1.0% pet
Diethylthiourea (DETU)	1.0% pet
Dibutylthiourea (DBTU)	1.0% pet
Dodecylmercaptan	0.1% pet
N-(Cyclohexylthio)-phthalimide	1.0% pet

[a] Available from Chemotechnique Diagnostics AB, Malmö, Sweden.
[b] *Conc* concentration; *veh* vehicle; *pet* petrolatum.

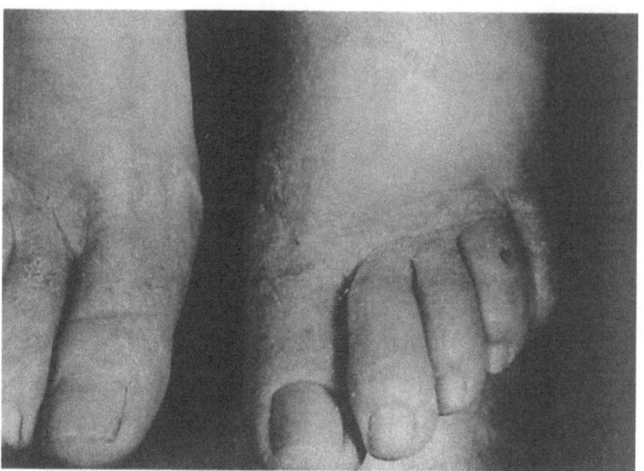

Fig 1. Subacute allergic contact dermatitis of the dorsal foot in an athletic director allergic to several thioureas and to 2-mercaptobenzothiazole. Although the manufacturer declined to verify the components of these shoes, patch tests to rubber portions of the "box" of the shoe were positive. Thioureas, which are frequently present in rubber manufactured for use in sporting equipment and clothes, were probably the more relevant allergens. (Reproduced with the permission of Donald V. Belsito, M.D., Division of Dermatology, University of Kansas Medical Center, Kansas City, KS)

for allergy to the "black rubber" anti-oxidants. In one study, all IPPD sensitive patients reacted to CPPD, but only 37% cross-reacted with PPD (Hervé-Bazin et al. 1977).

Although the amine anti-oxidants, especially IPPD, are strong sensitizers and cause acute, severe eczemas, the accelerators tend to provoke a more subacute to chronic appearing eczema (Fig. 1). In addition to an eczematous dermatitis, ACD to rubber can present as hyperkeratosis, purpura, achromia, urticaria or other, less frequently observed, clinical manifestations. The primary reason for such differing forms of cutaneous disease is the multitude of different allergens present in rubber.

ACD to rubber may be sharply demarcated, giving a clear indication of the object or garment causing the dermatitis (Fig. 2). Allergic reactions to rubber can also appear scattered over the body including the face, flexural areas of the arms and legs, torso and/or genitalia, and thus can simulate an endogenous dermatitis. Such disease patterns may result from indirect manual transfer of the allergen or from multiple different sources of exposure to the allergen. In addition, the possibility of airborne contact dermatitis (Dooms-Goossens et al. 1986) or systemic contact dermatitis due to ingestion of rubber accelerators that have migrated into food substances stored in rubber containers (Stankevich et al 1980) should also be considered.

"Bleached rubber syndrome" is an interesting allergic reaction to rubber accelerators (Blancas-Espinosa et al. 2000). Although the eczematous appearance of the eruption strongly implicates its allergic cause, standard patch tests are negative. Testing with a piece of the elasticized rubber from the offending bleached garment will yield a positive reaction. The allergen is *N,N*-dibenzylcarbamyl

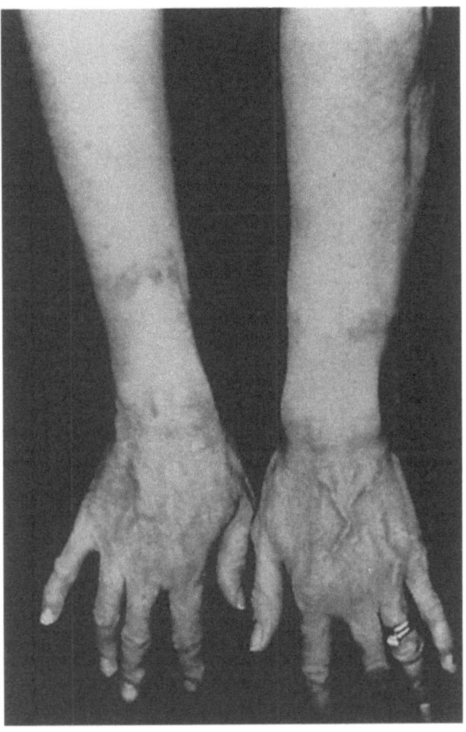

Fig. 2. Allergic contact dermatitis to a rubber glove. A middle-aged woman presented with dyshidrotic eczema of the fingers and was advised to wear rubber gloves for household work. Several months later, she developed this erythematous, scaling dermatitis of the dorsal hands. Note the demarcation at the wrists with patches of dermatitis about the midforearm. Patch testing revealed allergic reactions to both thiuram and carba mixes. Her dermatitis cleared with the use of cotton liners and vinyl gloves. (Reproduced with the permission of the Ronald O. Perelman Department of Dermatology, New York University School of Medicine, New York, NY)

chloride, which is produced by the effect of chlorine on zinc dibenzyldithiocarbamate (Jordan and Bourlas 1975).

"Pompholyx" or dyshidrotic-like eczema is found in bank employees and other workers with frequent exposure to rubber bands. The dermatitis principally affects the dorsolateral aspects of the digits of the dominant hand. The chief sensitizers are thiurams and thiazoles (Condé-Salazar, 1990b).

Hyperkeratotic lesions due to rubber appear mainly over the palmar and plantar surfaces and initially start as dryness with minimal scaling. With continued cutaneous contact to the allergen, the process intensifies and hyperkeratotic fissures, simulating psoriasis and/or mycotic disease, develop (Fig. 3). Patch tests can be diagnostic. An important characteristic of allergic reactions is the relatively rapid improvement when the patient stops using the offending object. Although palmoplantar hyperkeratosis could be attributable to the effects of any allergen on the thick horny layer, it is more frequent with allergy to the amine

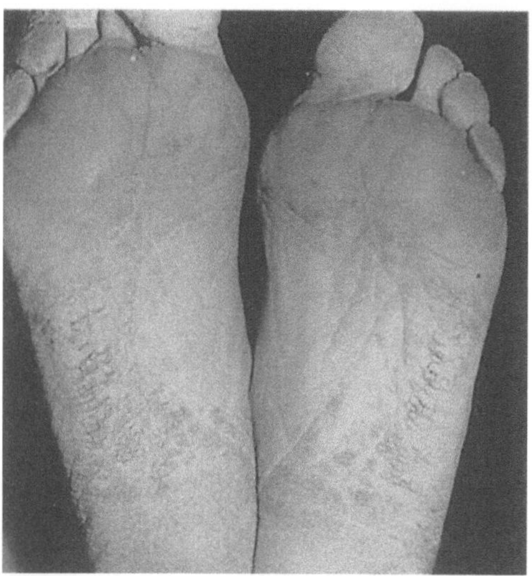

Fig. 3. Allergic contact dermatitis to black rubber in a work boot. Note the hyperkeratotic scaling dermatitis most pronounced over the metatarsal area and tips of the toes. This pattern, together with sparing of the interdigital webs, the toe creases and the arch of the foot should suggest the diagnosis. Patch tests were positive to IPPD and black rubber mix. (Reproduced with the permission of Donald V. Belsito, M.D., Division of Dermatology, University of Kansas Medical Center, Kansas City, KS)

anti-oxidants, where it has been termed "black rubber hands/feet" (Condé-Salazar, 1990b).

Leukoderma from rubber products is largely due to hydroquinone and its derivatives. These chemicals were previously used in the rubber industry as anti-oxidants and stabilizers. The first cases of occupational leukoderma were caused by monobenzylether of hydroquinone (Oliver et al. 1939). Monobenzylether of hydroquinone also caused an intense allergy. Nowadays, such reactions are rare since derivatives of hydroquinone are seldom used as anti-oxidants in rubber, although they are still extensively used in the photographic industry. Nonetheless, one occasionally sees a confetti-like hypopigmentation over the dorsal hands and forearms in individuals with glove allergies. Whether this is due to chemical leukoderma or post-inflammatory hypopigmentation following the allergy is often unclear.

Purpuric reactions to rubber were first described by Fisher (1974). He called the syndrome PPPP since it was characterized by the appearance of purpura, petechiae, and pruritus. Lesions localize to the area in contact with the rubber object. The causative factor is typically IPPD as demonstrated by a positive patch test that may also be purpuric (Romaguera and Grimalt 1977). Thiuram-derivatives have also been reported to induce purpuric ACD (Burrows 1972).

Other clinical forms of allergic reactions to rubber have also been described, albeit rarely. Calnan (1971) and Ancona, et al (1982) described *lichenoid contact dermatitis* produced by IPPD. Pecegueiro and Brandão (1984) reported *plantar pustulosis* due to MBT and its derivatives. Dooms-Goossens et al. (1985) described a *pustular reaction* from hexafluorosilicate, a component used in the manufacture of foam rubber. Eun et al. (1985) noted an epidemic of *pitted keratolysis* in building workers using rubber boots. Cases of *erythema multiforme* caused by allergy to IPPD present in a black rubber watchband (Foussereau et al 1988) and to natural rubber latex in gloves (Bourrain et al. 1996) have been described. Finally, *pyoderma gangrenosum* from anti-oxidants and accelerants in a stomal bag has also been reported (Lenane et al 1998).

Irritant Contact Dermatitis (ICD)

Powder in gloves, as well as the trapping of sweat under gloves and other occlusive rubberized materials, are not unusual causes of irritant dermatitis from rubber. However, ACD is more common than ICD among users of rubber products (Heese et al 1991).

Allergic Contact Urticaria (ACU)

Nutter (1979) first called attention to ACU induced by rubber. Since then, hundreds of additional cases have been reported. For a more complete discussion of ACU to latex, see Turjanmaa et al. (2000).

Diagnosis

The only useful and reliable method for the diagnosis of ACD remains the patch test. In recognition of the significant number of individuals allergic to rubber-related chemicals, five of the allergens available on the American "standard screening" kit are rubber-related. In fact, four of five are mixes (thiuram mix, mercapto mix, black rubber mix and carba mix) and, therefore, 14 rubber additives are tested. In the European standard series, carba mix is no longer tested; while, in Japan, only the mixes are used and 2-MBT is not routinely tested as an individual allergen. In addition, *p*-tert-butylphenol formaldehyde resin (PTBFR) and epoxy resin, plasticizers that can be added to specialty rubber items, are also included in most standard trays.

Given the vast number of additives in a given rubber product, practitioners interested in fully evaluating at least some patients with ACD to rubber must be prepared to perform tests with the patient's own materials. In so doing, pieces of the suspected materials should be cut to conform to the desired size of the patch; it is frequently helpful to soak the material in water for 15 min prior to testing. Furthermore, when testing for a rubber material as is, it may be necessary to leave the patch in place for longer than 48 h, perhaps up to 1 week. Alternatively, one may elect to use ultrasonic bath extracts of the suspected rubber product to improve the yield of patch testing (Bruze et al. 1992). Patients unreactive to the rubber allergens on the standard tray who react to their own product will often require testing to an expanded rubber series either obtained commercially (Table 10) or privately. For physicians compounding their own allergens, texts detailing appropriate concentrations and vehicles are available (de Groot 1994).

Treatment and Prevention

The treatment of ACD lies in correctly identifying its cause and in properly instructing the patient in avoidance of the responsible allergen(s). However, it can be difficult to offer adequate advice, since rubber is widely used in many different substances, which are rarely labeled with their chemical composition. Furthermore, the ingredients of a given rubber product can change from lot to lot. Patients must be warned that the term "hypoallergenic" when applied to rubber is meaningless unless they know the actual chemical constituents. Most hypoallergenic latex products contain carbamates, which have been regarded as less sensitizing than thiuram or thiazole derivatives (Fisher 1975). These materials would be very allergenic for the individual with ACD to carbamates or with ACU to latex.

For many needs, plastic substitutes are available. When in doubt, the patient can contact the manufacturer, who may be able to supply information. Guidance is generally needed in selecting the following:

Gloves are available for individuals reacting to the various allergens in rubber. Table 11 is a partial list that should be sufficient for most patients. A more detailed listing can be found elsewhere (Heese et al. 1991; Rich et al. 1991).

Shoes present a particular problem since tracking the individual ingredients of commercially available shoes is difficult. Specialty shoe manufacturers can customize shoes (Table 12). Although expensive, custom-made shoes are the easiest way to avoid relevant allergens. Alternatively, one can patch test to all components of a patient's existing shoes and, if negative, have the patient "use test" only this pair for a period of several weeks. Assuming the "use test" is negative, then the shoe is presumptively free of relevant allergens. Although not guaranteed, by purchasing the same make and model of shoe in the future, the patient may be able to avoid recurrent dermatitis. Patients with persistent dermatitis despite avoidance of allergens in shoes should be advised to purchase new socks, since at least one investigator has found that, even when thoroughly washed, socks can harbor the allergens (Rietschel 1984).

Medical devices pose a particular problem for rubber allergic individuals. Guidance in choosing contraceptive devices is especially needed; Table 13 lists some alternatives. These individuals must also warn physicians/dentists against performing examinations with gloves to which they might react. Finally, there are a vast number of other medical devices containing rubber that patients, especially those with ACU to latex, need to avoid. The Spina Bifida Association of America (4950 MacArthur Blvd., N.W., Suite 250, Washington, D.C. 20007–4226; Tel.: 800-6213141; http://www.sbaa.org/html/sbaa_latex.html) has a brochure that lists many of the potential exposures to latex in hospital and home environments and also offers acceptable non-latex alternatives.

Table 11. A partial listing of available gloves and their ingredients[a]

Brand name	Components[b]					
	Polymer	MBT	TH	CAR	TU	Powder
Sterile surgical						
Dermaguard Plus[c]	Latex	–	–	+	–	+CS
Pristine[d]	Latex	–	+	–	+	–
Safeskin PFS[e]	Latex	–	–	+	–	–
Dermaprene[c]	Neoprene	+	–	–	+	+
Neolon[f]	Neoprene	–	–	+	–	+LAC
Purple Nitrile Sterile[e*]	Nitrile	–	–	+	–	–
Non-sterile exam						
Safeskin LPE/PFE[e*]	Latex	–	–	+	–	±[k]
Tru-Touch[f]	Polyvinyl chloride	–	–	–	–	+CS
SensiCare[f]	Polyvinyl chloride/ plastic hybrid	–	–	–	–	+CS
Purple Nitrile[e*]	Nitrile	–	–	+	–	–
Household						
Bluette[g]	Neoprene	–	–	+	–	–
Allerderm vinyl[h]	Polyvinyl chloride	–	–	–	–	–
Industrial						
Purple-Nitrile-Xtra[e*]	Nitrile	+	–	+	–	–
N-Dex[i]	Nitrile	+	–	–	–	±[k]
Nitrile Glove[g]	Nitrile	+	–	+	–	–
4-H Gloves[j]	Polyethylene/ethyl-vinyl alcohol	–	–	–	–	–

[a] The accuracy of components was verified in September, 2001. The components of individual brands may have changed since then.

[b] *MBT* 2-mercaptobenzothiazole and related thiazoles, *TH* tetramethylthiurams and related thiurams, *CAR* carbamates; *TU* thioureas; *CS* corn starch *LAC* lactose.

[c] Ansell-Perry, Tel.: +1-800-3219752. Dermaguard Plus has a polyurethane inner lining; Dermaprene contains a *p*-cresol antioxidant.

[d] World Medical Supply, Tel.: +1-800-5455475.

[e] Safeskin Corp, Tel.: +1-800-4629989.

[f] Maxxim Medical, Tel.: +1-813-8552290.

[g] MAPA Professional, Tel.: +1-800-6522002. To order Bluette Gloves, Tel.: +1-800-4423855.

[h] Allerderm, Tel.: +1-800-3656868.

[i] Best Co, Tel.: +1-800-2410323.

[j] Safety 4, Inc. North Safety Products, Tel.: +1-800-4304110.

[k] Available in both powdered (LPE, corn starch) and non-powdered (PFE) models.

* Chemical extractions performed on the Safeskin PFS, PFE and Purple Nitrile glove using buffered saline extraction for 6 hours at 37 °C failed to detect ZDMC, ZDEC or ZDBC down to a limit of 0.025%. Nevertheless, carbamates are used as accelerants and the company cautions against use of the Safeskin glove by individuals extremely allergic to carbamates.

Table 12. Manufacturers of specialty shoes

Company	Shoe Types
The Cordwainer Shop P.O. Box 110 Deerfield, NH 03037 Tel.: +1-603-4637742	Men's and women's dress shoes and sandals
P.W. Minor & Son, Inc. P.O. Box 678 Batavia, NY 14021-0678, USA Tel.: +1-716-3431500, +1-800-828-8157	Men's workboots; orthopedic shoes
Loveless Orthopedic Appliance 2434 SW 29 St. Oklahoma City, OK 73119, USA Tel.: +1-800-6379731, +1-405-6319731	Men's dress shoes and women's dress flats (no heels); Men's and women's Western-style and hunting boots
Fontana's Shoe Sales and Repair 401 Eddy St. Ithaca, NY 14850, USA Tel.: +1-607-2727463	Women's comfort shoes and fashion shoes in leather
Birkenstock Sandals http://www.birkenstock.com/1.htm	Sandal-style shoe in leather with cork inner sole. No rubber products. Bard glues
LaCrosse Footwear, Inc. P.O. Box 1328 LaCrosse, WI 54602, USA Tel.: +1-800-4511806	PVC workboot with steel toe

Table 13. Contraceptive devices for rubber sensitive individuals[a]

Device	Comments
Condoms	
Natural lamb skin brands	Made from processed sheep intestines; no rubber-related allergens; not completely effective in blocking transmission of HIV
Avanti condom	Thermoplastic elastomer free of latex and rubber additives. Adequately prevents transmission of HIV.
Latex condom	Natural latex and must be avoided by patient with ACU; Trojan brands contain carbamates but no thiazoles, thiurams, or anti-oxidants[b]. Adequately prevents transmission of HIV.
Reality female condom	Vaginal condom made of polyurethane. No latex, thiazoles, thiurams, carbamates or thioureas. Adequately prevents transmission of HIV.
Diaphragms	
Wide Seal	Silicone diaphragm free of natural latex rubber, thiazoles, thiurams, carbamates or thioureas.

[a] The accuracy of components was verified in September, 2001. The components of individual brands may have changed since then.
[b] Information obtained from Taylor (1986). The manufacturer declined to confirm the components for unknown reasons and the reliability of this information cannot be assured.

To lessen sensitization to rubber and its additives, attempts have been made to substitute or lower the concentration of some of the more allergenic chemicals used in its production. Avoiding the use of highly sensitizing chemicals in gloves, boots, and other items in close contact with the skin is prudent. Another alternative is to use plastic, especially for gloves and shoes.

Non-rubber materials containing rubber-related allergens must also be avoided. 2-MBT and related thiazoles (Table 5) can be found in fungicides and algicides, cutting oils, antifreeze, photographic emulsions, and veterinarian products (Fregert and Skog 1962; Rudzki et al. 1981; Adams 1974). Thiurams (Table 4) are extensively used as animal repellents and fungicides (Shelley 1964), and are also the active ingredient in Antabuse. The carbamates (Table 6) are widely used as lawn and garden fungicides (Nater et al. 1979), as well as in the plastic industry (Rietschel and Fowler 2001). *p*-Phenylenediamine derivatives may cross react with PPD in hair dyes and can be used in acrylic products (Table 9). Finally, the thioureas (Table 7) are found in detergents (Anderson 1983), plastic-based adhesives (Fregert et al. 1982), photocopy paper (van der Leun et al. 1977), and paint/glue removers (Kanerva et al. 1984).

Summary and Highlights

Sensitization to rubber components often accompanies allergic or non-allergic hand eczemas. However, without patch testing, the diagnosis can be missed. Furthermore, since sensitizing rubber products may contain multiple allergens, individuals are often allergic to several chemicals. The existence of multiple sensitivities may also be due to cross-reactivity (thiurams with carbamates).

The allergens in rubber vary greatly depending upon the product and the country of origin. The composition of the same rubber product may change from lot to lot without the consumer being aware of any differences in the final product. In general, the rubber accelerators, especially the thiurams, cause the greatest amount of sensitivity among users of rubber. In contrast, workers involved in the manufacture of rubber are more likely allergic to the amine anti-oxidants.

The amine anti-oxidants, especially IPPD, are highly sensitizing and positive patch tests are typically intense. Palmoplantar reactions to the amine anti-oxidants often present with hyperkeratosis simulating psoriasis. The dermatitis clears quickly when contact is avoided. Fortunately, the majority of rubber products containing IPPD and its derivatives are black, which helps the individual to identify them.

An individual sensitized to components of rubber must take precautions not only with rubberized products used at work (gloves, masks, rubber bands, etc.), but also with personal products (elasticized garments, condoms, shoes, sporting equipment, etc.) and with non-rubber sources of the allergen(s), such as insecticides, fungicides, and medicaments. For many workers, it is particularly important to identify specific gloves and shoes, which are free of their allergens. Tables 11 and 12 are helpful in this regard.

References

Adams RM (1974) Mercaptobenzothiazole in veterinary medications. Contact Dermatitis Newsletter 16:514

Adams RM (1983) Occupational skin disease. New York: Grune-Stratton, pp 1–26, 289–312

Alfonzo C (1979) Allergic contact dermatitis to isopropylaminodiphenylamine (IPPD). Contact Dermatitis 5:145–147

Ancona A, Monroy F, Fernandez-Diez J (1982) Occupational dermatitis from IPPD in tyres. Contact Dermatitis 8:91–94

Andersen KE (1983) Diethylthiourea contact dermatitis from an acidic detergent. Contact Dermatitis 9:146

Blancas-Espinosa R, Ancona-Alayon A, Arevalo-Lopez A (2000) Allergic contact dermatitis to socks presenting as bleached rubber syndrome. Am J Contact Dermat 11:97–98

Bourrain JL, Woodward C, Dumas V, et al (1996) Natural rubber latex contact dermatitis with features of erythema multiforme. Contact Dermatitis 35:55–56

Brandão FM (1990) Rubber. In: Adams RM (ed). Occupational skin disease. Philadelphia, Saunders, pp 462–485

Bruze M, Trulsson L, Bendsöe N (1992) Patch testing with ultrasonic bath extracts. Am J Contact Dermatitis 3:133–137

Burrows D (1972) Thiuram dermatitis and purpura. Contact Dermatitis Newsletter 12:333

Calnan CD (1971) Lichenoid dermatitis from isopropylaminodiphenylamine. Contact Dermatitis Newsletter 10:237

Calnan CD (1978) Dermatology and industry. Prosser White Oration 1977. Clin Exp Dermatol 3:1–16

Condé-Salazar L (1987) Dermatosis por gomas y derivados. In: Tratado de dermatosis profesionales. Garcia Perez A, Condé-Salazar L, Camarasa JM (eds). Madrid: Eudema, pp 157–181

Condé-Salazar L (1990a) Sensibilidad profesional a componentes de las gomas. Doctoral thesis, University of Madrid

Condé-Salazar L (1990b) Rubber dermatitis: Clinical forms. Dermatol Clin 8:49–55

Condé-Salazar L, del Rio E, Guimaraens D, et al (1993) Type IV allergy to rubber additives. A 10-year study of 686 cases. J Am Acad Dermatol 29:176–180

Condé-Salazar L, Guimaraens D, Villegas C, et al (1995) Occupational allergic contact dermatitis in construction workers. Contact Dermatitis 33:226–230

Cronin E (1980) Rubber. In: Cronin E (ed) Contact dermatitis. Churchill Livingstone, Edinburgh, pp 714–770

de Groot AC (1994) Patch Testing: Test Concentrations and Vehicles for 3700 Chemicals, 2nd edn. Elsevier, Amsterdam

de Meester C (1988) Genotoxic properties of 1,3-butadiene. Mutat Res 195:273–281

Dooms-Goossens A, Loncke J, Michiels JL, et al (1985) Pustular reactions to hexafluorosilicate in foam rubber. Contact Dermatitis 12:42–47

Dooms-Goossens A, Debusschere KM, Gevers DM, et al (1986) Contact dermatitis caused by airborne agents: a review and case reports. J Am Acad Dermatol 15:1–10

Duarte I, Terumi-Nakono J, Lazzarini R (1998) Hand eczema: evaluation of 250 patients. Am J Contact Dermat 9:216–223

Estlander T (1990) Occupational skin disease in Finland. Observations made during 1974–1988 at the Institute of Occupational Health, Helsinki. Acta Derm Venereol Suppl (Stockh) 155:1–85

Estlander T, Jolanki R, Kanerva L (1986) Dermatitis and urticaria from rubber and plastic gloves. Contact Dermatitis 14:20–25

Eun HC, Park HB, Chun YH (1985) Occupational pitted keratolysis. Contact Dermatitis 12:122

Fajen JM, Roberts DR, Ungers LJ, et al (1990) Occupational exposure of workers to 1,3-butadiene. Environ Health Perspect 86:11–18

Feinman SE (1987) Sensitivity to rubber chemicals. J Toxicol Cut Ocular Toxicol 6:117–153

Fishbein L (1992) Exposure from occupational versus other sources. Scand J Work Environ Health 18 (Suppl 1):5–16

Fisher AA (1974) Allergic petechial and purpuric rubber dermatitis: The PPPP syndrome. Cutis 14:25–27

Fisher AA (1975) "Hypoallergenic" surgical gloves and gloves for special situations. Cutis 15:797–811

Foussereau J, Cavelier C, Protois JC, et al (1988) A case of erythema multiforme with allergy to isopropyl-p-phenylenediamine of rubber. Contact Dermatitis 18:183

Fregert S (1975) Occupational dermatitis in a 10-year material. Contact Dermatitis 1:96–107

Fregert S (1981) Manual of Contact Dermatitis, 2nd edn. Munksgaard, Copenhagen, pp 46–48

Fregert S, Skog E (1962) Allergic contact dermatitis from mercaptobenzothiazole in cutting oil. Acta Derm Venereol (Stockh) 42:235–238

Fregert S, Trulsson L, Zimerson E (1982) Contact allergic reactions to diphenylthiourea and phenylisothiocyanate in PVC adhesive tape. Contact Dermatitis 8:38–42

Gibbon KL, McFadden JP, Rycroft RJ et al (2001) Changing frequency of thiuram allergy in healthcare workers with hand dermatitis. Br J Dermatol 144:347–350

Hansson C (1994) Allergic contact dermatitis from N-(1,3-dimethylbutyl)-N'-phenyl-p-phenylenediamine and from compounds in polymerized 2,2,4-trimethyl-1,2-dihydroquinoline. Contact Dermatitis 30:114–115

Heese A, van Hintzenstern J, Peters KP, et al (1991) Allergic and irritant reactions to rubber gloves in medical health services. J Am Acad Dermatol 25:831–839

Helland S, Nyfors A, Utne L (1983) Contact dermatitis to Synthaderm®. Contact Dermatitis 9:504–506

Hervé-Bazin B, Gradiski D, Duprat P, et al (1977) Occupational eczema from N-isopropyl-N'-phenylparaphenylenediamine (IPPD) and N-dimethy-1,3-butyl-N'-phenylparaphenylenediamine (DMPPD) in tyres. Contact Dermatitis 3:1–15

International Agency for Research on Cancer (IARC, 1979) Some monomers, plastics and synthetic elastomers, and acrolein. In: IARC monographs on the evaluation of carcinogenic risk of chemicals to humans 19:231

International Agency for Research on Cancer (IARC, 1986) Some chemicals used in plastics and elastomers. In: IARC monographs on the evaluation of carcinogenic risk of chemicals to humans 39:155

Jordan WP Jr, Bourlas MC (1975) Allergic contact dermatitis to underwear elastic. Arch Dermatol 111:593–595

Kanerva L, Jolanki R, Plosila M, et al (1984) Contact dermatitis from dibutylthiourea. Contact Dermatitis 10:158–162

Kanerva L, Estlander T, Jolanki R (1996) Allergic patch test reactions caused by the rubber chemical cyclohexyl thiophthalimide. Contact Dermatitis 34:23–26

Kaniwa MA, Isama K, Nakamura A, et al (1994a) Identification of causative chemicals of allergic contact dermatitis using a combination of patch testing in patients and chemical analysis: Application to cases from rubber footwear. Contact Dermatitis 30:26–34

Kaniwa MA, Isama K, Nakamura A, et al (1994b) Identification of causative chemicals of allergic contact dermatitis using a combination of patch testing in patients and chemical analysis: Application to cases from rubber gloves. Contact Dermatitis 31:65–71

Kilpikari I (1982) Occupational contact dermatitis among rubber workers. Contact Dermatitis 8:359–362

Kilpikari I, Halme H (1983) Contact allergy to Hypalon® rubber. Contact Dermatitis 9:529

Knudsen BB, Menné T (1996) Contact allergy and exposure patterns to thiurams and carbamates in consecutive patients. Contact Dermatitis 35:97–99

Knudsen BB, Hametner C, Seycek O et al (2000) Allergologically relevant rubber accelerators in single-use medical gloves. Contact Dermatitis 43:9–15

Ko D, Leow YH, Goh CL (2001) Occupational allergic contact dermatitis in Singapore. Sci Total Environ 270:97–101

Lammintausta K, Kalimo K (1985) Sensitivity to rubber. Study with rubber mixes and individual rubber chemicals. Dermatosen 33:204–208

Lenane P, McKenna D, Murphy GM (1998) Pyoderma gangrenosum secondary to allergic contact dermatitis from rubber. Contact Dermatitis 38:238

Magnusson B, Möller H (1979) Contact allergy without skin disease. Acta Derm Venereol (Stockh) 59 (Suppl):113–115

Marks JG, Belsito DV, DeLeo VA, et al (1995) North American Contact Dermatitis Group standard tray patch test results (1992 to 1994). Am J Cont Derm 6:160–165

Marks JG, Belsito DV, DeLeo VA, et al (1998) North American Contact Dermatitis Group patch test results for the detection of delayed-type hypersensitivity to topical allergens. J Am Acad Dermatol 38:911–918

Marks JG, Belsito DV, DeLeo, VA et al (2000) North American ontact Dermatitis Group Patch Test Results: 1996–1998. Arch Dermatol 136:272–273

Mitchell JM, Rook A (1979) Botanical dermatology. Vancouver, Greengrass, p 286

Nater JP, Terpstra H, Bleumink F (1979) Allergic contact sensitization to the fungicide Maneb. Contact Dermatitis 5:24–26

National Institute for Occupational Safety and Health (NIOSH, 1984) 1,3-Butadiene. In: Current Intelligence Bulletin; no 41, publication no 84–105. Cincinnati, OH. US Department of Health and Human Services, NIOSH

Nethercott JR (1982) Results of routine patch testing of 200 patients in Toronto. Contact Dermatitis 8:389–395

Nethercott JR, Holness DL, Adams RM, et al (1991) Patch testing with a routine screening tray in North America, 1985 through 1989: I. Frequency of response. Am J Contact Dermatitis 2:122–129

Norris P, Storrs FJ (1990) Allergic contact dermatitis to adhesive bandages. Dermatol Clin 8:147–152

Nurse DS (1979) Rubber sensitivity. Austr J Dermatol 20:31–33

Nutter AF (1979) Contact urticaria to rubber. Br J Dermatol 101:597–598

Oliver EA, Schwartz L, Warren LH (1939) Occupational leukoderma: Preliminary report. JAMA 113:927–928

Pecegueiro S, Brandão F (1984) Contact plantar pustulosis. Contact Dermatitis 11:126–127

Plotnick HB (1978) Carcinogenesis in rats of combined ethylene dibromide and disulfiram. JAMA 239:1609

Plotnick H, Birmingham DJ (1993) Disulfiram alcohol facial flush in rubber industry. Abstracts: American Contact Dermatitis Society Annual Meeting, Washington, DC, p 11

Rich P, Belozer ML, Norris P, et al (1991) Allergic contact dermatitis to two antioxidants in latex gloves: 4,4'-thiobis(6-tert-butyl-meta-cresol) (Lowinox 44S36) and butylhydroxyanisole: Allergic alternatives for glove-allergic patients. J Am Acad Dermatol 24:37–43

Rietschel RL (1984) Role of socks in shoe dermatitis. Arch Dermatol 120:398

Rietschel RL, Fowler JF, Jr. (2001) Fisher's contact dermatitis, 5th edn. Lippincott William and Wilkins, Philadelphia

Rodriguez E, Reynolds GW, Thompson JA (1981) Potent contact allergen in the rubber plant guayule (Parthenium argentatum). Science 21:1444–1445

Rogers TH, Jr (1974) Natural Rubber. In: Chemical and process technology encyclopedia. Considine DM (ed). New York, McGraw-Hill. p 984

Romaguera C, Grimalt F (1977) PPPP syndrome. Contact Dermatitis 3:102–103

Rubber World Magazine's Blue Book (2001). Lippincott and Peto, Inc., Philadelphia. PA

Rudner EJ, Clendenning WE, Epstein E, et al (1975) The frequency of contact sensitivity in North America 1972–1974. Contact Dermatitis 1:277–280

Rudzki E, Napiorkowska T, Czerwinska-Dihm I (1981) Dermatitis from 2-mercaptobenzothiazole in photographic films. Contact Dermatitis 7:43

Shackelford KE, Belsito DV (2002) The etiology of allergic-appearing foot dermatitis: a 5-year retrospective study. J Am Acad Dermatol 47:715–721

Shelley WB (1964) Golf-course dermatitis due to thiram fungicide. JAMA 188:415–417

Sidi E, Hincky M (1954) Les eczemas aux gants de caout. Presse Med 62:1305–1307

Stankevich VV, Vlasiuk MG, Prokof'eva LG (1980) Hygienic assessment of organosulfur accelerators for vulcanization of rubbers for the food industry. Gig Sanit 10:88–89

Storrs FJ, Rosenthal LE, Adams RM, et al (1989) Prevalence and relevance of allergic reactions in patients patch tested in North America - 1984 to 1985. J Am Acad Dermatol 20:1038-1045

Taylor JS (1986) Rubber. In: Contact Dermatitis. Fisher AA (ed). Lea and Febiger, Philadelphia, pp 603-643

Themido R, Brandão FM (1984) Contact allergy to thiurams. Contact Dermatitis 10:251

Turjanmaa K, Alenius H, Mäkinen-Kiljunen S, Reunala T, Palosuo T (2000) Natural rubber latex allergy. In: Kanerva L, Elsner P, Wahlberg JE, Maibach HI (eds) Handbook of occupational dermatology. Springer, Heidelberg Berlin New York, pp 719-729

Toeppen-Sprigg B (1999) Management of dermatitis in the rubber manufacturing industry. Occup Med 14:797-818

van der Leun JC, deKreek EJ, Deenstra-vanLeeuwen M, et al (1977) Photosensitivity owing to thiourea. Arch Dermatol 113:1611

Varigos GA, Dunt DR (1981) Occupational dermatitis. An epidemiological study in the rubber and cement industries. Contact Dermatitis 7:105-110

Vestey JP, Gawkrodger DJ, Wong WK, et al (1986) An analysis of 501 consecutive contact clinic consultations. Contact Dermatitis 15:119-125

von Hintzenstern J, Heese A, Koch HU, et al (1991) Frequency, spectrum and occupational relevance of type IV allergies to rubber chemicals. Contact Dermatitis 24:244-252

White IR (1988) Dermatitis in rubber manufacturing industries. Dermatologic Clinics 6:53-59

Wilkinson SM, Beck MH (1993) Allergic contact dermatitis from sealants containing polysulphide polymers (Thiokol®). Contact Dermatitis 29:273-274

Wilkinson SM, Beck MH (1996) Allergic contact dermatitis from latex rubber. Br J of Dermatol 134:910-914

Wilson HT (1960) Rubber-glove dermatitis. Br Med J 2:21-23

World Health Organization (WHO 1983). Styrene. In: Environmental Health Criteria; no 26, WHO, Geneva

Wyss M, Elsner P, Wuthrich B, et al (1993) Allergic contact dermatitis from natural latex without contact urticaria. Contact Dermatitis 28:154-156

CHAPTER 40

Hairdressers

40

H. VAN DER WALLE

Introduction

In the Western world, customer desires and the marketing strategies of hair cosmetic producers have created a dynamic interaction, leading to changes in shape, colour and length of the hair almost every year.

Hair cosmetic producers provide the hairdresser with a great variety of chemicals to fulfil stylist and customer desires. Hand eczema is a well-recognized, and potentially severe drawback to the hairdressing profession. Hand eczema frequently leads to worker disability.

Epidemiology

Hand eczema is a well-known, and potentially severe, drawback to the hairdressing profession (Borelli 1965). In the 1990s several epidemiological studies confirmed this common knowledge. In 1991, Budde and Schwanitz reported the outcome of a questionnaire-based study among hairdressers' apprentices. The questionnaire was sent to 8256 apprentices, 4208 (48.5%) responded and 70% reported skin damage during apprenticeship with severe skin changes in 30% of cases.

The Schwanitz group (1997) followed 2351 hairdressing apprentices in a prospective cohort study. Eight hundred and forty-four (35.9%) showed signs of irritant contact dermatitis, mostly (80%) located interdigitally. In Germany, the data of insurance institutions and state medical authorities were used to calculate the 1 year incidence rate of occupational skin diseases in the period 1990–1999: for hairdressers it was 97.4/10,000; the overall incidence rate for all occupations was 6.7/10,000 (Dickel 2001). Schaad et al. (1992) evaluated the reasons why 872 dropouts from hairdressing schools stopped their hairdressing apprenticeship. In this study 486 responded (56%), and of these, 39% reported that skin disease was the reason.

Occupational dermatitis may cause sick leave. Data from the branch organization that monitors the administration of sick leave in the Netherlands showed that with approximately 23,000 registered hairdressers the number of sick leave days due to hairdresser's eczema increased from 21,050 in 1986 to 54,293 in 1991 (Schopman 1992).

All these studies confirm that dermatitis is a very common disease among hairdressers. The majority of the cases are affected by a slight chronic irritant contact dermatitis, but severe hand dermatitis is not uncommon and may cause sick leave or force hairdressers to give up their jobs.

Hairdressing Procedures

The main causes of contact dermatitis are water, irritants and allergens used as ingredients in professional hair cosmetics. Hairdressers perform the following procedures (Corbett 1991; Draelos 1995; Gershon 1972; Lee 1988; Umbach 1995).

Cleaning

- Aim 1. Removal of sebum, sweat components, scales of stratum corneum, hair styling products and dirt.
- Aim 2. Improvement of conditioning properties, shine, vitality, volume and elasticity.
- Product: Shampoos.
- Ingredients: Detergents, foaming agents, thickeners, fragrances, conditioners, softeners, preservatives.

Cutting

- Aim. Hygienic or styling.
- Instrument. Scissors and comb.
- Composition. Scissors – metal alloys, grips may be coated with synthetic polymers. Some alloys release significant amounts of nickel.

Permanent Waving

- Aim. Creation of long lasting curls or waves.
- Product. Perm solution. Depending on the hair characteristics and desired result the hairdresser can make a choice between different types of perm waving solutions: acid cold wave, acid heat activated, self regulated, exothermic, alkaline, buffered alkaline sulphite.
  - The perming process is based on reduction/oxidation of the cysteine-disulphide linkages in the hair keratin filament.
  - Breaking of the disulphide linkages by reducing agents enables the re-arrangement of the keratin filament by winding. Subsequent restoring of the disulphide linkages by oxidation, fixes the filaments in their new position, creating a (semi) permanent wave or curl.

- Ingredients:
  - Reducing agents: ammonium thioglycolate, diammonium thioglycolate, glyceryl thioglycolate, thiolactic acid, cysteamin, potassium sulphate, thioglycolic acid.
  - Oxidation agents: hydrogen peroxide, sodium bromate.
  - Alkaline and buffering agents: ammonium hydroxide, triethanolamine, ethanolamine, ammonium carbonate.
  - Various: wetting agents, conditioners, opacifiers, chelating agents, stabilizers, preservatives and perfumes.

Hair Colouring

- Aim. Hair dyes are used to cover grey hair, add coloured highlights, lighten or darken the original hair, or create fancy colours.
- Product. Dyes or dye precursors may be used in gels, mousses, shampoos or lotions. The colouring effect may be gradual, temporary, semi permanent or permanent, depending on the formulation of the product. Gradual and temporary colouring products deposit hair dyes on the hair shaft, semi permanent dyes penetrate the hair shaft and are retained by weak, polar and Van der Waals forces. Permanent colouring is achieved by oxidation and coupling of hair dye precursors in the hair shaft.
- Ingredients:
  - Gradual. Lead acetate, sulphur.
  - Temporary. Many dyes and pigments, e.g. CI acid yellow 1, CI acid red 33, CI acid brown 19, CI basic blue 99, ferric ferrocyanide.
  - Semi permanent. A long list of dyes may be used, e.g. 4-nitro-2-phenylene diamine, 2-amino-3-nitrophenol, 1,4 diamino anthraquinone.
  - Permanent. Primary intermediates, e.g. 4-phenylene diamine, 2,5-diamino toluene sulphate, 4-aminophenol and couplers f.e. resorcinol, 2,4-diamino phenoxyethanol, 1-naphthol, 3-aminophenol.

Bleaching

- Aim. Highlighting or blonding of hair.
- Products. Blonding lotions, creams or powders.
- Ingredients. Hydrogen peroxide to damage the hair melanin pigment by oxidation. The effect can be boosted by mixing hydrogen peroxide with sodium-, potassium- or ammonium persulphate.

Conditioning

- Aim. Damaged hair is harsh, brittle and difficult to comb. Conditioners restore the softness, glossy aspect and manageability of hair.

■ Products. Lotions, creams, blow drying lotions, liquids and rinses.
■ Ingredients. Alkanol amides, glycols, lipids, hydrolysed animal and vegetable proteins, quaternary ammonium compounds and surfactants.

Styling

■ Aim. Support a desired hairstyle.
■ Products. Sprays, mousses, gels, brilliantines, pomades.
■ Ingredients:
  - Sprays. E.g. polyvinylpyrolidone, phenyl acetate, copolymers of phenyl methyl ether and maleic acid hemi esters. Added are plasticisers, humectants, solvents, conditioners.
  - Gels. Contain merely the same ingredients as sprays. Synthetic colours may be added.
  - Mousse. Is a copolymer hair gel released under pressure from an aerosolised can. Colours may be added for highlights.
  - Brilliantines, pomades. Contain e.g. petrolatum, wax, mineral oil, lanolin, vegetable oil, silicone.

Clinical Picture

The clinical picture is the visual outcome of the dynamic interaction between the chemical, physical and mechanical properties of the irritant, the sensitising capacities of the allergens, and the biological make-up of the exposed skin. A great variety of factors, either belonging to the irritant, allergen or the involved skin, are responsible for the degree of damage. The clinical picture is modified by duration and medical treatment. The spectrum of the clinical picture varies from subjective symptoms such as stinging, burning and itching to clinical signs such as erythema, scaling, vesicles, rhagades, dermatitis and severe eczema.

Chronic Irritant Contact Dermatitis

Interdigital (web) dermatitis is often the first sign of skin damage and affects many apprentices during their first months in the profession. The dermatitis may gradually spread to the back of the hands and fingers and wrists. Unfavourable weather conditions may boost this aggravation. Fissures and rhagades may appear, especially in the folds on the dorsum of the fingers. Reactive oedema and pain can complicate the picture and impair the mobility of the fingers. The barrier function of the skin is damaged, enabling irritants and allergens easier access to the deeper parts of the skin, thus aggravating the dermatitis. In the early stages of irritant contact dermatitis, a hardening process may stop the progress of the dermatitis and eventually "repair" the dermatitis without medical treatment.

Mechanical Contact Dermatitis

Repetitive low-grade friction induces hyperkeratosis. Small circumscribed hyperkeratotic plaques may be observed on those finger parts where the grips of the scissors and skin have long-lasting intimate contact.

Freshly cut hair parts may penetrate the skin and induce the forming of foreign body granuloma with sinuses.

Allergic Contact Dermatitis

The extension and severity of the allergic contact dermatitis show a great variety. At one end of the spectrum is the fingertip dermatitis on the dominant hand of the master hairdresser, exposing his/her fingertips to glyceryl thioglycolate during the checking of the quality of the curls (test curl) (Fig. 1). At the other end is an extensive and severe eczema on hands, wrists, forearms, neck, face and ears of a young hairdressing apprentice (Fig. 2) due to an allergy to hair dyes.

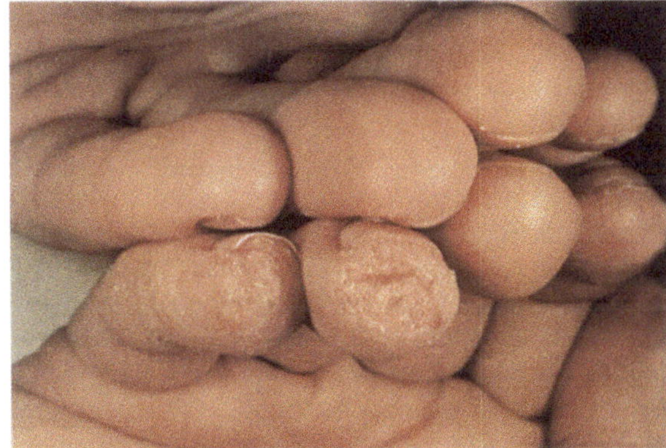

Fig. 1. Fingertip dermatitis on the dominant hand of a hairdresser caused by an allergy to glyceryl thioglycolate

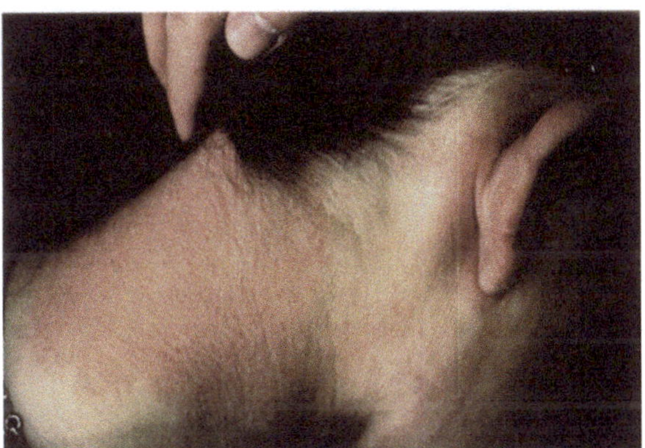

Fig. 2. Extensive dermatitis in a young hairdresser allergic to 4-phenylenediamine, after colouring her own hair

Allergic contact dermatitis may affect every part of the hands, with extension to wrists, underarm, neck and face. The localisation may sometimes give a clue to a specific allergen. Dermatitis of the second and third finger of the serving hand is often related to a hair dye allergy because these fingers grip the hair and present them to the scissors during cutting procedures after colouring. Dermatitis on the back of the hands and around the wrists may indicate a latex allergy caused by a latex protective glove. Glyceryl thioglycolate sensitised hairdressers may show a wide spread dermatitis involving hands, wrists, underarms, neck and face. Ammonium persulphate sensitised hairdressers often complain of both skin and respiratory symptoms.

Direct Contact Reaction

Direct contact reaction is an underestimated cause of hand dermatitis among hairdressers. Many hairdressers report stinging, itching and swelling while cutting greasy, un-shampooed hair. Prick tests with human dander are nearly always negative in these cases. The symptoms suggest that the mechanism is a (non-immunological) direct contact reaction.

Immunological direct contact reactions may be caused by type I allergies to latex proteins, hydrolysed animal proteins (ingredients of the styling products) and persulphates in blonding products. Type I allergies to latex and persulphates may cause reactions not only on the skin, but also on the conjunctivae and the respiratory tract.

Atopic Dermatitis

A history of or present atopic dermatitis is an important risk factor for the development of a work-related hand dermatitis. Hairdressing is a wet work profession par excellence and an atopic skin is an important factor in the development of hand dermatitis in hairdressers.

Nail Changes

Brown discoloration may be caused by hair dyes in hairdressers who neglect to use protective gloves. Transverse ridging, onycholysis and infiltrated nail folds occur in fingertip dermatitis. Nails may become soft and macerated by exposure to water, detergents and perm wave solutions. Sharp cut-hair parts may become implanted under the nails.

Hybrids

Chronic irritant, allergic and atopic factors may all contribute to the development of hand dermatitis. One factor can replace another during the course of a dermatitis, for example, irritant dermatitis in the beginning of the apprenticeship, later on replaced by type IV allergies. Severe cases of chronic hand eczema are in most cases hybrids.

Skin Damaging Factors

Water

The term hydration dermatitis refers to the important role of water in the development of irritant dermatitis (Kligman 1996.) Water penetrates the stratum corneum barrier, is retained in the horny cells and increases by swelling the thickness of the stratum corneum by a factor of 4 to 6. After exposure the water gradually evaporates.

By this alternating process of swelling and shrinking cytokines are released. Inflammation is induced and the proliferation and differentiation of the keratinocytes is disturbed, further impairing the barrier and giving easier access to water, irritants and allergens.

Irritants

Professional hair cosmetic products contain many ingredients with a capacity to irritate the skin. Important irritants are detergents in shampoos, hydrogen peroxide as an oxidizing agent in perm solutions, colouring and blonding products, thioglycolates in perm wave solutions and persulphates used in blonding products.

Dry Air

Hot-air dryers expose the skin of the hairdresser during styling procedures and may cause dehydration of the stratum corneum.

Friction

Handling of instruments (hand shower, dryer, scissors), handling of hair, opening of packages, dry blotting of hair with towels and wearing of gloves may all cause low grade repetitive frictional forces that contribute to the course of a dermatitis.

Gloves

The use of protective gloves may contribute to the development or chronicity of a dermatitis by friction, and the occlusive effect and exposure of the skin to allergens present in the glove material.

Allergens

The skin of the hairdresser is exposed to allergens during all hairdressing procedures and even the use of protective gloves may, unintentionally, expose the skin to allergens.

The major sensitizers are; (Table 1) (Storrs 1984; Straube 1996; Conde-Salazar 1995; Frosch 1993; Guerra 1992; Peters 1994; van der Walle 1997; Cronin 1979; Leino 1998; Kellett 1985; de Groot 1995; Niinimäki 1994; Pasche-Koo 1996; van der Walle 1995; Van der Burg 1986; Pilz 1994; Uter 2000).

■ *Reducing agents*
  - Glyceryl thioglycolate (GTG), a reducing agent in perm solutions with a pH 5 to 6; "acid perms".
  - Ammonium thioglycolate (ATG). Its use dates back to the thirties as the first reducing agent in cold wave solutions, alkaline perms in the range of pH 8–9. Has a low sensitising capacity.

Table 1. Allergens

Allergens	Test concentration/ vehiculum	Type I	Type IV
Glyceryl thioglycolate	1.0% pet.		×
Ammonium thioglycolate	1.0% pet.		×
Cysteamin	0.5% pet.		×
Thiolactic acid	0.3% pet.		×
4-Phenylene diamine	1.0% pet.		×
2,5-Diaminotoluene sulphate	1.0% pet.		×
2-Nitro-4-phenylene diamine	1.0% pet.		×
3-Aminophenol	1.0% pet.	–	×
4-Aminophenol	1.0% pet.	–	×
4-Aminodiphenylamine	0.25% pet.	–	×
Henna	1.0% aq/1.0% pet.	×	×
Ammonium persulphate	2.5% aq/2.5% pet.	×	×
Potassium persulphate	1.0% pet.	–	×
Sodium coco hydrolysed animal protein	2.0% aq/2.0% pet.	×	×
Resorcinol	1.0% pet.	–	×
Cocamidopropyl betain	1.0% aq	–	×
3-Dimethylaminopropylamine	1.0% aq	–	×
Formaldehyde	1.0% aq	–	×
Paraben mix	16.0% pet.	–	×
Methyldibromo glutaronitrile	0.5% pet.	–	×
2-Bromo-2-nitropropane-1,3-diol	0.5% pet.	–	×
2,5-Diazolidinyl urea	2.0% pet.	–	×
Imidazolidinyl urea	2.0% pet.	–	×
Quaternium 15	1.0% pet.	–	×
Methylchloroisothiazolinone and methylisothiazolinone	0.01% aq	–	×
Thiuram mix	1.0% pet.	–	×
Latex	5 mg/ml/pure	×	×
Human dander	5 mg/ml	×	–
Nickel sulphate	5.0% pet.	–	×
Fragrance mix	8.0% pet.	–	×

- Thiolactic acid, becoming popular as a replacement for GTG. Used by a few producers.
- Cysteamin. Increasingly popular as replacement for GTG and ATG.
- Thioglycolic acid, becoming popular as a replacement for GTG.
- *Hair dyes.* Allergies have been ascribed to:
  - 4-phenylene diamine
  - 2,5-diamino toluene sulphate
  - 2-nitro-4-phenylene diamine
  - 3-aminophenol
  - 4-aminophenol
  - 4-aminodiphenylamine
  - Resorcinol
- *Henna.* Hair dye derived form the dried leaves of Lawsonia inermis. May cause immunological direct contact reactions.
- *Blonding agents.* Ammonium and potassium persulphate.
- *Cocamidopropyl betain.* Amphoteric surfactant, ingredient of shampoos and liquid soaps.
- *Formaldehyde.* Most professional hair cosmetic products do not contain formaldehyde.
- *Fragrances.* It is difficult to determine if a fragrance allergy in a hairdresser is caused by professional or private exposure.
- *Preservatives.* Professional hair cosmetics contain the same range of preservatives as in non-professional skin care products.
- *Thiuram compounds.* Sensitisation is induced by thiuram compounds used in glove material.
- *Latex.* May induce type I and IV allergies.
- *Nickel.* The prevalence of nickel allergy among women is high and even higher for young women at the start of their apprenticeship as hairdresser. This higher prevalence is likely to be caused by their preference for jewellery at a young age. Hairdressers have no increased occupational exposure to nickel.
- *Hydrolysed animal and vegetable proteins.* These compound are used as hair conditioners
- *Human hair.* Type I allergies to human dander occur among hairdressers.
- *Various.* Allergic reactions have been reported to pyrogallol. This compound is not allowed anymore in hair colour products. The same holds true for Captan, a fungicide.

Allergy Tests

Allergens are an important factor in the development of dermatitis among hairdressers. In searching for the one single cause of the dermatitis, the importance of patch and prick tests can be easily overestimated by the doctor and the patient. Patch testing is obligatory in all cases of dermatitis, but the interpretation of the results should be done carefully with respect to relevant false-positive or negative results. Relevant positive reactions are important to design a tailor-made management and treatment plan for the patient and are a prerequisite for motivating or forcing producers to optimise the safety of their products.

Management and Treatment

Hand dermatitis in hairdressers is caused by a variety of skin damaging factors related to product ingredients, packages, application and preparation procedures, the use of protective gloves and skin care. To achieve long-lasting secondary prevention in cases of hand dermatitis the approach has to focus on reduction of skin damaging factors, rather than on medical treatment (van der Walle 1994a,b,c; Uter 1997).

The following strategy has proven to improve results (see also Table 2).

■ *Step 1.*
  a. Evaluate the burden of skin damaging factors.
  b. Evaluate the working conditions.
  c. Evaluate the use of protective gloves.
  d. Dermatological investigation.
  e. Evaluate the atopic constitution.
  f. Perform type I and type IV allergy tests.
■ *Step 2.* Make a diagnosis and create an order of major and minor causative factors and keep in mind that:
  a. In many cases irritant factors make a major contribution to the dermatitis in hairdressers.
  b. Not all positive patch tests are relevant for the management of the dermatitis.
■ *Step 3.* Combine the information of step 1 and step 2 and design a strategy that contains the following items:
  a. Reduction of irritants.
  b. Replacement or avoidance of allergens.
  c. Protection.
  d. Skin care.
■ *Step 4.* It takes time for the hairdresser and his/her employer to organize and implement all the good advice. In the meantime, medical treatment is required to support recovery of the skin damage. Consider the use of PUVA light therapy in this period.

Prevention and Prognosis

Safe hairdressing procedures are a prerequisite for successful "treatment". The motivation and skills of the employee, the employer, colleagues, doctor and staff are modifying factors. Focusing mainly on medical treatment contributes to a worse prognosis as was confirmed in a follow-up study among 150 hairdressers. Schopman et al. evaluated (1992) the outcome among 150 hairdressers in the Netherlands on sick leave due to occupational hand eczema and under treatment

Table 2. Safe hairdressing practice. Take notice of the following instructions and help each other to practise them! (1) Skin care of the hands before, during and after work. (2) Protection of the hands during work. (3) Wearing of jewellery. (4) Cleaning of instruments and materials. Be cooperative and help each other in the salon to follow the instructions. You will get used to it in no time!

1. Skin care of the hands	Wash the hands as little as possible, in most cases rinsing with water will be sufficient; afterwards drying with a dry towel, not with a hot-air drier. The same at home Use a water-resistant skin cream every morning before going to work. Use the ointment several times during the morning and afternoon for extra protection Dry your hands regularly. Use a dry towel or tissue Use a skin-care cream in the evening
2. Protection of the hands during work. Hands have to be protected with gloves during certain activities. Wear the gloves briefly and do not use them twice. Never let water get into the glove. When this accidentally happens, pull off the glove, dry your hands and pull on a new glove!	Use gloves for: Hair washing Preparation, applying and washing out hair bleach Preparation, applying and washing out hair dyes Setting a perm a. Mixing and applying the solutions. Take care to clear away the package first and pull off the gloves afterwards! b. Checking a test curl c. Washing out and neutralising
3. Wearing of jewellery	Many young women get nickel allergy by wearing metal earrings. In the hairdressing profession, an allergy to nickel may have serious consequences, so don't wear earrings that release nickel. Use earrings made of synthetic materials, stainless steel, silver or gold Get rid of jewellery, watches and metal parts of clothing (zippers, buttons) that cause dermatitis
4. Cleaning of instruments and materials	After every perm setting, rinse the washbowl, the taps and your tools carefully with water Remove the spoiled bleaching powder immediately with a moistened towel. Wear gloves! After work-time, clean the carriages, tools, work-baskets, wash-bowls, handles and control panels of the hair-dryers Use a mild household detergent for cleaning

by dermatologists. After one year 99 (66%) had left the profession due to the chronic character of their eczema.

Van der Walle and Brunsveld (1997) have published the results of a special hairdresser's clinic. This clinic was started by the Dutch organization of employers to improve the prognosis of hairdressers with hand dermatitis by focusing "treatment" on the introduction of safe hairdressing procedures in the salon. In the period from 1994 through 1999, 704 hairdressers visited the clinic. A follow-up after 6–12 month's was done in 666 hairdressers. In 468 (70%) recovery was achieved. The chance on a successful return to work for hairdressers with long-lasting sick leave due to hand eczema increased by a factor of 4 after consulting the clinic, compared to a group of hairdressers with severe hand eczema who did not visit the clinic (van Wijck 1996).

Primary prevention must focus on pre-hairdressing-school counselling (atopy!), introduction of safe hairdressing procedures, the use of protective gloves and continuing pressure on manufacturers to improve the safety of their products.

References

Borelli S, Moormann J, Dungemann H, Manok M (1965) Ergebnisse einer vierjährige Untersuchungsreihe bei Berufsanfängern des Friseurgewerbes. Berufsdermatosen 13:216–238

Budde von U, Schwanitz HJ (1991) Kontaktdermatiden bei Auszubildenden des Friseurhandwerks in Niedersachsen. Dermatosen 39:41–47

Burg van der CKH, Bruynzeel DP, Vreeburg KJJ, et al (1986) Hand eczema in hairdressers and nurses: a prospective study. Contact Dermatitis 14:275–279

Conde-Salazar L, Baz M, Guimaraens D, et al (1995) Contact dermatitis in hairdressers: patch test results in 379 hairdressers (1980–1993). Am J Contact Dermatitis 6:19–23

Corbett JF (1991) Hair coloring processes. Cosmetics Toiletries 106:53–57

Cronin E (1979) Immediate-type hypersensitivity to henna. Contact Dermatitis 5:198–199

Dickel H, Kuss O, Blesius CR, Schmidt A, Diepgen TL (2001) Report from the register of occupational skin diseases in northern Bavaria (BKH-N). Contact Dermatitis 44:258–259

Draelos ZD (1995) Cosmetics in dermatology. Churchill Livingstone

Frosch PJ, Burrows D, Camarasa JG, et al (1993) Allergic reactions to a hairdressers' series: results from 9 European centres. Contact Dermatitis 28:180–183

Gershon SD et al (1972) Permanent waving. In: Balsam MS, Sagarin E (eds) Cosmetics science and technology, 2nd edn. Wiley-Interscience, pp 167–233

Groot de AC, Van der Walle HB, Weyland JW (1995) Contact allergy to cocamidopropyl betaine. Contact Dermatitis 33:419–422

Guerra L, Tosti A, Bardazzi F, et al (1992) Contact dermatitis in hairdressers: the Italian experience. Contact Dermatitis 26:101–107

Kellett JK, Beck MH (1985) Ammonium persulphate sensitivity in hairdressers. Contact Dermatitis 13:26–28

Kligman AM (1996) Hydration injury to human skin. In: Valk van der PGM, Maibach HI (eds) The irritant contact dermatitis syndrome. CRC Press, pp 187–194

Lee AE, Bozza JB, Huff S, et al (1988) Permanent waves: An overview. Cosmetics Toiletries 103:37–56

Leino T, Estlander T, Kanerva L (1998) Occupational allergic dermatoses in hairdressers. Contact Dermatitis 38:166–167

Niinimäki A, Hannuksela M, Moilanen M (1994) Protein hydrolysates of hair cosmetic products as causes of contact urticaria in hairdressers. In: Abstracts of Second Congress of the European Society of Contact Dermatitis, 6–8 October 1994, Barcelona, p 57

Pasche-Koo F, Claeys M, Hauser C (1996) Contact urticaria with systemic symptoms caused by bovine collagen in a hair conditioner. Am J Contact Dermatitis 7:56–57

Peters KP, Frosch PJ, Uter W, et al (1994) Typ IV-Allergien auf Friseurberufstoffe. Dermatosen 42:50–57

Pilz B, Peschel H, Frosch PJ (1994) Lack of occupational exposure to nickel in hairdressers. In: Abstracts of Second Congress of the European Society of Contact Dermatitis, 6–8 October 1994, Barcelona, p 47

Schaad J, Jonge de JFM (1992) Te vroeg uit de kappersopleiding. TNO, Leiden
Schopman C, Taal EM, Waegemakers T (1992) De handen in het haar. Een onderzoek naar kapperseczeem. Detam, Nederland
Schwanitz HJ, Uter W (1997) Interdigital eczema: sentinel skin damage in wet work occupations. Exp Dermatol 6:255
Storrs FJ (1984) Permanent wave contact dermatitis: Contact allergy to glyceryl monothioglycolate. J Am Acad Dermatol 11:74–85
Straube M, Uter W, Schwanitz HJ (1996) Occupational allergic contact dermatitis from thiolactic acid contained in 'ester-free' permanent-waving solutions. Contact Dermatitis 34:229–230
Umbach W (1995) Kosmetik. Entwicklung, Herstellung und Anwendung kosmetischer Mittel. Georg Thieme Verlag, Stuttgart
Uter W, Wulfhorst B, Pilz B, et al (1997) Anamnese-Auxilium für das Friseurgewerbe – Dermatologisches Risikoprofil. Dermatosen 45:165–169
Uter W, Geier J, Schnuch A (2000) Current pattern and trends in sensitization to hairdressers allergens in Germany. Dermatol Beruf Umwelt 48:55–59
Walle van der HB (1994a) Hairdressing and hand eczema. 1. Current problems and causes. Cosmetics Toiletries 109:35–36
Walle van der HB (1994b) Hairdressing and hand eczema. 2. Tips to minimize sensitizing exposure. Cosmetics Toiletries 109:27–28
Walle van der HB (1994c) Dermatitis in hairdressers. 2. Management and prevention. Contact Dermatitis 30:265–270
Walle van der HB (1997) De Kapperspoli: een andere aanpak van handeczeem bij kapsters. Nederlands Tijdschrift voor Dermatologie & Venereologie 7:42–46
Walle van der HB, Brunsveld VM (1995) Latex allergy among hairdressers. Contact Dermatitis 32:177–178
Wijck van HJH (1996) Kapperseczeem and Kapperspoli Een effectmeting. TNO Preventie en Gezondheid divisie Arbeid en Gezondheid sector Opleidingen, Leiden

CHAPTER 41

Manicurists

41

P.G. ENGASSER, J.S. TAYLOR, H.I. MAIBACH

Manicurists (nail technicians) give manicures caring for the hands and finger-nails and also perform pedicures. Many reports document adverse reactions to nail cosmetics among consumers as well as manicurists. Although Hemmer et al. (1996) considered operators applying acrylic nails to be at lower risk than their clients, we agree with Guin et al. (1998) that this needs to be proved. Reviewing nail cosmetics that have been reported to cause adverse reactions allows us to identify the hazardous exposures for this occupation. These cosmetics include nail hardeners, nail polish (nail enamel or lacquers), and artificial nails (nail-elongating cosmetics).

Nail Cosmetics

In the 5-year study of contact dermatitis conducted by the North American Contact Dermatitis Group, 5.4% of the cases were caused by cosmetics. Nail cosmetics ranked fourth, causing 8% of these reactions (Adams and Maibach 1985).

Nail Polish (Nail Enamel, Nail Lacquer, Nail Varnish)

Nail polishes, including base coats and top coats, are usually of similar composition, containing some or all of the following types of ingredients: (Schlossman 1980; Schoon 1998)
1. Film formers or polymers: nitrocellulose forms a hard, strong film that does not adhere well and is inelastic.
2. Polymer resins: tosylamide/formaldehyde resin, alkyd resins, acrylics, vinyls, polyesters, arylalkylsulfonyl urethanes, glyceryl tribenzoate, and tosylamide epoxy resin. These improve adhesion and gloss. Tosylamide/formaldehyde resin is the official name for toluene sulfonamide formaldehyde resin (TSFR), used in labeling cosmetics. In California, toluene is a restricted substance listed in that state's Proposition 65, and this may have prompted the official name change (Schlossman and Wimmer 1992).
3. Plasticizers, including: camphor; dibutyl, dioctyl, and diphenyl phthalate; tricresyl and tiphenylphosphate; and glyceryl triacetate. These improve film flexibility (Schlossman 1979; Schlossman and Wimmer 1992).

4. Solvents and diluents, including ethyl, butyl, and isopropyl alcohol, butyl, ethyl, and amyl acetate, and toluene, improve viscosity.
5. Colorants (organic dyes) must be approved by the Food and Drug Administration (FDA) in the United States. So-called cream enamels contain insoluble organic dyes and titanium oxide or iron oxide; a few soluble organic dyes are used to tint "colorless" polishes. The nacreous pigments guanine, bismuth oxychloride, or mica are added to pearlized polishes.
6. The suspending agent stearalkonium hectorite, prevents pigment settling.

It is estimated that 6–13% of the adverse reactions to cosmetics relate to nail polish, and most of these reactions are attributed to TSFR (Hausen et al. 1995). Samplings of 20 brands of polish sold in Europe in 1995 showed that all contained TSFR at 0.08–11.0% concentrations, and 14 brands had detectable formaldehyde levels, which varied from 0.02–0.5% (Sainio et al. 1997). So-called "hypoallergenic" brands generally eliminate this ingredient. California legislation has prohibited the use of the solvent, toluene, and cosmetic manufacturers in a legal settlement agreed to reformulate nail polish in most cases eliminating toluene and TSFR. Salon distributed products may still contain TSFR (Schoon 1996). In the 1990s, a major manufacturer reformulated its nail polishes, eliminating TSFR, toluene, and dibutylphthalate, utilizing glyceryl tribenzoate and glyceryl triacetate without sacrificing durability (Levy, personal communication 1994). Top-coats may contain UV-absorbing material, such as benzophenones to prevent photodamage to colors. Some top-coats are not traditional evaporative coatings but UV-cured acrylate oligomer blends that act as protective shields (Schoon 1998).

Anatomic sites for nail polish allergic reactions are frequently ectopic, appearing away from the hands and nails, on places such as the eyelids, lips, or neck. In an interesting report (Liden et al. 1993), 18 patients who were suspected of occupational contact dermatitis proved instead to be allergic to TSFR in nail polish. This article stated that 17 of the 18 patients with patch test positive reactions to TSFR were positive on testing the dry nail polish itself. There have been rare reports of reactions to other allergens in nail polish, e.g., nitrocellulose (Castelain et al. 1997), methyl acrylate (Kanerva et al. 1995), benzalkonium (Guin and Wilson 1999), and phthallic anhydride/trimellite/glycol copolymer (Moffitt and Sansom 2001).

Patch Testing. The following components of nail polishes may be patch tested:
- Nail polish may be patch tested as is, open or closed (after thorough drying)
- Tosylamide formaldehyde resin, 10% in petrolatum (pet)
- Nitrocellulose 10%, in isopropyl alcohol
- Dibutyl phthalate, 5% in pet
- Formaldehyde, 1% aqueous
- Methyl acrylate, 1.5% in pet
- Benzalkonium chloride, 0.01–0.1% aqueous (0.1% is a marginal irritant)
- Guanine, as is
- Phthallic anhydride/trimellite/glycol copolymer, 1% in pet.

Nail Hardeners

There are two distinct types of hardeners. One contains free formaldehyde, commonly responsible for irritant and allergic reactions; these hardeners are only sold periodically, when popular (Norton 1991). In the United States, the FDA regulations require that they contain no more than 5% formaldehyde, have a protective shield for the nail, be applied only to the free end of the nail, and be labeled with warnings of side effects (Food and Drug Administration 1994). The second type of hardener encompasses nail enamels marketed as hardeners. They may have a high resin content, decreased amount of plasticizer, and additions, such as collagen, calcium, or minute fibers.

Patch Testing. The following component of nail hardeners may be patch tested:
- Formaldehyde, 1.0% aqueous

Artificial Nail Products and Techniques

Artificial nails, also referred to as acrylic nails, nail elongators, nail extenders, or liquid nails, generally involve the use of one of two types of acrylic resins: (1) acrylic or methacrylic acids and their esters and (2) cyanoacrylic acid and its esters (Quenon 1989; Bjorkner 1995; Koppula et al. 1995; Kanerva et al. 1996). Acrylics are thermoplastic resins that polymerize either at room temperature or by heating. Initiators, accelerators, and catalysts may be added to speed up the process. Ultraviolet (UV) light polymerization or curing can be used when no initiators are necessary (Bjorkner 1995). Manicurists (nail technicians) commonly use seven different techniques to elongate and enhance nails.

Sculptured Nails
Sculptured nails are custom-made by the manicurist on a template attached to the natural nail plate. The nail plate is sanded; a template is fit beneath the distal end of the nail and surrounds the other sides of the nail. The nail is coated with a primer that contains methacrylic acid. The liquid monomer and powdered polymer are mixed and painted on the nail and template extension. The sculptured nail is sanded to the desired form. Jewels, decals, and decorative metal strips can be added. As the nails grow out, the manicurist must "fill" with the same chemicals at the base above the cuticle every 2–3 weeks. The components and examples of the chemicals included are (Quenon 1989; Freeman et al. 1995):
1. Liquid monomer: ethyl-, butyl-, isobutyl-, hydroxypropyl-, and tetrahydrofurfuryl methacrylate; ethylene glycol- and diethylene glycol dimethacrylate; trimethylolpropane trimethacrylate; other esters of methacrylic acid; 4-methoxyphenol, *N,N*-dimethyl-*p*-toluidine, hydroquinone, resorcinol, and *p*-dimethylamino-chlorbenzene
2. Powdered polymer: poly(ethyl/methyl) methacrylate, benzoyl peroxide, and titanium dioxide
3. Primer: methacrylic acid, MEK, hydroquinone, and 4-methoxyphenol

Sculptured acrylic nails formerly used methyl methacrylate monomer as an ingredient until seizure and recall actions by the U.S. FDA in 1974 and 1975 (Eiermann 1981; Food and Drug Administration 1994). However, periodically, methyl methacrylate appears in these products because it is less costly and easier to work.

Porcelain Nails

Porcelain sculptured nails are like plain sculptured nails with a three-component primer, liquid, and powder, except they employ a finely ground glass-like material in the powdered material.

Gels

Light-cured gels are applied in layers to form a solid nail. The original formulas were hardened with UV light; newer ones harden under ordinary room lighting ("white light"). Some gels use layers of different resins while others use a single resin (Quenon 1989; Draelos 1995; Kanerva et al. 1996). Gels include acrylic oligomers and monomers, modified cellulose, photo-initiators or activators (Guin 2000), amine co-initiators, and titanium dioxide. UV-curable resins for artificial nails resemble dental composite resins based on epoxy bisphenol A glycidyl methacrylate (BIS-GMA) or acrylated urethane as the matrix monomers in combination with mono- and polyfunctional cross-linking monomers. Hemmer et al. (1996) tested patients using photo-bonded nail-cosmetic chemicals, and they patch tested positive to triethyleneglycol dimethacrylate (TREGDMA), ethyleneglycol dimethacrylate (EGDMA), 2-hydroxyethyl methacrylate (2-HEMA), 2-hydroxy propyl methacrylate (2-HPMA), aliphatic urethane diacrylate, and urethane dimethacrylate but not to methacrylated epoxy resins.

Sculptured Nails with Dips

We have seen an acrylic nail technician demonstrate a "dip". After initial nail preparation and application of liquid acrylic, the client then dipped her nails in the polymethylmethacrylate powder.

Wrapping

The nail's free edge is splinted with strips of silk, linen, paper, or fiberglass that strengthen the nail. These strips are fixed in layers with cyanoacrylate glue. The glues also contain a catalyst, N,N-dimethyl-p-toluidine, and hydroquinone (Baran and Schoon 1998). Material strips may also be used with sculpturing (Draelos 1995).

Artificial Tips

Artificial tips are popular with manicurists, because they do not require as much skill as sculpturing nails. The pre-formed tips extend half way down the nail and are fixed with a cyanoacrylate glue. Overlays with silk or fiberglass wraps are usually added; occasionally, sculpturing acrylics are blended (Engasser 1997).

Artificial Pre-formed Nails

Artificial pre-formed plastic nails come in press-on, pre-glued forms or those requiring glue application; the latter use either mono- or multi-functional acrylic resins (Draelos 1995). Patients use these as prostheses. Burrows and Rycroft (1981) report allergy developing to the *p*-tert-butylphenol formaldehyde resin adhesive and tricresyl ethyl phthalate in the plastic nail. For decorative purposes, some of these nails include gold metal (Quenon 1989).

Nail removal can be accomplished by soaking in acetone for about 15 min. Many artificial nail removers contain acetonitrile, which has caused deaths in children who accidentally ingested the nail remover because the containers did not have safety caps (Caravati and Litovitz 1988). Methacrylic acid, used in primers, is corrosive. Acetone cannot be used to remove photobonded nails, and this is a disadvantage if contact allergies develop (Baran and Schoon 1998).

Occupationally Related Skin Disorders in Manicurists

Manicurists should be aware of the sensitizing potential of the mono(meth)acrylates and use no-touch techniques for the skin before the acrylates become polymerized (Kanerva et al. 1996). Occupational sensitization has not been commonly reported. Hemmer's group (1996) estimated that only 10–15% of the reported cases of acrylic nail allergy were occupationally related, in contrast to dentistry, where most cases are occupational. They postulate "that sensitization is not primarily caused by the uncured gel or monomer but by the remaining monomers in the cured plastic nail and the filing dust that is produced when the nail is smoothed or polished".

Acrylic nails evolved from similarly composed products supplied to dentists (Eiermann 1981). In California, cottage industries supplying acrylic nails sprouted from dental-supply manufacturers as well as from other companies, such as automobile-body fiberglass-fender repair shops. Although acrylic nails did not become popular until the 1970s, Canizares (1956) reported methyl methacrylate allergy in a manicurist with dermatitis localized to her left hand, and Fisher and associates (1957) reported another occupationally acquired case. Schubert et al. (1992) reported a nail modeller who became sensitized and developed allergic contact dermatitis on the left hand from sculpturing the not-yet-hardened resin with a file in the right hand. Baran (1982) identified the manicurist's thumb and third finger of the left hand as being constantly exposed to the acrylics when the customer's fingers are held during the process. Similarly a manicurist allergic to cyanoacrylate glue with hand eczema also presented with an initial eruption on those fingers (Belsito 1987). Many manicurists also wear wraps, overlays, or sculptured nails, and presentation of allergy often includes the face, neck and other areas, as well as the hands and fingers (Goodwin 1976; Conde-Salazar et al. 1986; Marks 1990; Fitzgerald et al. 1995; Freeman et al. 1995; Jacobs and Rycroft 1995; Hemmer et al. 1996; Kanerva et al. 1996).

Paresthesias from acrylic monomers have been noted in orthopedic surgeons and dentists. Severe and prolonged paresthesias have also been reported by Fisher (1989) and Baran and Schibli (1990) in individuals wearing sculptured nails, as well as in individuals wearing photobonded nails (Fisher 1990). This subject was reviewed by Fisher and Baran (1991). It is maintained that the side effect of paresthesias may rarely occur in the absence of allergic sensitization if the acrylic monomer contacts injured skin that allows penetration and exposure of the nerves.

Nail-elongating chemicals reported to cause allergic contact dermatitis and their patch-test concentrations (Freeman et al. 1995; Koppula et al. 1995; Hemmer et al. 1996; Kanerva et al. 1996; Guin 2000) include:

- Cyanoacrylics, as is; dry before application
- *p*-Tert-butylphenol formaldehyde resin, 1% pet
- Tricresyl ethyl phthalate plasticizer, 5% pet
- Mono- and multifunctional esters of methacrylic acid, 0.1–2.0% pet
- Methyl acrylate, 1.5% pet
- Methyl methacrylate, 2% pet
- Ethyl methacrylate, 2–5% pet
- Ethyl acrylate, 0.1% pet
- Ethylene glycol dimethacrylate (EGDMA), 2–5% pet
- Triethylene glycol dimethacrylate (TEGDMA), 1–2% pet
- Triethylene glycol diacrylate (TEGDA), 0.1%–5% pet
- 2-Hydroxyethylacrylate (2-HEA), 0.5% pet
- 2-Hydroxyethyl methacrylate (2-HEMA), 2% pet
- 2-Hydroxypropyl methacrylate (2-HPMA), 2% pet
- BIS-GMA, 2% pet
- Bisphenol A methacrylate, 2% pet
- Bisphenol A ethoxymethacrylate, 1% pet
- Butyl acrylate, 0.1–0.5% pet
- Urethane diacrylate (aliphatic), 0.1% pet
- Urethane diacrylate (aromatic), 0.1% pet
- Methacrylic acid, 0.1–1% pet
- Benzoyl peroxide, 1% pet
- Dimethyl-*p*-toluidine, 2% pet
- Hydroquinone, 1% pet
- Benzophenone-3 and -4 10% pet

HPMA – In a Cleveland Clinic series acrylic nail users most frequently were patch test positive to HPMA (Sood and Taylor).

Note that the appropriate non-irritating concentration sufficient to identify delayed sensitivity needs further documentation for some of these materials.

Manicurists may sustain minor skin injuries working with sharp instruments, such as scissors, files, or drills. They are at risk of skin infections, and hygienic practices should be part of their practice for their own protection and that of their clients. UV light sources should be properly filtered, shielded, and maintained.

Occupationally Related Mucosal Irritation of Eyes, Mouth, and Throat in Manicurists

Mucosal irritation of eyes, mouth, and throat have been reported following industrial acrylic monomer exposure (Lozewicz et al. 1985), and this can potentially occur during a manicure. Other chemicals used in creating acrylic nails are potential occupational mucosal irritants depending on the extent of exposure and on individual susceptibility (Quenon 1989). These include acetone, diethyl-*p*-toluidine, ethyl acetate, hydroquinone, and methyl ethyl ketone. Industrial hygiene measurements with personal and area samplers in six different sculptured-nail salons recorded measurable levels of various organic vapors and methacrylate dusts. Throat irritation was the only statistically significant health effect noted among the nail technicians, although nose and skin irritation, drowsiness, dizzy spells, and trembling of the hands were reported more often among nail technicians than among the control group (Hiipakka and Samimi 1987).

Prevention

Prevention strategies for manicurists have been identified by Quenon (1989), Hiipakka and Samimi (1987) and the National Institute for Occupational Safety and Health (NIOSH) (1999). These include:

1. Substitution. Harmful chemicals should be avoided, including acrylic preparations with irritating vapors.
2. Engineering controls. Local exhaust ventilation systems, such as table systems, capture and remove contaminated air to the outdoors. A properly ventilated table is necessary (National Institute for Occupational Safety and Health 1999), and dust masks should be used if, for some reason, the exhaust system is not functioning.
3. Good work practices. Keep dispenser bottles closed. Soaked gauze should be disposed of in sealed bags. Wash exposed skin several times each day to remove dust. Adopt a "no-touch system" with liquid monomers.
4. Manicurists should wear protective clothing with long sleeves and glasses. Glasses are needed to prevent eye damage when nails are being clipped into pieces at removal. NIOSH suggests gloves to protect from dust but does not specify type. 4H laminate gloves (Safety 4A/S Lyngby, Denmark) are resistant to acrylates. The fingertips of the 4H gloves can be cut off and worn under a vinyl glove to minimize the bulkiness of the 4H glove.

References

Adams RM, Maibach HI (1985) A five-year study of cosmetic reactions. J Am Acad Dermatol 13:1062–1069
Baran RL (1982) Pathology induced by the application of cosmetics to the nail. In: Frost P, Horwitz SN (eds) Principles of cosmetics for the dermatologist. Mosby, St. Louis, pp 181–184
Baran RL, Schibli H (1990) Permanent paresthesia to sculptured nails. A distressing problem. Dermatol Clin 8:139–141
Baran RL, Schoon D (1998) Cosmetics for abnormal and pathological nails. In: Baran R, Maibach HI (eds) Textbook of cosmetic dermatology. Martin Dunitz, London, pp 233–244

Belsito DV (1987) Contact dermatitis to ethyl-cyanoacrylate-containing glue. Contact Dermatitis 17:234–236

Bjorkner B (1995) Plastic materials. In: Rycroft RJG, Menne T, Frosch PJ (eds) Textbook of contact dermatitis, 2nd edn. Springer, Berlin Heidelberg New York, pp 539–572

Burrows D, Rycroft RJG (1981) Contact dermatitis from PTBP resin and tricresyl ethyl phthalate in a plastic nail adhesive. Contact Dermatitis 7:336–337

Canizares O (1956) Contact dermatitis due to the acrylic materials used in artificial nails. Arch Dermatol 74:141–143

Caravati EM, Litovitz TL (1988) Pediatric cyanide intoxication and death from an acetonitrile containing cosmetic. JAMA 260:3470–3473

Castelain M, Veyrat S, Laine G, Montastier C (1997) Contact dermatitis from nitrocelluose in nail varnish. Contact Dermatitis 36:266–267

Conde-Salazar L, Guimaraens D, Romero LV, et al (1986) Occupational allergic contact dermatitis to artificial nails. Contact Dermatitis 15:242

Draelos ZD (1995) Cosmetics in dermatology, 2nd edn. Churchill Livingstone, New York

Eiermann H (1981) Methacrylate nail builders. Fact sheet. Food and Drug Administration Division of Cosmetics Technology, Rockville

Engasser PG (1997) Nail cosmetics. In: Scher RK, Daniel CR III (eds) Nails: therapy, diagnosis, surgery, 2nd edn. Saunders, Philadelphia, pp 276–281

Fisher AA (1989) Permanent loss of fingernails due to allergic reaction to an acrylic nail preparation: a sixteen-year follow-up study. Cutis 43:404–406

Fisher AA (1990) Adverse nail reactions and paresthesia from "photobonded acrylate 'sculptured' nails". Cutis 45:293–294

Fisher AA, Baran RL (1991) Adverse reactions to acrylate sculptured nails with particular reference to prolonged parethesia. Am J Contact Dermat 2:38–42

Fisher AA, Frank A, Glicks A (1957) Allergic sensitization of the skin and nails to acrylic plastic nails. J Allergy 28:84–88

Fitzgerald DA, Bhaggoe R, English JSC (1995) Contact sensitivity to cyanoacrylate nail-adhesive with dermatitis at remote sites. Contact Dermatitis 32:175–176

Food and Drug Administration (1994) (HFS-565) Department of Health and Human Services,Washington, p 13

Freeman S, Lee M-S, Gudmundsen K (1995) Adverse contact reactions to sculptured nails: 4 case reports and a literature review. Contact Dermatitis 33:381–385

Goodwin P (1976) Onycholysis due to acrylic nail applications. Clin Exp Dermatol 1:191–192

Guin JD (2000) Eyelid dermatitis from benzophenone use in nail enhancement. Contact Dermatitis 43:308–309

Guin JD, Wilson P (1999) Onycholysis from nail lacquer: a complication of nail enhancement? Am J Contact Dermat 10:34–36

Guin JG, Baas K, Nelson-Adesokan P (1998) Contact sensitization to cyanoacrylate adhesive as a cause of severe onychodystrophy. Int J Dermatol 37:31–36

Hausen BM, Milbrodt M, Koenig WA (1995) The allergens of nail polish. I. Allergenic constituents of common nail polish and toluenesulfonamide-formaldehyde resin (TSFR). Contact Dermatitis 33:157–164

Hemmer W, Focke M, Wantke F, Gotz M, Jarish R (1996) Allergic contact dermatitis to artificial fingernails prepared from UV light-cured acrylates. J Am Acad Dermatol 35:377–380

Hiipakka D, Samimi B (1987) Exposure of acrylic fingernail sculptors to organic vapors and methacrylate dusts. Am Ind Hyg Assoc J 48:230–237

Jacobs MC, Rycroft RJG (1995) Allergic contact dermatitis from cyanoacrylate? Contact Dermatitis 33:71

Kanerva L, Lauerma A, Jolanki R, Estlander T (1995) Methyl acrylate: a new sensitizer in nail lacquer. Contact Dermatitis 33:203–204

Kanerva L, Lauerma A, Estlander T, Alanko K, Henriks-Eckerman M-L, Jolanki R (1996) Occupational allergic contact dermatitis caused by photobonded sculptured nails and a review of (meth)acrylates in nail cosmetics. Am J Contact Dermat 7:109–115

Koppula SV, Fellman JH, Storrs FJ (1995) Screening allergens for acrylate dermatitis associated with artificial nails. Am J Contact Dermat 6:78–85

Liden C, Berg M, Farm G, Wrangsjo K (1993) Nail varnish allergy with far-reaching consequences. Br J Dermatol 128:57–62

Lozewicz S, Davidson AG, Hopkirk A, et al (1985) Occupational asthma due to methyl methacrylate and cyanoacrylates. Thorax 40:836–839

Marks JG (1990) Cosmetics. In: Adams RM (ed) Occupational skin disease, 2nd edn. Saunders, Philadelphia pp 326–348

National Institute for Occupational Safety and Health (1999) Controlling chemical hazards during the application of artificial fingernails. Department of Health and Human Services, Washington, pp 99–112

Moffitt DL, Sansom JE (2001) Allergy to phthallic anhydride/trimellite/glycol copolymer, a component of nail varnish. Br J Derm 145 [Suppl 59]:100

Norton LA (1991) Common and uncommon reactions to formaldehyde-containing nail hardeners. Semin Dermatol10:29–33

Quenon S (1989) Artificial fingernail products: a guide to chemical exposures in the nail salon. California Department of Health Services, Berkeley

Sainio E-L, Engstrom K, Henriks-Eckerman ML, Kanerva L (1997) Allergenic ingredients in nail polishes. Contact Dermatitis 37:155–162

Schlossman ML (1979) Nail-enamel resins. Cosmet Tech 1:52–55

Schlossman ML (1980) Modern nail enamel technology. J Soc Cosmet Chem 31:29–36

Schlossman ML, Wimmer E (1992) Advances in nail enamel technology. J Soc Cosmet Chem 43:331–337

Schoon DD (1996) Milady's nail structure and product chemistry. Milady Publishing, Albany New York

Schoon D (1998) Nail varnish formulation. In: Baran R, Maibach HI (eds) Textbook of cosmetic dermatology, 2nd edn. Martin Dunitz, London, pp 213–218

Schubert HJ, Lindner K, Prater E (1992) Kontakallergie im Nagelstudio. Z Hautkr 67:1067–1069

Sood A, Taylor JS (2003) Acrylic nail reactions: Review of 56 cases. Am J Contact Dermat 14:113 (abstract as presented at the American Contact Dermatitis Annual Meeting 2003)

CHAPTER 42

Patch-Test Concentrations and Vehicles for Testing Contact Allergens

42

A. C. De Groot

Introduction

Patch testing is a sound, relatively safe and reasonably reliable method of identifying contact allergens in patients with allergic contact dermatitis. It has been clearly shown that patch testing is necessary in the majority of patient with eczema (Rycroft 1990). The technique of patch testing is described in Chaps. 16 and 17 (this book).

All patients are tested with the European or American standard series, containing the most frequent contact allergens. Often, standard series patch testing is not enough, and additional allergens or potential allergens need to be tested, based on the patient's history and clinical examination. Examples are products and chemicals to which the patient is exposed occupationally or in his home environment. Test series containing the most frequent allergens in certain products (preservatives, fragrances, dental materials, plastics and glues, medicaments) or in certain occupations (hairdressing, pesticides, oil and cooling fluid) are very helpful. Approximately 500 patch test materials are commercially available from Hermal, Chemotechnique Diagnostics and Brial Allergen GmbH.

Hermal	Chemotechnique Diagnostics	Brial GmbH
Scholtzstrasse 3	42 Tygelsjö. P.O. Box 80	Bövemannstrasse 8
D-21462 Reinbek	S-230, Malmö	D-48268 Greven
Deutschland	Sweden	Deutschland
Tel: +494072704266	Tel: +4640466077	Tel: +49257193970
Fax: +494072704317	Fax: +4640466700	Fax: +492571939720
E-mail: info@hermal.de	E-mail: info@chemotechnique.se	E-mail: info@brial.com
www.hermal.de	www.chemotechnique.se	www.brial.com

More detailed information on these test materials can be found in Niklasson (2000).

For other chemicals and products, the investigator must decide how to apply them as a patch test. Chemicals usually need to be diluted, and it is of the utmost importance to use an appropriate patch test concentration and vehicle to avoid both false-negative and false-positive (irritant) reactions. The most useful reference source for documented test concentrations and vehicles of chemicals, groups

Table 1. Test concentrations, vehicles and commercial availability of contact allergens

Allergen	Test concentration and vehicle	Supplier		
		Trolab	Chemo	Brial
Abietic acid	10% pet.	+		+
Abitol	*see* Hydroabietyl alcohol			
Acamelin	1% pet.			
Acebutolol hydrochloride	2% pet.			+
Acetaldehyde 2-phenyl-2,4-pentanediol acetal	*see* Floropal®			
Acetone	10% o.o.			
Acetylcedrene (Vertofix®)	1%–5% pet.			
5-Acetyl-1,1,2,3,3,6-hexamethylindan (Phantolide®)	3% pet.			
Acetylsalicylic acid	10% pet.			+
Achillea millefolium (yarrow extract)	1% pet.	+	+	
Acid red 14 (azorubine)				0.1% aq.
Acid yellow 36 (CI 13065, metanil yellow)	1% pet.	+	+	+
Acid yellow 61	5% pet.		+	
Acriflavine (ph)	0.1%–1% pet.			
Acrylamide (pts)	1% pet.			
Acrylated aliphatic polyurethane	0.1% pet.			
Acrylonitrile	0.1% pet.			
Alachlor	1% pet.			
Alantolactone (cu)	0.1% pet		+	
Albendazole (cu)	1%–5% pet.			
Alcohol, ethyl (cu)	10% aq. – pure			
Alimemazine tartrate	*see* Trimeprazine tartrate			
Allantoin	0.5% aq.			
Allopurinol	0.01% pet.			
Allyl glycidyl ether	0.05%–0.5% acet. or pet.			
Allyl isothiocyanate (mustard oil)	0.1% pet.			
Aloe vera	10% pet.			
Alprenolol	0.125%–0.25%–0.5%–1% aq.			
Aluminum			Pure	

Aluminum chloride hexahydrate	2% pet.		+	
Amalgam		5% pet.		
Amalgam alloying metals	20% pet.	+		+
Amalgam non gamma 2				5% pet.
Amaranth	0.1% aqua			+
Amcinonide	1% alc.	0.1% pet.		0.1% pet.
Amerchol® L 101	*See* Lanolin alcohol and paraffinum liquidum			
Amethocaine	*See* Tetracaine hydrochloride			
4-Aminoantipyrine	*see* Ampyrone			
p-Aminoazobenzene (solvent yellow 1, CI 11000)	0.25%–1% pet.	1% pet.	0.25% pet.	1% pet.
4-Amino-*α*-bromo-3,5-dichloroacetophenone	0.5% and 1% pet.			
p-Aminocyclohexylamine	1% pet.			
Amino-4-*N*,*N*-diethylaniline sulfate (TSS Agfa®)			1% pet.	
p-Aminodiphenylamine	*see* *N*-Phenyl-*p*-phenylenediamine			
Amino-4-*N*-ethyl-*N*-(methanesulfonaminoethyl)-*m*-toluidine (CD 3)	1%–2% pet.	1% pet.	1% pet.	
5[(2-Aminoethyl)thiomethyl]-*N*,*N*-dimethyl-2-furan-methanamine	1% aq.			
1,4-*bis*(Aminomethyl)-2,3,5,6-tetrafluorobenzene (TFX diamine)	0.01% pet.			
m-Aminophenol	1% pet.	+	+	+
p-Aminophenol (CI 76550) (cu)	1% pet.	+	+	+
2-Aminophenyl disulfide	1% alc.			
2-Aminothiophenol	0.001%–0.01%–0.1% pet.			
Ammoniated mercury	1% pet.	+	+	+
Ammonium bituminosulfonate	*see* Ichthammol			
Ammonium fluoride	2% pet.			
Ammonium heptamolybdate				1% aq.
Ammonium hexachloroplatinate (cu)	0.1% aq.		+	
Ammonium persulfate (cu)	2.5% pet.	+	+	+
Ammonium tetrachloroplatinate (cu)	0.25% aq.	0.25% pet.	+	0.25% pet.
Ammonium thioglycolate	1% pet.	+	2.5% aq.	+

A. C. De Groot

Table 1 (continued)

Allergen	Test concentration and vehicle	Supplier		
		Trolab	Chemo	Brial
Ampicillin (cu)	5% pet.			+
Ampyrone (4-aminoantipyrine)				10% pet.
α-Amylcinnamaldehyde (cu)	2%–5% pet.	1% pet.	2% pet.	1% pet.
α-Amylcinnamic alcohol	5% pet.			
Amyl cinnamate	8% pet.			
Amylocaine hydrochloride	5% pet.		+	
Amyl salicylate	5% pet.			
Anethole	2%–5% pet.		5% pet.	
Aniline	1% pet.			+
Aniline blue	5% pet.			
Anisyl alcohol (cu)	5% pet.			
Anisylidene acetone	2% pet.			
Anthemis nobilis (chamomilla romana)	1% pet.		+	
Anthotecol	1% pet.			
Anthraquinone (ph)	2% pet.			
Antimony chloride	2% pet.			
ANTU (α-naphthyl thiourea)	1% pet.			
Apomorphine	0.01%–1% aq.			
Arnica montana (arnica extract)	0.5% pet.	+	+	
Arsenate sodium	*see* Sodium arsenate			
Arsenic	1% pet.			
Aspartame	0.1% coca			+
Atranorin (ph)	0.5% pet.		0.1% pet.	
Atrazine	1% pet.			
Atropine sulfate	1% aq. or pet.	1% aq.		1% aq.
Avoparcin	1% aq.			
Azathioprine	0.1% and 1% pet.			
Azidamfenicol	2%–5% pet.			
Aziridine cross-linker Cx 100	0.1% aq.			
Azodiisobutyrodinitrile			1% pet.	

Substance				
Azorubine	*see* Acid red 14			
Bacitracin (cu)	5%–20% pet.	20% pet.	5% pet.	20% pet.
Balsam of Peru	*see* Myroxylon Pereirae			
Balsam of Tolu	*see* Myroxylon toluiferum			
Barban	1% pet.			
Basic brown 1	*see* Bismark Brown			
Basic red 46			1% pet.	
Beech tar	*see* Fagus sylvatica			
Befunolol			1% aq.	
Benomyl	0.1% pet.			
Benzaldehyde (cu)	5% pet.	+		+
Benzaldehyde glycol methacrylate	2% pet.			
Benzalkonium chloride (BAK)	0.01%–0.1% aq.	0.1% pet.	0.1% aq.	0.1% pet.
Benzethonium chloride	0.1% aq.			
Benzidine	1% pet.			
2-Benzimidazolethiol (2-mercaptobenzimidazole)				1% pet.
Benzisothiazolinone (BIT) (ph)	0.05%–0.1% pet.	0.1% pet.	0.05% pet.	0.5% pet.
Benzocaine (cu)	5% pet.	+	+	+
Benzoic acid (cu) (ph)			5% pet.	5% pet. and 1% alc.
Benzoin resin	*see* Styrax benzoin			
Benzoin tincture (cu)	10% alc.			
Benzophenone	1% pet.			
Benzophenone-3 (oxybenzone) (ph)	10% pet.	+	10% pet.	+
Benzophenone-4 (sulisobenzone) (ph)	10% pet.	+	10% pet.	+
Benzophenone-10 (mexenone) (ph)	10% pet.		10% pet.	
IH-Benzotriazole	1% pet.	+	+	+
Benzoxonium chloride	0.05% aq.			
Benzoyl peroxide (cu)	1% pet.	+	+	+
Benzydamine hydrochloride (ph)	0.5% aq.			
Benzyl acetate	5% pet.			
Benzyl alcohol (cu)	1%–10% pet.	1% pet.	1% pet.	1% pet.
Benzylamine	0.1% alc.			

Table 1 (continued)

Allergen	Test concentration and vehicle	Supplier		
		Trolab	Chemo	Brial
Benzyl-1-amino-3-chloro-2-hydroxypropane	0.1% alc.			
Benzyl benzoate (cu)	5% pet.			
o-Benzyl-p-chlorophenol	see Clorophene			
Benzyl cinnamate	5% pet.	5% pet.		
N-Benzyl-N,N-dihydroxyethyl-N-cocosalkyl ammonium chloride	0.01% aq.			
Benzylhemiformal	1% pet.	1% pet.		
Benzylidene acetone	0.5% pet.			
Benzylparaben			3% pet.	
1-Benzyl-5-phenylbarbiturate	0.5% pet.			
Benzyl salicylate	1%–5% pet.	1% pet.	2% pet.	1% pet.
Bergamot oil	see Citrus bergamia			
Beryllium chloride	1% pet.			
Beryllium sulfate	1% pet.			
Betamethasone-17-valerate	1% alc.	0.12% pet.	1% pet.	0.12% pet.
Betula alba (birch tar)			3% pet.	
BHA (butylated hydroxyanisole) (cu)	2% pet.	+	+	+ and 2% alc.
BHT (butylated hydroxytolune) (cu)	2% pet.	+	+	+ and 1% alc.
Bioban® CS-1135	1% pet.	+	+	+
Bioban® CS-1246	1% pet.	+	+	+
Bioban® P 1487	1% pet.	1% pet.	0.5% pet.	1% pet.
Biperiden	1% pet.			
Biphenyl dimethacrylate	2% pet.			
Birch tar	see Betula alba			
BIS-EMA	1% pet.		+	
BIS-GA	0.5% pet.			

Allergen	Patch-test concentration			
BIS-GMA	2% pet.	+	+	+
BIS-MA	2% pet.		+	
Bismarck Brown (vesuvine brown, basic brown 1, CI 21000)	0.5% pet.	+		+
Bisphenol A	*see* 4,4′-Isopropylidenediphenol			
Bisphenol A diglycidyl ether (DGEBA)	1% pet.			
Bisphenol A dimethacrylate				2% pet.
BIS-PMA	2% pet.			
Bithionol (ph)	1% pet.	+	+	+
Black rubber mix (*N*-isopropyl-*N*-phenyl-*p*-phenylenediamine, *N*-cyclohexyl-*N*-phenyl-*p*-phenylenediamine, *N*,*N*-diphenyl-*p*-phenylenediamine)			0.25% pet.	
Borax	*see* Sodium borate			
Brillaint black				0.1% aq.
Brilliant lake red R (D&C red 31, CI 15800) (ph)	1% pet.			
4-Bromoacetoacet-2,4-dimethylaniline	0.1% and 1% pet.			
1-Bromo-3-chloro-5,5-dimethylhydantoin	1% aq.			
Bromochlorophene	2% pet.			
5-Bromo-4′-chlorosalicylanilide (ph)		1% pet.		
4-Bromomethyl-6,8-dimethyl-2(1H)-quinolone	0.1% and 1% pet.			
α-Bromomethyl-*p*-tolysulfone	0.01% alc.			
5-Bromo-5-nitro-1,3-dioxane	0.5% pet.			
2-Bromo-2-nitropropane-1,3-diol (cu)	0.5% pet.	0.5% pet.	0.25% pet.	0.5% pet.
Budesonide	0.1% pet.	+	0.01% pet.	+
Bufexamac	5% pet.	+		+
Bumetanide	1% pet.			
Bupirimate	0.01%–1% pet.			
1,4-Butanediol diacrylate (BUDA)	0.1% pet.		+	
1,4-Butanediol dimethacrylate (BUDMA)	2% pet.	+	+	+
2,3-Butanedione	*see* Diacetyl			
Butoxyethyl-4-dimethyl aminobenzoate	10% pet.			
Butyl acetate	5%–25% o.o.			
Butyl acrylate (BA)	0.1% pet.		+	+
Butylated hydroxyanisole	*see* BHA			
Butylated hydroxytoluene	*see* BHT			

Table 1 (continued)

Allergen	Test concentration and vehicle	Supplier		
		Trolab	Chemo	Brial
5-Butyl barbiturate	0.5% pet.			
4-*tert*-Butylbenzoic acid			1% pet.	
p-tert-Butylcatechol (PTBC)	1% pet.	1% pet.	0.25% pet.	1% pet.
1,3-Butyleneglycol diacrylate	0.1% pet.			
t-Butyl hydroquinone	1% pet.	+	+	+
n-Butyl methacrylate (BMA)	2% pet.		+	
Butyl methoxydibenzoylmethane (ph)	5% pet.	10% pet.	10% pet.	10% pet.
p-tert-Butyl-α-methylhydrocinnamic aldehyde	*see* Lilial			
Butylparaben (cu)	3% pet.	+	+	+
p-tert-Butylphenol	1% pet.	+	+	+
p-tert-Butylphenol formaldehyde resin (PTBT)	1% pet.	+	+	+
Cacodylic acid	0.1% aq.			
Cadmium chloride (ph)	1% aq.		1% aq.	0.5% pet.
Caine mix I (procaine hydrochloride, dibucaine hydrochoride)			3.5% pet.	
Caine mix II (dibucaine hydrochloride, lidocaine, tetracaine)			10% pet.	
Caine mix III (benzocaine, dibucaine hydrochloride, amethocaine)	10% pet.		+	
Caine mix IV (amylocaine, lidocaine, prilocaine)	10% pet.		+	
Cajeputol	*see* Eucalyptol			
Camphor (cu)	10% pet.			1% pet.
Camphor oil	10% pet.			
Camphoroquinone	2% pet.		1% pet.	
Cananga odorata (cananga oil, ylang-ylang oil)	1%–5% pet.		2% pet.	
Capsicum oil	1% alc.			
Captafol®	*see* Difolatan			
Captan	0.5% aq.		0.5% pet.	
Captopril	10% pet.			
Carba mix (*N,N*-diphenylguanidine, zinc dibutyldithiocarbamate, zinc diethyldithiocarbamate)			3% pet.	

Substance				
Carbenicillin	20% pet.			
Carbimazole (ph)	10%–25%–50% pet.			
2(*p*-Carboxyphenol) 4,5 diphenylimidazole	as is (?);		1% pet.	
Cardamom oil	2% pet.			
Carnauba wax	50% pet.			
Carvacrol (isothymol)	5% pet.			
Cashew nut formaldehyde resin	1%–5% pet.			
Cashew nut shell oil	3% alc.			
Cashmeran (6,7-dihydro-1,1,2,3,3-pentamethyl-4(5H)-indanone)	5% pet.			
CD 2 (colour developer 2)	*see* Methyl-3-amino-4-*N,N*-diethyl-aniline			
CD 3 (colour developer 3)	*see* Amino-4-*N*-ethyl-*N*(methane-sulfon-aminoethyl)-*m*-toluidine			
CD 4 (colour developer 4)	*see* 4-(*N*-Ethyl-*N*-2-hydroxyethyl)-2-methylphenylenediamine sulfate			
Cedarwood oil	*see* Cedrus atlantica			
Cedramber (cedrol methyl ether)	5% pet.			
Cedrol methyl ether	*see* Cedramber			
Cedrus atlantica (cedarwood oil) (ph)	10% pet.	+		+
Cefamandole	5% aq.			
Cefazolin	1% and 5% aq.			
Ceftiofur	1% aq.			
Cellulase (cu)	3.3%, 1% and 0.33% in aq. and pet.			
Cephalotin	1% and 5% aq.			
Cephradine	20% pet.			
Cesium chloride	5% pet.			
Cetalkonium chloride	0.1% aq.			0.1% pet.
Cetrimonium bromide	0.01%–0.1% aq.			
Cetyl alcohol (cu)	5% pet.		+	
Cetyl alcohol, stearyl alcohol	20% pet.	+		+
Cetylpyridinium chloride	0.05% aq.	0.1% pet.		0.1% pet.
Chamomilla recutita (chamomile extract) (cu)		2.5% pet.		
Chamomilla romana	*see* Anthemis nobilis			

Table 1 (continued)

Allergen	Test concentration and vehicle	Supplier		
		Trolab	Chemo	Brial
Chinacridone B	1% pet.			
Chloramine-T (cu)	0.05% aq.			
Chloramphenicol (cu)	5% pet.	+	+	10% pet.
Chlorhexidine diacetate (cu) (ph)			0.5% aq.	
Chlorhexidine digluconate (cu) (ph)	0.5% aq.	+	+	+
Chloracetamide	0.2% pet.	+	+	+
T-Chloroacetophenone (pts)	0.1% alc.			
Bis-(4-Chlorobenzoyl) peroxide	1% pet.			
N-(a-Chlorobenzylidene)phenyl-hydrazine (pts)	0.01% acet.			
4-Chloro-5-chlorosulfonyl benzoic acid	1% pet.			
4-Chloro-5-chlorosulfonyl-3-nitro-benzoic acid	1% pet.			
p-Chloro-*m*-cresol (PCMC) (cu)	1% pet.	+	+	+
Chlorodiazepoxide	1% pet.			
1-(4-(2-Chloroethyl)phenyl)-2-chloro-ethanol	1% MEK			
4-Chloromethyl-2-guanidinothiazole-nitrochloride	1% aq.			
Chloromethyl imidazoline	0.001% and 0.0001% aq.			
Chloromethylisothiazolinone, methylisothiazolinone	0.01% aq.	+	+	+
5-Chloro-1-methyl-4-nitroimidazole	0.01%–0.1%–1%–10% pet.			
Chloro-*p*-nitroaniline red	2% pet.			
4-Chloro-7-nitrobenzofurazan	0.01%–0.05%–0.1% pet.			
4-Chloro-3-nitro-5-sulfonyl benzoic acid	1% pet.			
Bis-(4-Chlorophenyl)-methyl chloride	1% chloroform			
Chlorophorin	10% pet.			
Chloroquine (diphosphate) (ph)	1%–5% aq. or pet.			
Chlorothalonil (TCPN, tetrachloro-isophthalonitrile) (cu)	0.01% acet.			
Chlorothymol	1% aq.; 2% pet.			
5-(1-Chlorovinyl)-2,4-dichlorpyrimidine	1% aq.			
Chloroxylenol (PCMX)		1% pet.	0.5% pet.	1% pet.
Chlorpheniramine maleate	5% pet.			+
Chlorpromazine hydrochloride (cu) (ph)	0.1% pet.	+	+	1% pet.

Chlorquinaldol	5% pet.		+	+	+
Chromic chloride					1% pet.
Chromic oxide	25% aq.				
Chromic potassium sulfate					2% pet.
Chromic sulfate					0.5% pet.
Chromium trioxide	0.5% pet.				
Chromonar	1% aq.				
Chrysanthemum cinerariaefolium (pyrethrum) (cu)		1% pet.			
Chrysanthemum parthenium (feverfew flower extract)	1% pet.	+			
CI 11000	*see* p-Aminoazobenzene				
CI 10375	*see* Disperse yellow 9				
CI 11080	*see* Disperse orange 1				
CI 11005	*see* Disperse orange 3				
CI 11110	*see* Disperse red 1				
CI 11153	*see* Disperse brown 1				
CI 11210	*see* Disperse red 17				
CI 11370	*see* Disperse blue 85				
CI 11855	*see* Disperse yellow 3				
CI 12070	*see* Para red				
CI 13065	*see* Acid yellow 36				
CI 15585	*see* Pigment red 53, barium lake				
CI 15800	*see* Brilliant lake red R				
CI 21000	*see* Bismarck brown				
CI 21115	*see* Pigment orange 34				
CI 37505	*see* Napthol AS				
CI 61505	*see* Disperse blue 3				
CI 62015	*see* Disperse red 11				
CI 64500	*see* Disperse blue 1				
CI 68210	*see* Helio Red R				
CI 76550	*see* p-Aminophenol				
Cinchocaine®	*see* Dibucaine hydrochloride				
1,8-Cineole	*see* Eucalyptol				
Cinnamal (cinnamic aldehyde) (ph) (cu)	1% pet.		+	2% pet.	+
Cinnamic acid (cu)					5% pet.

Table 1 (continued)

Allergen	Test concentration and vehicle	Supplier		
		Trolab	Chemo	Brial
Cinnamonum cassia (cinnamon oil) (ph)	1% pet.			0.5% pet.
Cinnamyl alcohol (cu)	3%–5% pet.	1% pet.	2% pet.	1% pet.
Cinnamyl benzoate	5% pet.			
Cinnamyl cinnamate (cu)	5% pet.			
Cinoxate (ph)	1% pet.			
Cistoran	0.5% pet.			
Citral	2% pet.			
Citronellal				2% pet.
Citronella oil	1% pet.			
Citronellol	5% pet.			
Citrus aurantium dulcis (neroli oil) (ph)	2% pet.	+		+
Citrus bergamia (bergamot oil) (ph)				2% pet.
Citrus dulcis (orange oil) (ph)	2% pet.	+		
Citrus limonum (lemon oil) (ph)	2% pet.	+		+
Clenbuterol	0.5% pet.			
Clioquinol	5% pet.	+	+	+
Clobetasol-17-propionate (cu)	1% alc.	0.25% pet.	1% pet.	0.25% pet.
Clorophene (*o*-benzyl-*p*-chlorophenol)	1% pet.			
Clotrimazole	5% pet.; 1% alc.	5% pet.		5% pet.
Clove oil	*see* Eugenia caryophyllus			
Cloxacillin	1% and 20% pet.			
Coal tar	*see* Pix ex carbone			
Cobalt chloride (ph) (cu)	1% pet.	+	+	+
Cobaltous sulfate (ph)				2.5% pet.
Cocamide DEA	0.5% pet.	+	+	+
Cocamidopropyl betaine	1% aq.	+	+	+
Codeine	1%–10% alc.		Codeine phosphate hydro-chloride	1% aq. or pet.

Cold cream				pure
Coleon O	0.1% pet.			
Colistin	1,000,000 U/gr. pet.			
Colophonium (rosin) (ph) (cu)	20% pet.	+	+	+
Columbium chloride	2% pet.			
Compositae mix		5% pet.		
Congo red	2% pet.			
Copper acetylacetone	5% pet.			
Copper naphthenate	1% pet.			
Copper oxide	see Cupric oxide			
Copper sulfate	see Cupric sulfate			
Cordiachromes A and E	0.1% pet. (1%–10% pet.??)			
Corticosteroid mix (budesonide, tixocortol pivalate, hydrocortisone-17-butyrate)	2.1% pet.		+	
Costunolide			0.033% pet.	
Coumarin (ph)	5% pet.			1% pet.
Cresyl glycidyl ether	0.25% pet.	+		+
Cromoglycate sodium	see Cromolyn			
Cromolyn (cromoglycate sodium) (cu)	2% aq.			2% pet.
Cuminaldehyde	5% pet.			
Cupric oxide (copper oxide)			5% pet.	2% pet.
Cupric sulfate (copper sulfate) (cu)	1%–2% pet.		2% pet.	10% aq.
Cyanamide (pts at 5%)	0.1%–5% aq.			
Cyanocobalamine	10% pet.			
Cyclacet®	see Tricyclodecen-4-yl 8-acetate			
Cyclohexanone peroxide	0.5% pet. or acet.			
Cyclohexanone resin			1% pet.	
N-Cyclohexylbenzothiazyl sulfenamide (CBS)	1% pet.	+	+	+
N-Cyclohexyl-N-phenyl-p-phenylenediamine (CPPD)			1% pet.	
Cyclohexyl thiophthalimide	1% pet.	+	+	+
Cymbopogon Schoenanthus (lemon grass oil) (ph)	2% pet.	+		+
Cysteamine	0.5% pet.			
Cytarabine intermediate	0.1%–0.5%–1% aq.			

A.C. De Groot

Table 1 (continued)

Allergen	Test concentration and vehicle	Supplier		
		Trolab	Chemo	Brial
Cytosine arabinoside	0.1%–0.5% aq.			
Dandelion	*see* Taraxacum officinale			
Dapsone (4,4′-diaminodiphenyl sulfone)	1% pet.			
Dazomet	0.1% pet.			
D & C red 31	*see* Brilliant lake red R			
DD	1% acet.			
DDT	1% pet.			
Decamethylene dimethacrylate (DMDMA)	2% pet.			
1,10-Decanediol dimethacrylate	2% pet.			
Dehydroacetic acid	0.1% and 1% pet.			
Dehydrocostus lactone			0.033% pet.	
Dehydro-isoeugenol	test Cananga odorata			
Deoxylapachol	0.01% pet.			
Dequalinium chloride	0.01% aq.			
Dexamethasone				0.5% pet.
Dexamethasone 21-phosphate disodium salt			1% pet.	
Dexpanthenol	see Panthenol			
2-Diamino-ethylene-amino-thiazolyl-methylenethiourea dichloride	1% aq.			
Diacetyl (2,3-butanedione)	1% aq.			
Diallyl disulfide	1%–5% pet.		1% pet.	
2,4-Diamino-6-chloromethylpteridine hydrochloride	0.01%–0.1%–01% pet.			
4,4′-Diaminodiphenylmethane (DDM) (ph)	0.5% pet.	+	+	+
4,4′-Diaminodiphenyl sulfone	*see* Dapsone			
2-Diamino-ethylene-aminothiazolyl-methylene-urea dichloride	1% aq.			
2,4-Diaminophenol	2% pet.			
Diazolidinyl urea	2% pet.	+	+	+
Dibenzothiazyl disulfide (MBTS)	1% pet.	+	+	+

1,2-Dibromo-2,4-dicyanobutane	*see* Methyldibromo glutaronitrile			
Dibromopropamidine isethionate	5% pet.			
Dibucaine hydrochloride (Cinchocaine®) (ph)	5% pet.	+	+	+
bis(Dibutyldithiocarbamato) zinc	1% pet.	+		+
Dibutyl phthalate	5% pet.	+	+	+
Dibutylthiourea	1% pet.	+	+	+
3,4-Dicarbethoxyhexane-2,5-dione	0.01% acet.			
3,4-Dicarboxyhexane-2,5-dione	0.03%–0.1%–1% acet.			
Dichlorobenzyl alcohol	2% pet.			
Dichlorophene (ph)	1% pet.	0.5% pet.	+	0.5% pet.
2,6-Dichloropurine	1% pet.			
4,7-Dichloroquinoline	5% pet.			
Diclofenac sodium	1% pet.			5% pet.
Dicyclohexylcarbodiimide	0.1% acet. or pet.			
Dieldrin	1% pet.			
Diethanolamine	2% pet.	+		+
Diethyl-β-chloroethylamine	pure(?); (0.01% pet., open test)			
Diethylene glycol	2% aq.			
Diethyleneglycol diacrylate (DEGDA)	0.1% pet.		+	
Diethyleneglycol dimethacrylate	2% pet.			
Diethylenetriamine (DETA)	1% pet.	0.5% pet.	+	
Di-2-ethylhexyl phthalate (DEHP)	*see* Dioctyl phthalate			
Diethyl maleate	2% pet.			
N,N-Diethyl-p-phenylediamine	0.25% pet.			
Diethyl phthalate				5% pet.
Diethylthiourea	1% pet.		+	
Diffractaic acid (in oak moss)	1% pet.			
Difolatan (Captafol®)	0.1% pet.			
o-Diglycidyl phthalate	1% pet.			
Dihydrocoumarin	5% pet.			
6,7-Dihydro-1,1,2,3,4-pentamethyl-4(5H)-indanone	*see* Cashmeran			
4,4'-Dihydroxydiphenyl				0.1% pet.

Table 1 (continued)

Allergen	Test concentration and vehicle	Supplier		
		Trolab	Chemo	Brial
7,8-Dihydroxy-2,4,5-trimethoxyisoflavan	1% pet.			
1,3-Diiodo-2-hydroxypropane	see Iothion			
Diisopropyl carbodiimide	0.2% acet.			
2,6-Dimethoxybenzoquinone	10% pet.			
[R]-3,4-Dimethoxydalbergion	0.01% pet.			
N,N-Dimethylaminoethyl methacrylate			0.2% pet.	
3-Dimethylaminopropylamine			1% aq.	
Dimethylbenzyl carbinyl acetate (DMBCA)	3% pet.			
Dimethyl citraconate	10% pet.			
Dimethyl dihydroxyethylene urea	4.5% aq.		+	
2,2-Dimethyl-3-(3-methylphenyl)propanol	see Majantol			
Dimethylol dihydroxyethyleneurea			5% aq.	
Dimethylol propylene urea			5% aq.	
Dimethoxane (Dioxin®) (ph)	0.1%–1% pet.; 2.5% o.o.			
N,N'-Dimethyl-p-phenylenediamine	1% pet.	0.25% pet.		
Dimethyl phthalate	5% pet.	+		+
2,2-Dimethyl-1,3-propane diamine	2% pet.			
N,N-Dimethyl-p-toluidine	2% pet.	+	5% pet.	+
N,N-Di-β-naphthyl-p-phenylenediamine (DBNPD)			1% pet.	
2,4-Dinitrochlorobenzene (DNCB) (cu)	0.01%–0.1% aq. or acet.			
4,6-Dinitro-o-cresol (DNOC)	0.5% aq.			
2,4-Dinitroflurobenzene	10% aq.			
Dinitrophthalene	2% pet.			
Dinitrotoluene	2% pet.			
Dinocap	0.5% pet.			
Dioctyl phthalate (di-2-ethylhexyl phthalate)	5% pet.	5% pet.	2% pet.	5% pet.
Dioctyl trioctyl ethylenetriamine (Tego® diocto S)	1% pet.			
Dioxane	1% aq.			

3,6-Dioxaoctamethylene dimethacrylate	2% pet.			
Dioxin®	*see* Dimethoxane			
Dipentamethylenethiuram disulfide		0.25% pet.	1% pet.	0.25% pet.
Dipentamethylenethiuram tetrasulfide				0.25% pet.
Dipentene (d-limonene)		2% pet.	1% pet.	2% pet.
Diphencyprone	*see* Diphenylcyclopropenone			
Diphenhydramine hydrochloride (ph)	1% pet.		+	
Diphenylcyclopropenone (diphencyprone) (cu) (pts)	0.01% acet.			
1,3-Diphenylguanidine (DPG) (cu)	1% pet.	+	+	+
Diphenylmethane 4,4-diisocyanate (MDI)	1%–2% pet.	1% pet.	2% pet.	1% pet.
Diphenyloxazole	2% MEK			
N,N'-Diphenyl-*p*-phenylenediamine (DPPD)	1% pet.	0.25% pet.	1% pet.	0.25% pet.
Diphenylthiourea (DPTU)	1% pet.	+	+	+
Dipyrone (metimazol) (cu)	10% pet.			1% pet.
Disodium EDTA (edetic acid disodium salt)	1% pet.	+	+	+
Disperse blue 1 (CI 64500)	1% pet.	+		+
Disperse blue 3 (CI 61505)	1% pet.	+	+	+
Disperse blue 35 (ph)	1% pet.		+	
Disperse blue 85 (CI 11370)	1% pet.		+	
Disperse blue 106	1% pet.		+	
Disperse blue 124	1% pet.		+	
Disperse blue 153	1% pet.		+	
Disperse blue mix (124/106)	1% pet.	+		
Disperse brown 1 (CI 11153)	1% pet.		+	
Disperse orange 1 (CI 11080)	1% pet.		+	
Disperse orange 3 (CI 11005)	1% pet.	+	+	+
Disperse orange 13	1% pet.		+	
Disperse red 1 (CI 11110)	1% pet.	+	+	+
Disperse red 11(CI 62015)	1% pet.	+		+
Disperse red 17 (CI 11210)	1% pet.	+	+	+
Disperse yellow 3 (CI 11855)	1% pet.	+	+	+
Disperse yellow 9 (CI 10375)	1% pet.	+	+	+
Dithianone	1% pet.			
Diurethane dimethacrylate		2% pet.		

Table 1 (continued)

Allergen	Test concentration and vehicle	Supplier		
		Trolab	Chemo	Brial
DMDM hydantoin	2% aq.	+	+	+
1,12-Dodecanediol dimethacrylate	2% pet.			
Dodecyldi(aminoethyl)glycine (DDAG)	0.1%–1% aq.			
Dodecyl dimethyl ammonium chloride	0.01%–0.1% aq.			
Dodecyl gallate (lauryl gallate)	0.1%–0.25%pet.	0.3% pet.	0.25% pet.	0.3% pet.
Dodecyl mercaptan	0.1% pet.		+	+
Dodecyl succinyl anhydride	0.5% acet.			
Domiphen bromide	0.01% aq.			
Doxycycline	10% pet.			
Drometrizole (2-(2'-hydroxy-5'-methylphenyl) benzotriazole)	1% pet.		+	
Econazole nitrate	1% alc.		+	
Edetic acid disodium salt	*see* Disodium EDTA			
Eosine (ph)	50% pet.			+
Epichlorohydrin	0.001% aq.; 0.1% pet.		0.1% pet.	
Epoxy acrylate	0.5%–1% pet.		0.5% pet.	
Epoxylated epoxy oligomer	1% pet.			
Epoxypropyl trimethyl ammonium chloride	0.2%–0.5% pet.			
Epoxy resin (cu)	1% pet.	+	+	+
Epoxy resin, cycloaliphatic	0.5% pet.		+	
Erythromycin (base and salts)	1% pet.	+		+
Erythrosine (ph)				0.25% pet. and alc.
Estrontium chloride	2% pet.			
Ethacridine (ph)	1%–2% pet.			
Ethanolamine (monoethanolamine)	2% pet.	+		+
Ethoxylated acrylate	0.1% acet.			
Ethoxymethylenemalonitrile	0.01% pet.			
Ethoxyquin (ph)	0.5% pet.		+	
Ethyl acetate	10% pet.			

Allergen				
Ethyl-5-acetoxy-6-bromo-2-(bromomethyl)-1-methyl indole-3-carboxylate	0.1% pet.			
Ethyl acrylate (EA)	0.1% pet.		+	
Ethyl alcohol	10% aq. – pure			
Ethyl anisate	4% pet.			
Ethyl-2-bromo-*p*-methoxyphenyl acetate	0.01%–0.1%–1%–10% alc.			
Ethyl chlorooximido acetate	0.1% pet.			
Ethyl cyanoacrylate	2%–10% pet.		10% pet.	
Ethylenediamine dihydrochloride (cu) (ph)	1% pet.	+	+	+
Ethylene glycol	2.5% aq.			
Ethyleneglycol diglycidyl ether	0.25% pet.			
Ethyleneglycol dimethacrylate (EGDMA)	2% pet.	+	+	+
Ethylene glycol dinitrate	0.1%–0.5% pet.			
Ethylene urea	*see* 2-Imidazolidinone			
Ethyleneurea + melamineformaldehyde			5% pet.	
Ethyl ethoxymethylene cyanoacetate	0.01% pet.			
2-Ethylhexyl acrylate (EHA)	0.1% pet.		+	+
2-Ethylhexyl-*p*-dimethylaminobenzoate	*see* Octyl dimethyl PABA			
2-Ethylhexyl-*p*-methoxycinnamate	*see* Octyl methoxcinnamate			
Bis-(2-Ethylhexyl)phthalate	5% pet.			+
4-(*N*-Ethyl-*N*-2-hydroxyethyl)-2-methyl-phenylenediamine sulfate (CD 4)	1% pet.	+	+	
Ethyl methacrylate (EMA)	2% pet.		+	
Ethylparaben (cu)	3% pet.	+	+	+
N-Ethyl-4-toluenesulfonamide	0.1% alc.		0.1% pet.	
Eucalyptol (1,8-cineole, cajeputol)	5% pet.			
Eucalyptus globulus (eucalyptus oil)	1%–2% pet.	2% pet.	2% pet.	2% pet.
Eucerin, anhydrous (lanolin)	Pure			+
Eugenia caryophyllus (clove oil)	2% pet.	+		+
Eugenol (cu) (ph)	3%–5% pet.	1% pet.	2% pet.	1% pet.
Euxyl® K 400	1% pet.	+	1.5% pet.	+
Evernia prunastri (oak moss absolute) (ph)	3%–5% pet.	1% pet.	2% pet.	2% pet.
Evernic acid (ph)	0.1%–1% pet. or 0.1% acet.		0.1% pet.	
Fagus sylvatica (beech tar)			3% pet.	

Table 1 (continued)

Allergen	Test concentration and vehicle	Supplier		
		Trolab	Chemo	Brial
Falcarinol	0.1% pet.			
Famotidine	1% aq.			
Farnesol	5% pet.			
Fentichlor (ph)	1% pet.		+	
Fenticonazole	1% alc.			
Ferric chloride	2% pet.			
Ferrous chloride				2% alc.
Ferrous sulfate				5% pet.
Feverfew flower extract	*see* Chrysanthemum parthenium			
Fixolide	3% pet.			
Floropal® (acetaldehyde 2-phenyl-2,4-pentanediol acetal)	5% pet.			
Fluazinam	0.5% pet.			
Folpet	0.1% pet.			
Formaldehyde (ph) (cu)	1% aq.	+	+	1% pet.
Formic acid				1% aq.
Fragrance mix (ph) (cinnamic alcohol, cinnamal, hydroxy-citronellal, α-amyl-cinnamaldehyde, geraniol, eugenol, isoeugenol, oakmoss absolute)	8% pet.	+	+	+
Frullanolide (pts)	0.1% pet.			
Fumarprotocetraric acid	0.1% pet.			
Fusidic acid sodium salt	2% pet.	+	+	+
Galaxolide®	*see* 1,3,4,6,7,8-Hexahydro-4,6,6,7,8,8-hexamethylcyclopenta-γ-2-benzopyran			
Galbanum resin	2% pet.			
Gallium chloride	5% pet.			
Gallium oxide				1% pet.
Gentamicin sulfate (cu)	20% pet.	+	+	+
Gentian violet (cu)	2% aq.			

Geranial	1%–5% pet.			
Geraniol (cu)	3%–5% pet.	1% pet.	2% pet.	1% pet.
Geranyl geranylhydroquinone (pts)	0.5% pet.			
Geranyl hydroquinone (pts)	0.5% pet.			
Geranium oil, Bourbon			2% pet.	
Ginger oil (ph)	4% pet.			
Glutaral	0.2%–0.3% pet.	0.3% pet.	0.2% pet.	0.3% pet.
Glycerylphosphate dimethacrylate	2% pet.			
Glyceryl thioglycolate	1% pet.	+	+	+
Glyceryl triacetate	1% and 10% alc.			
Glycidyl methacrylate	0.1% pet.			
4-Glycidyloxy-*N,N*-diglycidylaniline (GDODGA)	1% pet.			
Glyoxal	1% pet./aq.; 2% aq.	1% pet.		1% pet.
Gold sodium thiomalate	0.1%–5% pet.			
Gold sodium thiosulfate	0.5% pet.	0.25% pet.	0.5% pet. and 2% aq.	
Grapeseed oil	Pure			
Grevillol	0.1% pet.			
Grotan® BK	*see* 1,3,5-Tris (2-hydroxyethyl)-hexahydro-triazine			
Grotan® OD	*see* Methylene-*bis*-oxazolidine			
Guanine	Pure			
Gum arabic	50% aq.			
Helional (*a*-methyl-3,4-methylene dioxy-hydrocinnamic aldehyde)	5% pet.			
Helio Red R (CI 68210)	2% pet.			
Heliotropin	5% pet.			
Hexachlorophene (ph)	1% pet	+	+	+ and 0.5% pet.
1,3,4,6,7,8-Hexahydro-4,6,6,7,8,8-hexamethylcyclopenta-*y*-2-benzopyran (Galaxolide®)	15% pet.			
Hexamethylene diisocyanate (HDI)	0.1% pet.		+	

Table 1 (continued)

Allergen	Test concentration and vehicle	Supplier		
		Trolab	Chemo	Brial
Hexamethylenetetramine	*see* Methenamine			
Hexamidine isethionate (cu) (ph)	0.15% aq.			
1,6-Hexanediol diacrylate (HDDA, HDODA)	0.1% pet.		+	
Hexanitrodiphenylamine	0.1% pet.			
Hexantriol (cu)	5% aq.			
cis-3-Hexenyl salicylate	3% pet.			
Hexetidine	0.1% pet.			
α-Hexylcinnamic aldehyde	10% pet.			
Hexylresorcinol	0.1%–0.25% pet.	0.25% pet.		0.25% pet.
Hexyl salicylate	12% pet.			
Homosalate (ph)	5% pet.		+	
Hyacinthin	*see* Phenylacetaldehyde			
Hydrangenol	0.1% pet.			
Hydrazine (sulfate)	1% pet.		+	+
Hydroabietyl alcohol (abitol)	1%–10% pet.	1% pet.	10% pet.	
Hydrochlorothiazide (ph)	1%–20% pet.			
Hydrocortisone (ph)	1% alc./pet.	1% pet.		1% pet.
Hydrocortisone-17-butyrate	1% alc.	0.1% pet.	+	0.1% pet.
Hydrogen peroxide			3% aq.	
Hydroquinone (HQ)	1% pet.	+	+	+
Hydroquinone monobenzylether	*see* Monobenzone			
Hydroquinone monomethyl ether (HQME)	2% pet.			
Hydroxycitronellal (ph)	2%–5% pet.	1% pet.	2% pet.	1% pet.
2-Hydroxyethyl acrylate (2-HEA)	0.1% pet.		+	+
2-Hydroxyethyl methacrylate (HEMA)	2% pet.	1% pet.	+	0.1% and 1% pet.
Hydroxylamine sulfate	0.1% aq.			
Hydroxylammonium chrloride	0.1% aq.		+	
Hydroxylammonium sulfate	0.1% aq.		+	

2-Hydroxymethyl-2-nitro-1,3-propanediol		1% pet.		1% pet.
2-(2′-Hydroxy-5′-methylphenyl)benzotriazole	*see* Drometrizole			
N-Hydroxyphthalimide	0.001%–0.1% alc.			
2-Hydroxypropyl acrylate (HPA)	0.1% pet.		+	
2-Hydroxypropyl methacrylate (HPMA)	2% pet.		+	+
Hypericum perforatum (hypericum oil)				0.5% pet.
Ichthammol (ammonium bituminosulfonate)	10% pet.			+
Idoxuridine	1% pet.		+	+
2-Imidazolidinone (ethylene urea)			1% pet.	
Imidazolidinyl urea	2% pet.	+	+	+
Indigo (blue)	5% pet.			
Indium chloride	5% pet.			1% pet.
Indomethacin	5% pet.			1% pet.
Iodine (cu)	0.5% alc.			0.5% pet.
Iodoform	5% pet.			
Iodopropynyl butyl carbamate			0.1% pet.	
Ionone	8% pet.			
Iothion (1,3-diiodo-2-hydroxypropane) (cu)	0.05% alc.			
Irgalite Orange F2G	*see* Pigment orange 34			
Iridium chloride (cu)	1% pet.			
Isoamyl-*p*-methoxycinnamate (ph)	10% pet.	+		+
Isobornyl cyclohexanol (synthetic sandalwood)	2% pet.	*see also* Sandela		
Isobutyl methacrylate	2% pet.			
3-*trans*-Isocamphyl cyclohexanol	*see* Sandela			
Iso E Super®	*see* 1,1,6,7-Tetramethyl-6-acetyl decalene (isomers)			
Isoeugeol	3%–5% pet.	1% pet.	2% pet.	1% pet.
Isoniazid	2.5% aq.			
Isophorone diamine (IPD) (cu)	0.1% pet.	0.5% pet.	0.1% pet.	0.5% pet.
Isophorone diisocyanate (IPDI)			1% pet.	
Isopropyl alcohol (cu)	5%–10% aq.; 1% alc.			
Isopropyl dibenzoylmethane (cu) (ph)				10% pet.

Table 1 (continued)

Allergen	Test concentration and vehicle	Supplier		
		Trolab	Chemo	Brial
4,4'-Isopropylidenediphenol (bisphenol A)	1% pet.	+	+	+
Isopropyl myristate		10% pet.	20% pet.	10% pet.
N-Isopropyl-N'-phenyl-p-phenylenediamine (IPPD)	0.1% pet.	+	+	+
Isopulegol	5% pet.			
Isothymol	see Carvacrol			
Jasminum officinale (jasmine absolute, synthetic)	5%–10% pet.		2% pet.	
Jojoba oil	20% o.o.			
Juniperus (juniper tar)			3% pet.	
Kanamycin sulfate	10% pet.	+	+	+
Ketoprofen (ph)	2.5%–5% pet.			
Kitasamycin (leukomycin)	Pure			
Kitasamycin tartrate (leukomycin tartrate)	4% aq.			
Lanolin				30% pet.
Lanolin alcohol (wool alchols) (cu)	30% pet.	+	+	+
Lanolin alcohol and paraffinum liqidum (Amerchol® L 101) (cu)	50% pet.	+	+	+
Lake Red C	see Pigment red 53			
Lapachol	1% pet.			
Laurus nobilis (laurel oil)	2% pet.	+		+
Lauryl gallate	see Dodecyl gallate			
Lavandula angustifolia (lavender, absolute, lavender oil) (ph)			2% pet.	
Lemon grass oil	see Cymbopogon Schoenanthus			
Lemon oil	see Citrus limonum			
Leukomycins	see Kitasamycin (tartrate)			
Levobunolol hydrochloride			1% aq.	
Lichen acid mix (atranorin, evernic acid, usnic acid)			0.3% pet.	
Lidocaine hydrochloride (cu)	5% pet.	15% pet.	+	15% pet.
Ligustral (methyl-(2,4(3,5)-dimethyl-3-cyclohexen-1-yl)-methylene anthranilate)	5% pet.			

Lilial (lily aldehyde, *p-tert*-butyl-α-methylhydrocinnamic aldehyde)	5% pet.			
Lily aldehyde	*see* Lilial			
D-Limonene	*see* Dipentene			
Linalool	2%–30% pet.			
Lindane (cu)	1% pet.			
Linseed oil acrylates	1% pet.			
Lyral	5% pet.			
Lysergol	7% alc.			
Macassar quinone	1% pet.			
Mafenide	10% pet.			+
Magnesium chloride	5% pet.			
Majantol (2,2-dimethyl-3-(3-methylphenyl)-propanol)	5% pet.			
Malathion	0.5% pet.			
Maltol	1% pet.			
Mancozeb	1% pet.			
Maneb (ph)	0.5% pet.			
Manganese chloride	5% pet.			
Mansonone A	0.1% pet.			
Mansonone X	3% pet.			
Mechlorethamine hydrochloride (cu)	0.02% aq.			
Mecillinam	1% and 10% pet.			
Melacacidin	1% pet.			
Melaleuca alternifolia (tea tree oil)	1% pet.		5% pet.	
Melamine formaldehyde resin			7% pet.	
Menadiol (vitamin K4)	0.1% o.o.			
Menadione (vitamin K3)	0.1% o.o.			
Mentha piperitia (peppermint oil) (cu)	1%–2% pet.	2% pet.		2% pet.
Menthol (cu)	1%–2% pet.	1% pet.	2% pet.	1% pet.
Mepivacaine	1% pet.			+
Merbromin (mercurochrome) (cu)	0.1%–2% aq.; 2% pet.			
2-Mercaptobenzimidazole	*see* 2-Benzimidazolethiol			
Mercaptobenzothiazole (MBT) (cu)	2% pet.	+	+	+

Table 1 (continued)

Allergen	Test concentration and vehicle	Supplier		
		Trolab	Chemo	Brial
2-Mercaptoethane sulfonate	0.1%–20% aq.			
Mercapto mix (mercaptobenzothiazole, dibenzothiazyl disulfide, morpholinyl mercaptobenzothiazole, *N*-cyclohexyl-benzothiazyl sufenamide)		1% pet.	2% pet.	1% pet.
Mercuric chloride	0.1%–0.5% pet.		0.1% pet.	
Mercurochrome	*see* Merbromin			
Mercury	0.5%–1% pet.		0.5% pet.	0.5% pet.
Mesna	1% aq.			
Metanil yellow	*see* Acid yellow 36			
Metaproterenol	2.5% aq.			
Methacrylic acid	2% pet.			
Methacycline	10% pet.			
Methenamine (hexamethylenetetramine)		1% pet.	2% pet.	1% pet.
Methotrexate	0.1% pet.			
o-Methoxycinnamic aldehyde	4% pet.			
Methoxycitronellal	10% pet.			
[R]-4-Methoxydalbergion	1% pet.			
10-*α*-Methoxy-dihydrolysergol	7% alc.			
4-Methoxyphenol	2% pet.			
1-Methylamine-1-methylthio-2-nitro-ethylene	0.5% and 1% pet.			
Methyl-3-amino-4-*N*,*N*-diethyl-aniline (CD 2)		1% pet.	1% pet.	
p-Methylaminophenol sulfate (Metol®)		1% pet.	1% pet.	
3-Methylaminopropylamine	1% aq. or pet.			
Methyl anisate	4% pet.			
Methyl anthranilate (ph)	5% pet.		+	
4-Methylbenzylidene camphor (ph)	10% pet.	+	10% pet.	+
3-Methyl-2-butenyl caffeate	0.1% pet.			
Methylchloroisothiazolinone, methyl-isothiazolinone (cu)	0.01% aq.	+	+ and 0.02% aq.	+
Methylcoumarin (6-MC) (ph)	1% alc.		1% pet.	

Allergen	Vehicle			
Methyldibromo glutaronitrile (1,2-dibromo-2,4-dicyanobutane)	0.5% pet.	0.3% pet.	0.3% pet.	1% pet.
Methyldichlorobenzene sulfonate	0.1% pet. or alc.			
Methyl diisocyanate (MDI)	1% pet.			
Methyl-(2,4(3,5)-dimethyl-3-cyclohexen-1-yl)-methylene anthranilate	see Ligustral			
N,N-Methylenebisacrylamid (MBAA)	1% pet.		+	
Methylene-bis(methyloxazolidine)		1% pet.		
Methylene-bis-oxazolidine (Grotan® OD)	1% pet.			
α-Methylene-γ-butyrolactone (tulipaline)	0.01% pet.		+	
Methyl 2,3 epoxy-3-(4-methoxyphenyl)-propionate	1% alc.			
Methyl ethyl ketone (cu)	Pure			
Methyl ethyl ketone peroxide	1% pet.			
Methyl heptine carbonate	0.5% pet; 1% MEK			
Methylhydroquinone (MHQ)			1% pet.	
2-(4(5)-Methyl-5(4)-imidazolylmethylthio)-C13	0.1% and 1% aq. or pet.			
Methylionone (cu)	10% pet.			
Methyl methacrylate (MMA)	2% pet.	+	+	+
1N-Methyl-10-α-methoxy dihydrolysergol	7% alc.			
trans-Methyl-3-(4-methoxyphenyl)-glycidate	0.5%–1%–10% pet.			
α-Methyl-3,4-methylene dioxyhydrocinnamic aldehyde	see Helional			
N-Methyl-N-nitroso-p-toluenesulfonamide	0.01% pet.			
Methyl octine carbonate	1% MEK			
N-Methylochlorocetamide			0.1% pet.	
Methyl orange	2% pet.			
Methylparaben (cu)	3% pet.	+	+	+
Methyl-ter-pyridine	0.01% acet.			
1-Methylquinoxalinium-p-toluene sulfonate	1% aq.			
Methyl salicylate (oil of wintergreen) (cu)	2% pet.			+
2-Methyl-4,5-trimethylene-4-isothiazolin-3-one	0.01% aq.			
Methyl violet				0.5% pet.
Metol®	see p-Methylaminophenol sulfate			
Metopropol			3% aq.	
Metronidazole	1% pet.			+

Table 1 (continued)

Allergen	Test concentration and vehicle	Supplier		
		Trolab	Chemo	Brial
Mexenone	*see* Benzophenone-10			
Miconazole nitrate	1% alc.		+	
Midecamycin	Pure			
Minoxidil (ph)	2% aq.			
Monobenzone (monobenzylether of hydroquinone)	1% pet.		+	+
Monobenzylether of hydroquinone	*see* Monobenzone			
Monoethanolamine	*see* Ethanolamine			
2-Monomethylol phenol			1% pet.	
Morantel	1% and 5% pet.			
Morantel tartrate	1% pet.			
Morphine	1% alc.			
Morpholinyl mercaptobenzothiazole (MOR) (cu)		0.5% pet.	1% pet.	1% pet.
Musk ambrette (ph)	5% pet.	+		+
Musk ketone (ph)			1% pet.	
Musk mix (xylene, moskene, ketone)			3% pet.	
Musk moskene (ph)			1% pet.	
Musk xylene (ph)	5% pet.		1% pet.	
Mustard oil	*see* Allyl isothiocyanate			
Myristyl alcohol	5% pet.			
Myroxylon Pereirae (balsam of Peru) (cu) (ph)	25% pet.	+	+	+
Myroxylon toluiferum (balsam of Tolu)		20% pet.	10% alc.	20% pet.
Myrrh (cu)	10% pet.			
Naled	1% pet.			
1- and 2-Naphthol	0.1% pet.; 5% o.o.			
Naphthol AS (CI 37505)	5% aq.; 0.01% pet.	1% pet.		1% pet.
Naphthylaminoazobenzol (Sudan brown)	2% pet.			
α-Naphthylisothiocyanate	0.01% acet.			
Naphthyl mix (*N,N*-di-*β*-naphthyl-*p*-phenylenediamine, *N*-phenyl-2-naphthylamine)			1% pet.	
α-Naphthylthiourea (ANTU)	1% pet.			

Narcissus jonquilla (absolute)			2% pet.	
Narcissus oil	2% pet.			
Neomycin sulfate (cu)	20% pet.	+	+	+
Neral	2% pet.			
Neroli oil	*see* Citrus aurantium dulcis			
Nicergoline	7% alc.			
Nickel sulfate	5% pet.	+	+	+
Nicotine	1%–2% aq. or alc.			
Nicotine sulfate (cu)	5% aq.			
Nigrosine	1% pet.		+	
Nitramine (Tetryl®)	0.1% pet.			
p-Nitroacetamidoacetophenone	1% alc.			
p-Nitroacetamidohydroxypropiophenone	0.5% alc.			
p-Nitroaminoacetophenone	1% MEK			
p-Nitrobenzoyl chloride	1% and 3% pet.			
p-Nitrobenzyl bromide	0.001% pet.			
p-Nitrobromacetophenone	0.1% alc.			
Nitrocellulose	10% isopropyl alc.			
Nitrofurazone	1% pet.		+	+
Nitroglycerin (cu)	2% pet.; 0.02% aq.			
4-Nitrophenyl-*N*-(2-chloroethyl)carbamate	0.0001%–0.001%–0.01% acet. or aq.			
4-Nitrophenyl-*N*-(2-chloroethyl)-*N*-nitrosocarbamate	0.001% and 0.01% acet or aq.			
2-Nitro-*p*-phenylenediamine (ONPPD)	1% pet.		+	+
Nitrosourea	0.001% aq.			
Nopyl acetate	10% pet.			
Nystatin	2% pet.	+		+
Oak moss absolute	*see* Evernia prunastri			
Obtusaquinone	1% and 10% pet.			
Octyl dimethyl PABA (2-ethylhexyl-*p*-dimethylaminobenzoate) (ph)	5%–10% pet.	10% pet.	10% pet.	10% pet.
Octyl gallate	0.25% pet.	0.3% pet.	0.25% pet.	0.3% pet.
Octylisothiazolinone	0.025%–0.1% pet.	0.025% pet.	0.1% pet.	
Octyl methoxycinnamate (2-ethylhexyl-*p*-methoxycinnamate) (ph)	10% pet.	+	10% pet.	+

Table 1 (continued)

Allergen	Test concentration and vehicle	Supplier		
		Trolab	Chemo	Brial
Octyl salicylate (ph)	5% pet.			
Oil of wintergreen	see Methyl salicylate			
Olaquindox (ph)		1% pet.		
Olea Europeae (olive oil)	Pure			+
Oleamidopropyl dimethylamine				0.1% aq.
Oligotriacrylate 480	0.1% pet.			+
Olive oil	see Olea Europeae			
Omeprazole	0.25%–1% pet.; 0.1%–1% alc.			
Orange oil	see Citrus dulcis			
Oxolamine (tannate)	0.1% and 0.5% aq. + alc.			
Oxprenolol hydrochloride	1% pet.			
Oxyayanin A and B	1% pet.			
Oxybenone	see Benzophenone-3			
Oxyphenbutazone	1%–5% pet.			10% pet.
Oxytetracycline	3%–10% pet.	3% pet.		3% pet.
PABA (ph)	5%–10% pet.; 5% alc.	10% pet.	10% pet.	10% pet.
Palladium chloride	1.5% pet.	1% pet.	2% pet.	1% pet.
Panthenol (dexpanthenol)	50% aq.	5% pet.		5% pet.
Papain	1% pet.			+
Paraben mix (butyl, ethyl, methyl, propyl-paraben) (cu)		16% pet.	16% pet.	16% pet.
Paracetamol				10% pet.
Paraquat	0.1% pet.			
Para red (CI 12070)	2% pet.			
Parathion	1% alc.			
Paromomycin	20% pet.			
Parthenolide			0.1% pet.	
Patchouli oil	2% pet.			
Patent blue VF				0.25% coca

PBA-1 (persulfate bleach accelerator)	0.1% aq. or pet.			
Pectin				1% coca
PEG 6 (and) PEG 32 (polyethylene glycol ointment)	Pure	+		+
PEG 400				Pure
Penicillin G (cu)	3.000.000 U/gr. pet.; 1% and 10% pet.			
Penicillin V	1% and 10% pet.			
Pentachloronitrobenzene (PNCB)	1% pet.			
Pentachlorophenol (PCP) (cu)	1% pet. or aq.			
Pentadecyl resorcinol	0.1% pet.			
Pentaerythritol triacrylate (PETA)	0.1% pet.		+	
Peppermint oil	*see* Mentha piperita			
Perphenazine (ph)	0.01% pet.			
Petrolatum, white	Pure	+	+	+
Phantolide®	*see* 5-Acetyl-1,1,2,3,3,6-hexamethylindan			
Phenacetin				10% pet.
Phenazone	*see* Antipyrine			
Phenidone®	*see* 1-Phenyl-3-pyrazolidinone			
Phenol (cu)	0.5%–1% aq.			
Phenol formaldehyde resin (P-F-R-2)	1%–10% pet.	5% pet.	1% pet.	5% pet.
Phenolphthalein				0.5% pet.
Phenoxybenzamine	1% aq.			
Phenoxyethanol	1% pet.	+	+	+
Phenylacetaldehyde (hyacinthin)	0.5% pet.			
Phenylbenzimidazol sulfonic acid (ph)	10% pet.	+	+	+
Phenylbutazone (cu)	1%–5% pet.			10% pet.
Phenyldichloroarsine	0.1% alc., open test			
p-Phenylenediamine free base (cu) (ph)	1% pet.	+	+	+
Phenylephrine hydrochloride	10% aq.	+		10% coca
Phenylethyl alcohol	5% pet.			
Phenyl glycidyl ether (pts)	0.25% pet.		0.25% pet.	
Phenylhydrazine	2% pet.			
a-Phenylindole			2% pet.	
Phenyl isocyanate				0.1% pet.
Phenylmercuric acetate (cu)	0.01% aq.; 0.05% pet.	0.05% pet.	0.01% aq.	0.05% pet.

Table 1 (continued)

Allergen	Test concentration and vehicle	Supplier		
		Trolab	Chemo	Brial
Phenylmercuric borate	0.05% pet.			
Phenylmercuric nitrate (cu)	0.01%–0.05% pet.			0.01% pet.
Phenyl-β-naphthylamine (PBN)	1% pet.	+	+	+
o-Phenylphenol (ph)	1% pet.		+	
N-Phenyl-p-phenylenediamine (p-aminodiphenylamine)	0.25% pet.			+
1-Phenyl-3-pyrazolidinone (Phenidone®)	1% pet.	+	+	
Phenyl salicylate	1% pet.	+	+	+
Phenylsalicylate glycidyl methacrylate	2% pet.			
Phenyl tetralone tosylhydrazone	0.5% MEK			
Phosphorus sesquisulfide (cu)			0.5% pet.	
Phthalic anhydride (cu)	1% alc. or pet.			
Physodalic acid	0.1% pet.			
Physodes acid	0.1% pet.			
Picric acid (2,4,6-trinitrophenol)	1%–2% pet.; 5% aq.			
Pigment orange 34 (CI 21115, Irgalite F2G)	0.5%–2% pet.			
Pigment red 53, barium lake (lake Red C, CI 15585)	2% pet.			
Piketoprofen	2.5% pet.			
Pilocarpine hydrochloride	1% pet.	1% aq.	1% aq.	1% alc./glyc.
Pindolol				2% pet.
α-Pinene				15% pet.
β-Pinene	15% pet.			
Pinus (pine tar) (cu)	3% pet.		+	+
Piperazine	0.1%–0.5%–1% pet.			
Piperazine diacrylamide	0.1% pet.			
Pix ex carbone (coal tar) (cu) (ph)	5% pet.		+	+
Pivampicillin (base)	5% pet.			
Pivmecillinam	10% pet.			
Platinic chloride (cu)	1% aq. or pet.			
Polidocanol	3% pet.	+		+

Polyethylene glycol ointment	*see* PEG 6 (and) PEG 32			
Polyethyleneglycol-400 dimethacrylate	2% pet.			
Polymyxin B sulfate	3% pet.	+	5% pet.	+
Polyoxyethylene sorbitan monooleate	*see* Polysorbate 80			
Polyoxyethylene sorbitan monopalmitate	*see* Polysorbate 40			
Polysorbate 40 (polyoxyethylene sorbitan monopalminate)	5% pet.			10% pet.
Polysorbate 80 (polyoxyethylene sorbitan monooleate)	5% pet.		+	10% pet.
Potassium chloride	0.075%–0.3% aq.			
Potassium dichromate (ph)	0.5% pet.	+ and 0.25% pet.	+	+
Potassium dicyanoaurate		0.002% aq.	0.1% aq.	0.002% pet.
Potassium metabisulfite	1%–5% pet.; 1% aq.			
Potassium persulfate	1% pet.			
Potassium sorbate	5% pet.			
Povidone-iodine	5%–10% aq. or pet.			10% aq.
Prednisolone	1% alc.	1% pet.		0.5% pet.
Prilocaine hydrochloride	5% pet.		+	
Primin	0.01% pet.	+	+	+
Procaine hydrochloride (cu) (ph)	1%–2% pet.		1% pet.	2% pet.
Proflavine dihydrochloride	0.1%–1% pet.			
Promethazine hydrochloride (cu) (ph)	1%–10% pet.	0.1% pet.	1% pet.	2% pet.
Propacetamol	10%–50% aq.			
Propanidid	0.1% aq.			
Propantheline bromide	5% aq. or pet.			5% pet.
Propionic acid			3% pet.	
Propolis	10% pet.	+	+	+
Propoxylated glycerol triacrylate	0.1% pet.			
Propranolol	1% pet.			
Propranolol hydrochloride	10%–20% pet.			
Propylene glycol (cu)	5%–10% aq.; 4% pet.	5% pet. and 20% aq.	5% pet.	20% pet.
Propylene oxide	0.1%–1% alc.			
Propylidene phthalide	2% pet.			
Propyl gallate	1% pet.	0.5% pet.	1% pet.	0.5% pet.

Table 1 (continued)

Allergen	Test concentration and vehicle	Supplier		
		Trolab	Chemo	Brial
Propylparaben (cu)	3% pet.	+	+	+
Propyphenazone				1% pet.
Pyrazinobutazone	1% and 5% pet.			
Pyrethrum	*see* Chrysanthemum cinerariaefolium			
Pyridine (ph)	Pure			
Pyridoxine	2% aq.			
Pyritinol (ph)	2% aq.			
Pyrocatechol	2% pet.			
Pyrogallol	1% pet.	+		+
Quaternium-15	1% pet.	+	+	+
Quinazoline oxide	1% pet.			
Quinidine sulfate (ph)	0.5%–1% pet.	1% pet.		1% pet.
Quinine alkaloid	1% pet.			
Quinine dihydrochloride (ph)	1% aq.			
Quinine sulfate (ph)	1% pet.		+	25% pet.
Quinoline mix (clioquinol, chlorquinaldol)			6% pet.	
4-Quinolines (ph)	10% pet.			
Quinoline yellow	1% pet.			0.1% aq.
Ranitidine	1%–10% pet.			
Reactive black 1	1% pet.		+	
Reactive blue 21	1% pet.		+	
Reactive blue 238	1% pet.		+	
Reactive orange 107	1% pet.		+	
Reactive red 123	1% pet.		+	
Reactive red 228	1% pet.		+	
Reactive red 238	1% pet.		+	
Reactive violet 5	1% pet.		+	
Resorcinol (cu)	1%–2% pet.		1% pet.	1% pet.

Resorcinol-formaldehyde resin	5% pet.			+
Resorcinol monobenzoate			1% pet.	
Retinyl acetate	0.1% and 0.5% pet.			
Rhodinol (mixture of 1-citronellol and geraniol)	3% pet.			
Rhodium chloride	3% pet.			
Rhutenium oxide	2% pet.			0.1% pet.
1-Rodan-2,4-dinitrobenzene	1% pet.			
Rosa (rose oil)	2% pet.			0.5% pet.
Rosa centifolia (rose oil, Bulgarian)	2% pet.	+		
Rosin	*see* Colophonium			
Rotenone	1% pet.; 5% talcum powder			
Ruthenium				0.1% pet.
Saccharin				0.1% coca
Salicylaldehyde	2% pet.	+		+
Salicylic acid	1% pet.			5% pet.
Sandalore (5-(2,2,3-trimethyl-3-cyclopentenyl)-3-methyl-pentan-2-ol)	5% pet.			
Sandalwood oil	*see* Santalum album			
Sandalwood, synthetic	*see* Isobornyl cyclohexanol			
Sandela (isobornyl cyclohexanol + 3-*trans*-isocamphyl cyclohexanol)	5% pet.			
Santalol	2% pet.			
Santalum album (sandalwood oil) (ph)	2%–10% pet.		2% pet.	
Sesamum indicum (sesame oil)	10% pet.			
Sesquiterpene lactone mix (alantolactone, costunolide, dehydrocostus lactone)	0.1% pet.	+	+	
Silicon tetrachloride	2% pet.			
Silver colloidal				0.1% pet.
Silver nitrate (ph)	0.5% pet.		1% aq.	
Silver protein				3% pet.
Sodium alginate				1% coca
Sodium amidotrizoate	25% aq.			
Sodium arsenate (arsenate sodium)	1% aq.			
Sodium benzoate (cu)	5% pet.	+	+	+

Table 1 (continued)

Allergen	Test concentration and vehicle	Supplier		
		Trolab	Chemo	Brial
Sodium borate (borax)	Saturated aq. solution			
Sodiun *N*-chloro-*p*-toluenesulfonamide	1% pet.			
Sodium coco hydrolysed animal protein	2% aq. or pet.			
Sodium diphosphate				1% coca
Sodium disulfide				1% pet. and coca
Sodium formate				2% coca
Sodium glutamate				1% coca
Sodium hypochlorite (cu)	0.1%–1% aq.			
Sodium lauryl sulfate	0.1% aq. or pet.			
Sodium metabisulfite	1% aq.	1% pet.		
Sodium nitrite				2% aq.
Sodium omadine	*see* Sodium pyrithione			
Sodium pyrithione (sodium omadine)	0.1% aq.		+	
Sodium selenite	0.1% pet. or aq.			
Sodium sulfite				1% coca
Sodium thiosulfoaurate		0.25% pet.		0.25% pet.
Solvent blue 36	5% o.o.			
Solvent red 23 (Sudan III)	2% pet.			1% pet.
Solvent red 24 (Sudan IV)	2% pet.			
Solvent yellow 1	*see p*-Aminoazobenzene			
Sorbic acid (cu)	2% pet.	+	+	+ and 2% alc.
Sorbitan oleate (Span® 80)	5% aq.		5% pet.	
Sorbitan sesquioleate (cu)	20% pet.	+	+	+
Spearmint oil	1% pet.			
Spironolactone	1% alc.			
Squaric acid dibutyl ester (cu)	0.02% pet.			
Stannous chloride (tin chloride)				0.5% pet.
Stearyl alcohol (cu)	30% pet.		+	

Stitic acid (ph)	0.1% pet.			
Streptomycin (sulfate) (cu)	1% and 10% pet.			5% pet.
Styrax benzoin (benzoin resin)	2% pet.		+	10% mixture
Sudan III	*see* Solvent red 23			
Sudan IV	*see* Solvent red 24			
Sudan brown	*see* Naphthylaminoazobenzol			
Sulfanilamide (ph)	5% pet.	+	+	+
Sulfiram (tetraethylthiuram monosulfide)	1% pet.			
Sulfur dioxide (cu)				2% aq.
Sulfur (precipitated) (cu)	5% pet.			10% pet.
Sulisobenzone	*see* Benzophenone-4			
Tanacetum vulgare (tansy extract)	1% pet.	+	+	
Tansy extract	*see* Tanacetum vulgare			
Tantalum				1% pet.
Tantalum chloride	1% pet.			
Taraxacum officinale (dandelion)			2.5% pet.	
Tartrazine (cu)	2% pet.			1% coca
Tea tree oil	*see* Melaleuca alternifolia			
Tego® 103 G	0.1%–1% aq.			
Tego® diocto S	*see* Dioctyl trioctyl ethylenetriamine			
Tellurium dioxide	2% pet.			
γ-Terpinene	2% pet.			
α-Terpineol	5% pet.			
Tetracaine hydrochloride (amethocaine)	5% pet.	1% pet.	+	1% pet.
Tetrachlorosalicylanilide (TSCA) (ph)			0.1% pet.	
Tetrachloroisophthalonitrile	*see* Chlorothalonil			
Tetracycline hydrochloride (cu)	10% pet.	2% pet.		2% pet.
Tetraethylene glycol dimethacrylate			2% pet.	2% pet.
Tetraethylthiuram disulfide (TETD)		0.25% pet.	1% pet.	0.25% pet.
Tetraethylthiuram monosulfide (sulfiram)	1% pet.			
Tetrafluoroterephthalonitrile	0.01% pet.			
Tetrafluoropropyl methacrylate (TFPMA)	2% pet.			
Tetraglycidyl-4,4'-methylene dianiline (TGMDA)	1% pet.			

Table 1 (continued)

Allergen	Test concentration and vehicle	Supplier		
		Trolab	Chemo	Brial
Tetrahydrofurfuryl methacrylate (THFMA)	2% pet.			
1,1,6,7-Tetramethyl-6-acetyl decalene (isomers) (Iso E Super®)	1%–5% pet.			+
Tetramethylbenzidine			0.1% pet.	
Tetramethylol acetylenediurea			5% aq.	
Tetramethylthiuram disulfide (TMTD, thiram)	1% pet.	0.25% pet.	1% pet.	0.25% pet.
Tetramethylthiuram monosulfide (TMTM)		0.25% pet.	+	0.25% pet.
Tetrazepam (ph)	1%–10% pet.			
Tetryl®	*see* Nitramine			
Thebaine	5% alc.			
Thiabendazole	1% pet.			
Thiamine	5% and 10% aq.			
Thimerosal (cu)	0.1% pet.	+	+	+
Thioglycerol	5% pet.; 10% aq.			
Thiolactic acid	0.3% pet.			
Thiothiamine	1% and 5% aq.			
Thiourea (ph)	0.1% pet.	+	+	+
Thiram	*see* Tetramethylthiuram disulfide			
Thiuram mix (tetramethylthiuram monosulfide, tetra-methylthiuram disulfide, tetraethylthiuram disulfide, dipenta-methylenethiuram disulfide)	1% pet.	+	+	+
Thymol	1% pet.			
Thymoquinone	0.1% pet.			
Timolol			0.5% aq.	
Tin			50% pet.	
Tin chloride	*see* Stannous chloride			
Titanium dioxide	0.1% pet. – pure			
Titanium oxide	5% pet.			0.5% pet.
Tixocortol pivalate	0.1% pet.		+	
Toluene-2,5-diamine (*p*-toluenediamine) (PTD)	1% pet.	+	+	+

Toluene diisocyanate (TDI)	1% pet.	+	2% pet.	+
Toluenesulfonamide/formaldehyde resin	*see* Tosylamine/formaldehyde resin			
p-Toluenesulfonyl chloride (tosyl chloride)	1% alc.			
4-Tolyldiethanolamine	2% alc.		2% pet.	
N-Tolylglycine glycidyl methacrylate	2% pet.			
Tosylamide/formaldehyde resin (toluenesulfonamide/formaldehyde resin)	10% pet.	+	+	+
Tosyl chloride	*see p*-Toluenesulfonyl chloride			
Tragacanth gum	1% aq.	·		
Tree moss absolute	5% pet.			
Triamcinolone acetonide	1% alc.	0.1% pet.	1% pet.	0.1% pet.
Triazine	0.5% aq.			
Tribromsalan (TBS) (ph)	1% pet.	+	+	
Trichlorocarbanilide	*see* Triclocarban			
3,4,6-Trichloropyridazine (pts!!!)	<<<1% pet.			
Triclocarban (trichlorocarbanilide) (TCC) (ph)	1% pet.		+	+
Triclosan (ph)	2% pet.	+	+	+
Tricresyl phosphate	2%–5% pet.	5% pet.	5% pet.	5% pet.
Tricyclodecen-4-yl 8-acetate (Cyclacet®)	5% pet.			
Tridecyl resorcinol	0.1% pet.			
2,4,6-Tri(dimethylaminomethyl)phenol	0.1% pet.			
Triethanolamine	2%–2.5% pet.	2.5% pet.	2% pet.	2.5% pet.
Triethylenediamine	0.5% pet.			
Triethyleneglycol diacrylate (TREGDA)	0.1% pet.		+	
Triethyleneglycol dimethacrylate (TREGDMA)	2% pet.	+	+	+
Triethylenetetramine (TETA)	0.5%–1% pet.	0.5% pet.	0.5% pet.	0.5% pet.
Trifluorothymidine			5% pet.	
Triforine	0.02% aq.			
Triglycidyl isocyanurate (TGIC)	0.5% pet.			
7,8,3-Trihydroxy-2,4-dimethoxyisoflavan	1% pet.			
Trimeprazine tartrate (alimemazine tartrate)				1% pet.
5-(2,2,3-Trimethyl-3-cyclopentenyl)-3-methyl-pentan-2-ol	*see* Sandalore			
2,2,4-Trimethyl-1,2-dihydroquinoline			1% pet.	
Trimethylolpropane triacrylate (TMPTA)	0.1–2% pet.		0.1% pet.	

Table 1 (continued)

Allergen	Test concentration and vehicle	Supplier		
		Trolab	Chemo	Brial
Trimethylolpropane trimethacrylate	2% pet.			
Trinitroanisole	1% pet.			
2,4,6-Trinitrophenol	see Picric acid			
Triphenyl phosphate	5% pet.	+	+	+
Triphenyl phosphite	0.1% pet.			
Tripropyleneglycol acrylate	0.1% pet.			
Tripropyleneglycol diacrylate (TPGDA)	0.01%–1% pet.		0.1% pet.	
2,4,6-Tris-(dimethylaminomethyl)phenol (tris-DMP)	0.5%–1% pet.			
1,3,5-Tris(2-hydroxyethyl)-hexahydrotriazine (Grotan® BK)	1% pet.	+	1% aq.	
Tris-(2-hydroxyethyl)isocyanurate triacrylate (Tris-HEICA)	0.1% pet.			
Tris(hydroxymethyl)nitromethane (tris nitro)	1% pet.		+	
Tris nitro	see Tris(hydroxymethyl)nitro-methane			
Trolamine	see Triethanolamine			
Tropicamide (cu)	1% pet.			
TSS Agfa®	see Amino-4-N,N-diethylaniline sulfate			
Tulipaline	see α-Methylene-γ-butyrolactone			
Tungsten (metal)	5% pet.			
Turpentine oil (cu)	10% pet.	+		+ and 20% pet.
Turpentine peroxides (cu)	0.3% o.o.		+	0.3% pet.
Undecylenamide DEA	1% aq.			
Undecylenic acid	2%–5% pet.			
Urea-formaldehyde resin	10% pet.		+	
Urethane acrylate (UA)	0.1% pet.			
Urethane diacrylate (aliphatic)	0.1% pet.		+	
Urethane diacrylate (aromatic)	0.05% pet.		+	
Urethane dimethacrylate (UEDMA)	2% pet.		+	+
Urethane methacrylate	2% pet.			
Urushiol	Do not test			
Usnic acid (ph)	0.1%–1% pet.	0.1% pet.	0.1% pet.	0.1% pet.
Vanadium chloride	1% pet.			

Vanilla	Pure			
Vanillin (cu)	10% pet.	+	+	+
Vertofix®	*see* Acetylcedrene			
Vesuvine brown	*see* Bismarck brown			
Vincamine tartrate	1% aq.			
Vinyl cyclohexene diepoxide	0.25% pet.			
Vinyl pyridine (cu) (pts)	0.1% isopropyl alc.			
Violet leaves absolute	2% pet.			
Virginiamycin (cu)	5% pet.			
Vitamin K3	*see* Menadione			
Vitamin K3 sodium bisulfite	0.1% pet.			
Vitamin K4	*see* Menadiol			
Warfarin	0.5% pet.			
Wheat germ oil	20% pet.			
Wolframium metal (powder)	5% pet.			
Wood tar mix (pine, spruce, birch, teak) (ph)			20% pet.	12% pet.
Wool alcohols	*see* Lanolin alcohol			
Xylanase (cu)	3.3%, 1% and 0.33% in aq. and pet.			
Yarrow	*see* Achillea millefolium			
Ylang-ylang oil	*see* Cananga odorata			
Ytterbium sulfate	2% pet.			
Yttrium oxide	2% pet.			
Zinc chloride	2% pet.		+	1% pet.
Zinc dibutyldithiocarbamate (ZBC) (cu)	1% pet.		+	
Zinc diethyldithiocarbamate (ZDC) (cu)	1% pet.	+	+	
Zinc dimethyldithiocarbamate (cu)			1% pet.	
Zinc ethylenebis(dithiocarbamate)	*see* Zineb			
Zinc (powder)			2.5% pet.	1% pet.
Zinc pyrithione (ph)	1% pet.		+	0.1% pet.
Zineb (zinc ethylenebis(dithiocarbamate)) (ph)	1% pet.		+	+
Ziram	1% pet.			
Zirconium oxide				0.1% pet.

® Registered trade name *alc.* alcohol, *aq.* water, *DMSO* dimethyl sulfoxide, *glyc.* glycerin, *MEK* methyl ethyl ketone, *o.o.* olive oil, *pet.* petrolatum, *prop. glyc.* propylene glycol, *cu* contact urticaria reported, *ph* photosensitivity (toxicity/allergy) reported, *pts* risk of patch test sensitisation.

of chemicals and products is the book *Patch Testing* (De Groot 1994). Other useful lists are provided in recent textbooks on contact dermatitis (Adams 1990; De Groot et al. 1994; Rietschel and Fowler 1995; Rycroft et al. 2000).

Guidelines for testing patients' own materials are provided in Chap. 17.

Table 1 lists alphabetically all chemicals mentioned in this book with their test concentrations and vehicles (sometimes two or more concentrations are suggested when insufficient data is available) as suggested by the various authors. All allergens commercially available are also listed with their supplier(s), their test concentrations and vehicles as supplied. It should be appreciated that, for some allergens, the concentrations vary between suppliers.

References

Adams RM (1990) Occupational skin disease, 2nd edn. Saunders, Philadelphia

De Groot AC (1994) Patch testing. Test concentrations and vehicles for 3700 chemicals, 2nd edn. Elsevier, Amsterdam

De Groot AC, Weijland JW, Nater JP (1994) Unwanted effects of cosmetics and drugs used in dermatology, 3rd edn. Elsevier, Amsterdam

Niklasson BJ (2000) List of Patch-Test Allergens. In: Kanerva L, Elsner P, Wahlberg JE, Maibach HI (eds) Handbook of occupational dermatology. Springer, Heidelberg Berlin New York, pp 1192–1256

Rietschel RL, Fowler JF Jr (eds) (1995) Fisher's contact dermatitis, 4th edn. Williams and Wilkins, Baltimore

Rycroft RJG (1990) Is patch testing necessary? In: Champion RH, Pye RJ (eds) Recent advances in dermatology, vol 8. Churchill Livingstone, Edinburgh, pp 101–111

Rycroft RJG, Menné T, Frosch PJ (eds) (2000) Textbook of contact dermatitis, 3rd edn. Springer, Berlin Heidelberg New York

Printing: Druckhaus Berlin-Mitte GmbH
Binding: Buchbinderei Stein & Lehmann, Berlin